MW00563283

Medical Microbiology and Immunology for Dentistry

Medical Microbiology and Immunology for Dentistry

Nejat Düzgüneş, PhD

Professor of Biomedical Sciences
Arthur A. Dugoni School of Dentistry
University of the Pacific
San Francisco, California

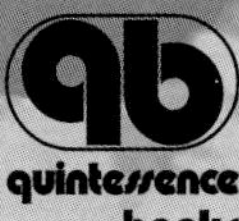

Quintessence Publishing Co, Inc

Chicago, Berlin, Tokyo, London, Paris, Milan, Barcelona, Istanbul, Moscow, New Delhi, Prague, São Paulo, Seoul, and Warsaw

Library of Congress Cataloging-in-Publication Data

Düzgüneş, Nejat, author.
Medical microbiology and immunology for dentistry / Nejat Düzgüneş.
p. ; cm.
Includes bibliographical references and index.
ISBN 978-0-86715-647-8
I. Title.
[DNLM: 1. Stomatognathic Diseases--immunology. 2. Stomatognathic Diseases--microbiology. 3. Dentistry--methods. WU 140]
QR47
617.5'22--dc23
2015031156

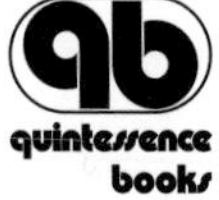

Quintessence Publishing Co, Inc
4350 Chandler Drive
Hanover Park, IL 60133
www.quintpub.com

5 4 3 2 1

Editor: Leah Huffman
Editorial Intern: Cassidy Olson
Design: Ted Pereda
Production: Angelina Sanchez

Printed in the USA

Contents

Dedication

To Maxine, Avery, and Diana
for all the wonderful experiences you have brought into my life, for your love,
and for asking many, many questions
and
to the memories of my cousin Professor Ferruh Ertürk and my aunt Sevim Uygurer,
who were always there for me

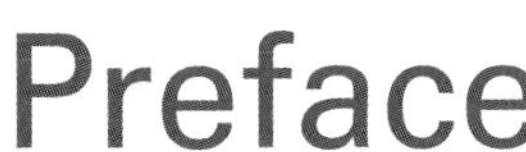

Preface

This book is the outcome of my teaching the Microbiology course at the University of the Pacific Arthur A. Dugoni School of Dentistry in San Francisco. In my 25 years of teaching this course, I have relied on medical microbiology texts that cover all areas quite extensively, are written by numerous experts, and are excellent reference books; however, all of them are too detailed for instructional purposes. Therefore, I decided to write this textbook and tailor the information specifically for dental students. Practicing dentists and other dental professionals, as well as students in other health professions, may also benefit from the didactic, succinct, yet thorough coverage of the field.

Dentists are "physicians of the mouth" and thus need to have a basic understanding of medical microbiology and immunology. Most of the conditions treated by general dentists and specialists are the result of bacterial infection, including caries, periodontal disease, and endodontic infections. The response of the immune system to these infections may also contribute to their pathology. Caries and periodontal disease are initiated by changes in the oral bacterial ecosystem, and understanding the microbiology of these diseases is essential for their treatment.

Dentists need to be able to diagnose oral infections, such as denture stomatitis caused by *Candida* species, as well as obvious systemic medical conditions whose medical implications may be lost on patients. They should also understand the nature and complications of any infectious disease their patients may have, including HIV/AIDS, hepatitis, tuberculosis, and emerging diseases such as SARS and MERS. Members of the dental care team as well as other patients must be protected from these infectious diseases, and dentists should be able to answer questions, address patient concerns, and allay their fears about cross infection. Finally, dentists are health care providers who can influence decisions on public health issues such as the importance of vaccinations, fluoridation of water sources, and funding for biomedical research by the National Institutes of Health. Therefore, understanding microbiology and immunology and their roles in the initiation, progression, and treatment of disease is pertinent for any practicing dentist.

The book starts with chapters on immunology and proceeds with chapters on bacterial structure, genetics, and diseases, with intervening chapters on microbial identification and control as well as antimicrobial chemotherapy. Oral microbiology is covered in two major chapters, and these are followed by a discussion of fungal structure, pathogenesis and diseases, and antifungal chemotherapy. The book continues with chapters on virus structure, antiviral chemotherapy, and viral diseases, including HIV, hepatitis, and influenza as well as viruses that are much less prevalent. Prions and parasitic diseases conclude the didactic part of the book. The appendix includes cases in medical microbiology that allow readers the opportunity to integrate their knowledge of the field to diagnose cases.

The chapters also highlight some of the exciting discoveries in microbiology, immunology, and molecular biology and pose research questions to stimulate the reader to further inquiry and thinking. Each chapter concludes with take-home messages that will be useful for reviewing the material for an examination. The reader is encouraged to consult some of the references in the bibliography for more detailed information on a given subject. Microbiology affects every aspect of dental practice, so it is paramount that today's students understand the processes at work in the mouth as well as in the rest of the body.

Acknowledgments

I have benefited greatly from the contributions to the Microbiology course by past and present colleagues Dr Ken Snowdowne, Dr Krystyna Konopka, Dr Taka Chino, Dr Matt Milnes, and Dr Ove Peters.

I am grateful to the staff at Quintessence, particularly Lisa Bywaters for enthusiastically supporting the project and moving it along and Leah Huffman for being a very helpful and competent editor. Jeanne Robertson also did a superb job with the illustrations.

I am fortunate to have a supportive and loving family who are all interested in science and who made sure I was working on the book when I had other obligations.

Chapter Opener Image Credits

1 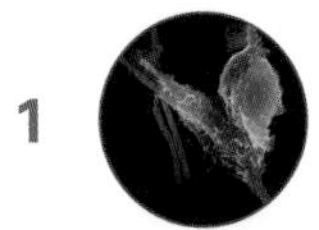 SEM of a neutrophil engulfing *Bacillus anthracis*. (Courtesy of PLoS Pathogens and Volker Brinkman.)

2 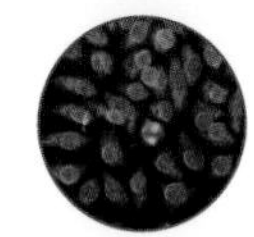 SEM of HeLa cells stained with anti-nuclear pore complex antibody and chicken anti-vimentin. (Courtesy of antibodies-online.com.)

3 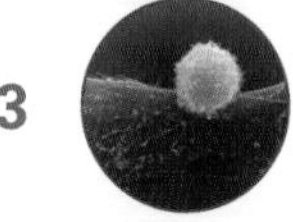 SEM of a cytotoxic T cell and a somatic cell. (Courtesy of G. Wanner.)

4 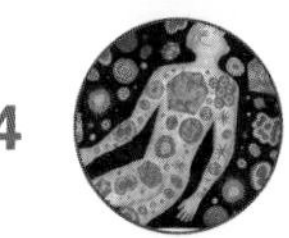 Artist rendering of the immune system from "The Body on Fire." (Courtesy of J. Flaherty.)

5 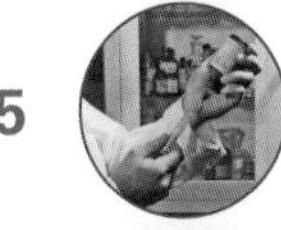 Photograph of a scientist filling a syringe with a rabies vaccine. (PHIL image 8326, courtesy of the CDC.)

6 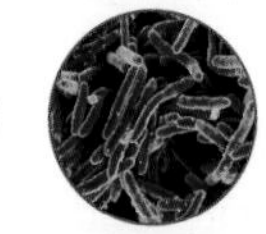 SEM of rod-shaped *Mycobacterium tuberculosis*. (PHIL image 18138, courtesy of the NIAID.)

7 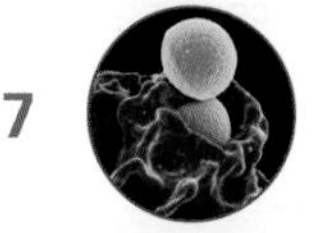 SEM of spherical MRSA interacting with a white blood cell. (PHIL image 18168, courtesy of the NIAID.)

8 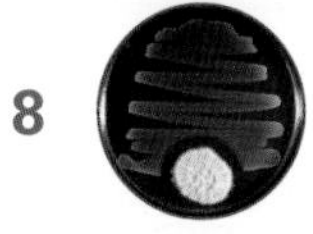 Penicillin inhibiting growth of *Staphylococcus aureus*. (Courtesy of Christine Case, Skyline College.)

9 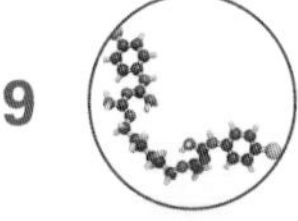 Chemical structure of chlorhexidine.

10 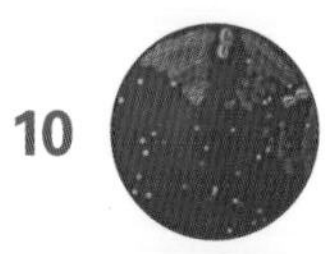 Petri dish with *Streptococcus pyogenes*–inoculated trypticase soy agar. (PHIL image 8170, courtesy of Dr Richard Facklam.)

11 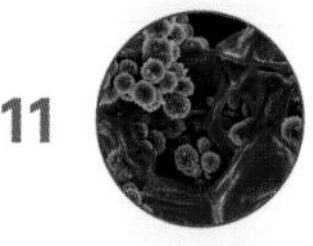 SEM of spheroid-shaped MRSA enmeshed within the pseudopodia of a human white blood cell. (PHIL image 18125, courtesy of the NIAID.)

12 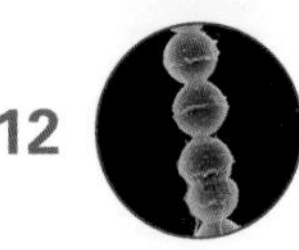 *Streptococcus*. (Courtesy of Tina Carvalho, University of Hawaii at Manoa.)

13 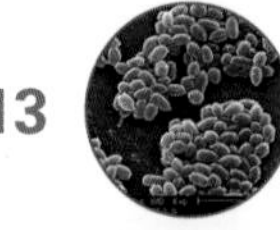 SEM of spores from the Sterne strain of *Bacillus anthracis*. (PHIL image 10122, courtesy of Janice Haney Carr.)

14 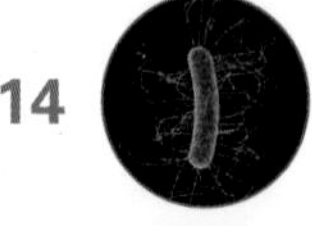 Illustration of *Clostridium difficile*. (PHIL image 16786, courtesy of Melissa Brower.)

15 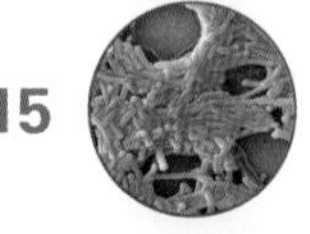 SEM of *Legionella pneumophila*. (PHIL image 11147, courtesy of Janice Haney Carr.)

16 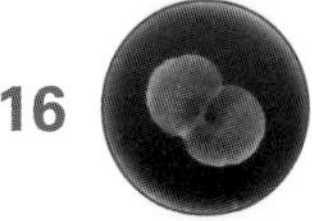 TEM of a diplococcal pair of *Neisseria gonorrhoeae*. (PHIL image 14493, courtesy of Dr Wiesner at the CDC.)

17 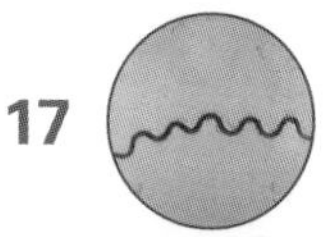 Photomicrograph of *Treponema pallidum*. (PHIL image 14969, courtesy of Susan Lindsley.)

18 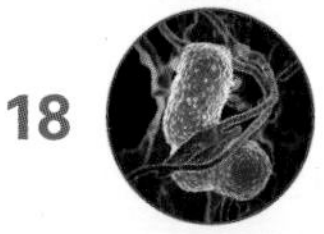 SEM of a human white blood cell interacting with *Klebsiella pneumoniae*. (PHIL image 18170, courtesy of the NIAID.)

19 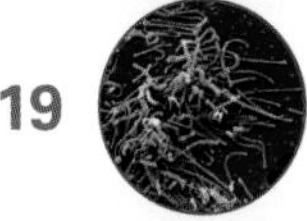 SEM of *Mycoplasma pneumoniae* on the surface of a cell. (Courtesy of Dr David M. Phillips.)

20 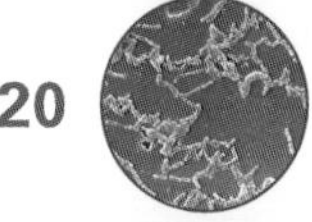 SEM of *Mycobacterium chelonae*. (PHIL image 227, courtesy of Janice Haney Carr.)

21 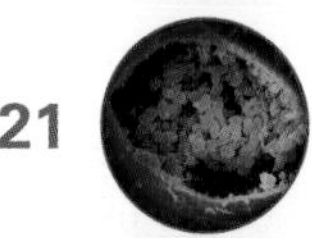 SEM of *Coxiella burnetii* undergoing rapid replication in an opened vacuole of a dry-fractured Vero cell. (PHIL image 18164, courtesy of the NIAID.)

22 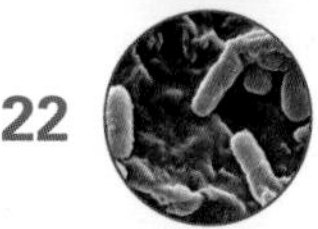 SEM of *Pseudomonas aeruginosa*. (PHIL image 10043, courtesy of Janice Haney Carr.)

23 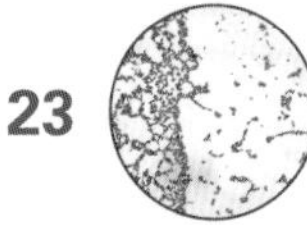 Photomicrograph of *Streptococcus mutans* with Gram stain. (PHIL image 1070, courtesy of Dr Richard Facklam.)

24 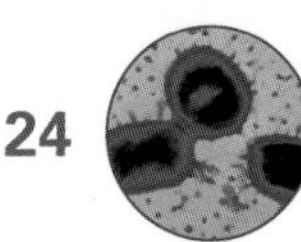 *Porphyromonas gingivalis*. (Courtesy of Tsute Chen, PhD.)

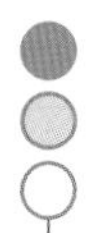

25 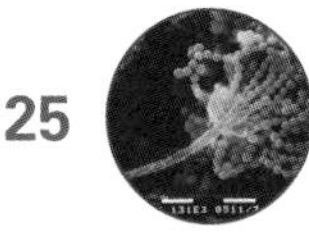 SEM close-up of an asexual *Aspergillus* species fungal fruiting body. (PHIL image 13367, courtesy of Janice Haney Carr.)

26 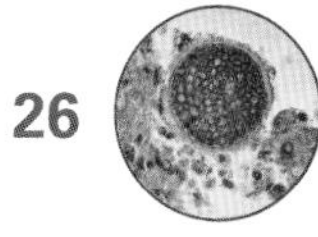 Spherule of a *Coccidioides* fungal organism. (PHIL image 14499, courtesy of the CDC.)

27 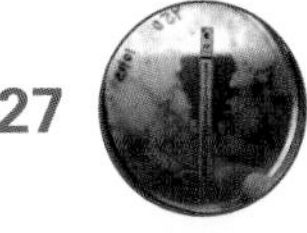 Susceptibility testing to the antifungal amphotericin B. (PHIL image 15147, courtesy of James Gathany.)

28 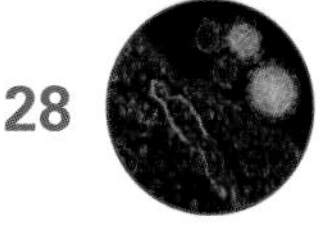 TEM of spherical MERS coronavirus virions. (PHIL image 18113, courtesy of the NIAID.)

29 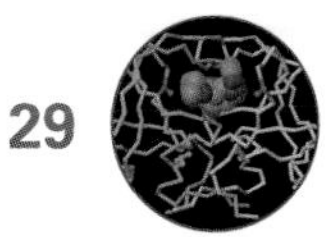 An HIV-1 protease inhibitor interacting with a mutant protease. (Courtesy of Nature.com and the Protein Data Bank.)

30 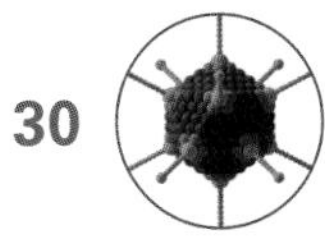 A simplified 3D-generated structure of adenovirus. (Courtesy of Thomas Splettstoesser.)

31 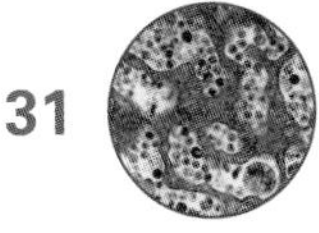 Electron micrograph of monocytic THP-1 cells infected with HIV-1 cells. (Reprinted with permission from Konopka et al.*)

32 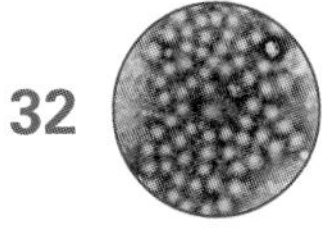 TEM showing numerous hepatitis virions of an unknown strain. (PHIL image 8153, courtesy of E. H. Cook, Jr.)

33 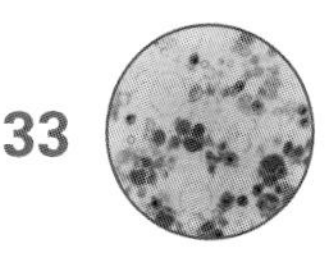 TEM depicting cytomegalovirus virions. (PHIL image 14429, courtesy of the CDC.)

34 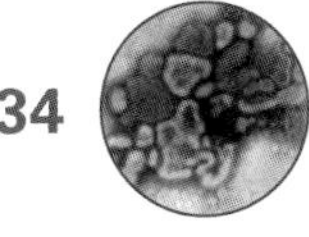 TEM depicting a strain of swine flu (A/New Jersey/76 [Hsw1N1]) virus in a chicken egg. (PHIL image 1246, courtesy of Dr E. Palmer and R. E. Bates.)

35 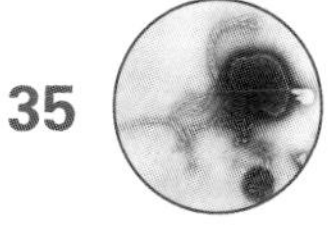 TEM of parainfluenza virus. (PHIL image 236, courtesy of Dr Erskine Palmer.)

36 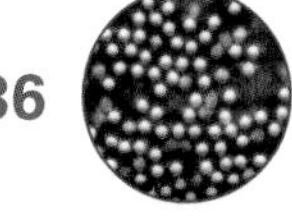 TEM of poliovirus. (Courtesy of Graham Beards.)

37 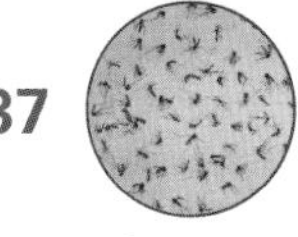 Deceased mosquitos about to undergo laboratory testing. (PHIL image 14887, courtesy of James Stewart.)

38 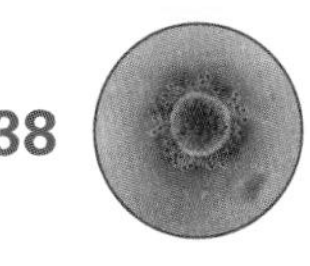 TEM highlighting the particle envelope of a single MERS coronavirus virion through the process of immunolabeling the envelope proteins. (PHIL image 18108, courtesy of the NIAID.)

39 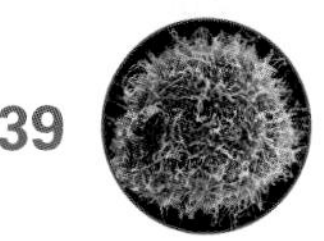 SEM of numerous Ebola virus particles budding from a chronically infected Vero E6 cell. (PHIL image 17768, courtesy of the NIAID.)

40 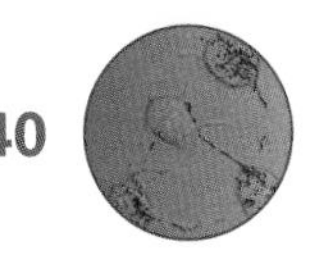 Photomicrograph of a neural tissue specimen harvested from a scrapie-affected mouse showing the presence of prion protein. (PHIL image 18131, courtesy of the NIAID.)

41 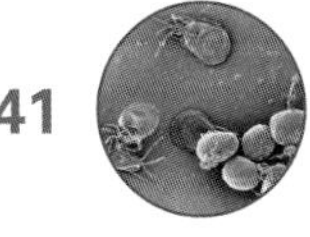 SEM of an in vitro *Giardia lamblia* culture. (PHIL image 11636, courtesy of Dr Stan Erlandsen.)

*Konopka K, Pretzer E, Plowman B, Düzgüneş N. Long-term noncytopathic productive infection of the human monocytic leukemia cell line THP-1 by human immunodeficiency virus type 1 (HIV-1IIIB). Virology 1993;193:877–887.

CDC, Centers for Disease Control and Prevention; MERS, Middle East respiratory syndrome; MRSA, methicillin-resistant *Staphylococcus aureus*; NIAID, National Institute of Allergy and Infectious Diseases; PHIL, Public Health Image Library (of the CDC); SEM, scanning electron micrograph; TEM, transmission electron micrograph.

1 The Immune System

The protective responses of the immune system against invading microorganisms consist of natural barriers (eg, skin, mucosa, tears); nonspecific, innate immunity (eg, response of neutrophils and interferons); and antigen-specific immunity (eg, antibodies and cell-mediated immunity). The soluble mediators of the immune response include cytokines, interferons, and chemokines. All of these components of the immune system work together in harmony, much like a symphony orchestra does.

Organs and Tissues of the Immune System

The immune system functions within all the organs and tissues of the body to protect it from invading microorganisms. The main avenues of the immune system, however, are in the lymphatic system, which consists of the primary and secondary lymphoid organs. The primary lymphoid organs are the bone marrow and the thymus, where B cells and T cells mature, respectively. Cellular and humoral immune responses take place in the secondary lymphoid organs and tissues (Box 1-1). These include bronchus-associated and urogenital lymphoid tissues, bone marrow, the spleen, mesenteric and other lymph nodes, Peyer's patches, and Waldeyer's ring (including tonsils and adenoids).

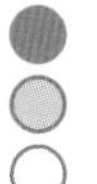

Box 1-1 Primary and secondary lymphoid organs

B cells and T cells mature in the bone marrow and thymus, respectively. Cellular and humoral immune responses occur in the secondary lymphoid organs.

Primary lymphoid organs
- Bone marrow
- Thymus

Secondary lymphoid organs and tissues
- Waldeyer's ring (tonsils, adenoids, and lymph nodes)
- Bronchus-associated lymphoid tissue
- Mesenteric lymph nodes
- Other lymph nodes
- Peyer's patches
- Bone marrow
- Spleen

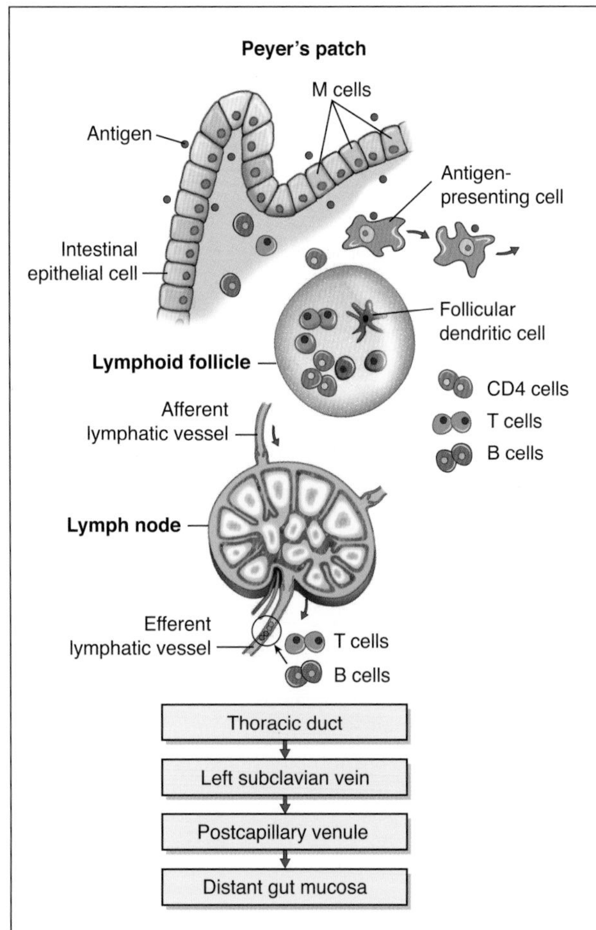

Fig 1-1 Trafficking of B cells and T cells following activation at the Peyer's patch.

Peyer's patches are differentiated lymphoid tissues along the intestines that are involved in antigen internalization and that facilitate the encounter of the antigen with lymphocytes, macrophages, and dendritic cells (Fig 1-1). The M cells along the intestinal lumen transcytose antigens from the apical to the basolateral side of the cells. B and T lymphocytes that encounter the antigens migrate to the local lymphoid follicle. Follicular dendritic cells in the lymphoid follicle facilitate the activation of the lymphocytes. Some of the activated lymphocytes enter an afferent lymphatic vessel and a local lymph node. Antigen-presenting cells (APCs)—such as macrophages, dendritic cells, and B cells—and T cells in the lymph node further activate the lymphocytes. These lymphocytes enter the efferent lymphatic vessel, the thoracic duct, and peripheral blood. The lymphocytes can then enter distal sites at postcapillary venules.

In the oral cavity, the lymphoid tissues include lingual tonsils, palatine tonsils, and pharyngeal tonsils (also called *adenoids*).

Lymph nodes consist of the cortex (the outer layer), the paracortex, and the medulla (the inner layer) (Fig 1-2). In the cortex, B cells and macrophages are arranged in clusters called *follicles*. In the paracortex, dendritic cells present antigens to T cells to initiate the specific immune response. The medulla contains T cells and B cells and antibody-producing plasma cells. Following activation of lymphocytes by microbial antigens, they alter the expression of their receptors for chemokines (chemoattractant cytokines). This results in the migration of T cells and B cells to meet at the edge of the follicles, with helper T (T_h) cells interacting with B cells to induce the differentiation of the B cells into antibody-producing cells (plasma cells).

Lymphocytes enter the node from the circulation through postcapillary venules called *high endothelial venules*. Lymphocytes and antigens from adjacent tissues or lymph nodes enter the node via the afferent lymphatic vessel. Activated lymphocytes leave the lymph node via the efferent lymphatic vessels and may enter the circulation and travel to the sites of infection.

RESEARCH

What facilitates the localization of B cells in follicles and T cells in the paracortex?

Cells of the Immune System

The different types of cells that constitute the immune system are generated by the differentiation of hematopoietic cells. Self-renewing stem cells differentiate into pluripotent stem cells, which can in turn differentiate into either myeloid progenitors or lymphoid progenitors (Fig 1-3). The myeloid progenitors then differentiate to produce erythroid colony-forming units (CFUs), megakaryocytes, basophil CFUs, eosinophil CFUs, and granulocyte-monocyte CFUs.

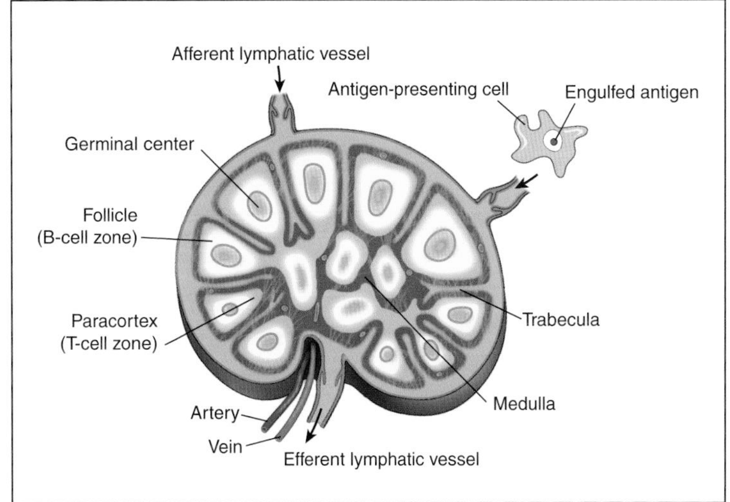

Fig 1-2 Schematic cross section of a lymph node. Note the cortex (which includes the germinal center and follicle), paracortex, medulla, and the germinal centers.

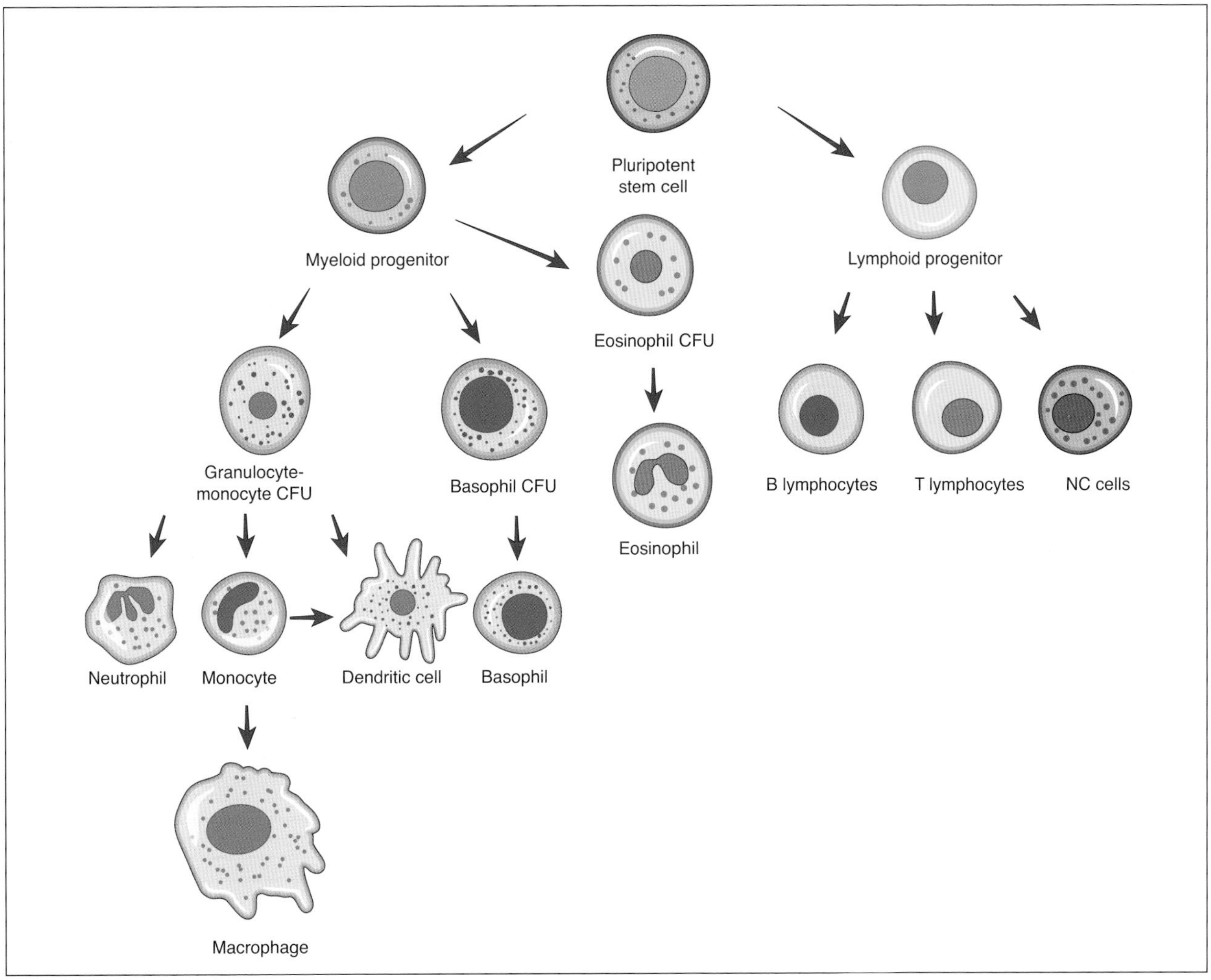

Pluripotent stem cell
Myeloid progenitor
Eosinophil CFU
Lymphoid progenitor
Granulocyte-monocyte CFU
Basophil CFU
Eosinophil
B lymphocytes
T lymphocytes
NC cells
Neutrophil
Monocyte
Dendritic cell
Basophil
Macrophage

Fig 1-3 Differentiation of self-renewing stem cells into the cells of the immune system. CFU, colony-forming unit (to be distinguished from the CFU of bacteria grown on nutrient agar). Myeloid progenitors can also differentiate into megakaryocytes and erthyroid CFUs (not shown). NC, natural cytotoxic (also known as *natural killer*).

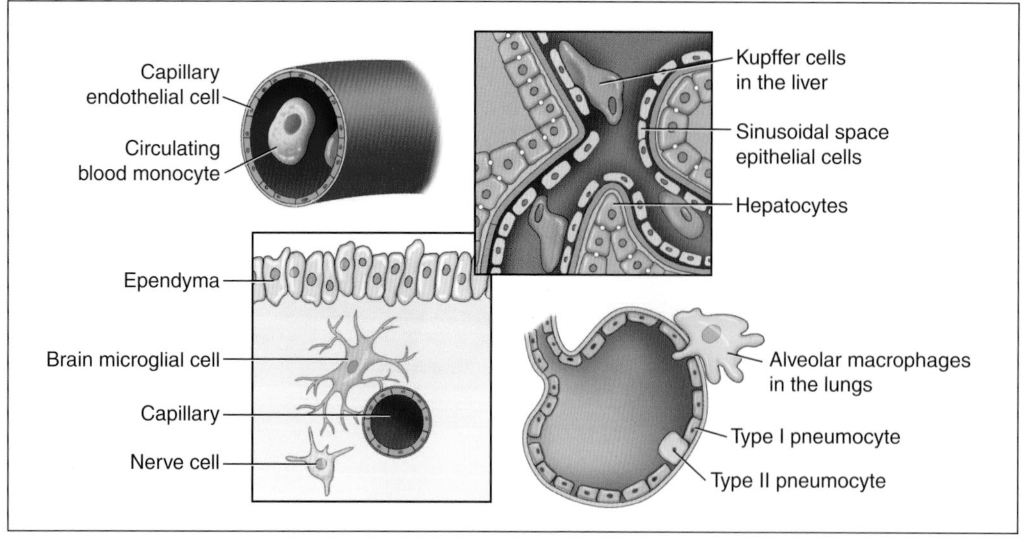

Fig 1-4 Resident macrophages in various tissues.

The erythroid CFUs form erythrocytes, megakaryocytes form platelets, basophil CFUs form basophils, and eosinophil CFUs form eosinophils. The granulocyte-monocyte CFUs can differentiate into neutrophils, monocytes, and dendritic cells. Monocytes, in turn, can differentiate into macrophages as well as dendritic cells.

The lymphoid progenitors can differentiate into B lymphocytes, T lymphocytes, and natural killer cells (the author prefers the term *natural cytotoxic cells*).

RESEARCH

What makes a myeloid progenitor cell differentiate into a granulocyte-monocyte CFU and not into an erythroid CFU?

Macrophages are phagocytotic cells that are derived via the differentiation of circulating monocytes that have entered tissues. They become Kupffer cells in the liver, histiocytes in connective tissue, dendritic cells in various tissues, microglial cells in neural tissue, alveolar macrophages in the lung, osteoclasts in bone, and sinusoidal lining cells in the spleen (Fig 1-4). Macrophages engulf bacteria, fungi, and viruses in endocytotic vesicles called *phagosomes* and destroy them following the fusion of the phagosomes with lysosomes. Lysosomes contain numerous enzymes (acid hydrolases) that degrade proteins, nucleic acids, polysaccharides, and lipids at acidic pH. Attachment of bacteria to the macrophage membrane is facilitated by the binding of the complement component C3b or specific antibodies to the bacterial membrane. The macrophage, in turn, binds these molecules via its C3b receptor (CR1) and Fc receptor (FcR), respectively. The bacteria are internalized in phagosomes, and the enzyme nicotinamide adenine dinucleotide phosphate (NADPH) oxidase is activated to produce superoxide anion, resulting in the consumption of excess oxygen by the cells, a process called the **respiratory burst**. The superoxide anion can damage bacterial cell membranes.

Macrophages can also bind bacteria via their lipopolysaccharide (LPS) receptors, mannose receptors, and glycan receptors. Macrophages can be activated by receptors on their surface for the cytokines tumor necrosis factor-alpha (TNF-α) and interferon gamma (IFN-γ) as well as for **pathogen-associated molecular patterns**. The receptors for the latter—including lipoarabinomannan (from mycobacteria), flagellin (from bacterial flagella), LPS, heat shock protein (Hsp60), CpG DNA (characteristic of bacterial DNA), lipoteichoic acid, and peptidoglycan—are called **pattern-recognition receptors** or **Toll-like receptors** (called as such because of their homology to Toll receptors involved in *Drosophila* development) (Fig 1-5).

Another major role for macrophages is to be a central part of the specific immune responses. Macrophages present antigens on their surface to helper T lymphocytes to help the immune system select the most appropriate T lymphocytes to be stimulated to proliferate in response to a specific antigen. The antigen is presented to the outside world after it is associated with a **major histocompatibility complex class II (MHC II)** molecule embedded in the plasma membrane. Other membrane proteins such as B7 act as co-stimulatory molecules, and leukocyte function antigen-3 (LFA-3) and intercellular adhesion molecule-1 (ICAM-1) facilitate adhesion between the macrophage and the T_h cell.

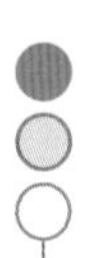

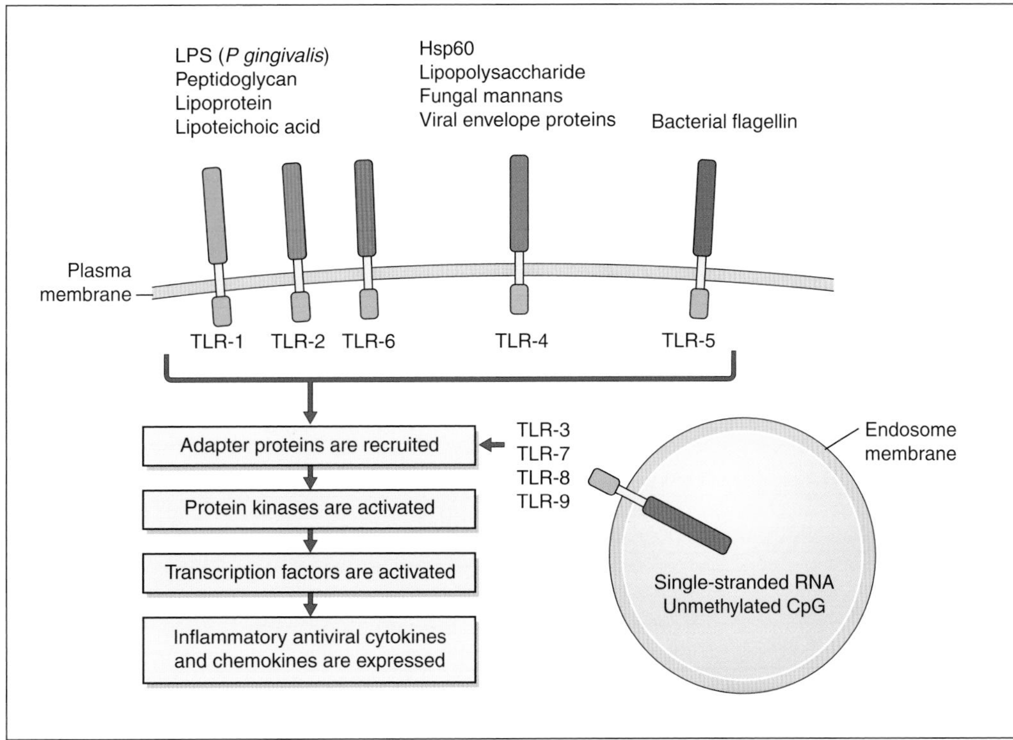

Fig 1-5 Pattern-recognition receptors (Toll-like receptors [TLRs]).

Granulocytes consist of neutrophils, basophils, and eosinophils. Between 50% and 70% of white blood cells (leukocytes) are neutrophils, 1% to 3% are eosinophils, and less than 1% are basophils. During infection, the number of circulating neutrophils increases, a condition termed leukocytosis. Neutrophils are the initial phagocytotic defense against bacterial infection. Their primary (azurophilic) granules contain myeloperoxidase, elastase, and cathepsin G. The secondary (specific) granules contain lysozyme and lactoferrin. Neutrophils can migrate from the circulation into tissues by squeezing in between vascular endothelial cells in a process termed diapedesis. They recognize endothelial cells that have been activated by TNF-α and histamine produced as a result of the infection of the tissue. Activation of the endothelial cells involves the expression of ICAM-1 and E-selectin molecules on the cell surface. In response to TNF-α and histamine, neutrophils express integrins, L-selectin, and LFA-1 on their cell membrane. The initial binding of the neutrophil to the endothelial cell is facilitated by its mucin-like cell adhesion molecule (CAM), or selectin ligand, to the E-selectin on the endothelial cell. The chemokine/chemoattractant receptor on the neutrophil responds to chemokines like interleukin-8 (IL-8; also termed CXCL8 because it acts as a chemokine) secreted by the endothelial cell. This results in the conformational change of the integrin on the neutrophil to a high-affinity state, facilitating strong binding to the integrin ligand on the endothelial cells. This is followed by migration through the endothelium (Fig 1-6).

Eosinophils are involved in defense against parasitic infections. Basophils are not phagocytotic but release pharmacologically active molecules.

T lymphocytes are generated from T-cell progenitors that can differentiate into $CD4^+$ $T_h$cells, $CD8^+$ cytotoxic T cells, and CD8 suppressor T cells ($CD8^+$ T_{reg} cells). The $CD4^+$ cells can differentiate further into T_h1, T_h2, T_h3, T_h17, and regulatory T_{reg} cells. The designation CD refers to cluster of differentiation and is used to identify specific molecules on the surface of immune cells that are characteristic of the state of differentiation of the cells. For example, T cells have the CD3 molecule as part of the T-cell receptor complex, the set of molecules that recognize foreign antigens.

T-cell differentiation takes place in the thymus. If a developing T cell reacts with a protein made by its host before it matures, it will die via apoptosis (programmed cell death), thereby eliminating many T cells that have the potential to attack the body.

RESEARCH

How is the T cell programmed so it "knows" that it should undergo apoptosis when it encounters a "self" antigen while undergoing differentiation?

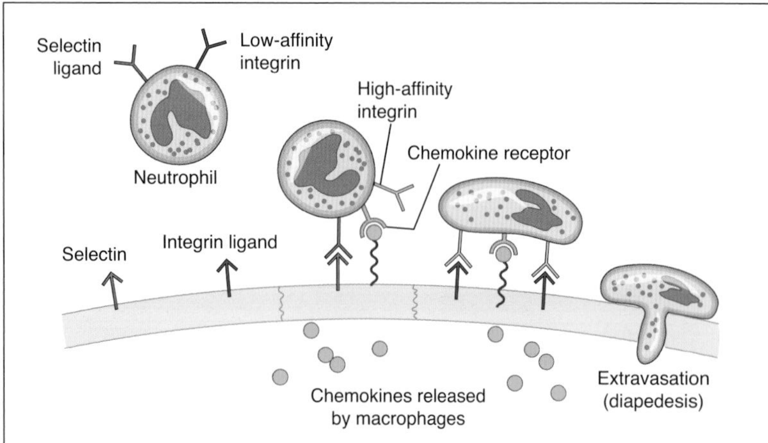

Fig 1-6 Leukocyte recruitment to and migration through the endothelium. (Adapted from Abbas et al.)

T_h1 cells promote local initial defenses and delayed-type hypersensitivity responses (as in the tuberculin skin test for tuberculosis). T_h2 cells promote antibody production, whereas T_h3 cells facilitate immunoglobulin A (IgA) production. T_h17 cells are involved in inflammation. They produce IL-17, which induces chemokine and cytokine production in other cells, resulting in the recruitment of neutrophils. Their numbers increase in multiple sclerosis, inflammatory bowel disease, and rheumatoid arthritis. T_{reg} (T-regulator) cells control the immune response.

Lymphocytes differentiate into B cells in the bone marrow and gut-associated lymphoid tissue. In the antigen-independent phase, progenitor B cells (with the CD45R surface marker) undergo Ig gene rearrangement and selection and become mature (but still naïve) B cells with IgM and IgD on their surface. They express MHC II molecules on their surface and thus are also APCs. Following exposure to a particular antigen and to T_h cells that have been presented to the antigen by APCs, the naïve B cells become activated to differentiate into plasma cells that secrete antibodies that recognize the antigen (in the peripheral lymphoid tissues) (Fig 1-7). If the naïve B cells do not encounter antigen and T_h cells, they undergo apoptosis. **Antibody class switching** also occurs at this stage, where the plasma cells switch from producing **IgM** antibodies (the type of antibodies that are produced initially) to producing **IgG** antibodies. A subset of the B cells differentiate into **memory cells** that facilitate the anamnestic response (the rapid response upon re-exposure to the antigen).

RESEARCH

How were T_h17 and T_{reg} cells discovered?

Lymphocyte progenitors can also differentiate into large granular lymphocytes, known as **natural killer (NK) cells**. Because of the anthropomorphic connotation of violence of the term *killer*, this monograph introduces the designation **natural cytotoxic (NC) cells**. These cells can also act as antibody-dependent cellular cytotoxicity cells by means of the **Fc receptors** that bind the Fc regions of antibodies that recognize antigens on foreign cells.

The common myeloid progenitor cells can differentiate into **Langerhans cells** and **interstitial dendritic cells**. The progenitor cells can also differentiate into monocytes, which in turn differentiate into **myeloid dendritic cells**. The common lymphoid progenitor can also be transformed into **lymphoid dendritic cells**. Long ignored, dendritic cells are now recognized as the most potent APC. They are found in very small numbers in blood (less than 0.1% of leukocytes). Dendritic cells are also called *veiled cells* because of their ruffled membrane. Langerhans cells are the dendritic cells in the skin. In draining lymph nodes, dendritic cells become **interdigitating cells**, carrying antigen to the T-cell regions of the node.

DISCOVERY

In the early 1970s, Ralph Steinman and Zanvil Cohn were studying spleen cells to understand the induction of immune responses in the mouse at Rockefeller University. They knew from previous research that the development of immunity by the spleen required lymphocytes as well as other cells of uncertain function called *accessory cells*. Although these cells were initially thought to be macrophages, Steinman and Cohn focused on cells with unusual treelike or "dendritic" shapes and processes. Steinman therefore named them *dendritic cells*. These cells had little resemblance to the macrophages, lacked a membrane enzyme that was typical of macrophages, detached from culture surfaces, had poor viability, and had a rapid turnover in the spleen. In contrast to macrophages, dendritic cells had few digestive bodies or lysosomes, lacked Fc receptors for particles opsonized with antibodies, and were not highly phagocytotic in vivo and in vitro. The previous experience of Steinman and Cohn with the cell biology of macrophages enabled them to readily identify dendritic cells as a new type of cell with distinct functions in the immune system.

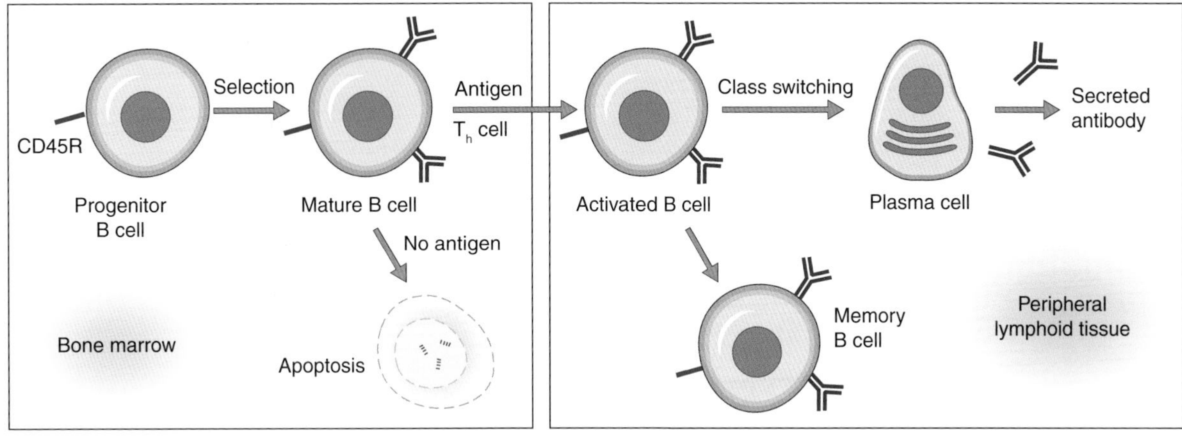

Fig 1-7 Differentiation of B cells. CD, cluster of differentiation; Ag, antigen; Ab, antibody.

Take-Home Messages

- The primary lymphoid organs are the bone marrow and the thymus, where B cells and T cells mature, respectively.
- Cellular and humoral immune responses take place in the secondary lymphoid organs and tissues.
- T cells and B cells meet in the lymph nodes, where T_h cells interact with B cells to induce their differentiation into antibody-producing plasma cells.
- Self-renewing stem cells differentiate into pluripotent stem cells, which can in turn differentiate into either myeloid progenitors or lymphoid progenitors.
- Macrophages engulf bacteria, fungi, and viruses in endocytotic vesicles called *phagosomes* and destroy them following the fusion of the phagosomes with lysosomes.
- Macrophages, dendritic cells, and B cells present antigens on their surface to helper T lymphocytes that can recognize the antigen and proliferate in response to a specific antigen.
- Neutrophils are the initial phagocytotic defense against bacterial infection; they can migrate from the circulation into tissues through endothelial cells via diapedesis.
- T-cell progenitors generate T lymphocytes that can differentiate into $CD4^+$ helper cells, $CD8^+$ cytotoxic cells, and $CD8^+$ suppressor cells. The $CD4^+$ cells can differentiate further into T_h1, T_h2, T_h3, T_h17, and regulatory T_{reg} cells.
- Progenitor B cells undergo Ig gene rearrangement and selection and become mature (but still naïve) B cells with specific IgM and IgD on their surface.
- Lymphocyte progenitors can also differentiate into large granular lymphocytes, known as *natural killer (NK)* or *natural cytotoxic (NC) cells*.

Bibliography

Abbas AK, Lichtman AH. Basic Immunology: Functions and Disorders of the Immune System, ed 3. Philadelphia: Saunders/Elsevier, 2011.

Abbas AK, Lightman AH, Pillai S. Cellular and Molecular Immunology, ed 6. Philadelphia: Saunders/Elsevier, 2010.

Coico R, Sunshine G. Immunology: A Short Course, ed 6. Hoboken, NJ: John Wiley & Sons, 2009.

Goldsby RA, Kindt TJ, Osborne BA, Kuby J. Immunology, ed 5. New York: WH Freeman and Company, 2003.

Murray PR, Rosenthal KS, Pfaller MA. Medical Microbiology, ed 6. Philadelphia: Mosby/Elsevier, 2009.

Pier GB, Lyczak JB, Wetzler LM. Immunology, Infection and Immunity. Washington: ASM Press, 2004.

Rockefeller University/International Society for Dendritic Cell and Vaccine Science. Introduction to Dendritic Cells. lab.rockefeller.edu/steinman/dendritic_intro/discovery. Accessed 14 April 2015.

Roitt I, Brostoff J, Male D. Immunology, ed 5. London: Mosby, 2008.

Antibodies and Complement

2

Antibodies are produced by the humoral immune system. This system comprises stem cells, B lymphocyte precursors, immature B lymphocytes that undergo gene rearrangement to produce mature B cells, B cells that proliferate upon interaction with a particular antigen that they are programmed to recognize, plasma cells that differentiate from the latter cells and start producing large amounts of antibody, and memory B cells that facilitate the anamnestic response.

The Clonal Selection Theory

The Australian immunologist Frank Macfarlane Burnet proposed the clonal selection theory to explain the proliferation of B lymphocytes specific for an invading antigen or a vaccine. According to this theory, each set of lymphocytes (a clone) arises from a single precursor and can recognize a particular epitope, or antigenic determinant, via specific antibodies on the B-cell surface. This B cell is thus activated to proliferate, and the proliferating cells differentiate into plasma cells that produce antibodies with the same specificity as that of the antibodies on the particular B cell. Some of the proliferating cells differentiate into memory B cells.

A similar clonal selection takes place for T cells. Stem cells differentiate into a pre–T cell, which then forms cells that are both $CD4^+$ and $CD8^+$. If these cells interact weakly with major histocompatibility complex class II (MHC II) molecules, they differentiate into $CD4^+$ cells, which will eventually have to recognize MHC II molecules during antigen presentation by antigen-presenting cells. If the cells weakly recognize the MHC I molecules, they become $CD8^+$ cells, which will eventually have to recognize MHC I molecules during antigen presentation by infected cells. The strong recognition of MHC I or MHC II molecules by the $CD4^+$ and $CD8^+$ cells results in the apoptosis of the cells, thereby providing tolerance for self-antigens. If the cells do not recognize the MHC molecules together with the peptides they present, this also results in apoptosis, providing the basis for clonal deletion.

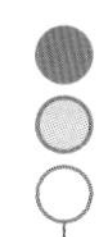

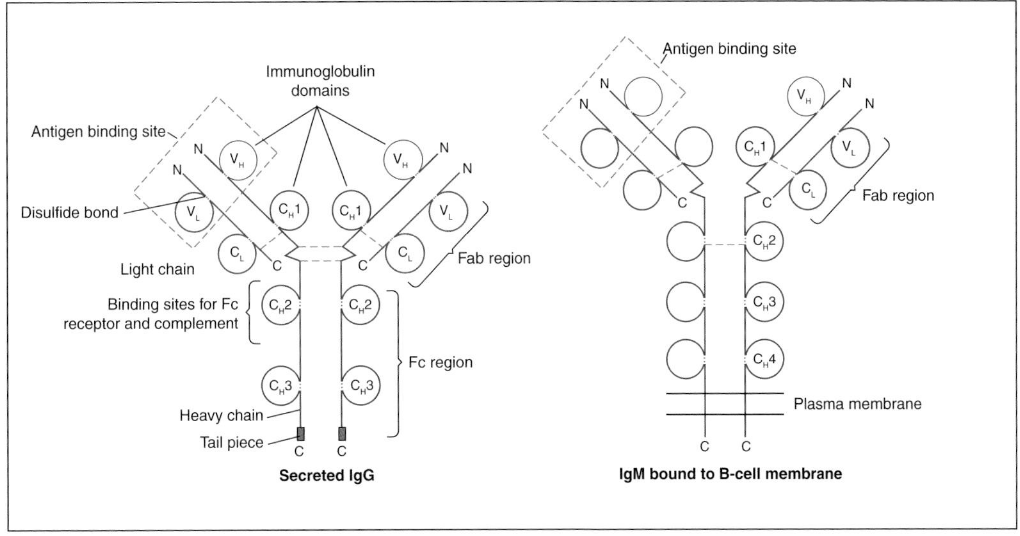

Fig 2-1 The schematic structures of IgG and membrane-bound IgM. The heavy chains are in *blue*, and the light chains are in *red*. Disulfide bonds are shown as *dotted lines*. The approximate binding sites for complement and the Fc receptor within the Fc region are also indicated. (Adapted from Abbas and Lichtman.)

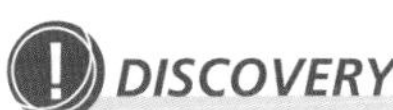

DISCOVERY

The German scientist Paul Ehrlich postulated in 1900 that the surface of white blood cells has receptors that can bind foreign molecules and that this interaction leads to the proliferation of the cells and the production of more of the receptors. This "selective theory" did not receive scientific recognition at the time. Niels Jerne introduced the clonality concept, in which the host has a small number of antibodies against potential antigens, and the complex of the antibody and antigen interacts with white blood cells and results in the production of the same antibody. David Talmadge proposed that the cells that produce a particular antibody start proliferating when their antibody interacts with the antigen. Frank Macfarlane Burnet theorized that one cell produces just one kind of antibody and that the interaction of an antigen with the cell surface–bound antibody induces the cell to proliferate and produce more of the same antibody. Burnet described this scheme as the clonal selection theory. This theory also explained immunologic tolerance, whereby clones of antibody-producing cells reacting with self-antigens would be eliminated during fetal development, as shown by Peter Medawar.

Antibody Structure

Antibodies are the main elements of the humoral immune response and belong to the immunoglobulin (Ig) superfamily of proteins. They neutralize toxins and microorganisms, or "opsonize" microorganisms to help their efficient internalization by phagocytes. An antibody "monomer" consists of four polypeptide chains: two light chains, which are designated kappa (κ) and lambda (λ), and two heavy chains (Fig 2-1).

The structure generated by the N termini of one light chain and one heavy chain constitutes the variable region of the antibody and recognizes an epitope (a molecular structure recognized by an antibody) on an antigen (a molecule that interacts with the products of a specific immune response). Epitopes can be linear (ie, a continuous sequence of amino acids on a protein) or conformational (ie, a three-dimensional structure consisting of different linear regions of the protein). The paratope is the region of the antibody that interacts with an epitope.

The region of the heavy chain that is invariant is termed the constant region (Fc, for the "crystallizable" fragment that could be used for determining the partial x-ray diffraction structure of the antibody molecule). There are five types of heavy chains that define the class of the antibody: IgG, IgM, IgA, IgE, and IgD. These heavy chains are known as γ, μ, α, ϵ, and δ, respectively, and constitute isotypes. These five classes of antibodies can be identified by antibodies directed against the Fc segment of the molecule. Allotypes are additional genetic features of immunoglobulins that vary among individuals. Idiotypes are antigenic determinants formed by the specific protein sequence in the variable region of an immunoglobulin that generate the large number of antigen-binding regions.

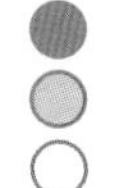

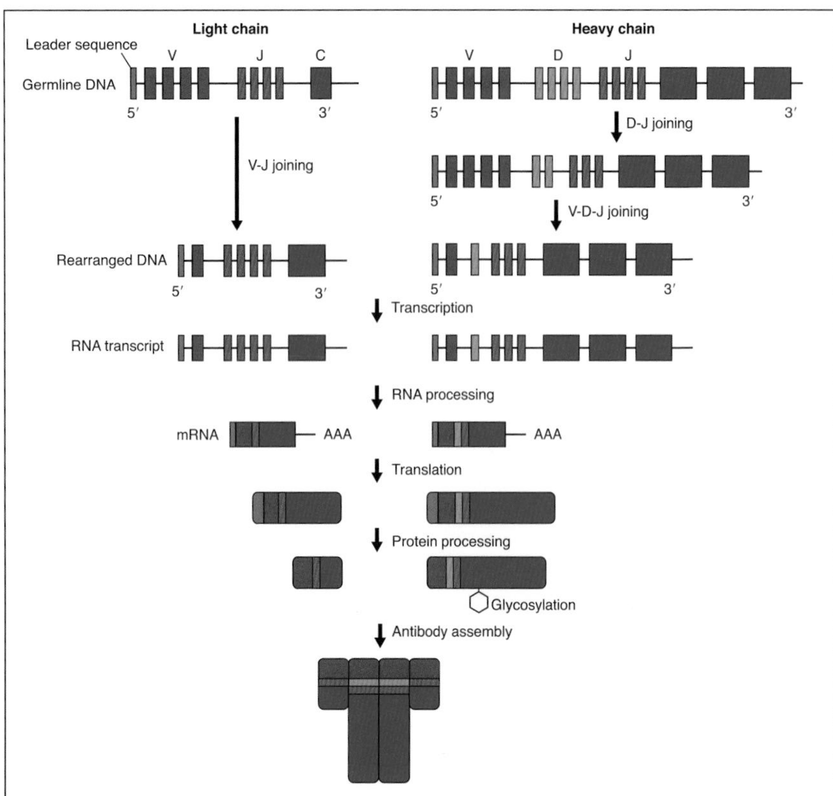

Fig 2-2 Recombination and expression of immunoglobulin genes.

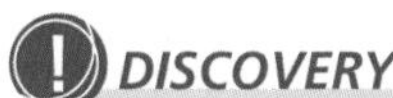

DISCOVERY

Immunologists have puzzled in the past over the specificity of antibodies for the antigens that they recognize. In the 19th century, Paul Ehrlich proposed that the answer to this specificity was in the molecular structure of the antibodies. However, methods to study the structure of large proteins became available only in the mid-20th century. After he joined the laboratory of Henry Kunkel at the Rockefeller Institute in 1958 as a graduate student, Gerald Edelman began working on the structure of antibodies. In Cambridge, England, Rodney Porter, using the enzyme papain, found that rabbit IgG is cleaved into three similarly sized pieces. The two Fab fragments retained their original antibody specificity, but the third fragment, Fc, crystallized. Porter and Edelman showed that immunoglobulin molecules comprise two kinds of polypeptides: the light (L) and heavy (H) chains. Edelman continued his work on IgG by sequencing the 1,300 amino acids of the macromolecule, the longest amino acid sequence to be worked out at that time. Edelman and Porter were awarded the Nobel Prize in 1972 "for their discoveries concerning the chemical structure of antibodies."

The immunogenicity of a molecule is its ability to induce a humoral and/or cell-mediated immune response. Proteins are the strongest immunogens. Pure polysaccharides and lipopolysaccharides are good immunogens. Nucleic acids are not effective in eliciting an immune response, except when they are single stranded or associated with proteins. The antigenicity of a molecule is its ability to combine specifically with the final products of the immune response (ie, antibodies and/or T-cell receptors specific for the molecule). Small molecules like penicillin, called haptens, are antigenic, but they are incapable of inducing a specific immune response by themselves; they become immunogenic if they are bound to peptides or proteins. Penicillin allergies are mediated by recognition by IgE antibodies as well as by T cells.

Antibody Diversity

Antibody diversity is generated by the rearrangement of DNA by recombinases and by RNA splicing. The light chain is encoded by V (variable region) and J (joining segment) genes (Fig 2-2). The heavy chain is encoded by V, D (diversity segment), and J genes. The DNA segments rearrange to make genes for chains that are different in each B cell. Thus, only a limited number of gene segments can generate the estimated 100 million distinct antibodies that the body can produce.

The κ light chain gene clusters on chromosome 2, the λ light chain genes on chromosome 22, and the heavy chain genes (α, δ, ϵ, γ, μ) on chromosome 14 encode the different components of antibodies. Certain nucleotide segments are removed at both the DNA and RNA levels, enabling the apposition of genes that were previously separated. A light chain gene is generated in a pre–B cell by combining one of 35 $V_L\kappa$ genes (or one of 30 $V_L\lambda$ genes) with one of 4 $J_L\kappa$ (or one of 5 $J_L\lambda$) light chain–joining segment genes and one constant segment gene ($C_L\kappa$ or $C_L\lambda$) (see Fig 2-2). An antibody can have either a κ chain or a λ chain.

A heavy chain gene is generated by the combination of one of about 100 variable segment genes (V_H), one of 23 diversity segment genes (D_H), one of 6 joining segment genes (J_H), and one constant region gene among the 5 genes encoding the different classes of antibody ($C_H\alpha$, $C_H\delta$, $C_H\epsilon$, $C_H\gamma$, and $C_H\mu$; IgA, IgD, IgE, IgG, and IgM antibodies, respectively). This recombination process can generate:

35 $V_L\kappa$ genes × 4 $J_L\kappa$ genes = 140 κ chain variable region genes

and

30 $V_L\lambda$ genes × 5 $J_L\lambda$ genes = 150 λ chain variable region genes

Because antibodies contain either a κ chain or a λ chain, and not both, there is the potential to generate 140 + 150 = 290 different light chains.

Recombination of the heavy chain genes can generate:

100 V_H genes × 23 D_H genes × 6 J_H genes = 13,800 heavy chain variable regions

Because the light chain and heavy chain variable regions together comprise the antigen-recognition site on the antibody, a B cell has the potential to create:

13,800 heavy chain variable regions × 290 light chains = 4,002,000 binding specificities.

Further specificities are added to the antibody genes by terminal deoxyribonucleotidyl transferase, an enzyme that adds or removes nucleotides between the different gene segments to create junctional diversity that increases the specificity of the variable region up to 10^{10}.

Immunoglobulin Isotypes

Immunoglobulin G (IgG) constitutes between 75% and 85% of antibodies in blood and has the longest half-life (23 days) among the immunoglobulins. It can opsonize antigens, activate complement, and cross the placenta during pregnancy. It also mediates antibody-dependent cellular cytotoxicity, where a cell coated with specific antibodies is killed by natural cytotoxic cells (also known as *natural killer cells*). There are four types of IgG, namely IgG_1, IgG_2, IgG_3, and IgG_4, with IgG_1 being the most abundant (about 9 mg/mL in serum).

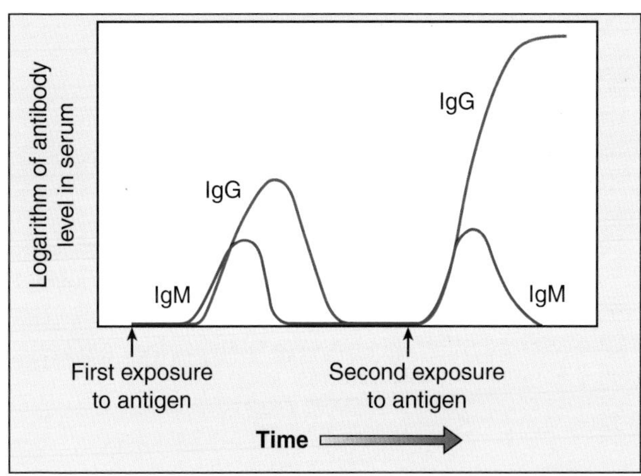

Fig 2-3 Primary and secondary antibody responses. (Adapted from Edgar.)

IgA makes up between 5% and 15% of blood antibodies and has a half-life of 6 days. It is found in blood, tears, colostrum, intestinal and respiratory secretions, and saliva. Secretory IgA consists of two antibodies joined by a J chain and the secretory component that helps the transport of the dimer through epithelial cells. Monomers of IgA are of two types: IgA_1 and IgA_2. The concentration of IgA in serum is about 3 mg/mL.

IgM antibodies have a unique, pentameric structure, with five immunoglobulin units connected via sulfhydryl bonds and a J chain. They constitute about 5% to 10% of blood antibodies (1.5 mg/mL in serum), have a half-life of 5 days, and are the first class of antibodies produced during the primary immune response following the introduction of an immunogen into the host. They are found on the plasma membrane of B cells, are the most efficient antibodies for binding complement, and are effective against polysaccharide antigens.

IgE antibodies are present at very low concentrations, constitute less than 1% of blood antibodies (0.00005 mg/mL in serum), and mediate anaphylactic, Type I hypersensitivity by binding to basophils and mast cells. Antigen-antibody binding and the clustering of Fc receptors on the cells results in cell activation and histamine secretion, giving rise to allergy symptoms. IgE antibodies also protect against parasitic infections.

IgD antibodies are found on B-cell membranes and, together with IgM, function as antigen receptors and activate B-cell growth.

Primary and Secondary Immune Responses

The primary immune response is generated as the production of antibodies by plasma cells after a 5- to 10-day lag period (Fig 2-3). The first class of antibodies produced are IgM antibodies. Immediately after this step, IgG antibodies are

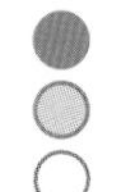

produced. After a few days of increased production, antibody levels decline. The primary immune response also leads to the production of memory cells in lymphoid tissues.

The secondary immune response is initiated when the antigen enters the blood or tissues again. Memory cells facilitate a quicker response to the antigen (3 to 5 days) than that in the primary immune response. The IgM response takes place over a shorter period, and IgG is produced sooner. During this anamnestic response, the antibodies are predominantly IgG, and the antibody levels, measured as the antibody titer, persist for a longer period compared with that in the primary immune response.

Antibody Class Switching

One V_H gene can associate sequentially with different C_H genes during the immune response to produce different classes of immunoglobulins. Whereas the initial antibodies produced are IgM, class switching generates IgG antibodies and eventually IgA antibodies. Class switching occurs only by the change in the heavy chains and not the light chains. The control of class switching depends on the concentration of interleukins. For example, interleukin-4 (IL-4) enhances the production of IgE, whereas IL-5 enhances IgA production.

Monoclonal Antibodies

Monoclonal antibodies recognize a single epitope on an antigen. They were first generated by Georges Köhler and César Milstein, who took lymphocytes from the spleen of mice immunized with a particular antigen and fused them with myeloma cells to produce hybridomas that could divide indefinitely, thus constituting an unlimited reservoir of antibody-producing cells. They could select a particular hybridoma by screening for its antibody product that would recognize the epitope of interest. Such antibodies would be of particular use in the construction of enzyme-linked immunosorbent assays (ELISAs) to detect or quantify particular antigens, since antibodies to different epitopes would be required: one to capture the antigen onto the plastic surface of the well of a microtiter plate and another to recognize the bound antibody. Monoclonal antibodies can also be used in therapeutics; for example, monoclonal antibodies against the epidermal growth factor receptor are used in the treatment of colorectal cancer and head and neck cancer. For this purpose, monoclonal antibodies are genetically engineered to produce chimeric antibodies with a murine variable region and a human constant region to reduce the immunogenicity of murine antibodies.

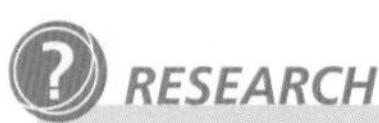

RESEARCH

How are chimeric and human antibodies genetically engineered?

The Complement System

The complement system enhances phagocytosis, facilitates inflammation, and can directly lyse certain microorganisms. There are three complement pathways: the classical, alternative, and lectin pathways (Fig 2-4). The three activation pathways of complement converge on a common point, which is the activation of the C3 component of complement by the enzyme C3 convertase.

In the classical complement pathway, two IgG antibody molecules or a single IgM antibody bound to the surface of a microorganism activates the first component of complement, the protein C1. Activated C1 splits the C2 component into C2a and C2b and the C4 component into C4a and C4b. C4b and C2b form C3 convertase, which cleaves the C3 component of complement into C3a and C3b. C3a is an inflammatory mediator that facilitates chemotaxis and histamine release (see Fig 2-4a). C3b participates in the formation of C5 convertase, which is composed of C4b, C2a, and C3b. C5 convertase splits the C5 component of complement into C5a and C5b. Like C3a, C5a causes chemotaxis and histamine release. C5b combines with C6, C7, C8, and eventually C9 to form a pore, called the *membrane attack complex*, in certain bacterial membranes, such as *Neisseria* species, resulting in cell lysis (see Fig 2-4a).

In the alternative pathway, spontaneously formed C3b binds components of the microbial cell surface (endotoxin or polysaccharides). Factor D (a serine protease) cleaves factor B (also a serine protease) bound to C3b, forming Bb (and Ba). The complexation of C3b and Bb forms C3 convertase, which produces C3b. C3b then binds to the membrane-bound C3b/Bb complex, resulting in the formation of C5 convertase (see Fig 2-4b). In the lectin pathway, the host's mannan-binding protein (MBP), also known as *mannose-binding lectin*, binds to various sugar residues on bacterial surfaces. This binding activates MBP-associated serine protease, which then cleaves C4 and C2 to form C3 convertase (composed of C4b and C2b) (see Fig 2-4c).

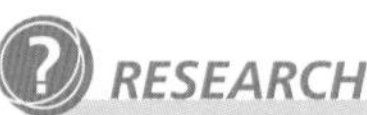

RESEARCH

What are lectins? What do lectins do when they bind cell membranes? Can lectins inhibit viral infection?

In its role as a stimulator of immune adherence, C3b also acts as an opsonin that facilitates the clearance of bacteria by the immune system. It binds to the bacterial cell membrane and stimulates phagocytosis by binding to CR1 (complement receptor 1) receptors on macrophages. The two components of the complement system that facilitate inflammation are C3a and C5a, which stimulate neutrophil and macrophage chemotaxis to the tissue of infection. These components also bind to mast cells and platelets, stimulating histamine release and enhancing vascular permeability and smooth muscle contraction.

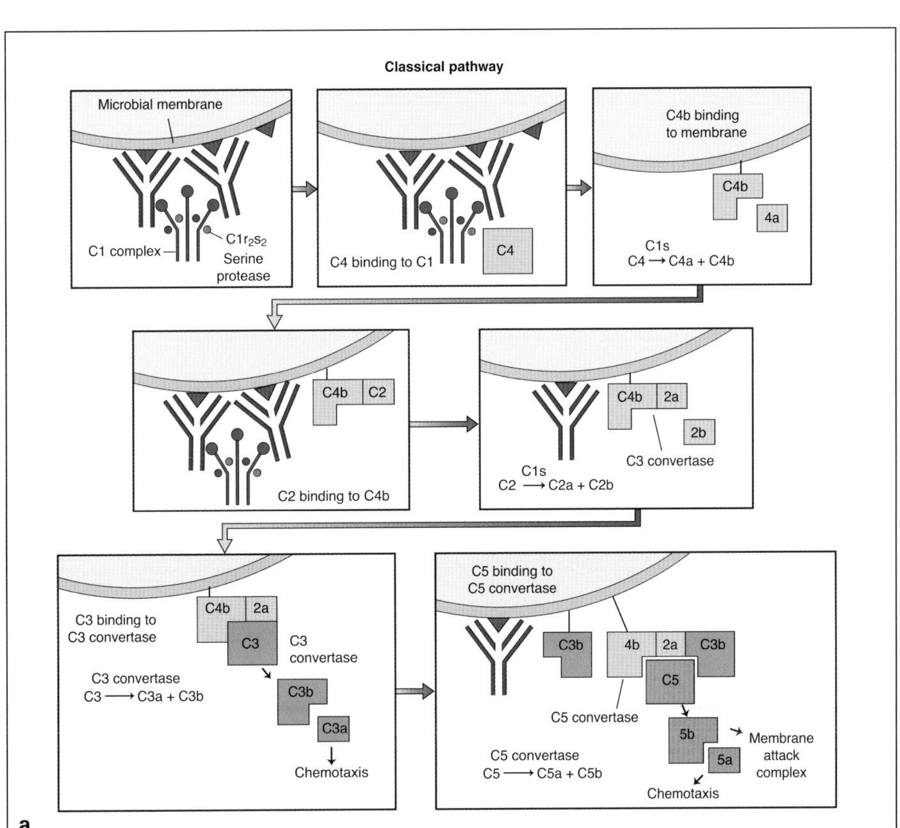

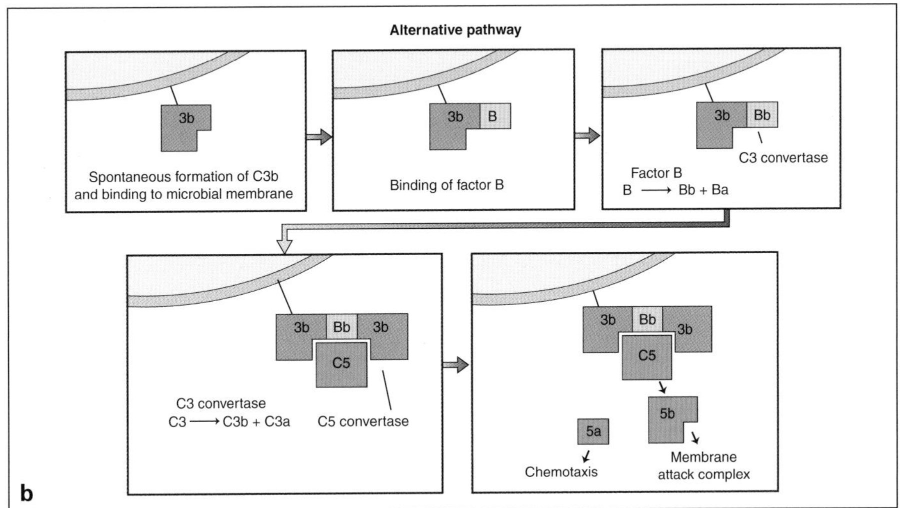

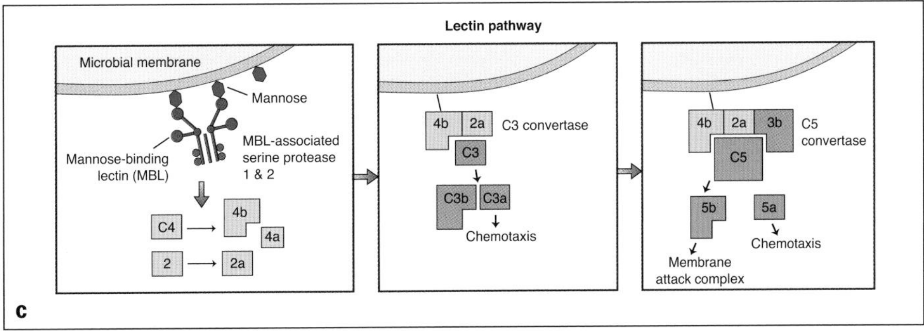

Fig 2-4 The three pathways of the complement system. *(a)* Classical pathway. *(b)* Alternative pathway. *(c)* Lectin pathway.

Take-Home Messages

- According to the clonal selection theory, each set of B lymphocytes (a clone) arises from a single precursor and can recognize a particular epitope via specific antibodies on the B-cell surface.
- A monomeric antibody molecule consists of four polypeptide chains: two light chains and two heavy chains.
- The structure generated by the N termini of one light chain and one heavy chain constitutes the variable region of the antibody and recognizes an epitope on an antigen.
- The immunogenicity of a molecule is its ability to induce a humoral and/or cell-mediated immune response. The antigenicity of a molecule is its ability to combine specifically with the final products of the immune response.
- Antibody diversity is generated by the rearrangement of DNA by recombinases and by RNA splicing.
- IgG constitutes between 75% and 85% of antibodies in blood and has the longest half-life (23 days) among the immunoglobulins.
- IgA makes up between 5% and 15% of blood antibodies and has a half-life of 6 days.
- Secretory IgA consists of two antibody monomers joined by a J chain and the secretory component.
- IgM antibodies have a pentameric structure, with five immunoglobulin units connected via sulfhydryl bonds and a J chain. They constitute about 5% to 10% of blood antibodies and have a half-life of 5 days.
- IgE antibodies mediate anaphylactic, Type I hypersensitivity by binding to basophils and mast cells. They are present at very low concentrations.
- The primary immune response is the production of antibodies by plasma cells after a 5- to 10-day lag period.
- The secondary immune response is initiated when the antigen enters the blood or tissues again and is quicker than the primary response.
- Monoclonal antibodies are generated by fusing lymphocytes from the spleen of immunized mice with myeloma cells to produce hybridomas. They recognize a single epitope on an antigen and are useful in ELISAs and therapeutics.
- The three pathways of complement—the classical, alternative, and lectin pathways—converge on a common point, the activation of the C3 component by the enzyme C3 convertase.
- C3a and C5a are inflammatory mediators. C3b acts as an opsonin, coating microbial surfaces and facilitating phagocytosis. C5b initiates the formation of the membrane attack complex.

Bibliography

Abbas AK, Lichtman AH. Basic Immunology: Functions and Disorders of the Immune System, ed 3. Philadelphia: Saunders/Elsevier, 2011.

Abbas AK, Lichtman AH, Pillai S. Cellular and Molecular Immunology, ed 7. Philadelphia: Saunders/Elsevier, 2012.

Coico R, Sunshine G. Immunology: A Short Course, ed 6. Hoboken, NJ: John Wiley & Sons, 2009.

Department of Biochemistry, University of Oxford. Rodney Porter Memorial Lectures. www.bioch.ox.ac.uk/glycob/rodney_porter_lectures/porter/history.html. Accessed 16 April 2015.

Edgar JD. Clinical immunology. Ulster Med J 2011;80:5–14.

Engleberg NC, DiRita V, Dermody TS. Mechanisms of Microbial Disease, ed 4. Baltimore: Lippincott Williams & Wilkins, 2009.

Mandal A. Antibody history. www.news-medical.net/health/Antibody-History.aspx. Accessed 16 April 2015.

Murray PR, Rosenthal KS, Pfaller MA. Medical Microbiology, ed 6. Philadelphia: Mosby/Elsevier, 2009.

Rockefeller University. Discovering the Molecular Structure of Antibodies and Elaborating the "Sciences of Recognition." centennial. rucares.org/index.php?page=Molecular_Structure_Antibodies. Accessed 16 April 2015.

Shetty N. Milestones in immunology. In: Immunology: Introductory Textbook. New Delhi: New Age International Publishers, 2005.

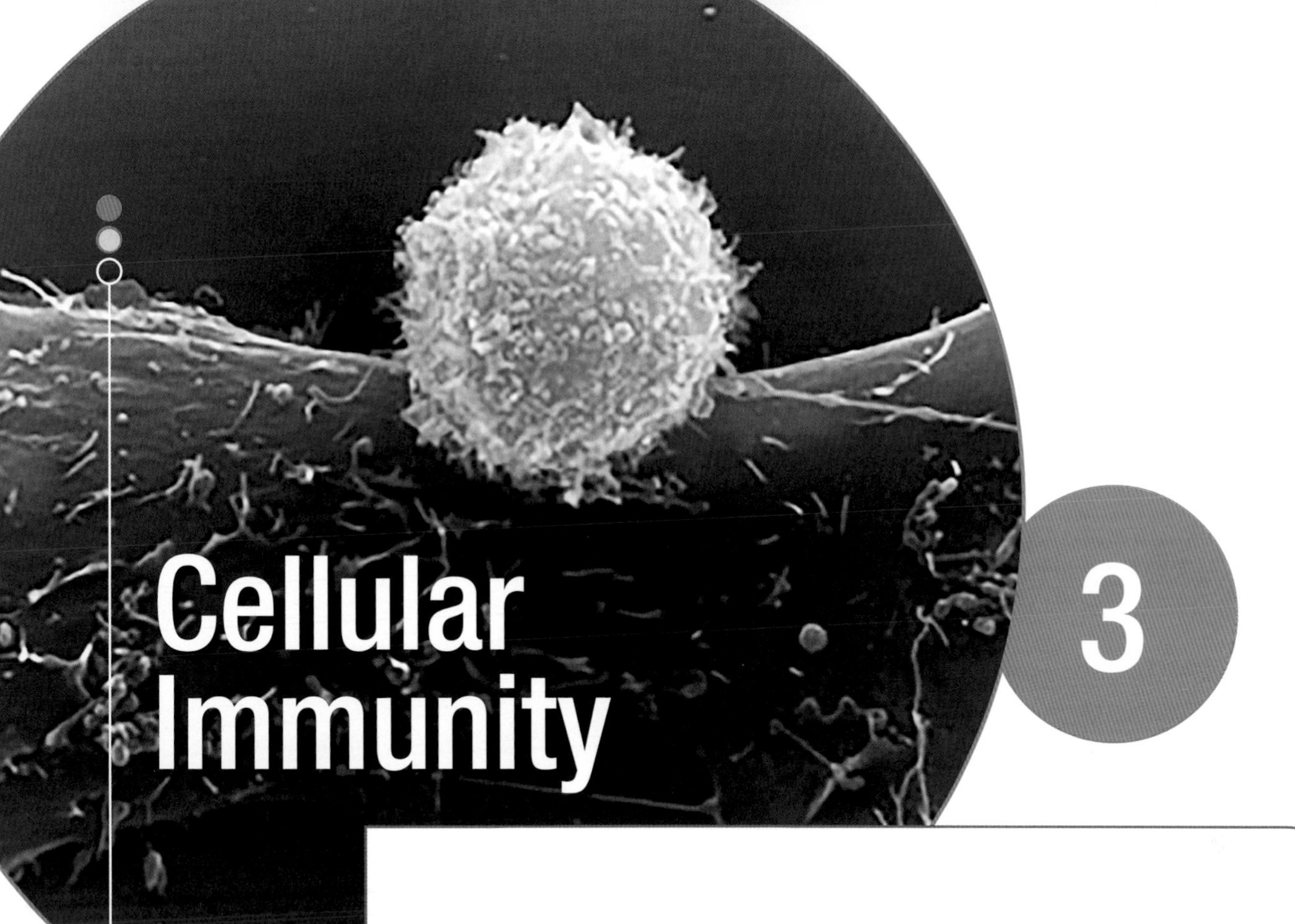

Cellular Immunity

3

Cellular immunity refers to the arm of the immune system by which foreign antigens are presented by antigen-presenting cells (APCs) to T cells, which then become activated to coordinate and carry out the "effector" immune response. This immune response involves cytotoxic T cells that attack infected host cells to try to confine the infection. The former function—coordination—involves helper T cells. The primary reason that human immunodeficiency virus infection causes immunodeficiency is that it infects helper T cells, which are slowly destroyed and decrease in number as the disease progresses.

Antigen Presentation

Major histocompatibility complex (MHC) class I and class II molecules on cell surfaces present antigens to cells of the immune system. MHC class I (MHC I) is the major determinant of "self" and is found in all nucleated cells in the human body. If the MHC I molecule that is presenting a foreign antigen is recognized by a cytotoxic T cell, the latter will be activated to kill the infected "self" cell.

MHC class II (MHC II) molecules are found on APCs, which engulf and digest pathogens and present peptide antigens in association with the MHC II. These antigens are recognized by helper T cells that also recognize the MHC II. Additional co-stimulatory signals are generated by the interaction of additional molecules on the surface of the APCs and the helper T cells.

In our current understanding of the immune response, APCs comprise dendritic cells, macrophages, and B cells.

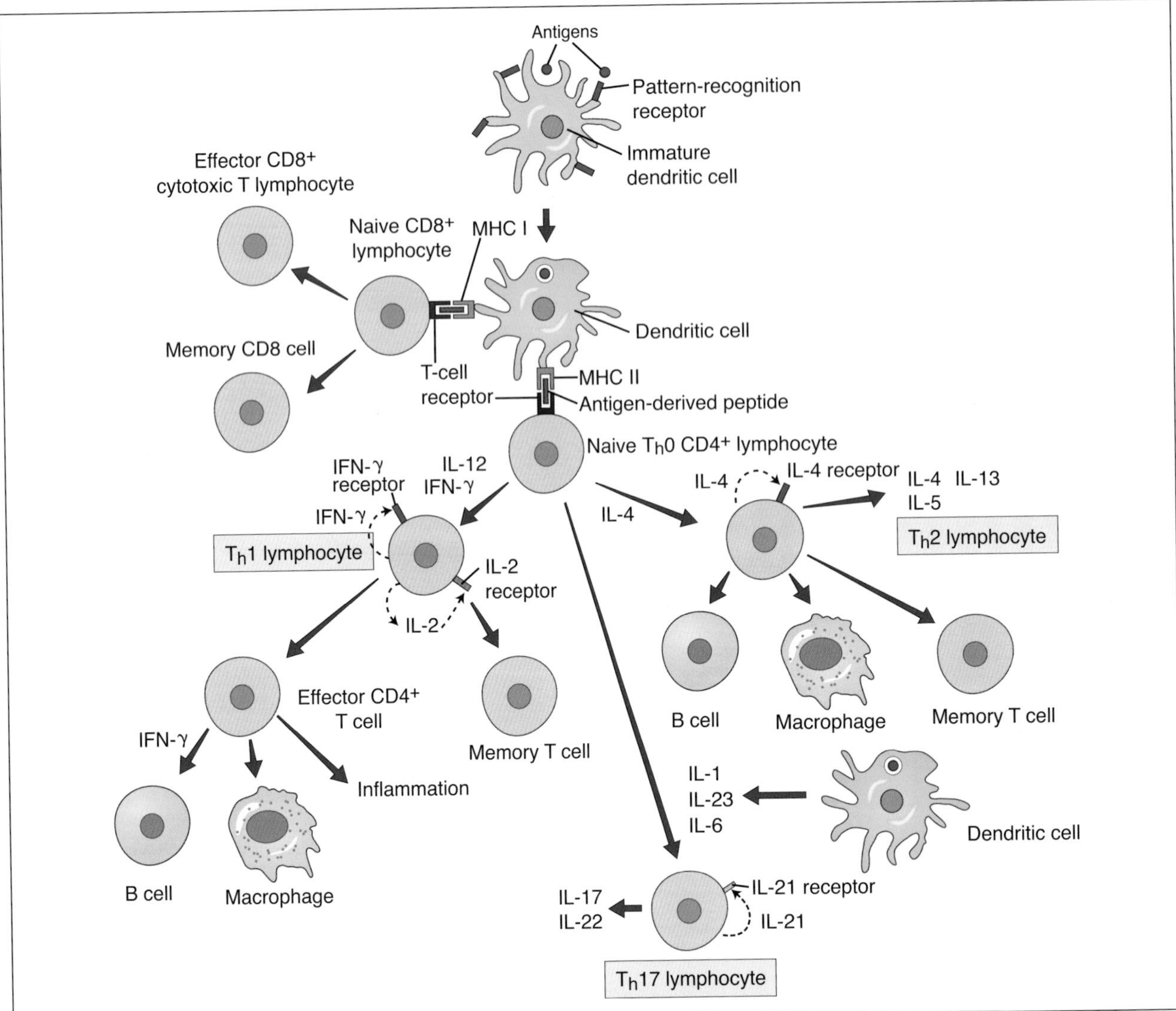

Fig 3-1 Activation of the immune system via antigen presentation by dendritic cells. Immature dendritic cells mature and present antigen to naïve T cells to initiate the antigen-specific responses. Naïve T cells differentiate into T_h1, T_h2, or T_h17 cells. T_h1 cells stimulate cell-mediated immune responses, T_h2 cells stimulate humoral immune responses, and T_h17 cells stimulate intestinal immunity to infection. During a secondary or memory response, B cells, macrophages, and dendritic cells present antigen to the memory T cells (not shown). IFN, interferon; IL, interleukin.

Dendritic cells

Immature dendritic cells release cytokines as an early warning system when they encounter pathogens (Fig 3-1). After ingesting the pathogens and degrading their macromolecules, they mature into dendritic cells and present antigens to T cells and B cells. They differentiate into Langerhans cells and dermal interstitial cells in the skin, interdigitating cells in the lymph nodes and spleen, and splenic marginal dendritic cells. They are also found in the liver, thymus, and germinal centers of lymph nodes, where they become follicular dendritic cells.

Dendritic cells present antigens on MHC I and MHC II to T cells. Follicular dendritic cells lack MHC II but capture antigens via lectins and present them to B cells. Dendritic cells express **Toll-like receptors (TLRs)** that recognize pathogen-associated molecular patterns. TLR recognition results in a cascade of protein kinases that activate immature dendritic cells into mature dendritic cells. After activation, they release cytokines and migrate to the lymph nodes.

Mature dendritic cells present antigens attached to CD1 and MHC I molecules on their surface to naïve CD8 cells and natural cytotoxic T cells (or *natural killer T cells*) to initiate the antigen-specific response. The antigens associated with MHC II molecules are presented to CD4 T cells.

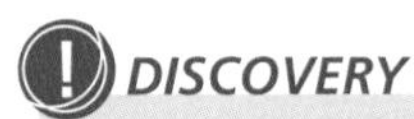

By 1973, it was known that the development of the immune response required "accessory cells" in addition to lymphocytes. At the time at Rockefeller University, Ralph Steinman and Zanvil Cohn were studying spleen cells and macrophages to understand how immune responses are induced. In this process, they discovered cells that had unusual movements and shapes with "dendritic" protrusions reminiscent of dendrites on nerve cells. The cells were therefore named *dendritic cells*.

Unlike macrophages, dendritic cells detached from culture plates, had few lysosomes, did not have Fc receptors that facilitate the uptake of antibody-coated particles, did not have a membrane-bound enzyme found on macrophages, and were poorly phagocytotic. Because Steinman and Cohn were experts in macrophage biology, they could readily identify dendritic cells as a new type of cell.

Steinman developed techniques to isolate pure dendritic cells and found that they stimulate immune function. Dendritic cells were found in different tissues in a variety of animals as well as in humans. They co-localized with the T-cell areas of the lymphatic system. Dendritic cells were found to develop in the bone marrow along a pathway common to macrophages and granulocytes. By 1992, methods were developed for producing a large number of dendritic cells from their progenitors, facilitating cellular and molecular biologic studies on these cells.

T lymphocytes

The T-cell receptor (TCR) complex on the surface of T lymphocytes (Fig 3-2) acts in a manner similar to that of the antigen receptor on B cells, except that it recognizes antigens that are bound to MHC I or MHC II molecules on APCs. Cell activation molecules (CD3) are part of the TCR complex and mediate signal transduction. The ability of TCRs to recognize diverse antigens is enabled by their generation via the combination of genes encoding V, D, and J regions. When the TCR is interacting with peptides presented by MHC molecules on APCs, CD4 or CD8 molecules on the T lymphocytes stabilize the interaction of the TCR with the MHC molecules.

Activation of the T cell during antigen presentation is also dependent on co-stimulatory signals, such as the binding of B7-1 or B7-2 molecules on the APC to CD28/CTLA-4 on the T cell. Lack of this signal leads to anergy (unresponsiveness) or apoptosis of the T cell. When B cells are presenting antigen, CD40L on T cells bind to CD40 on B cells. In addition to the co-stimulatory molecules, adhesion molecules—such as intercellular adhesion molecule on APCs and leukocyte function antigen-1 on T cells—facilitate the interaction of the two cells. The lymphokine receptor interleukin-2 receptor (IL-2R), binds IL-2 secreted by activated helper T cells and stimulates T-cell growth.

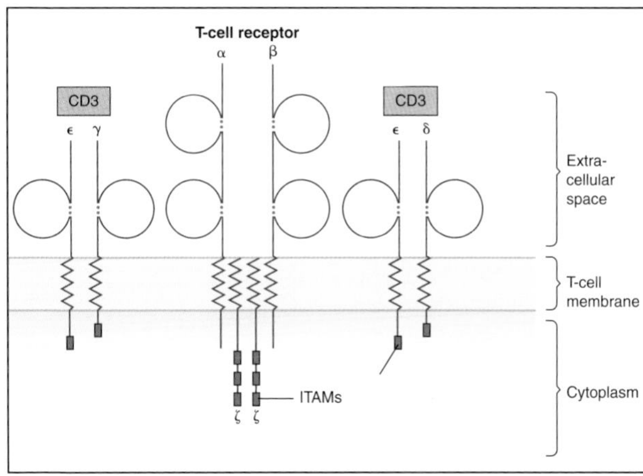

Fig 3-2 Components of the TCR complex. The TCR is composed of the α and β chains, which are linked noncovalently to the CD3 polypeptides ϵ, δ, γ, and ζ. The immunoreceptor tyrosine-based activating motifs (ITAMs) are found in the cytoplasmic domain of the proteins and are phosphorylated by Src family kinases when the receptors are activated.

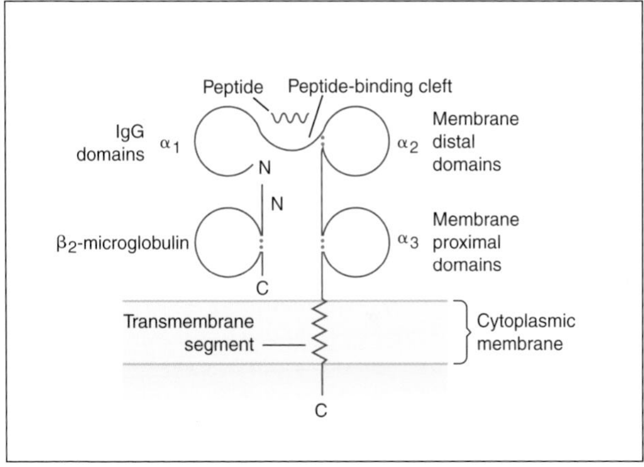

Fig 3-3 The schematic structure of an MHC I molecule, composed of a polymorphic α chain and the noncovalently attached β_2-microglobulin.

Antigen presentation by MHC I molecules

MHC I proteins, which are found on all nucleated cells, link with foreign antigens belonging to an infectious agent produced in an infected cell, or with mutated or overexpressed proteins in the cytosol of tumor cells, and present them on the cell surface (Fig 3-3). Although the antigens belong to the infectious agent, they are called *endogenous antigens* because they are synthesized by the infected cell. Alternatively, phagocytosed microbes or particulate antigens may enter the cytoplasm and may be processed for MHC I–mediated presentation. For example, *Listeria monocytogenes* may penetrate phagosomes and enter the cytoplasm. A small polypeptide called ubiquitin binds the damaged or improperly folded cytosolic protein antigens, enabling the targeting of the antigens to the proteasome, where they are digested proteolytically.

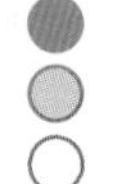

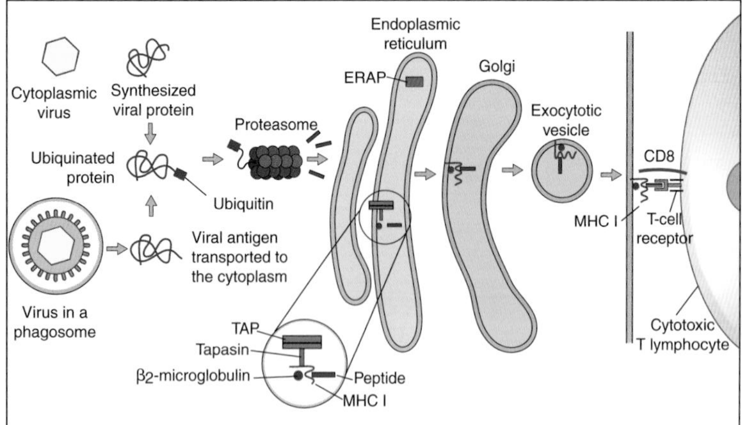

Fig 3-4 Antigen presentation via the MHC I pathway. ERAP, ER-resident aminopeptidase. (Adapted from Abbas et al.)

Peptides of 8 to 16 amino acids are transported into the endoplasmic reticulum (ER) by the protein transporter associated with antigen processing (TAP). In the lumen of the ER, the protein tapasin links TAP with an MHC I. The ER-resident aminopeptidase cleaves the TAP-transported peptide to fit into the peptide-binding cleft of the MHC I molecule (Fig 3-4). MHC I molecules can only hold relatively short peptides, because the binding site is closed off at the edges of the MHC molecule. The MHC I–peptide complex is transported to the Golgi apparatus and then in exocytotic (also called *exocytic*) vesicles to the plasma membrane. TCRs on $CD8^+$ cytotoxic T lymphocytes recognize this complex, with the CD8 co-receptor stabilizing this interaction. Accessory molecules on cytotoxic CD8 T cells include the Fas ligand that can recognize the Fas molecule on target cells and induce apoptosis of the infected cell.

Antigen presentation by MHC II molecules

MHC II molecules present peptides derived from exogenous antigens that are internalized by APCs in endocytotic (also called *endocytic*) vesicles (Fig 3-5). Macrophages and dendritic cells internalize pathogens that bind to receptors that recognize pathogen-associated molecular patterns. Macrophages have Fc receptors that recognize the constant region of antibodies and C3b receptors that recognize the complement component that binds to pathogens. The internalized antigens are digested in late endosomes or lysosomes with the action of proteolytic enzymes, the most abundant of which are the cathepsins.

The MHC II molecules assemble in the ER and are transported in exocytotic vesicles to the endosomes/lysosomes containing the degraded antigens with the help of the invariant chain (I_i). I_i facilitates the folding and assembly of the MHC II molecule and blocks the peptide-binding cleft from accepting degraded peptides until it reaches the compartments containing digested antigens. This protection also prevents peptides encountered in the ER from binding to the cleft. Parts of the I_i are degraded in this compartment, leaving a 24–amino acid peptide termed *class II–associated invariant chain peptide (CLIP)* in the cleft. The CLIP in turn is removed by the action of another MHC molecule called *HLA-DM*, enabling exogenous peptides to bind to the MHC II molecule (Fig 3-6). These peptides are trimmed by proteases to a length of 10 to 30 amino acids before they are transported to the cell surface attached to the MHC II. MHC II molecules can bind peptides of different length because the binding site is open at both ends. The peptides are then recognized by specific $CD4^+$ helper T lymphocytes that also recognize the MHC II molecules. The CD4 molecule interacts with the nonpolymorphic segments of the MHC II and stabilizes the interaction between the APC and $CD4^+$ cell.

In addition to the proteins that are internalized and degraded, proteins that are synthesized and destined for secretion in vesicles may also co-localize in the same compartment as the MHC II molecules and be presented at the cell surface. Membrane proteins that are internalized in the same vesicles as exogenous antigens may be processed similarly and presented with MHC II molecules. Likewise, viral membrane proteins expressed on the surface of infected cells may also be presented with MHC II to $CD4^+$ T cells. This process will thus generate viral antigen-specific helper T cells. In a process called autophagy, cytoplasmic proteins, including those belonging to intracellular microbes, may be trapped and processed in autophagosomes. These organelles may then deliver their contents to the MHC II–containing vesicles, thereby enabling digested peptides to be presented to $CD4^+$ T cells.

In the process of cross-presentation, dendritic cells ingest virus-infected or tumor cells, and peptides derived from these cells are transported from vesicles to the cytosol, where they can be processed by the proteasome for entry into the class I pathway. The peptides can then be presented to $CD8^+$ cells.

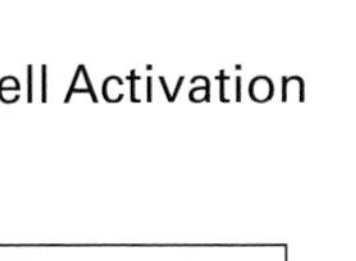

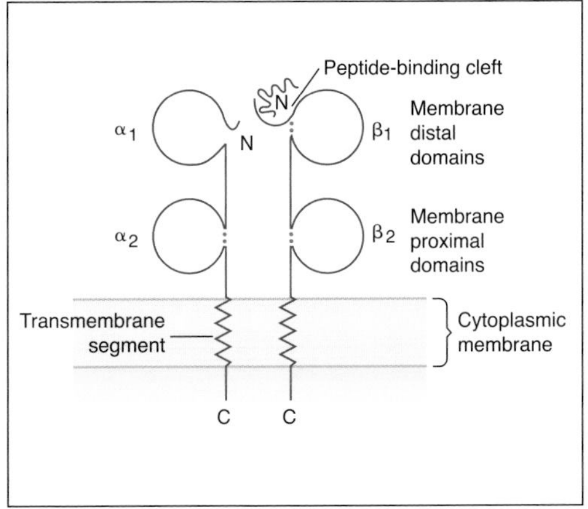

Fig 3-5 The schematic structure of an MHC II molecule, composed of a polymorphic α chain and a polymorphic β chain.

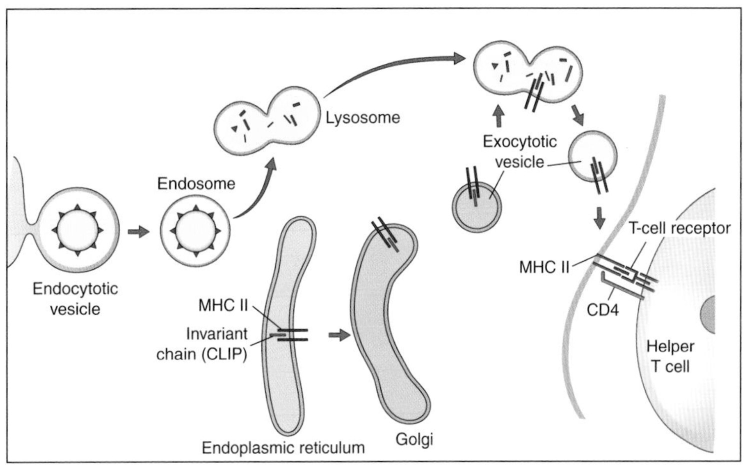

Fig 3-6 Antigen presentation via the MHC II pathway. (Adapted from Abbas et al.)

T-Cell Activation

The binding of the TCR to the MHC II–peptide complex (for CD4 cells) or the MHC I–peptide complex (for CD8 cells) initiates a series of signal transductions via the associated CD3 polypeptides. In simple terms, the T cell is activated to produce IL-2 and IL-2R. This process takes place via the activation of protein kinase C and small GTP-binding proteins and the release of intracellular calcium, all leading to the production of active transcription factors.

The more detailed steps of activation can be summarized as follows:

1. The lymphocyte kinase Lck attached to the cytoplasmic tail of CD4 phosphorylates the tyrosines in the immunoreceptor tyrosine-based activating motifs (ITAMs) on the ζ-chains of the TCR complex.
2. The protein kinase ζ-associated protein of 70 kDa (ZAP-70) binds to the phosphorylated ITAMS, gets phosphorylated by Lck, and is thereby activated.
3. Phosphorylated ZAP-70 phosphorylates a series of membrane-associated adaptor molecules, including Src homology (SH2) domain–containing leukocyte protein of 76 kDa (SLP-76) and linker of activated T cells (LAT).
4. Phospholipase C γ1 anchors to the adaptor molecule LAT, is phosphorylated, and cleaves the phospholipid phosphatidyl inositol bisphosphonate to produce diacylglycerol (DAG) and inositol triphosphate (IP_3).
5. DAG activates a membrane-bound protein kinase C (PKC), which phosphorylates IκB. Nonphosphorylated IκB prevents transcription factor NF-κB from entering the nucleus. The phosphorylation of IκB releases the NF-κB and enables it to enter the nucleus (Fig 3-7).
6. IP_3 induces the release of Ca^{2+} from intracellular stores. Ca^{2+} activates calmodulin, and together they associate with and activate Ca^{2+}/calmodulin–dependent calcineurin, which acts as a phosphatase. It removes a phosphate group from the transcription factor NFAT (nuclear factor of activated T cells), which can then be translocated into the nucleus.
7. NFAT and NF-κB transcriptionally activate several genes.
8. Phosphorylated LAT also mediates the activation of the Ras pathway by binding to and activating the guanine nucleotide exchange factor (GEF or Sos [*Son of sevenless* protein]). This factor catalyzes the exchange of guanosine 5′-triphosphate (GTP) for guanosine 5′-diphosphate (GDP) on the Ras protein, producing the active Ras-GTP.
9. Ras-GTP initiates the mitogen-activated protein kinase pathway, resulting in the activation of Elk, which is a transcription factor for the expression of Fos in the nucleus. Rac-GTP is also formed by the activation of GEF, and it activates a pathway that results in the phosphorylation of the protein Jun, which in turn complexes with Fos. This complex forms the transcription factor AP-1 (activator protein 1). AP-1 may interact with other transcription factors in expressing genes, including the IL-2 gene (see Fig 3-7).

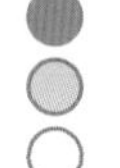

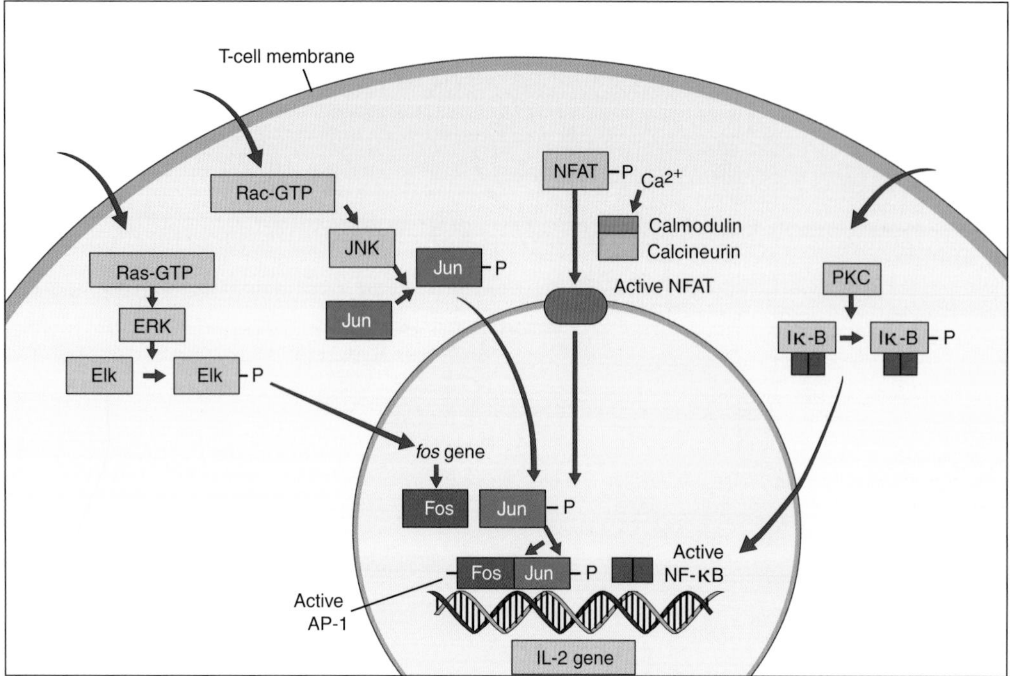

Fig 3-7 Activation of transcription factors in T cells. (Adapted from Abbas et al.)

CD4 Helper T Cells

Naïve CD4+ T cells can differentiate into helper T (T_h) cells—T_h1, T_h2, and T_h17 cells—which are involved in the immune reaction against different infections as well as in causing tissue injury in disease states. Other subsets of T_h cells include follicular T_h cells, which are involved in antibody responses, and regulatory T cells, although they tend to produce different sets of cytokines at different times and are difficult to classify into different populations. The different subsets of T_h cells are defined by the cytokines and transcription factors they express and the epigenetic changes in the cytokine genes. The characteristic cytokines secreted by these subsets are the following: T_h1 cells: interferon gamma (IFN-γ); T_h2 cells: IL-4, IL-5, and IL-13; and T_h17 cells: IL-17 and IL-22 (see Fig 3-1).

T_h1 cells

Precursor T_h cells are activated by interaction with MHC molecules via the immunological synapse to secrete certain cytokines and express cell surface receptors for cytokines. This initially activated cell is a T_h0 cell. If the APC is stimulated by bacterial lipopolysaccharide, it may secrete the cytokine IL-12, which induces the T_h0 cell to become committed to the pathway of T_h1 cells. These cells are produced first in an immune response and secrete IFN-γ (also known as *macrophage-activating factor*), IL-2, and tumor necrosis factor-beta (TNF-β; lymphotoxin), which stimulate local responses. IL-2 stimulates B cells, cytotoxic T lymphocytes, natural cytotoxic cells, and T_h1 cells (autocrine stimulation). IFN-γ activates B cells and macrophages, promoting IL-12 production by the macrophages, which in turn stimulates T_h1 cells.

The activation of macrophages, cytotoxic T cells (CD8+), and natural cytotoxic cells results in the enhancement of local inflammatory responses. These responses are involved in fighting intracellular infections by viruses and bacteria but can also result in autoimmune diseases, including multiple sclerosis and rheumatoid arthritis.

T_h2 cells

The production of IL-4 by follicular T_h cells in lymph nodes stimulates T_h0 cells to differentiate into T_h2 cells, which stimulate B-cell growth and their differentiation into plasma cells. This is achieved by the secretion of IL-4, IL-6, and IL-10. B-cell differentiation involves antibody class switching from immunoglobulin M (IgM) and IgD to IgG, IgE, and IgA. T_h2 cell responses can inhibit inflammatory and autoimmune conditions by limiting T_h1 cell responses, but this can also result in an inability to fight off intracellular infections.

Fig 3-8 The generation and functions of regulatory T cells. The regulation and survival of these cells require IL-2, TGF-β, and the transcription factor FoxP3. In peripheral tissues, T_{reg} cells suppress the activation and effector function of self-reactive lymphocytes that can cause autoimmunity. (Adapted from Abbas et al.)

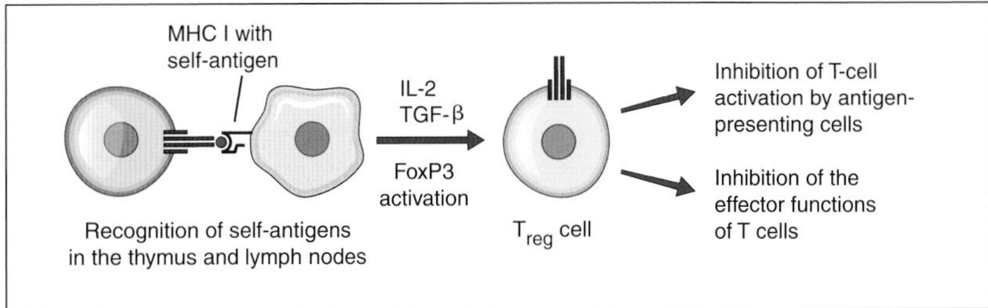

Fig 3-9 CTL-mediated lysis of target cells. Recognition of a foreign antigen presented on the MHC I molecule on the surface of an infected cell activates the CTL. It releases its granule contents (granzymes and perforin) in the vicinity of the immunological synapse. This leads to the death of the target cell.

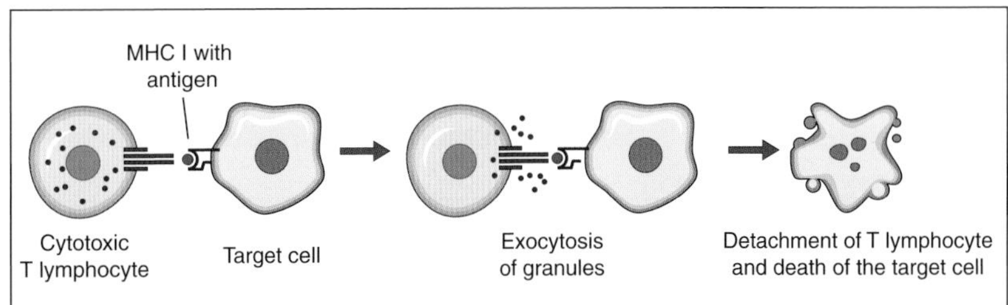

T_h17 cells

Dendritic cells stimulated by the presence of bacteria and fungi secrete IL-1, IL-6, and IL-23. CD4+ helper T cells exposed to these interleukins differentiate to become T_h17 cells. The anti-inflammatory cytokine TGF-β is thought to suppress the production of T_h1 and T_h2 cells and thus negate the inhibitory effect of the latter cells on the development of T_h17 cells. T_h17 cells produce the cytokines IL-17, IL-21, and IL-22. IL-17 induces the production of chemokines and other cytokines, including TNF, that attract neutrophils (and some monocytes) to the site where T cells are activated. IL-17 also stimulates the production of antimicrobial molecules such as defensins from different cell types. IL-21 is necessary for the generation of follicular T_h cells and stimulates germinal center B cells. IL-22 appears to support the barrier function of epithelial cells in the gut and skin and stimulate tissue-repair reactions.

T_{reg} cells

Certain self-reactive CD4+ T cells that can react with self-antigens are not deleted in the thymus, but they differentiate into regulatory T (T_{reg}) cells. After leaving the thymus, they block the potential activation of other T cells against self-tissues (Fig 3-8). The CTLA-4 molecule on T_{reg} cells binds to B7 molecules on APCs and blocks the proper interaction of B7 with T_h cells. T_{reg} cells produce IL-10 and TGF-β, which inhibit immune responses. TGF-β inhibits the activation of macrophages, neutrophils, and endothelial cells, thereby controlling immune and inflammatory responses. An interesting action of TGF-β is that it acts both to stimulate the production of proinflammatory T_h17 cells and to induce the production of T_{reg} cells, thereby suppressing immune and inflammatory responses. TGF-β also induces B cells to class switch to IgA production. IL-10 inhibits macrophages and dendritic cells. Because IL-10 is also produced by macrophages and dendritic cells, it provides a negative feedback regulation of the cells.

CD8+ T Cells

Activation of antigen-specific CD8+ cells is initiated by antigen presentation by MHC I proteins on infected APCs or by cross-presentation of an antigen by a dendritic cell that has acquired the antigen at the site of infection. The help of CD4+ T cells may not be required if the immune response is strong. However, if the immune response is weak, as in the case of latent viral infections, tumors, or organ transplants, help from CD4+ T cells may be required. In this case, cytokines secreted by T_h cells, such as IL-2, bind to IL-2Rs on the CD8+ cells and induce proliferation and differentiation into cytotoxic T lymphocytes (CTLs). During viral challenge in experimental animals, the number of CTLs increases by a factor of 10^5. Activated CD4+ T_h cells express CD40 ligand, which binds to CD40 in APCs, thereby rendering the APCs more efficient at stimulating the differentiation of CD8+ T cells.

The differentiation of CD8+ T cells into CTLs involves the development of cytoplasmic granules that contain the pore-forming protein perforin and granzymes, which are esterases. These granules localize near the immune synapse between the CTL and the infected target cell (Fig 3-9). Perforin forms holes in the target membrane and enables the granule contents to enter the infected cell and initiate programmed cell death (apoptosis). Apoptosis involves the breakdown of the DNA into fragments of about 200 base pairs, exposure of the anionic phospholipid phosphatidylserine on the outer leaflet of the cell membrane, and the formation of apoptotic bodies that are then engulfed by macrophages and dendritic cells. The interaction of Fas ligand on the CTL with Fas on the target cell can also initiate apoptosis. Activated CTLs secrete IFN-γ, which stimulates macrophages to kill intracellular microbes.

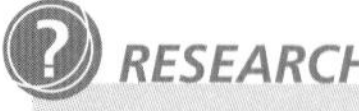

How are cytotoxic T cells protected from the lytic effects of the perforin they secrete?

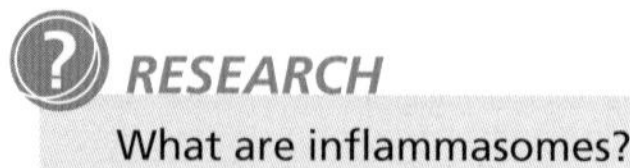

What are inflammasomes?

Take-Home Messages

- MHC I molecules are expressed on the cell surface of all nucleated cells in the human body and are the determinants of "self."
- MHC I molecules present in their peptide-binding cleft endogenous antigenic peptides from the self, described as protein "trash," as well as synthesized viral proteins.
- Following tissue transplantation, allotypes of heavy chains and different self peptides on MHC I molecules elicit a T-cell response.
- MHC II molecules are found on APCs and express exogenous antigenic peptides derived from ingested and degraded foreign proteins, such as those of bacteria.
- These peptides are recognized by the TCR, which can activate T cells through a series of reactions.

Bibliography

Abbas AK, Lichtman AH, Pillai S. Cellular and Molecular Immunology, ed 7. Philadelphia: Elsevier/Saunders, 2012.

Coico R, Sunshine G. Immunology: A Short Course, ed 6. Hoboken, NJ: John Wiley & Sons, 2009.

Goldsby RA, Kindt TJ, Osborne BA, Kuby J. Immunology, ed 5. New York: WH Freeman, 2003.

Murray PR, Rosenthal KS, Pfaller MA. Medical Microbiology, ed 7. Philadelphia: Mosby/Elsevier, 2013.

Rockefeller University. Introduction to Dendritic Cells. lab.rockefeller.edu/steinman/dendritic_intro/discovery. Accessed 20 April 2015.

The Immune Response to Pathogens and Immunopathogenesis

4

Inflammation

Inflammation is the body's initial response to tissue damage from injury, exposure to toxins, or infection, resulting in the extravascular localization of plasma proteins and leukocytes. Its manifestations include redness, swelling, heat, and pain. The term is derived from the Latin *inflammare*, meaning "set on fire." Inflammation can not only control infections and mediate tissue repair but also mediate tissue damage. It progresses through phases of acute inflammation, repair and regeneration, and chronic inflammation.

Acute (localized) inflammation

Macrophages that encounter microbes at the site of injury release interleukin-1 (IL-1) and tumor necrosis factor-alpha (TNF-α) at the site of infection. These molecules activate the local endothelial cells to express the cell surface molecules: selectins and ligands for integrins. The chemokines produced in the tissue (eg, by the complement system) or by the endothelial cells are displayed on their surface bound to heparan sulfate glycosaminoglycans (Fig 4-1). In acute (localized) inflammation, innate immune cells, including macrophages and neutrophils, are recruited from the local blood vessels to the site of injury. Smooth muscle contraction causes the local blood vessels to constrict, thus increasing the local blood pressure. Concomitantly, the local permeability of the vascular endothelium to plasma increases, and the increased blood pressure forces the plasma into the tissue, bringing complement components and antibodies. The loosening of the tight junctions also facilitates the extravasation of leukocytes from the blood into the tissue; this process is called diapedesis. The leukocytes initially roll along the capillary wall under the shear force of the blood flow. When leukocytes bind to the selectins and the proteoglycan-bound chemokines, their integrins are transformed into a high-affinity state and bind to the integrin receptors on the endothelial cells. After firm adhesion to the endothelial cells, the leukocytes migrate to the junctions between the endothelial cells and extravasate into the tissue.

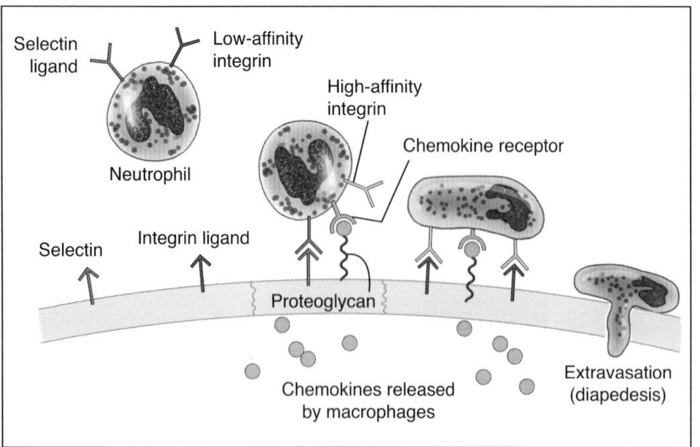

Fig 4-1 Interaction of leukocytes with endothelial cells during leukocyte recruitment into tissues. Macrophages that have encountered microbes release cytokines, including TNF-α and IL-1, at the site of infection. These molecules activate the local endothelial cells to express the cell surface molecules: selectins and ligands for integrins. The chemokines produced in the tissue (eg, by the complement system) or by the endothelial cells are displayed on their surface bound to heparan sulfate glycosaminoglycans ("proteoglycan" in the figure). The leukocytes initially roll along the capillary wall under the shear force of the blood flow. When leukocytes bind to the selectins and the chemokines, their integrins are transformed into a high-affinity state and bind to the integrin receptors on the endothelial cells. After firm adhesion to the endothelial cells, the leukocytes migrate to the junctions between the endothelial cells and extravasate into the tissue. (Adapted from Abbas et al.)

Acute inflammation is mediated by the chemotactic components of the complement system—C3a and C5a—the kinin and plasmin systems, histamine, prostaglandins, and leukotrienes. Histamine is released by activated mast cells. The **kinin system** generates the peptides kallidin and bradykinin; these molecules increase local vascular permeability. The **plasmin system** is involved in wound repair by remodeling the extracellular matrix. Prostaglandins are produced by the conversion of arachidonic acid (a fatty acid that is part of membrane phospholipids) by cyclooxygenase-2 (COX-2), and leukotrienes are generated likewise but with the action of 5-lipooxygenase.

Pathogen-associated molecular patterns (PAMPs) are molecules found on or in microbes that are essential for pathogenicity. PAMPs are recognized by host molecules called **pathogen recognition receptors (PRRs)**. When PAMPs are recognized by PRRs, inflammatory cytokines, chemokines, and type I interferons (IFN-α and IFN-β) are generated. Among PRRs are Toll-like receptors (TLRs), RIG-I-like receptors, the cytoplasmic peptidoglycan receptors (nucleotide-binding oligomerization domain 1 [NOD1] and NOD2 and cryopyrin), NOD-like receptors, and DNA receptors (cytosolic sensors for DNA).

The **inflammasome** is a complex of various proteins in macrophages, dendritic cells, epithelial cells, and other cells and is activated by adaptor proteins that are induced by the PRRs, intracellular infections, or tissue damage. Inflammasomes regulate host responses that are protective against infections. These responses include the secretion of the proinflammatory cytokines IL-1β and IL-18 and the induction of **pyroptosis**, which is a form of cytotoxicity resulting in the death of infected cells. Inflammasomes contain PRRs belonging to the NOD-like receptor family or the PYHIN protein family and the protease caspase-1. The release of the cytokines and the induction of pyroptosis protects against many pathogens.

During the **repair and regeneration phase**, chronically activated macrophages release cytokines that stimulate **fibroblast** proliferation and the production of collagen. Fibroblasts replace fibrin in the clot, and capillaries grow into the fibrin meshwork. The resulting tissue is called *granulation tissue*. **Chronic inflammation** occurs when the host cannot eliminate the inflammatory agent. A granuloma is formed by monocytes, histiocytes, lymphocytes, and plasma cells, and this condition is usually termed *granulomatous inflammation*. **Multinucleated giant cells** formed as a result of the fusion of activated macrophages are often found at the center of the granuloma. These are surrounded by flattened macrophages called **epithelioid cells**, because they resemble epithelial cells. IFN-γ, secreted by helper T (T_h1) cells, natural cytotoxic cells (also known as *natural killer cells*), and cytotoxic T cells, and TNF-α, secreted by activated macrophages, play an important role in the development of chronic inflammation. IFN-γ serves many different functions, among them the activation of macrophages, which then express higher levels of major histocompatibility complex class II (MHC II) molecules, secrete various cytokines (including TNF-α), and have increased microbicidal activity (Fig 4-2). Under chronic inflammatory conditions, macrophages can release reactive oxygen and nitrogen species and hydrolytic enzymes that can damage neighboring tissues.

Acute-phase response

The acute-phase response is triggered by macrophages in response to lipopolysaccharide (LPS) and other bacterial components. Macrophages release **IL-1** and **IL-6**, which then trigger hepatocytes in the liver to release **C-reactive protein**, **serum amyloid P** (both members of the pentraxin family of proteins), and **mannose-binding lectin** (a member of the collectin family of proteins). The acute-phase response also results in the production of adrenocorticotropic hormone (corticotropin), hydrocortisone, fever, and increased production of leukocytes. Elevated temperatures inhibit the growth of certain microbes and appear to facilitate the immune response (Fig 4-3).

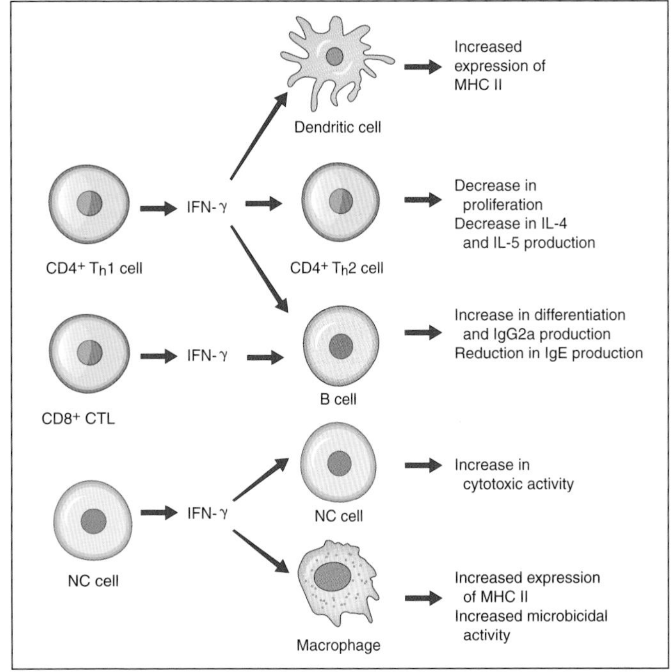

Fig 4-2 Different activities of IFN-γ, which is secreted by T_h1 cells, natural cytotoxic (NC) cells (known more commonly as *natural killer cells*), and cytotoxic T lymphocytes. Macrophage activation by IFN-γ is involved in chronic inflammation. CTL, cytotoxic T lymphocyte; Ig, immunoglobulin.

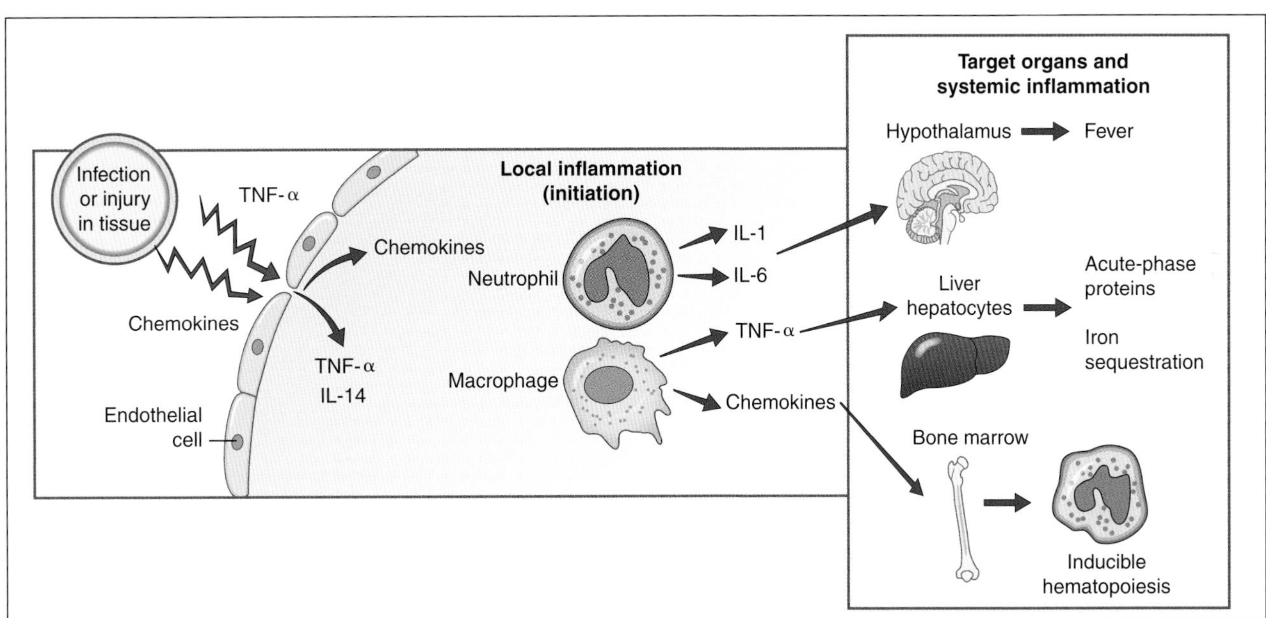

Fig 4-3 The acute-phase response: the systemic inflammatory response. This phase is initiated by the cytokines IL-1, IL-6, and TNF-α; leukemia inhibitory factor; and oncostatin M, which are produced at the initial site of infection and travel in the circulation to the hypothalamus, liver, and bone marrow. The brain responds by producing prostaglandins, which cause fever; the liver produces the acute-phase proteins C-reactive protein, fibrinogen, and complement; and the bone marrow responds by producing leukocytes such as neutrophils ("inducible hematopoiesis").

C-reactive protein complexes with bacterial and fungal "C" polysaccharides (C substance) and activates the complement pathway. The complement component C3b thus produced can opsonize microbes and facilitate their uptake by phagocytes via the C3b receptor.

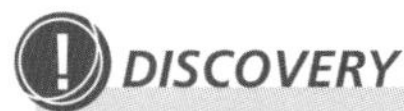

C-reactive protein was discovered in the laboratory of Oswald Avery at the Rockefeller Institute. It was termed *C-reactive* because it precipitated the "C polysaccharide" from the cell wall of pneumococci. William S. Tillett and Thomas Francis, Jr, had found a new antigen of *Streptococcus pneumoniae* and called it Fraction C. They tested its reaction with serum from patients with pneumonia and found that serum from patients during the acute stage of infection caused a strong precipitation reaction. As the patients recovered, the reaction diminished, and later it disappeared. The Fraction C reaction was not specific to pneumococcal infection; it precipitated a substance from the serum of patients with bacterial endocarditis and acute rheumatic fever. Some years later, Avery, Theodore J. Abernethy, and Colin MacLeod found that the C-reactive substance was a protein. Maclyn McCarty crystallized the protein in 1947. In the 1990s, it was recognized that inflammation contributes to the development of atherosclerosis, and C-reactive protein levels were analyzed to assess cardiovascular risk.

C-reactive protein not only may be a marker for inflammation but also may contribute to inflammatory diseases. Like other pentraxins, C-reactive protein consists of five identical subunits that are noncovalently attached to each other. The circulating pentameric C-reactive protein (pCRP) may dissociate to form monomers (mCRP). In vitro studies have indicated that activated platelets and apoptotic cells mediate the deposition of mCRP on inflamed surfaces.

Pentraxins can be considered as soluble pattern-recognition molecules that are involved in fighting pathogenic bacteria. They act as opsonins by binding to pathogens and activate the complement pathway, and they facilitate binding to Fcγ receptors on phagocytotic cells. These proteins recognize membrane phospholipids and nuclear molecules that may be exposed on damaged cells. C-reactive protein interacts with small nuclear ribonucleoproteins and phosphorylcholine (found on the cell wall or LPS of certain bacteria). Serum amyloid P recognizes DNA. C-reactive protein in blood is used widely as a marker of inflammation and infection.

Mannose-binding lectin binds to microbial cells that have terminal mannose and fucose on their glycoproteins and glycolipids, but not to mammalian cells. Mannose-binding lectin activates the lectin pathway of the complement system and, after opsonizing microbes, binds the C1q receptor on macrophages, thereby facilitating the phagocytosis of the microbe.

Fever

Body temperature is regulated by the hypothalamus. Pyrogens are molecules that can induce fever. The lysate from Gram-negative bacteria is a powerful exogenous pyrogen, the key component being LPS. The receptor for LPS was identified as TLR4 in the Toll-like receptor family. LPS-TLR4 binding induces a signal transduction cascade, resulting in the nuclear factor kappa B (NF-κB)–mediated synthesis of IL-1, TNF-α and COX-2. Following stimulation with exogenous pyrogen, endogenous messenger molecules must be released. Studies trying to identify endogenous pyrogen pointed to the cytokine IL-1, which turned out to be the lymphocyte-activating factor that other studies were trying to identify. The endogenous pyrogens IL-1, IL-6, and TNF-α are secreted by monocytes and macrophages. The levels of IL-1 in blood are very low in the absence of inflammation but increase 20- to 100-fold in response to the activation of TLRs by viruses or bacteria within 30 to 90 minutes.

Elevated temperature results in increased leukocyte adhesion to tissues mediated by the activation of L-selectin in lymphocytes, which is dependent on an unusual signaling mechanism called IL-6 trans-signaling, aided by the action of a soluble (ie, not membrane bound) IL-6 receptor. Lymphocytes adhere strongly to high endothelial venules in lymph nodes and Peyer's patches through this mechanism at elevated temperatures. They then extravasate to the underlying parenchyma. This mechanism greatly increases the likelihood that circulating lymphocytes encounter target antigens in lymphoid tissues and provides an answer to the question of how fever helps the immune system during inflammation and infection. An additional benefit of fever is that some pathogens do not replicate at high temperature.

Interferons

Interferons are low–molecular weight proteins (approximately 19.5 kDa) produced in response to viral infections (IFN-α and IFN-β) or upon activation of the immune response (IFN-γ). IFN-α is produced by B cells, monocytes, and macrophages, whereas IFN-β is made by fibroblasts and other cells. IFN-γ is produced by T cells and natural cytotoxic cells. IFN-α and -β are secreted by virally infected cells, bind to interferon receptors on neighboring cells, and induce an antiviral state (Fig 4-4). The antiviral state is accomplished by the inhibition of protein synthesis through the degradation of mRNA and inhibition of ribosome assembly. IFN-γ, which was originally called *macrophage-activating factor*, plays a significant stimulatory role in the T_h1 response.

Immunity to extracellular bacteria

Extracellular bacteria multiply in various locations in the body: the blood, the gastrointestinal tract, connective tissue, and the respiratory tract. These bacteria can cause inflammation or produce endotoxins or exotoxins. Innate immunity to these bacteria involves phagocytosis, inflam-

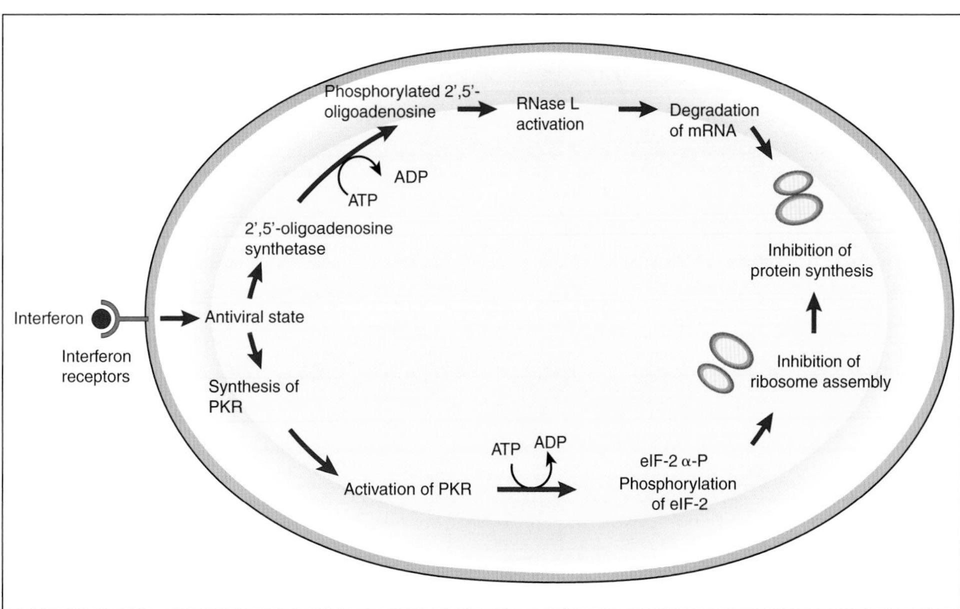

Fig 4-4 Two main pathways of IFN-α inhibition of viral protein synthesis. Interferon binding to its receptor results in the generation of the antiviral state. *Top pathway:* Entry of viral double-stranded RNA into the cytoplasm causes the activation of the 2',5'-oligoadenosine synthetase, producing an unusual nucleotide that activates ribonuclease L (RNase L). This enzyme then degrades mRNA. *Bottom pathway:* The antiviral state causes the production and activation of protein kinase R (PKR), which inactivates eukaryotic initiation factor (eIF-2) by phosphorylating it. This results in the inhibition of ribosome assembly and of protein synthesis. (Inspired by Murray et al.)

mation, and the complement system. Phagocytosis is facilitated by mannose and scavenger receptors as well as receptors for the Fc region of opsonizing antibodies and for complement components (eg, C3b) coating bacteria. The alternative complement pathway is activated by LPS and peptidoglycan, and the lectin pathway is activated by mannose on bacterial surfaces (see chapter 2). Activation leads to the formation of chemotactic components of complement and the membrane attack complex that can kill *Neisseria* species.

Adaptive immunity protects against bacteria by generating antibodies via the humoral immune response (Fig 4-5). The antibodies block infection, opsonize the bacteria to facilitate phagocytosis, initiate the classical complement cascade, and neutralize the exotoxins of bacteria. Bacterial polysaccharides are "thymus-independent" antigens, which humoral immunity recognizes and defends the host against polysaccharide-capsulated bacteria. The protein antigens of the bacteria are processed and presented by dendritic cells to CD4 helper T cells that then produce cytokines that stimulate antibody production, local inflammation, phagocytosis, and microbicidal action of macrophages and neutrophils. IL-17, TNF, and other cytokines mediate neutrophil and macrophage recruitment. IFN-γ secreted by the T cells activates macrophages to phagocytose and kill bacteria. Various cytokines stimulate the production of antibody isotypes that opsonize bacteria and activate complement.

Immunity to intracellular bacteria

Intracellular bacteria can survive and replicate in phagosomes or the cytoplasm of host cells. Thus, they are not accessible to antibody intervention, and cell-mediated immune responses are essential to control the infection. Innate immune responses to these bacteria involve neutrophils, macrophages, and natural cytotoxic (NC) cells. Bacterial products are recognized by TLRs and NOD-like receptor proteins in the cytoplasm, leading to phagocyte activation. NC cells are activated by the expression of certain NC cell ligands on the surface of the infected cells. Infected phagocytes secrete IL-12 that activates NC cells, which in turn produce IFN-γ to activate macrophages to kill the intracellular bacteria (Fig 4-6). The innate immune response is generally insufficient to eliminate all intracellular bacteria.

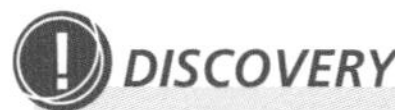

In the 1950s, it was shown that when mice were infected with a low dose of *Listeria monocytogenes*, they were immune to a challenge with lethal doses of the bacterium. The immunity could be transferred to untreated mice by injecting lymphocytes from the infected mice. Transferring serum, however, did not confer immunity, indicating that the humoral immune response was not involved in the killing of intracellular bacteria. In vitro experiments indicated that it was not T lymphocytes from the immune animals that killed intracellular bacteria but rather activated macrophages.

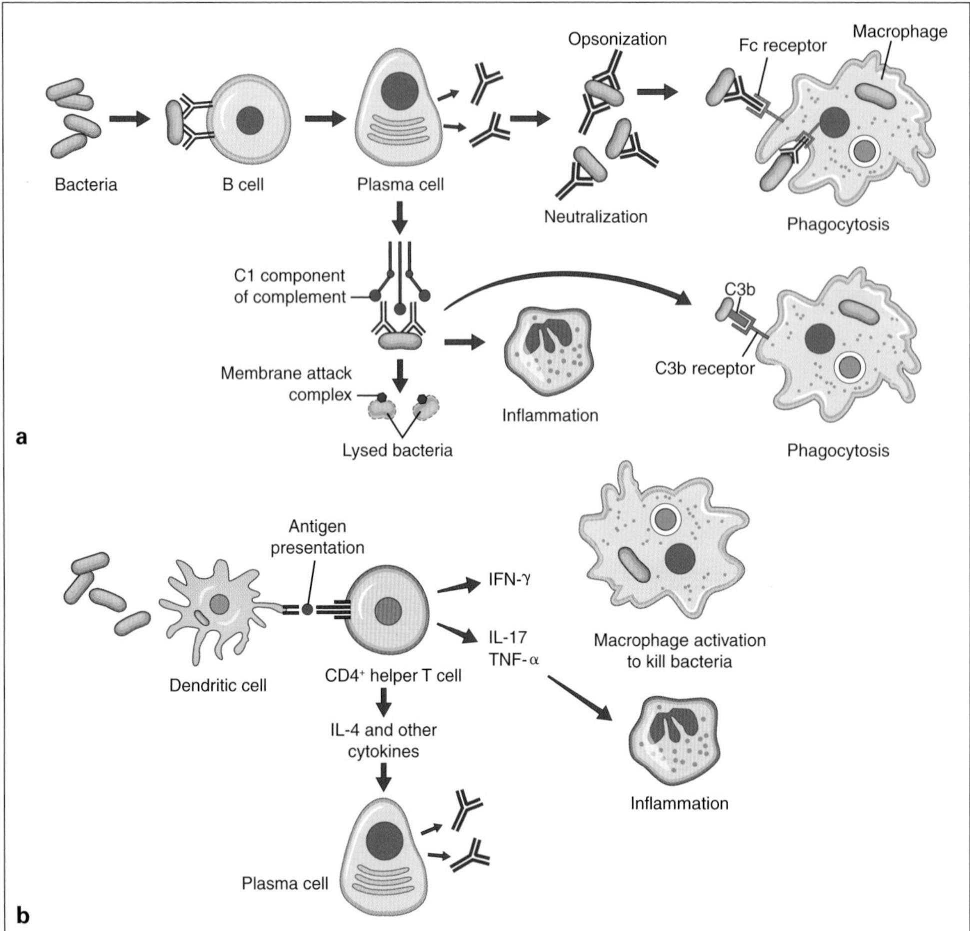

Fig 4-5 Adaptive immune responses to extracellular bacteria. *(a)* Antibody production. *(b)* Activation of CD4+ T_h cells. (Adapted from Abbas et al.)

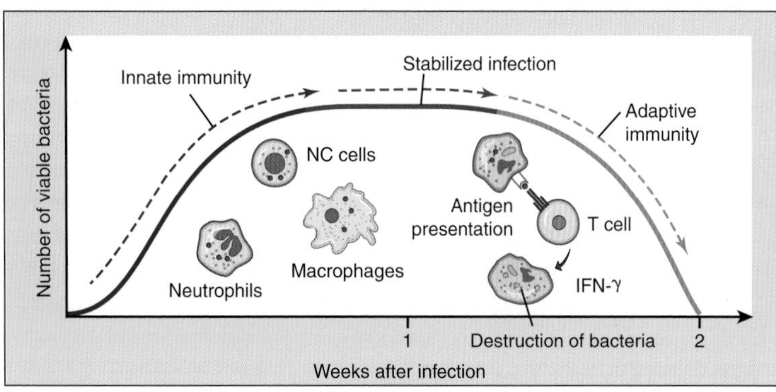

Fig 4-6 The time course of innate and adaptive immunity to intracellular bacteria. Innate immunity can control bacterial growth, but adaptive immunity is essential for eliminating the bacteria. (Inspired by Abbas et al.)

Eradication of intracellular bacteria requires the adaptive immune response. CD4+ T cells activated by antigen presentation in turn recruit and activate macrophages via the action of CD40 ligand and IFN-γ. The macrophages can then kill intracellular bacteria.

Immunity to viruses

Innate immunity to viruses involves the induction of type I IFNs and the killing of infected cells by NC cells (Fig 4-7). The plasmacytoid-type dendritic cells are the primary producer of type I IFNs, which induce an antiviral state in uninfected cells. NC cells can detect virus-infected cells where the virus prevents the surface expression of MHC I; this in turn deactivates the normal inhibitory state of the NC cells, enabling them to kill the infected cells.

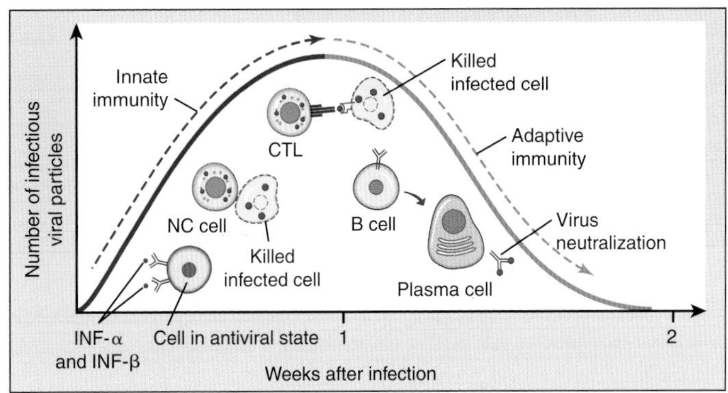

Fig 4-7 The time course of innate and adaptive immune responses to infection by a virus. CTL, cytotoxic T lymphocyte. (Inspired by Abbas et al.)

Adaptive immunity to viruses involves both humoral and cell-mediated responses. Antibodies can neutralize the virions, preventing their binding to host cell receptors. Secretory immunoglobulin A (sIgA) antibodies prevent viral infection along the respiratory and gastrointestinal tracts. Antibodies also act as opsonins to facilitate the phagocytosis and destruction of viruses. Once the virus enters its host cell, the humoral immune system is unable to eradicate the virus. Cytotoxic T lymphocytes (CTLs) recognize viral antigens synthesized in the infected cell and presented by the MHC I molecules. CTLs require cytokines secreted by CD4$^+$ T cells and co-stimulatory molecules expressed by the infected cell. Activated CTLs then kill the infected cell by the secretion of perforin, which facilitates the entry of granzymes into the cytoplasm of the target cell, either at the plasma membrane or following endocytosis of these molecules.

Viruses whose genome is sequestered in the nucleus of the host cell, such as Epstein-Barr virus or herpes simplex virus, can escape immune recognition unless they are activated to produce virions.

Immunity to fungi

Neutrophils and macrophages are the main mediators of innate immunity to fungal infections. Fungi are sensed by phagocytes and dendritic cells via TLRs and lectin-like receptors ("dectins"). Neutrophils phagocytose fungi and release reactive oxygen intermediates and lysosomal enzymes. Intracellular *Histoplasma capsulatum* is eliminated in a manner similar to that used against intracellular bacteria. *Cryptococcus neoformans* yeasts are eliminated by the cooperative action of CD4$^+$ and CD8$^+$ cells. Another indirect pathway for antifungal activity is the activation of dendritic cells via binding of fungal glucans to the dectin-1 receptor. The dendritic cells secrete IL-6 and IL-23, which activate T_h17 cells that in turn cause inflammation; the recruited neutrophils and monocytes kill the fungi. Cell-mediated immunity is thought to prevent the spread of *Candida* species from mucosal surfaces into tissues. Specific antibodies to fungi are also protective against fungal infections.

Immunity in the oral cavity

With the large numbers and different species of bacteria in the mouth, it is important to maintain the integrity of the oral mucosal surfaces. High–molecular weight salivary glycoproteins, called *mucins*, form a protective, viscous gel over the oral epithelium. Mucin glycoproteins 1 and 2 (MG1 and MG2) have branched oligosaccharide side chains with terminal sialic acid and fucose residues. Mucins are part of a series of nonspecific defense molecules that include defensins, histatins, and lysozyme (Table 4-1). They mediate the aggregation of oral bacteria, exogenous bacteria such as *Pseudomonas aeruginosa* and *Staphylococcus aureus*, and influenza virus. Inhibition of salivary flow in sedated patients in intensive care can result in the overgrowth of Gram-negative bacteria, which can lead to pulmonary infections. By contrast, saliva can also provide the molecules that form the acquired pellicle, including proline-rich proteins, amylase, and statherin, providing a surface to which initial colonizers can adhere.

Cationic antimicrobial peptides contain 15 to 20 amino acids, most of which are arginine, lysine, and histidine. Hydrophobic amino acids enable the peptides to interact strongly with bacterial membranes following electrostatic binding. They are active against Gram-positive and Gram-negative bacteria, fungi, parasites, and enveloped viruses, including human immunodeficiency virus (HIV) and herpesviruses. Defensins are cationic peptides with antibacterial, antiviral, and antifungal activity. Human β-defensins are involved in protecting mucosal surfaces in the mouth. They can associate with mucins and access the aggregated bacteria. They are found mainly in epithelial cells but have also been detected in monocytes, dendritic cells, and neutrophils. α-defensins are found in high concentrations in neutrophil granules and are involved in killing phagocytosed microbes. Cathelicidin is also a cationic peptide secreted by epithelial cells and neutrophils. Histatins are histidine-rich basic peptides secreted by parotid and submandibular/sublingual glands, and most of them are degradation products of histatins 1 and 3. Histatin 5 can kill yeast cells, even in biofilms. Histatins 5 and 8 inhibit the growth of *Streptococcus mutans* and induce the aggregation of other oral streptococci.

Table 4-1 Nonspecific and specific host defense factors of the mouth

Defense factor	Main function
Nonspecific	
Saliva flow	Physical removal of microorganisms
Mucin and agglutinins	Physical removal of microorganisms
Lysozyme and proteases	Cell lysis
Lactoferrin	Sequestration of iron
Apolactoferrin	Cell killing
Sialoperoxidase system	Hypothiocyanite production (at neutral pH); hypocyanous acid production (at low pH)
Histatins	Antifungal with some antibacterial activity
α- and β-defensins	Antimicrobial and immunomodulatory activity
Cystatins, SLPI, and TIMP	Inhibitors of cysteine-, serine-, and metalloproteases, respectively
Chitinase and chromogranin	Antifungals
Cathelicidin	Antimicrobial
Calprotectin	Antimicrobial
Neutrophils; macrophages*	Phagocytosis
Specific	
Intra-epithelial lymphocytes	Initiation of cellular immunity and Langerhans cells
Secretory IgA	Prevents microbial adhesion
IgG, IgM	Prevent microbial adhesion; opsonize pathogens; activate complement
Complement	Chemotaxis and activation of neutrophils

SLPI, secretory leukocyte protease inhibitors; TIMP, tissue inhibitor of metalloproteases.
*Phagocytosis of specific antibody-opsonized microorganisms may also be considered part of the specific defenses.
(Adapted from Marsh and Martin.)

Saliva also contains protease inhibitors, including cystatins, secretory leukocyte protease inhibitor (SLPI), and tissue inhibitor of metalloproteases (TIMP). Cystatins inhibit cysteine proteases of bacteria, for example the gingipains of *Porphyromonas gingivalis*. Cystatins can thus limit the ability of bacteria to degrade proteins for their nutrition and hence inhibit bacterial growth. Cystatins may counter the periodontal tissue destruction caused by human lysosomal cathepsins during local inflammation by inhibiting these enzymes. SLPI is a serine protease inhibitor; it is secreted by mucosal epithelial cells, and it has antibacterial, antifungal, and anti-inflammatory effects. Independent of its protease inhibitor activity, SLPI can also inhibit HIV entry into host cells.

Lysozyme can lyse bacteria by breaking down the peptidoglycan layer and can also aggregate bacteria. Monovalent anions enhance the activity of lysozyme at acidic pH. Lactoferrin binds iron with high affinity and limits the availability of iron for bacteria, which need it to generate nucleic acid precursors via the action of ribonucleotide reductase. Apolactoferrin, the protein without bound iron, is also bactericidal to some bacteria following binding to the bacterial cell surface.

Neutrophils are the first cells of the nonspecific immune system that are recruited to the subgingival space to counter bacteria. A gradient of chemokines such as IL-8 and cell adhesion molecules such as ICAM-1 induce the migration of neutrophils from the vasculature to the gingival crevice (Fig 4-8). The immune defense of periodontal tissues depends on the recruitment and proper functioning of neutrophils. Patients with neutropenia, leukocyte adhesion deficiencies, and Chédiak-Higashi and Papillon-Lefèvre syndromes (defects in bacterial killing) have increased susceptibility to periodontal disease. When neutrophils are recruited to the gingival crevice in high numbers, or their function is impaired by pathogens, they can cause destruction of host tissues.

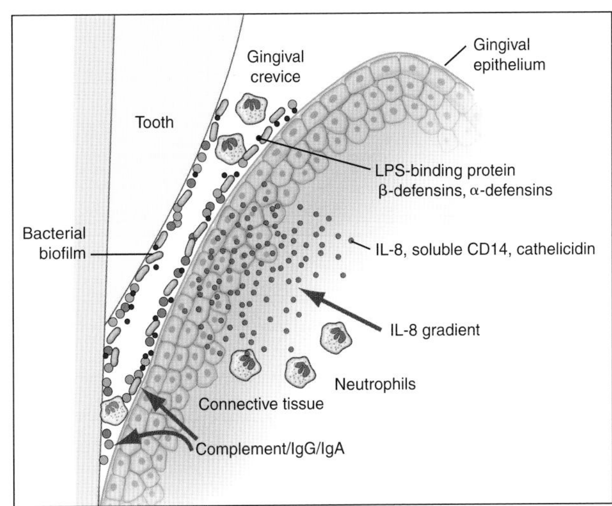

Fig 4-8 Significant host immune components in the gingival crevice. The subgingival biofilm of microorganisms induces the host immune response to control the bacteria. Neutrophils are recruited from the vasculature through the action of chemokines (IL-8) and cell adhesion molecules (ICAM-1). PRRs are overexpressed in the gingival epithelial layers exposed to the bacteria. These cells then secrete antimicrobial peptides, including β-defensins. Epithelial cells express IL-8, soluble CD14, and LPS-binding protein that may aid in bacterial clearance. Neutrophils and other leuokocytes in the junctional epithelium or the connective tissue secrete antimicrobial peptides that reach the gingival crevice. Complement components and IgG and IgA antibodies are also present in the crevice.

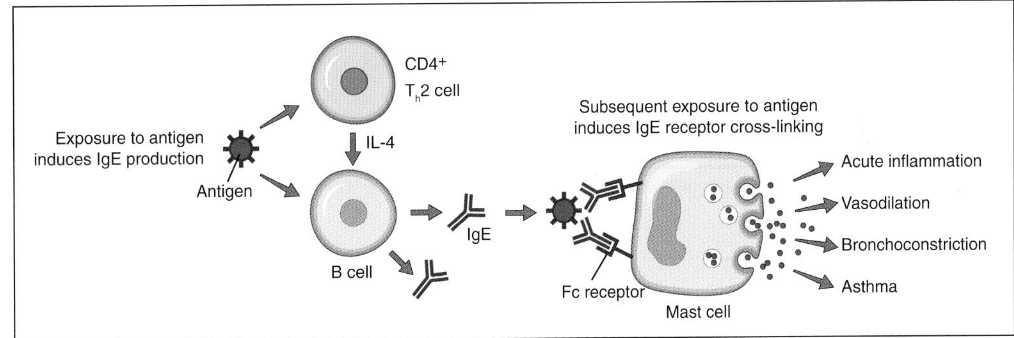

Fig 4-9 Mechanisms of anaphylactic (Type I) hypersensitivity.

Complement components C3a and C5a, which act as chemokines, are present in large numbers in the gingival crevicular fluid of periodontitis patients and in inflamed gingiva. Gingipains of *P gingivalis* mimic the C5 convertase of the complement system and generate large amounts of C5a. The interaction of C5a with TLR2 in leukocytes inhibits an antimicrobial pathway, which would be beneficial for the bacterium. C5a-induced vasodilation increases the flow of gingival crevicular fluid that is a source of hemin and protein fragments for *P gingivalis*.

The gingival mucosa is rich in CD4$^+$ T cells, B cells, and dendritic cells, which are involved in the adaptive immune response, including the T-cell effector response. This response may be both protective and destructive. T cells and B cells are primary sources of receptor activator of nuclear factor-κB ligand (RANKL), which interacts with RANK on osteoclasts and induces osteoclastogenesis and destruction of alveolar bone. The RANKL-RANK interaction can be inhibited by osteoprotegerin, and the ratio of RANKL to osteoprotegerin in gingival crevicular fluid is predictive of periodontitis. The T$_h$17 subset of CD4$^+$ T cells is thought to be involved in destructive inflammation as well as bone immunopathology. IL-17, which is secreted by T$_h$17 cells as well as innate immune cells, is found at increased levels in inflamed periodontal tissue. It induces RANKL in T cells and matrix metalloproteases in neutrophils and fibroblasts.

Hypersensitivity Responses

Immune responses can also cause tissue injury when they are not controlled adequately or when they are triggered by environmental antigens. These reactions are termed *hypersensitivity reactions* because the body is initially sensitized by exposure to a particular antigen and then can react strongly to that antigen. These reactions are classified as Type I (anaphylactic) hypersensitivity, Type II (antibody-mediated) hypersensitivity, Type III (immune complex–mediated) hypersensitivity, and Type IV (cell-mediated or delayed-type) hypersensitivity.

Anaphylactic (Type I) hypersensitivity reactions include hay fever, asthma, penicillin allergy, and reaction to bee stings. Anaphylactic hypersensitivity is caused by an initial sensitization to an allergen, which results in IgE production by B cells and IgE binding to Fc receptors on mast cells and basophils (Fig 4-9). Re-exposure to allergen causes IgE cross-linking on the cell surface that triggers degranulation, thereby releasing chemoattractants, activators, and spasmogens. Chemoattractants such as cytokines and leukotrienes attract eosinophils, neutrophils, and macrophages. Activators include histamine, platelet activating factor, tryptase, and kininogenase, which cause vasodilation and edema. Histamine, prostaglandin D2, and leukotrienes act as spasmo-

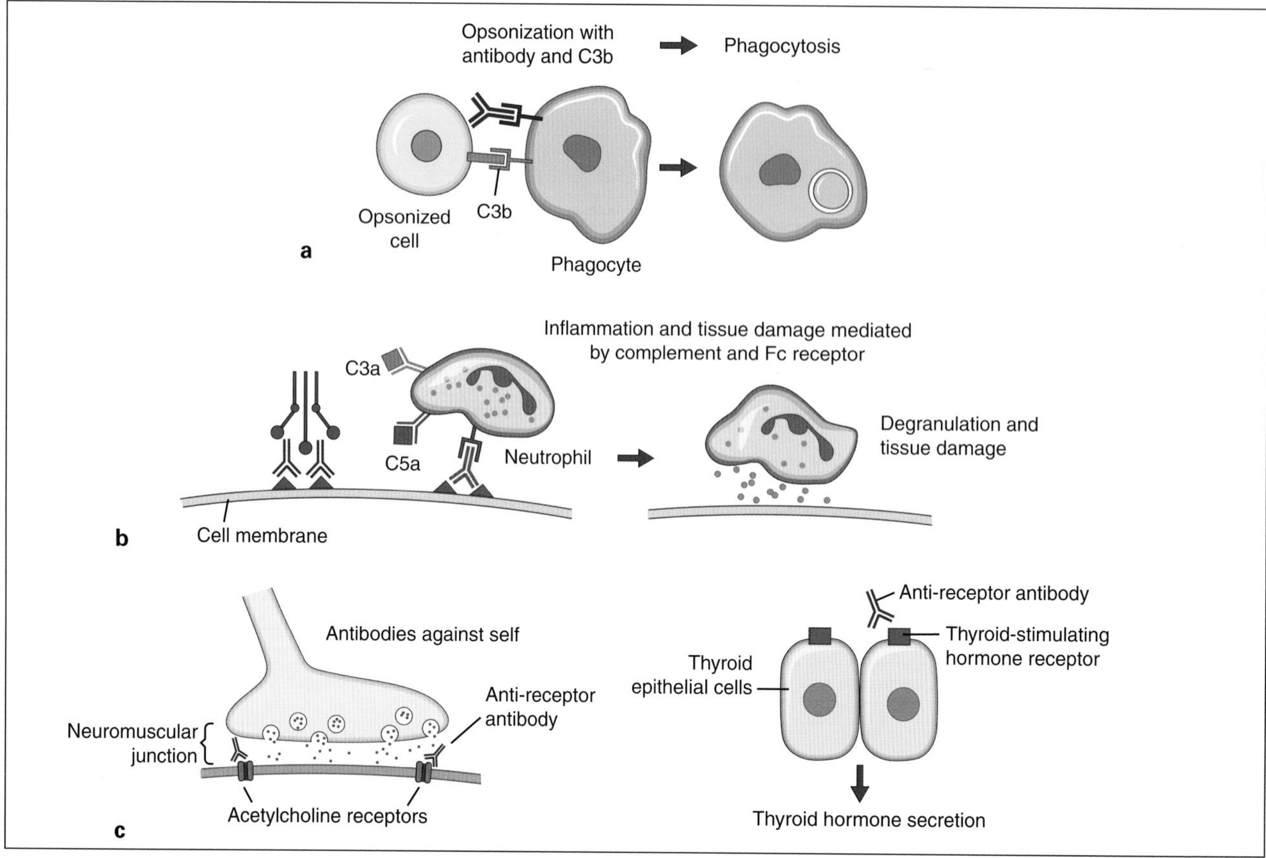

Fig 4-10 Antibody-mediated hypersensitivity. *(a)* Antibody opsonization of cells activates the complement system, whose components further opsonize cells. Fc and complement receptors on phagocytes mediate phagocytosis of the cell. *(b)* Leukocytes bind the Fc segment of bound antibodies, and complement components act as chemoattractants for leukocytes, leading to inflammation and tissue injury. *(c) Left panel:* Antibodies to the neurotransmitter acetylcholine may inhibit its binding to its receptor. *Right panel:* Antibodies to cell surface receptors for hormones, in this case thyroid-stimulating hormone, may stimulate the receptor without the natural ligand.

gens and mediate bronchial smooth muscle contraction and mucus secretion. Respiratory anaphylaxis is characterized by airway constriction and mucus secretion. Asthma is caused by inhaled or ingested allergens. Anaphylactic shock refers to the life-threatening drop in blood pressure. In such cases, epinephrine must be administered immediately to constrict blood vessels and relax smooth muscle.

Binding of IgG or IgM antibodies to specific cell surface antigens or the extracellular matrix activates the complement system, recruits effector cells, or inhibits cellular functions (Fig 4-10). This disorder is identified as antibody-mediated (Type II) hypersensitivity. In the autoimmune condition myasthenia gravis, antibodies bind acetylcholine receptors. Graves disease is characterized by the activation of thyroid-stimulating hormone receptors by antibodies to the receptor. In Goodpasture syndrome, antibodies are produced against the glomerular basement membrane in the kidneys. Some forms of diabetes may be caused by the blocking of insulin receptors by antibodies. The hemolytic disease of the newborn (Rh incompatibility) is caused by the generation of antibodies to the Rh factor on red blood cells of an Rh^+ fetus during birth. In a subsequent pregnancy, the mother's anti-Rh antibodies attack and destroy the red blood cells of the fetus.

In immune complex–mediated (Type III) hypersensitivity, large quantities of antigen present in blood react with antibodies, forming antibody-antigen complexes. These complexes can get trapped in capillaries and activate complement, resulting in local inflammation. Type III hypersensitivity may be caused by persistent infections, such as hepatitis B virus and malaria, or autoimmunity, as in the case of rheumatoid arthritis and systemic lupus erythematosus (Fig 4-11). In the case of hepatitis B, the large amounts of surface antigen produced leads to antibody-antigen complex formation and to glomerulonephritis. Type III hypersensitivity may also be induced by consistently inhaled antigens, such as mold. Extrinsic allergic alveolitis is a reaction to inhaled fungal antigens. Serum sickness is caused by the production of anti–horse serum protein antibodies following injection of horse anti-diphtheria toxin serum to prevent diphtheria.

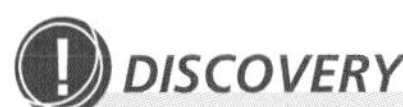

DISCOVERY

In the early 20th century, diphtheria infections were being treated with anti-diphtheria toxin serum from horses, a form of passive immunization. In 1911, the Austrian scientist and physician Clemens von Pirquet observed that rash, fever, and joint inflammation developed in patients who were administered the horse serum. The same type of response occurred in response to horse serum without the antitoxin. The reaction occurred at least a week after the initial injection, and it was more rapid if the injection was repeated. Dr Pirquet suggested that these conditions were caused by antibodies made by the host against horse serum proteins, so he called it *serum disease*. The symptoms are the result of antibody-antigen complexes and are now termed *serum sickness*.

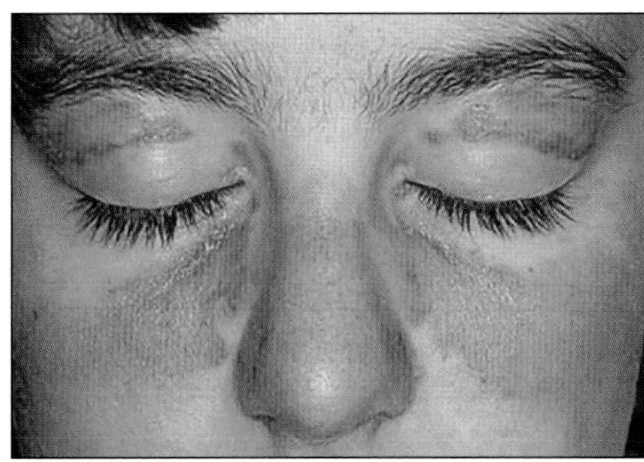

Fig 4-11 The facial rash, sometimes called "butterfly rash," characteristic of systemic lupus erythematosus. The shape of the rash reflects areas most exposed to sunlight, which exacerbates the condition. (Courtesy of Drs Riccardo Rondinone and Andrea Doria at the University of Padova, Italy.)

Cell-mediated (Type IV) hypersensitivity responses are delayed-type hypersensitivity (DTH) inflammatory responses mediated by $CD4^+$ cells that recognize presented antigens and become activated T_h1 cells. This process takes between 24 and 48 hours. These cells then activate macrophages at the site of infection. DTH responses are normally involved in controlling intracellular infections like tuberculosis, but they are also involved in the allergic response called contact dermatitis against cosmetics, nickel, and latex. Contact dermatitis can result in the formation of blisters in the epidermis. Response to poison ivy is also a DTH response to self-proteins modified by chemicals from the plant such as pentadecacatechol. In the tuberculin skin test for tuberculosis, bacterial antigens called *purified protein derivative* are injected in the dermis. The DTH response causes the formation of a firm induration 48 to 72 hours later in persons exposed to *Mycobacterium tuberculosis* or who have been vaccinated with the bacille Calmette-Guérin (BCG) vaccine. Granulomas are formed that consist of chronically infected macrophages, which in turn form flattened epithelioid cells, fused epithelioid cells, lymphocytes, and collagen deposits from fibroblasts. Such granuloma formation is seen in tuberculosis, leprosy, schistosomiasis, Crohn disease, and sarcoidosis.

Contact dermatitis in dentistry

Allergic contact dermatitis can result from frequent glove use (due to chemicals used during their manufacture) or from exposure to other chemicals used in dentistry (eg, hand hygiene products). It often appears as a rash beginning hours after contact, and it generally appears in the areas of contact; it is considered a Type IV hypersensitivity.

Type I hypersensitivity to latex proteins, known as *latex allergy*, is a more serious systemic allergic reaction. Usually the allergy begins soon after exposure, but sometimes it occurs much later, within a matter of hours. The symptoms include runny nose, sneezing, itchy eyes, itchy burning sensations, scratchy throat, and hives. There can be more severe symptoms, however, including difficulty breathing, coughing spells, wheezing, and cardiovascular and gastrointestinal manifestations. In rare cases, anaphylaxis and death may occur.

It is important that dental professionals who are allergic to latex take precautions against exposure to latex both at work and elsewhere. The National Institute for Occupational Health and Safety has published recommendations regarding latex allergy. These include *(1)* avoiding subsequent exposure to the protein and using only non-latex gloves, such as nitrile or vinyl; *(2)* ensuring that other staff in the dental practice wear either reduced-protein, powder-free latex gloves or non-latex gloves; *(3)* using synthetic or powder-free rubber dam; *(4)* changing ventilation filters and vacuum bags frequently; *(5)* cleaning work areas contaminated with latex dust; and *(6)* educating the staff on the symptoms of latex allergies.

Health care providers can become sensitized to latex proteins after repeated exposure. Latex proteins become attached to glove powder, and when powdered gloves are used, the skin is exposed to more latex proteins. Particles of latex protein powder become aerosolized when gloves are removed and can reach mucous membranes. Therefore, health care personnel as well as patients can show symptoms of cutaneous, respiratory, and conjunctival exposure. Patients who are allergic to latex should be treated in a latex-free environment.

Cytokine Storm

The *cytokine storm* refers to the stimulation of the immune system that results in the production of large quantities of cytokines that disrupt the normal functioning of the body. This condition can be initiated by Gram-negative bacteremia, the presence of Staphylococcus toxic shock syndrome toxin, infection with influenza virus, or rejection of transplanted tissue. Certain proteins of pathogens, called superantigens, can cause nonspecific binding of the T-cell receptor to the MHC II proteins on antigen-presenting cells and activate the T cells and macrophages to produce large amounts of cytokines. Pathogens can induce the secretion of acute-phase cytokines and type 1 interferons by plasmacytoid dendritic cells. TNF-α is one of the cytokines formed during a cytokine storm, and it induces increased vascular permeability and activates neutrophils. This leads to chills, aches, fever, elevation in liver enzymes, **initiation of the coagulation cascade**, loss of appetite, and weight loss, and it may result in shock.

Autoimmunity and Immunodeficiencies

Immune tolerance to self-antigens is normally acquired during development, where clones of T cells and B cells encountering self-antigens undergo apoptosis. Certain infections can initiate the production of antibodies that cross-react with self-antigens. In **rheumatic fever**, antibodies against group A streptococci react with myocardial proteins because of the molecular mimicry between the streptococcal antigens and myocardial proteins. **Rheumatoid arthritis** is thought to result from the interaction of autoantibodies (rheumatoid factors), usually IgM, with the Fc region of IgG, resulting in complexes that deposit in joints. In **multiple sclerosis**, $CD4^+$ T_h1 and T_h17 T-cell subsets react with the myelin sheath surrounding nerve axons and initiate local inflammation, with macrophages around the nerves. The destruction of pancreatic β cells in **type 1 diabetes** is mediated in part by $CD4^+$ T_h1 cells reacting with islet antigens, including insulin, cytotoxic T cell–mediated lysis of the islet cells, autoantibodies against the islet cells, and the local secretion of cytokines such as TNF-α. In **systemic lupus erythematosus**, autoantibodies to DNA, ribonucleoproteins, histones, and the nucleolus form immune complexes with their antigens and cause vasculitis in small arteries, arthritis, and glomerulonephritis. Genetic and environmental factors are involved in the breakdown of tolerance in B cells and T lymphocytes toward self-antigens. Blood cells in patients show gene-expression patterns indicative of exposure to IFN-α, presumably produced in large quantities by plasmacytoid dendritic cells.

Immunodeficiencies may be of genetic origin or may be induced by steroid treatment, cancer chemotherapy, or disease, such as HIV/AIDS. Immunosuppressive therapy may be employed to reduce inflammatory responses. Synthesis of inflammatory prostaglandins may be inhibited by aspirin or nonsteroidal anti-inflammatory drugs. Corticosteroids inhibit the production of TNF-α, IL-1, and IL-12 by macrophages. **Hereditary complement deficiencies** may result in the impairment of the innate immune function of the complement system. C3 deficiency may result in pyogenic bacterial infections, since it is involved centrally in opsonization, enhanced phagocytosis, and microbial killing. Properdin and factor D deficiencies may increase the susceptibility to pyogenic bacteria. Individuals with C2 and C4 deficiency are prone to systemic lupus erythematosus. C1-inhibitor deficiency can result in laryngeal edema and asphyxiation. In **chronic granulomatous disease**, phagocytes cannot produce superoxide anion.

Bibliography

Abbas AK, Lichtman AH, Pillai S. Cellular and Molecular Immunology, ed 7. Philadelphia: Elsevier/Saunders, 2012.

Bartfai T, Conti B. Fever. ScientificWorldJournal 2010;10:490–503.

Bauman RW. Microbiology with Diseases by Taxonomy, ed 4. Boston: Pearson, 2014.

Black S, Kushner I, Samols D. C-reactive protein. J Biol Chem 2004;279:48487–48490.

Centers for Disease Control. Infection Control in Dental Settings. www.cdc.gov/OralHealth/infectioncontrol/faq/latex.htm. Accessed 23 April 2015.

Du Clos TW. Pentraxins: Structure, function, and role in inflammation. ISRN Inflamm 2013:379040.

Eisenhardt SU, Thiele JR, Bannasch H, Stark GB, Peter K. C-reactive protein: How conformational changes influence inflammatory properties. Cell Cycle 2009;8:3885–3892.

Goldsby RA, Kindt TJ, Osborne BA, Kuby J. Immunology, ed 5. New York: WH Freeman, 2003.

Konopka K, Dorocka-Bobkowska B, Gebremedhin S, Düzgünes N. Susceptibility of *Candida* biofilms to histatin 5 and fluconazole. Antonie Van Leeuwenhoek 2010;97:413–417.

Kumar H, Kawai T, Akira S. Pathogen recognition by the innate immune system. Int Rev Immunol 2011;30:16–34.

Lamont RJ, Hajishengallis GN, Jenkinson HF. Oral Microbiology and Immunology, ed 2. Washington, DC: ASM Press, 2014.

Marsh PD, Martin MV. Oral Microbiology, ed 5. Edinburgh: Churchill Livingstone Elsevier, 2009.

Murray PR, Rosenthal KS, Pfaller MA. Medical Microbiology, ed 7. Philadelphia: Saunders, 2013.

Pier GB, Lyczak JB, Wetzler LM. Immunology, Infection, and Immunity. Washington, DC: ASM Press, 2004.

Rockefeller University. C-reactive Protein: From Pneumococcal Pneumonia to Cardiovascular Disease Risk. centennial.rucares.org/index.php?page=C-Reactive_Protein. Accessed 23 April 2015.

Sahoo M, Ceballos-Olvera I, del Barrio L, Re F. Role of the inflammasome IL-1b, and IL-18 in bacterial infections. ScientificWorldJournal 2011;11:2037–2050.

Shine N, Konopka K, Düzgünes N. The anti-HIV-1 activity associated with saliva. J Dent Res 1997;76:634–640.

Vardam TD, Zhou L, Appenheimer MM, et al. Regulation of a lymphocyte–endothelial–IL-6 trans-signaling axis by fever-range thermal stress: Hot spot of immune surveillance. Cytokine 2007;39:84–96.

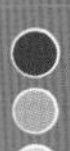

Take-Home Messages

- Acute (localized) inflammation involves the recruitment of innate immune cells, such as macrophages and neutrophils, from the local blood vessels to the site of injury, utilizing their integrins.
- PAMPs are found on or in microbes and are essential for pathogenicity. They are recognized by PRRs on host cells.
- The inflammasome is a complex of various proteins in macrophages, dendritic cells, epithelial cells, and other cells that is activated by adaptor proteins induced by the PRRs, intracellular infections, or tissue damage.
- The acute-phase response is triggered by macrophages in response to LPS and other bacterial components. In response, the liver releases C-reactive protein, which may be a marker for inflammation as well as a possible contributor to inflammation.
- Pyrogens are molecules that can induce fever. LPS is a powerful exogenous pyrogen. The endogenous pyrogens IL-1, IL-6, and TNF-α are secreted by monocytes and macrophages.
- IFNs are proteins produced in response to viral infections (IFN-α and IFN-β) or upon activation of the immune response (IFN-γ).
- Innate immunity to invading bacteria involves phagocytosis, inflammation, and the complement system. Adaptive immunity involves the generation of antibodies. Intracellular bacteria are not accessible to antibody intervention, but cell-mediated immune responses can control intracellular infections.
- Cytotoxic T lymphocytes (CTLs) recognize viral antigens synthesized in infected cells and presented by MHC molecules. CTLs need cytokines secreted by $CD4^+$ T cells and co-stimulatory molecules expressed by the infected cell.
- In the oral cavity, mucins are part of a series of nonspecific defense molecules that include defensins, histatins, and lysozyme.
- Cystatins inhibit cysteine proteases of bacteria, such as the gingipains of *P gingivalis*.
- RANKL is produced by T cells and B cells and interacts with RANK on osteoclasts, inducing osteoclastogenesis and destruction of alveolar bone.
- Anaphylactic (Type I) hypersensitivity reactions include hay fever, asthma, penicillin allergy, and reaction to bee stings. Anaphylactic shock is the life-threatening drop in blood pressure. Latex allergy is a serious systemic allergic reaction.
- In antibody-mediated (Type II) hypersensitivity, antibody binding to cell surface antigens activates the complement system, recruits effector cells, or inhibits cellular functions.
- In immune complex–mediated (Type III) hypersensitivity, large quantities of antigen in blood react with antibodies, forming antibody-antigen complexes that can get trapped in capillaries.
- Cell-mediated (Type IV) hypersensitivity responses are DTH inflammatory responses and are mediated by $CD4^+$ cells.

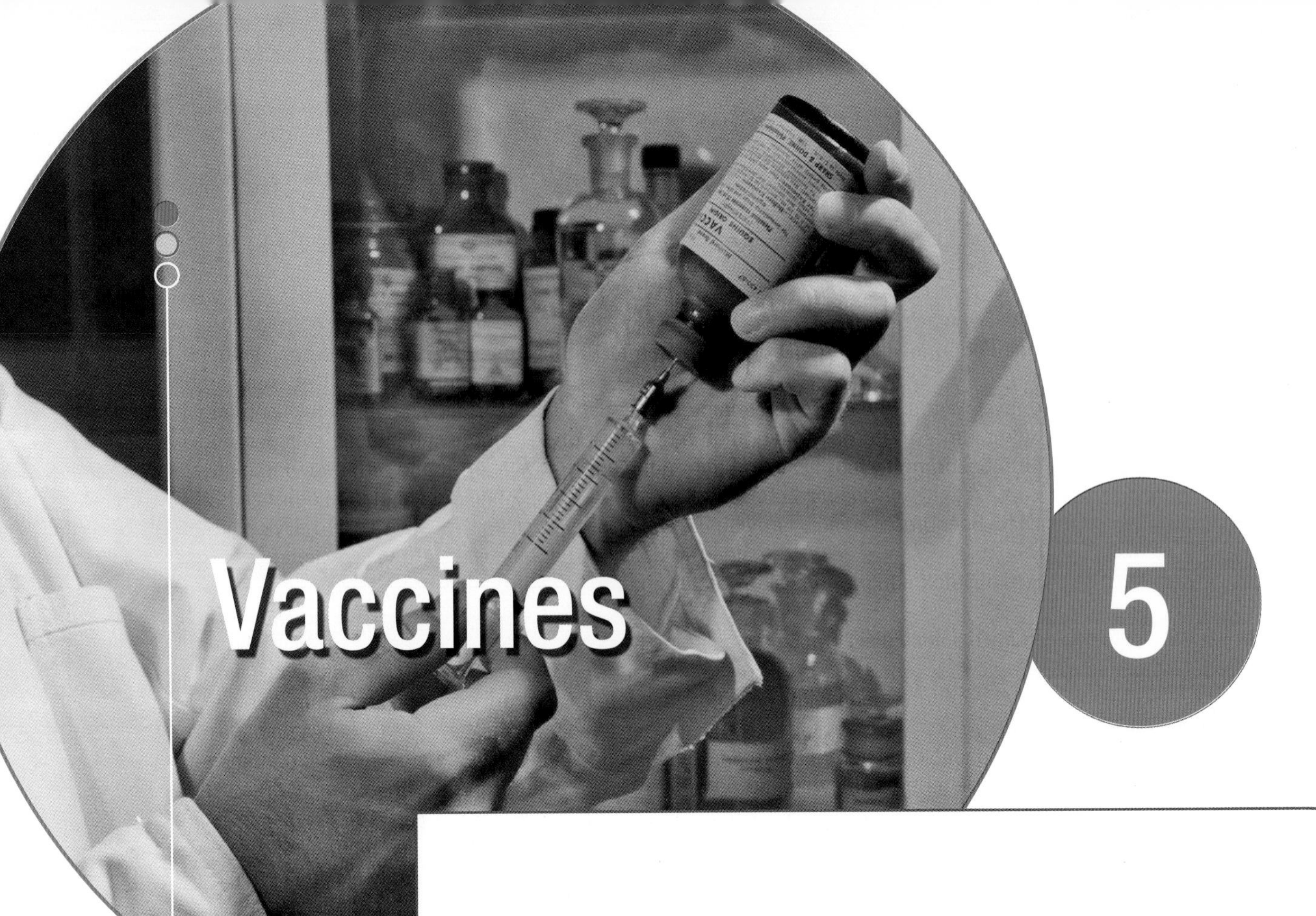

5 Vaccines

The essential concept of vaccination is to introduce into the host a non-infectious form of the pathogen, either killed or attenuated, or a protein or polysaccharide component of the microorganism that elicits a protective immune response against the live pathogen. Since the development of the smallpox vaccine by Edward Jenner in 1798, vaccines have been extremely successful in the complete or near complete eradication of many diseases. The World Health Organization announced in 1980 that smallpox has been eradicated through a vigorous vaccination campaign.

The highest number of reported diphtheria cases in the United States was 206,939 in 1921, but there were 0 cases reported in 2009. Measles cases declined from a maximum of 894,134 in 1941 to just 61 in 2009. However, outbreaks of measles in the United States have affected 173 individuals in 2015 and more than 600 people in 2014. Most of the patients had not been vaccinated against measles. The increase in the number of recent cases is attributable to a troubling decrease in the rate of vaccination of school-age children, resulting from parents' fears of potential side effects. Paralytic polio cases were reduced from a maximum of 21,269 in 1952 to 0 in 2009. Pertussis cases peaked at 265,269 in 1934 and were reduced to 13,506 in 2009, indicating that a better vaccine still needs to be developed.

Effective vaccines can be developed if certain criteria are met: *(1)* The infectious agent should not establish latency; for example, human immunodeficiency virus integrates its genome into the host chromosome and is not accessible to vaccine prevention when it is in this state. *(2)* The agent should not undergo antigenic variation. *(3)* The infectious agent should not interfere with the immune response.

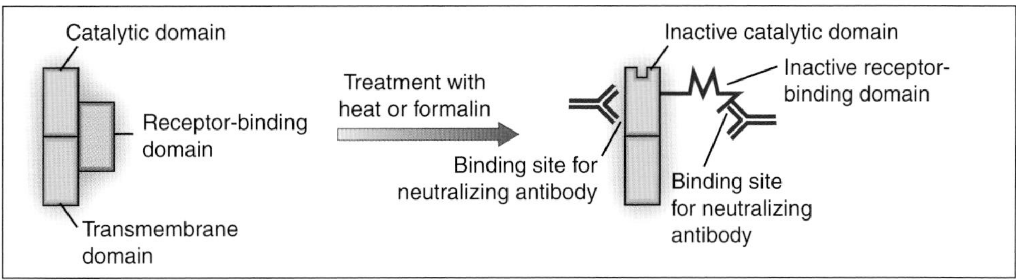

Fig 5-1 Toxoid vaccines. Bacterial exotoxins, such as the diphtheria toxin depicted here, are inactivated by physical or chemical treatments so that they are not toxic, but they still elicit neutralizing antibodies. The toxoids produced in this manner are used in vaccines against diphtheria and tetanus.

Attenuated Vaccines

Attenuated microbial vaccines induce innate, humoral, and cell-mediated responses that are similar to those induced by the pathogen itself. Attenuated vaccines are useful for eliciting an immune response against enveloped viruses that can be cleared by T-cell immune responses. Among the live bacterial vaccines are the bacille Calmette-Guérin (BCG) vaccine against tuberculosis, which is attenuated *Mycobacterium bovis*, and the live attenuated *Salmonella typhi* strain (Ty21a) vaccine against typhoid. The BCG vaccine is used around the world to vaccinate children but is not particularly effective in adults. The vaccine is not used in the United States because vaccinated individuals display a false-positive skin reaction to the purified protein derivative test for tuberculosis.

Attenuated virus vaccines are obtained by growing the virus in embryonated eggs or tissue culture cells at low temperatures (25°C to 34°C), avoiding the selective pressures of the host immune response. These viruses, called *low-temperature mutants*, grow more slowly at body temperature and are less virulent. Some viruses may not replicate efficiently in human cells and are called *host-range mutants*. Some attenuated viruses may replicate at a localized site, such as the gastrointestinal tract, but do not reach the target tissue where the disease occurs, for example neurons in the case of the live attenuated polio vaccine, developed by Albert Sabin. The Sabin vaccine has at least 57 mutations compared with the wild-type virus. The vaccine induces an immunoglobulin A (IgA) response along the gut and an IgG response in blood.

Other live viral vaccines include the measles, mumps, and rubella (MMR) vaccine and the varicella zoster vaccine. These vaccines must be administered after a child reaches 1 year of age, when a robust T-cell response can be elicited. A live attenuated influenza vaccine is administered intranasally to individuals in the age range 2 to 49 years, inducing T-cell and B-cell responses and mucosal immunity.

Inactivated Vaccines

Attenuated viruses and bacteria cannot be obtained in the case of many microorganisms; therefore, inactivated pathogens are used as vaccines. A prime example of an inactivated vaccine is the polio vaccine developed by Jonas Salk via formaldehyde treatment of poliovirus. An inactivated influenza vaccine is developed yearly to contain two influenza A and one influenza B virus strains that are expected to be most prevalent in the flu season. The viruses are grown in embryonated eggs and then inactivated; this poses a problem for recipients who may be allergic to eggs. Hepatitis A and rabies vaccines also use inactivated virions. The rabies vaccine is based on virus grown in human diploid cells in culture and subsequently inactivated. The vaccine can be administered soon after exposure, in a procedure called post-exposure prophylaxis, because the disease develops slowly and the elicited antibodies are protective.

Inactivated bacterial vaccines may consist of killed bacteria, inactivated toxins called *toxoids*, or protein or polysaccharide subunits of the bacteria. Killed bacterial vaccines include *Vibrio cholerae*, *Bacillus anthracis*, *Yersinia pestis*, and *Coxiella burnetii*. Commonly administered antibacterial vaccines are directed at the toxins produced by the bacteria (Fig 5-1). Diphtheria and tetanus vaccines consist of toxoids.

Inactivated vaccines have disadvantages in that *(1)* the induced immunity is usually just humoral and not long-lasting, *(2)* a local IgA response is not elicited, and *(3)* booster shots are required. The diphtheria and tetanus vaccines must be re-administered every 10 years.

Subunit Vaccines

Molecular components of bacteria or viruses can be used as vaccines. These include capsular polysaccharides and surface proteins of bacteria and viral envelope glycoproteins. These components are either isolated biochemically from the pathogen or synthesized by recombinant DNA technology. The current hepatitis B virus (HBV) vaccine consists of HBsAg, which is expressed in yeast from its gene. The expressed protein is purified, treated chemically, and combined with alum (potassium aluminum phosphate) as an adjuvant to boost the immune response. **Virus-like particles** are formed by the subunit proteins in the HBV vaccine and the **human papillomavirus (HPV) vaccine** and are more immunogenic than the individual antigens. Liposomes are also used as experimental adjuvants. HPV proteins 6, 11, 16, and 18 are combined with an adjuvant for the HPV vaccine. Because HPV 16 and 18 are linked with the initiation of cervical cancer (and, potentially, oropharyngeal cancer), the HPV vaccine is an anticancer vaccine.

Capsular polysaccharides are used as vaccines for 23 strains of *Streptococcus pneumoniae*, four major serotypes (A, C, Y, and W-135) of *Neisseria meningitidis*, and for *Haemophilis influenzae* B. Polysaccharides are T-independent antigens and usually elicit poor immunity. Their immunogenicity can be improved by conjugation to a protein carrier, such as diphtheria toxoid or *N meningitidis* outer membrane protein. These vaccines are called *conjugate vaccines*, and they work in a manner similar to hapten-carrier conjugates. They also illustrate the importance of T-cell and B-cell cooperation during the immune response.

Immunization Schedules

Current immunization schedules for individuals up to 18 years of age are given at the Centers for Disease Control website: www.cdc.gov/vaccines/schedules/hcp/imz/child-adolescent.html.

Note that the first vaccine given soon after birth is the **HBV vaccine**. This is followed at 2 months with vaccines for diphtheria, tetanus, acellular pertussis (DTaP); rotavirus; *H influenzae* B; the pneumococcal conjugate vaccine; and inactivated poliovirus. The hepatitis A vaccine, the MMR vaccine, and the varicella vaccine are given at 12 months. Inactivated influenza virus can be given yearly starting at 18 months, and the live attenuated influenza virus is administered yearly after age 2 years. The HPV vaccine and a different formulation of the DTaP vaccine called *Tdap* are administered at age 11 to 12 years.

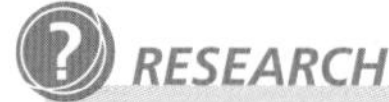

What were the scientific steps taken by Jonas Salk and his collaborators in the development of the first polio vaccine?

Take-Home Messages

- Live viral vaccines have numerous mutations that prevent them from being pathogenic. They include the Sabin polio vaccine, the MMR vaccine, and the varicella zoster vaccine.
- Inactivated vaccines include the Salk polio vaccine, influenza vaccines, the hepatitis A vaccine, and the diphtheria and tetanus toxoid vaccines.
- Subunit vaccines comprise molecular components of bacteria or viruses and include the HBV and HPV vaccines.
- The first vaccine given soon after birth is the HBV vaccine.

Bibliography

Abbas AK, Lichtman AH, Pillai S. Cellular and Molecular Immunology, ed 7. Philadelphia: Elsevier/Saunders, 2012.

Ingraham JL, Ingraham CA. Introduction to Microbiology: A Case History Approach. Pacific Grove, CA: Brooks/Cole (Thomson), 2004.

Krowka J, Stites D, Debs R, et al. Lymphocyte proliferative responses to soluble and liposome-conjugated envelope peptides of HIV-1. J Immunol 1990;144:2535–2540.

Murray PR, Rosenthal KS, Pfaller MA. Medical Microbiology, ed 7. Philadelphia: Saunders, 2013.

Bacterial Structure, Metabolism, and Genetics

6

Bacterial Structure

Bacteria have characteristic shapes. Spherical bacteria, termed *cocci*, can occur as single organisms or appear in pairs (diplococcus), chains (streptococcus), clusters (staphylococcus), tetrads, or sarcina (cube of eight cocci). Rod-shaped bacteria can be single (bacilli), double (diplobacilli), or in chains (streptobacilli). Some bacteria can have an intermediate shape between a coccus and a bacillus and are therefore termed *coccobacilli*. The bacteria that cause syphilis (*Treponema pallidum*) are spiral or corkscrew shaped, and those causing cholera (*Vibrio*) are comma shaped. *Corynebacteria* have a club shape, and certain bacilli, including *Bacillus anthracis*, can contain a spore.

These shapes are maintained by the cell wall of the bacteria composed of peptidoglycan. Bacteria do not have a nucleus surrounded by a membrane, but their chromosome forms a structure usually termed a *nucleoid*. They do not have membrane-bound organelles; however, they can have storage granules or invaginated plasma membrane inclusions. Their sizes are in the range of micrometers and are about one order of magnitude smaller than eukaryotic cells. However, a bacterium about 600 μm in length and 80 μm in diameter was discovered living in the intestinal tract of surgeonfish in 1993 and was named *Epulopiscium fishelsoni*.

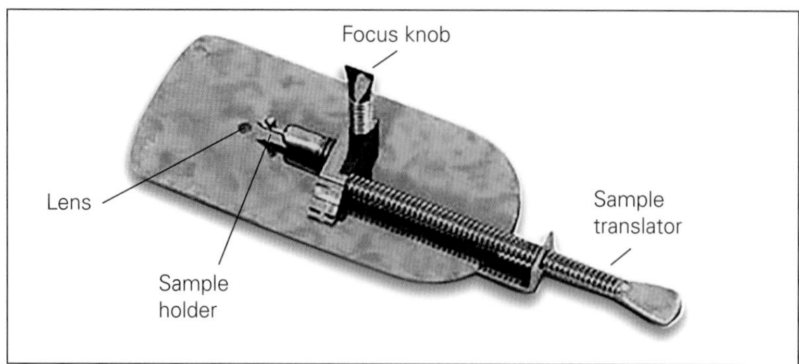

Fig 6-1 Antonie van Leeuwenhoek's microscope.

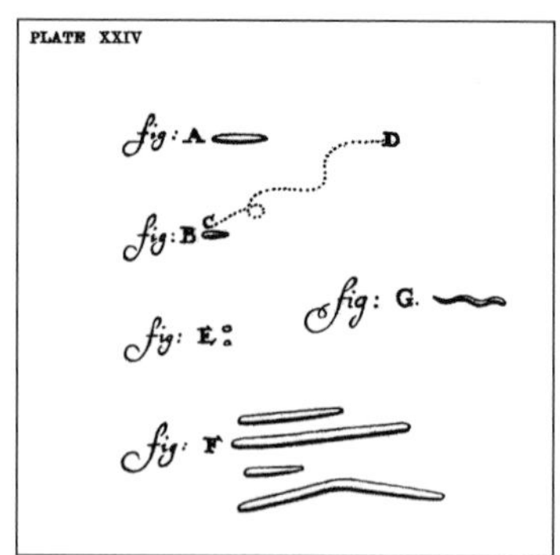

Fig 6-2 Leeuwenhoek's drawings of the bacteria he observed through his microscope.

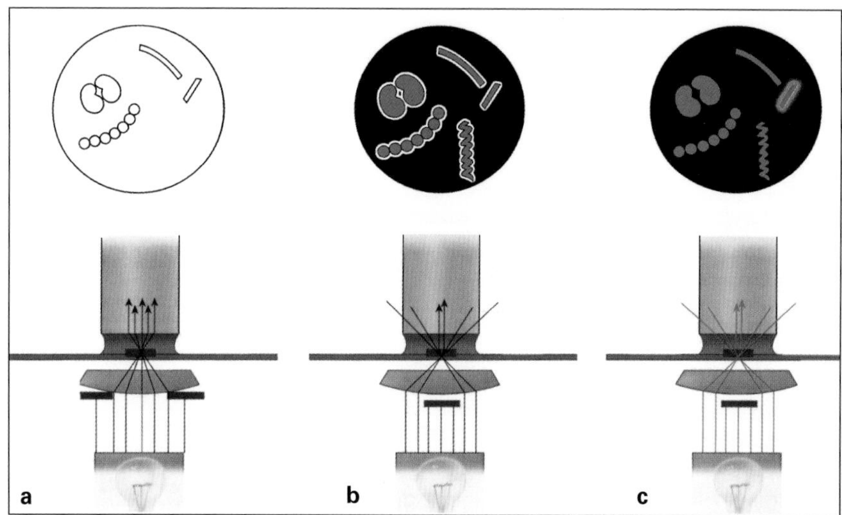

Fig 6-3 *(a)* Bright-field microscopy. *(b)* Dark-field microscopy. *(c)* Fluorescence microscopy. (Reprinted with permission from Ryan and Ray.)

DISCOVERY

The Dutch scientist Antonie van Leeuwenhoek (1632–1723) is considered to be the first to observe bacteria through his simple microscope. He was inspired by Robert Hooke's book, *Micrographia*, to develop a microscope with high enough magnification to examine objects not visible to the naked eye. He utilized a simple biconvex lens that he prepared by flaming soda-lime glass and placed it in between two metal plates. The sample was placed on a pointed metal holder and could be moved into focus by means of screws (Fig 6-1). Van Leeuwenhoek observed red blood cells, the alga *Spirogyra* from a pond, *Giardia* from a stool sample, and different bacteria from dental tartar (Fig 6-2). He wrote of his discoveries to the Royal Society in London, and after some initial skepticism, Society members confirmed them in 1673. He was elected as a full member of the Royal Society in 1680.

Bacteria and other microorganisms can be readily visualized by light microscopy. Because the resolution limit is about 0.2 μm, the optics must be optimized to obtain a clear image. A 100× oil-immersion objective, a 10× eyepiece, and optimal lighting are used to achieve this (Fig 6-3). In **bright-field microscopy**, it is difficult to visualize small bacteria, so specific dyes are used to stain the bacteria. In **dark-field microscopy**, a black background is created by blocking the light at the center of the visual field. The light at the periphery is collected by the objective only when it is reflected off the surface of an object, such as a bacterium. Dark-field microscopy is particularly suitable for observing spirochetes. In **fluorescence microscopy**, the microorganisms are stained with a fluorescent probe, such as a live-dead stain, or a fluorescent antibody. The incident light, which is usually ultraviolet, excites the fluorophore, which then emits light at a higher wavelength (and lower energy). Only the stained microorganisms are seen.

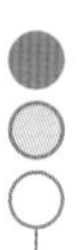

	Unstained	Crystal violet	Iodine	Decolorized	Safranin
Gram-positive					
Gram-negative					

Fig 6-4 The Gram staining procedure and the resulting appearance of Gram-positive and Gram-negative bacteria.

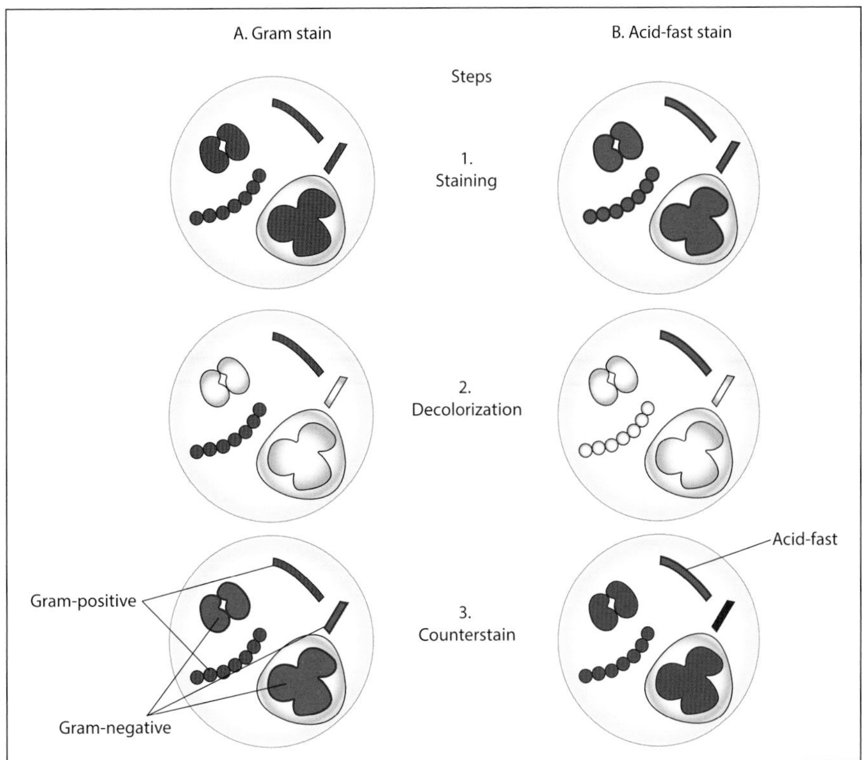

Fig 6-5 Comparison of the Gram stain and the acid-fast stain. Four types of bacteria and a neutrophil are shown at each stage of the procedure. In the Gram stain, they are all stained *purple* by crystal violet and iodine (used as a mordant) (A1). In the acid-fast stain, they are stained *red* by the carbol fuchsin (B1). After decolorization, Gram-positive bacteria retain the *purple* stain (A2) and the acid-fast bacteria their *red* stain (B2). Counterstaining enables the visualization of the other bacteria. In Gram-staining, safranin stains Gram-negative bacteria *red* (A3). In the acid-fast method, methylene blue stains the remaining organisms *blue* (B3). (Reprinted with permission from Ryan and Ray.)

Structurally, bacteria can be classified as being Gram-positive or Gram-negative, based on how they stain with the Gram stain procedure. This procedure was developed serendipitously by the Danish physician Christian Gram in 1884 when an iodine solution spilled over methyl violet-stained lung tissue sections from patients who had died of lobar pneumonia. The currently used procedure involves staining a bacterial sample with crystal violet, setting the dye with Gram's iodine, decolorizing with alcohol or acetone, and counterstaining with safranin (Fig 6-4). After the decolorization step, the Gram-positive bacteria retain the crystal violet that has been set by Gram's iodine, whereas the Gram-negative bacteria do not and appear transparent. The counterstain enables the visualization of the latter. A similar procedure is used to stain acid-fast bacteria, including *Mycobacterium tuberculosis* (Fig 6-5).

Gram-positive bacteria have a single lipid bilayer membrane surrounded by a thick layer of peptidoglycan (also called *mucopeptide* or *murein*), which is a mesh of linear polysaccharide co-polymer chains composed of N-acetylglucosamine (GlcNAc) and N-acetylmuramic acid (MurNAc). The chains are cross-linked by peptides (Fig 6-6). The organization of the peptidoglycan layer confers shape to the bacterium. The peptidoglycan also enables the bacterium to withstand osmotic pressure differences across the cytoplasmic membrane of

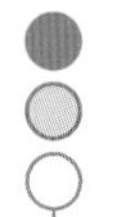

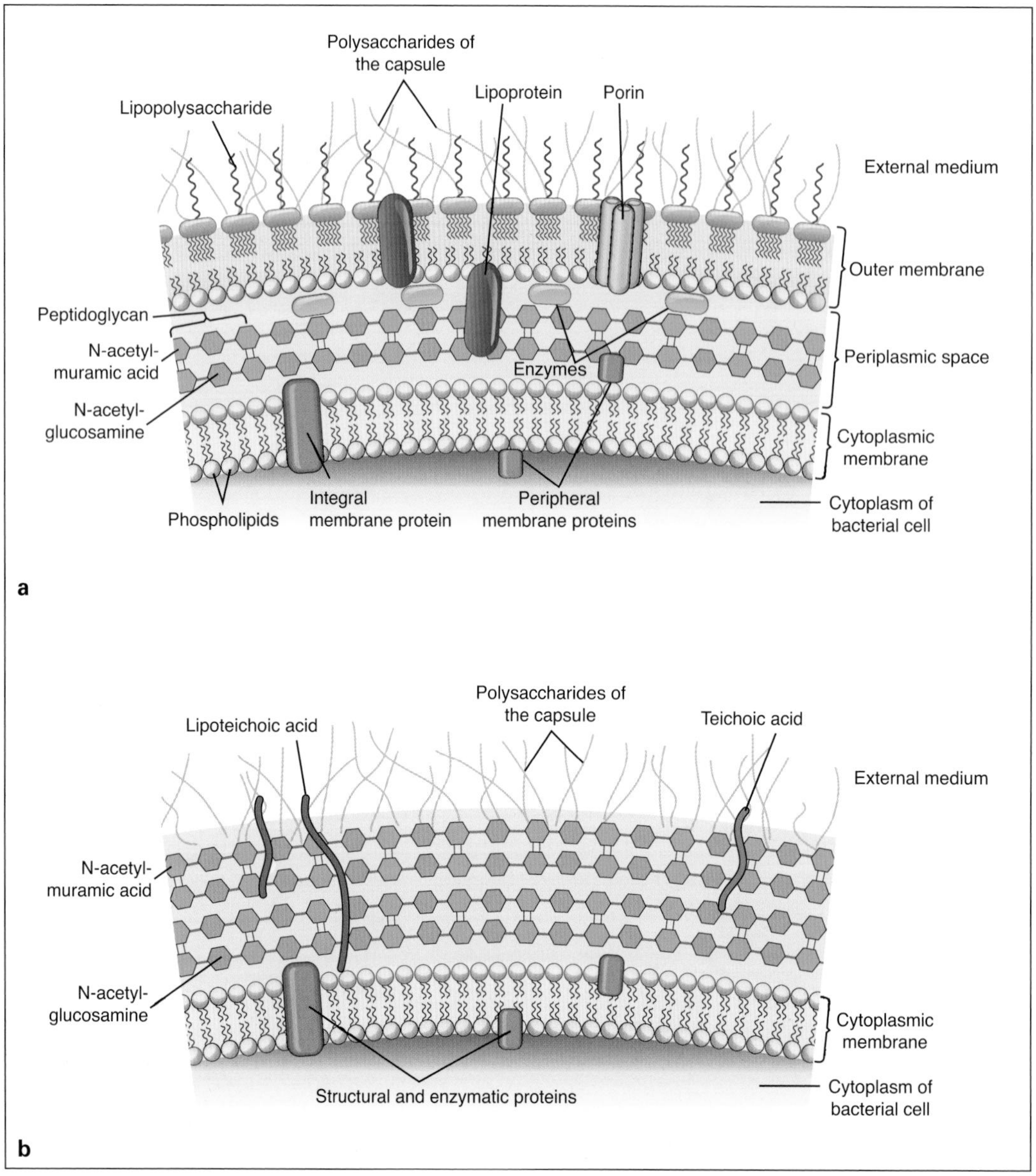

Fig 6-6 Schematic representation of the cell wall of Gram-negative *(a)* and Gram-positive *(b)* bacteria.

Gram-positive cells and the inner and outer membranes of Gram-negative cells. The β-1,4 glycosidic linkage between GlcNAc and MurNAc acid is the target of the enzyme **lysozyme** found in tears, saliva, and mucosal surfaces and is directly accessible to the enzyme in Gram-positive bacteria. In *Staphylococcus aureus*, a Gram-positive coccus, the peptide bridge consists of L-alanine–D-glutamine–L-lysine–D-alanine–D-alanine and is attached to MurNAc (Fig 6-7). The peptides from adjoining polysaccharides are linked by the action of membrane-bound **transpeptidases** via the **pentaglycine** bridge attached to the lysine in one peptide and the penultimate D-alanine in the peptide of the adjoining polysaccharide. The terminal D-alanine is removed by a carboxypeptidase. Transpeptidases are penicillin-binding proteins, and they are inhibited by the antibiotic.

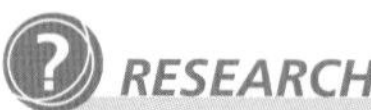

RESEARCH

If the components of peptidoglycan are synthesized inside the bacterial cell, how is peptidoglycan assembled outside the cytoplasmic membrane of bacteria?

The cell wall of Gram-positive bacteria also contains the polymers, teichoic acids, lipoteichoic acids, and complex (C) polysaccharides. **Teichoic acids** are polymers of glycerol phosphate or ribitol phosphate (Fig 6-8). Lipoteichoic acids

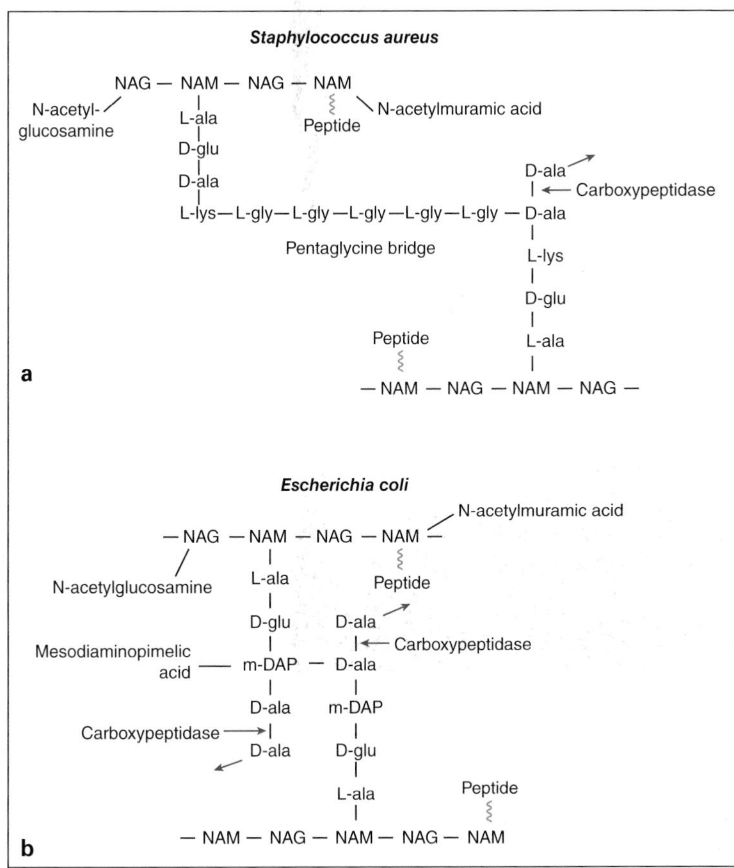

Fig 6-7 The peptidoglycan structure in representative *(a)* Gram-positive *(S aureus)* and *(b)* Gram-negative *(E coli)* bacteria. (Inspired by Greenwood et al.)

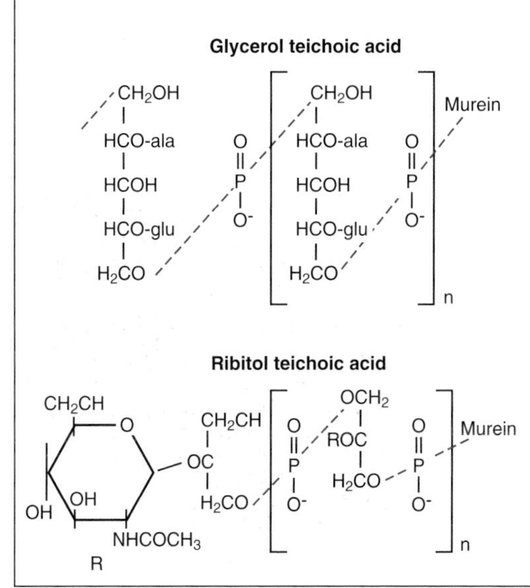

Fig 6-8 Glycerol and ribitol teichoic acid. Teichoic acid may be attached covalently to the peptidoglycan. Lipoteichoic acid is anchored covalently to lipids in the cytoplasmic membrane.

are poly(glycerol phosphates) linked to glycolipid anchors in the cytoplasmic membrane. These molecules facilitate interbacterial attachment and binding to mammalian cell surfaces. They also act as antigens that can be used to distinguish among different serotypes of the microorganism.

Gram-negative bacteria have both a cytoplasmic and an outer membrane with a thin peptidoglycan layer in between (see Fig 6-6). The peptides that link the polysaccharide polymers are slightly different than those in Gram-positive bacteria. The peptide sequence is L-alanine–D-glutamic acid–mesodiaminopimelic acid–D-alanine–D-alanine (see Fig 6-7). As the mesodiaminopimelic acid binds to the penultimate D-alanine of the other glycan chain, the terminal D-alanine on both of the peptides is cleaved off by a carboxypeptidase.

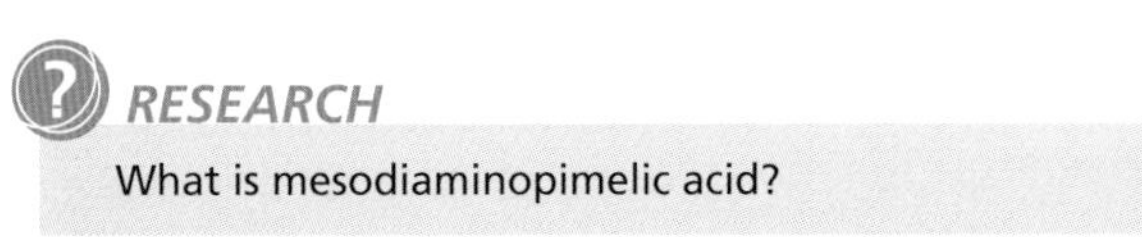

What is mesodiaminopimelic acid?

Peptidoglycan is synthesized via a series of biosynthetic reactions, starting with the intracellular synthesis of MurNAc, which is then activated energetically by reacting with uridine triphosphate, producing uridine diphosphate (UDP)–MurNAc. Five amino acids are added enzymatically to the UDP-MurNAc, and this conjugate is attached to a lipidic carrier called bactoprenol through a pyrophosphate (high-energy diphosphate) link, with the concomitant release of the UDP. Then GlcNAc is added, and the bactoprenol facilitates the transport of the disaccharide-peptide across the membrane. The MurNAc-GlcNAc is added to the growing peptidoglycan chain via transglycosylases that utilize the energy of the pyrophosphate on the bactoprenol. The antibiotic bacitracin blocks the recycling of the pyrophosphobactoprenol back to phosphobactoprenol, thereby inhibiting peptidoglycan synthesis. Peptides from adjacent peptidoglycan chains are linked covalently by transpeptidases.

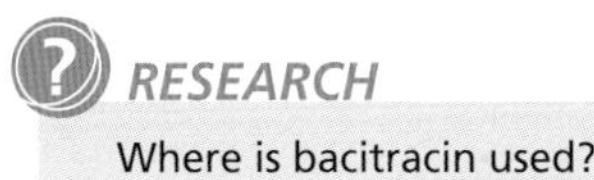

Where is bacitracin used?

Bacteria need to transport some of the proteins they synthesize across the cytoplasmic membrane, as well as the outer membrane in the case of Gram-negative bacteria. The general secretory pathway (Fig 6-9) transports pre-

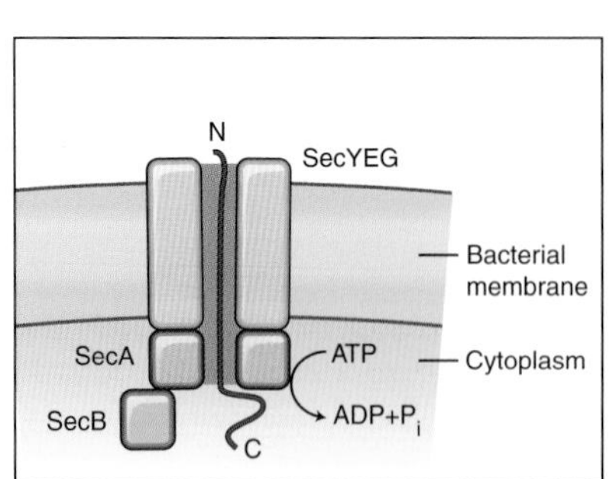

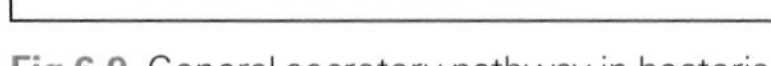
Fig 6-9 General secretory pathway in bacteria.

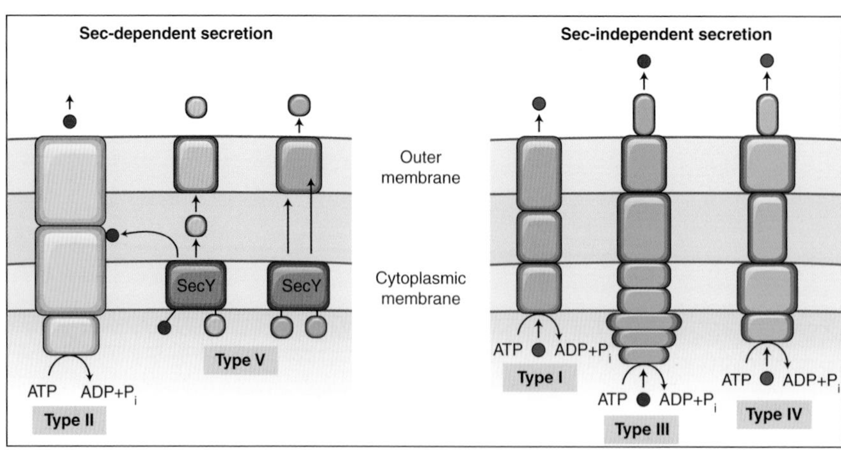

Fig 6-10 Secretion systems in Gram-negative bacteria. (Adapted from Fronzes et al.)

proteins, with signal peptides attached to their N-termini, through the channel formed by the proteins SecY, SecE, and SecG, with the help of the "chaperone" protein SecB and the propelling protein SecA. Once outside the membrane, the signal peptide is removed.

There are five additional secretion pathways in Gram-negative bacteria that enable the export of proteins through the outer membrane (Fig 6-10). The type III and type IV secretion systems enable cytoplasmic proteins such as exotoxins to traverse not only the two bacterial membranes but also the membrane of the host cell. The type IV system can also microinject DNA into the host cell. The type I secretion system enables the transport of proteins to the external medium through both bacterial membranes, whereas the type II and type V systems secrete proteins that have been transported by the general secretory pathway into the periplasmic space, the region between the inner and outer membranes. The periplasmic space contains various enzymes, including proteases, lipases, nucleases, phosphatases, and carbohydrate-degrading enzymes. It also contains the virulence factors of pathogenic bacteria, such as collagenases, hyaluronidases, proteases, and β-lactamase. The outer membrane is a permeability barrier to large molecules such as lysozyme. Its outer monolayer primarily comprises lipopolysaccharide (LPS), and its inner monolayer contains phospholipids normally found in bacterial membranes.

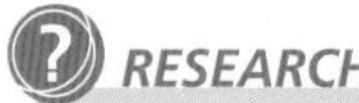

RESEARCH

What are the phospholipids normally found in bacterial membranes?

LPS has three structural domains (Fig 6-11):

1. Lipid A is necessary for bacterial viability and mediates the endotoxin activity of LPS. The two phosphates attached to the disaccharide region are necessary for this activity. Interestingly, monophosphoryl lipid A does not have endotoxin activity but can stimulate the immune system as a vaccine adjuvant.
2. The core polysaccharide consists of 9 to 12 sugars, including the unusual sugar 2-keto-3-deoxy-octanoate that links the core to lipid A. The core is conserved for a particular species of bacteria. A representative sequence of residues starting from the link to the O antigen may be: O antigen – [glucose–GlcNAc] – [galactose] – [glucose–galactose] – [L-glycero-D-mannoheptose] – [L-glycero–D-mannoheptose–diphosphoethanolamine] – [keto-deoxy-octanoate] – [keto-deoxy-octanoate–keto-deoxy-octanoate – phosphoethanolamine] – lipid A.
3. The O antigen is a long linear polysaccharide comprising a large number of repeating units (up to 40) of four to seven sugars per unit and is useful for the identification of different serotypes of a bacterial species. A repeat unit may be composed of [mannose-abequose] – [rhamnose] – [galactose], as in the case of *Salmonella*.

The outer membrane contains porins, which are trimeric protein channels that mediate the diffusion of hydrophilic molecules less than 700 D in molecular weight. The outer membrane is connected to the cytoplasmic membrane at adhesion sites that are membranous routes for the delivery of newly synthesized molecules to the outer membrane.

External structures include the capsule, which is composed of polysaccharides (in most species) that surround the bacterium and mediates the attachment of the bacterium to host tissues such as heart valves and to catheters (Fig 6-12). In some species, the capsule is composed of polypeptides. The capsule can inhibit phagocytosis by neutrophils and macrophages and is thus a virulence factor for some bacteria. *Streptococcus mutans*, one of the causative agents of dental caries, attaches to tooth surfaces via its capsule. The capsule is a determinant of serologic types within a bacterial species; for example, there are more than

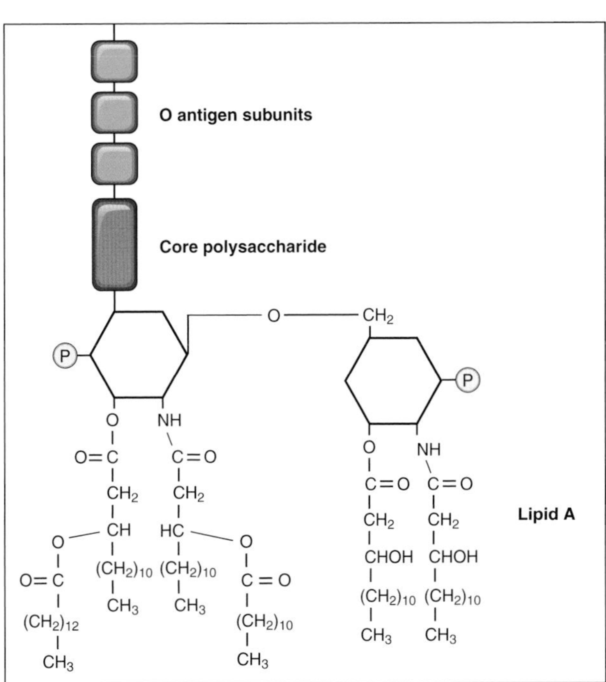

Fig 6-11 The structure of LPS. Note the two phosphate groups that are necessary for the endotoxin activity of lipid A.

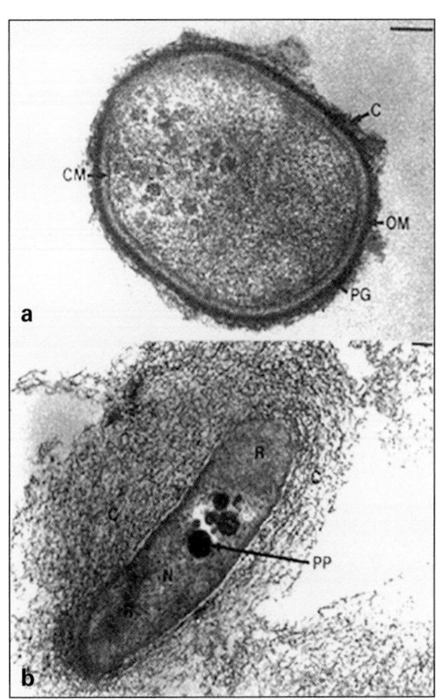

Fig 6-12 Electron micrographs of *Porphyromonas gingivalis (a)* and *Pseudomonas aeruginosa (b)* showing the capsule surrounding the bacteria. C, capsule; OM, outer membrane; PG, peptidoglycan; CM, cytoplasmic membrane; R, ribosome; PP, polyphosphate. Bar = 0.1 µm. (Reproduced from micro.digitalproteus.com/morphology2.php.)

80 serologic types of *Streptococcus pneumoniae*. The vaccine used against *Streptococcus pneumoniae* infection, Pneumovax23, contains 23 different purified capsular polysaccharides of the bacterium. Some bacteria may have a loosely adherent colloidal material that they secrete, usually similar to the capsular material; this material is called the slime layer.

Some bacteria have flagella whose external portion (the filament) is made up of protein subunits, flagellin, that coil helically and are connected to one of the most primitive molecular motors attached to the bacterial membrane. They are anchored in the outer and inner membranes via four basal bodies, which are discoidal, washer-like structures. As the molecular motor turns the shaft of the flagellum, the hook section of the flagellum right outside the cell membrane enables the entire structure to "whip" the medium, providing bacterial motility and chemotaxis toward nutrients. The flagella are also involved in the pathogenesis of *Escherichia coli* urinary tract infections. Flagella originating from the sides of elongated bacteria are classified as peritrichous, and those emanating from one or both ends are polar.

Pili (fimbriae) are filamentous structures on the outside of bacteria composed of protein subunits termed *pilin*. There are many more pili than flagella, and they mediate the attachment to receptors on human cells, such as those mediating the binding of *Neisseria gonorrhoeae* to mucosal epithelial cells. F pili mediate bacterial conjugation between fertility factor-positive (F^+) and F^- cells.

Bacteria multiply by binary fission. If *N* is the number of bacteria, and *t* is the time,

$$\Delta N/\Delta t = kN$$

where *k* is the growth rate constant. The law of growth is obtained by integrating this equation, resulting in:

$$N_t = N_0 e^{kt}$$

where N_t is the number of bacteria at time *t* and N_0 is the number of bacteria at t = 0 (ie, at the beginning of the experiment). This is a geometric progression, or exponential growth. The generation time is the time required for cells to divide, doubling the population. If *n* is the number of generations, and *N* is the number of cells, then

$$N = N_0 2^n$$

With exponential growth, an initial culture of 1,000 *E coli* organisms that divide every 20 minutes would produce about 10^6 cells in 200 minutes ($N = 2^{10}$).

The generation time is dependent on both the bacterium and environmental factors such as temperature and the availability of nutrients. *M tuberculosis* grows slowly, dividing about every 24 hours; therefore, identifying mycobacteria by culturing them can take several weeks. Growth in a closed, or batch, system—with no new nutrients being added to the culture—goes through the lag, exponential,

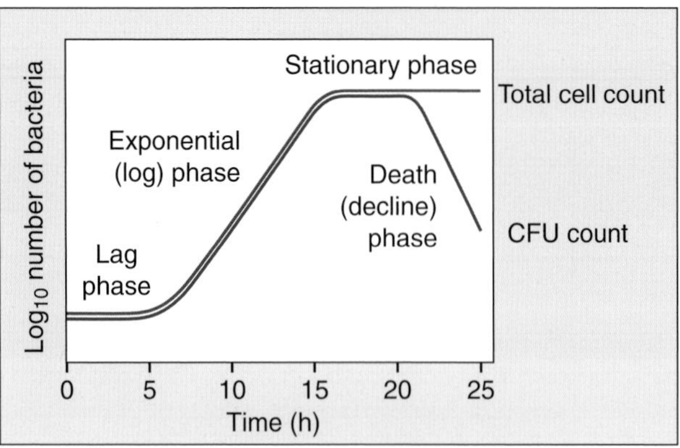

Fig 6-13 The growth of bacteria in a broth culture. CFU, colony-forming unit.

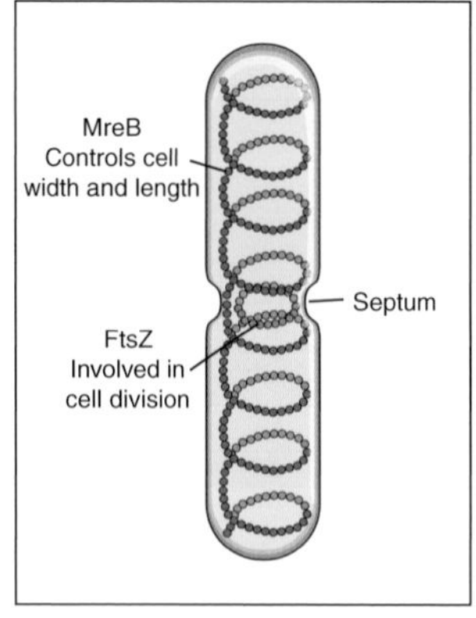

Fig 6-14 Cytoskeletal elements in bacteria.

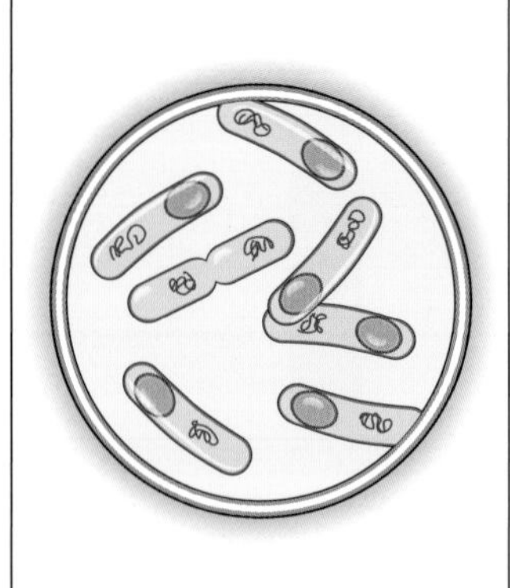

Fig 6-15 Schematic representation of fluorescence images of Gram-positive bacteria *(green)* that are producing spores *(purple)*. A dividing, non-sporulating cell with septum is also shown.

Box 6-1 Classification of medically relevant bacteria*

B12 Proteobacteria (largest bacterial phylum)
- Alphaproteobacteria (*Rickettsia*)
- Betaproteobacteria (*Bordetella, Neisseria*)
- Gammaproteobacteria (*Francisella, Legionella*)
- Epsilonproteobacteria (*Campylobacter, Helicobacter*)

B13 Firmicutes (low G+C, Gram-positive bacteria and mycoplasmas)
Clostridium, Mycoplasma, Bacillus, Listeria, Staphylococcus aureus, Lactobacillus, Streptococcus pneumoniae

B14 Actinobacteria (actinomycetes, mycobacteria)
Corynebacterium, Mycobacterium, Nocardia, Propionibacterium acnes, Streptomyces griseus (produces streptomycin)

B16 Chlamydiae
Chlamydia trachomatis

B17 Spirochaetes
Borrelia, Treponema, Leptospira

B20 Bacteroidetes
Porphyromonas gingivalis, Cytophaga

B21 Fusobacteria
Fusobacterium nucleatum

*A partial classification of bacteria adapted from Ingraham and Ingraham.

stationary, and decline (or death) phases (Fig 6-13). In a chemostat, in which fresh nutrients are added and waste products are removed, bacteria can grow in the exponential phase for prolonged periods. The oral cavity can be considered a chemostat where nutrients are replenished and products of metabolism are removed by saliva.

For cell division to occur, new components have to be incorporated into the cell wall and the membrane. When the cell expands to a sufficient stage, the cell wall in the middle of the growing structure invaginates to form a septum, most likely facilitated by tubulin-like contractile proteins called FtsZ (Fig 6-14). The two apposed faces of the cytoplasmic membrane fuse with each other, producing two "daughter" bacteria. Although the presence of cytoskeletal proteins is generally attributed to eukaryotic cells, studies in the last decade have indicated the presence of proteins like FtsZ as well as the actin-like protein MreB, which controls cell width and length. The two copies of DNA that are attached to the cytoplasmic membrane move apart as the two daughter cells move away from the region of the septum.

Certain Gram-positive bacteria form spores, especially under adverse environmental conditions (Fig 6-15). The spore consists of an inner core that includes the DNA and other essential molecules needed for reproduction; the inner membrane; the spore wall; the cortex, composed of a special form of peptidoglycan; the outer membrane; a cysteine-rich, keratin-like protein coat; and an exosporium composed of lipoprotein and carbohydrate. The core contains high concentrations of dipicolinic acid (pyridine dicarboxylic acid) that chelates calcium.

A simplified scheme of bacterial classification is shown in Box 6-1.

Bacterial Metabolism

Bacterial metabolism starts with the import of nutrients into the cell, which then act as substrates in a series of catabolic reactions that result in the formation of 12 precursor metabolites, adenosine triphosphate (ATP), and reducing power. Then the molecules necessary for cell function, including building blocks for macromolecules, are produced. These building blocks, such as amino acids and nucleosides, are synthesized into macromolecules that are then assembled into all the cellular structures. Catabolism is the set of reactions that break down complex molecules and release energy, which is captured in molecules like ATP that the cell can utilize. Anabolism refers to the set of reactions that use this energy to synthesize molecules such as carbohydrates, lipids, proteins, and nucleic acids necessary for the cells, utilizing sugars, fatty acids, amino acids, and other molecules as starting molecules.

Bacteria use three major pathways to metabolize glucose: *(1)* the glycolytic (Embden-Meyerhof-Parnas) pathway, *(2)* the pentose phosphate pathway, and *(3)* the tricarboxylic acid (Krebs) cycle. Glycolysis starts with the conversion of glucose to glucose-6-phosphate by the enzyme hexokinase and proceeds through a series of three enzymatic reactions to the production of the 3-carbon glyceraldehyde-3-phosphate, which is then converted through a set of five reactions to pyruvate. This pathway results in the net production of two ATP and two reduced nicotinamide adenine dinucleotide (NADH) molecules per molecule of glucose metabolized. ATP is formed from adenosine diphosphate (ADP) by the action of a kinase enzyme in a reaction termed substrate-level phosphorylation at two steps in glycolysis, one of these being the conversion of phosphoenolpyruvate to pyruvate in the last step of glycolysis. Glycolysis also produces the six precursor metabolites: glucose-6-phosphate, fructose-6-phosphate, triose phosphate, 3-phosphoglycerate, and phosphoenolpyruvate, in addition to pyruvate. Most heterotrophic organisms (which use organic molecules for their metabolism), whether aerobic or anaerobic, use glycolysis to break down carbohydrates.

The initial step in the pentose phosphate pathway is the conversion of glucose-6-phosphate from the glycolysis pathway to the pentose ribose-5-phosphate and to erythrose-4-phosphate, both of which are precursor metabolites. The pathway provides two reduced NADH phosphates needed for biosynthesis. The ribose-5-phosphate is involved in nucleic acid and coenzyme synthesis. This pathway also enables aerobic growth without the participation of Krebs cycle enzymes and the metabolism of external pentose sugars as carbon and energy sources.

Both glycolysis and the pentose phosphate pathway can take place under both aerobic and anaerobic conditions. Fermentation takes place under anaerobic conditions and involves the conversion of pyruvate to various end products such as ethanol and lactic acid, depending on the bacterial species. Lactobacilli, streptococci, and mammalian cells convert pyruvate to lactic acid. The reduction of pyruvate to the end products results in the oxidation of NADH to NAD^+, which then continues to participate in glycolysis, where it is converted back to the reduced NADH.

Under aerobic conditions, the pyruvate produced at the end of glycolysis reacts with coenzyme A (CoA) and NAD^+ to produce acetyl CoA, CO_2 and NADH. Acetyl CoA then enters the tricarboxylic acid (Krebs) cycle by interacting with oxalate, resulting in the formation of citrate, which then undergoes a series of enzyme-catalyzed reactions to form oxaloacetate, thus completing the cycle. As the cycle proceeds, two molecules of CO_2, three molecules of NADH, one molecule of reduced flavin adenine dinucleotide ($FADH_2$), and one molecule of guanosine 5′-triphosphate (GTP) are produced. The GTP is then converted to ATP. The Krebs cycle also generates four precursor metabolites: acetyl CoA, alpha-ketoglutarate, succinyl CoA, and oxaloacetate.

$FADH_2$ and NADH formed in glycolysis, the Krebs cycle, and fatty acid oxidation are energy-rich molecules that can each donate a pair of electrons to oxygen, thereby liberating a large amount of free energy that can be used to form ATP. This is accomplished via oxidative phosphorylation, in which electrons are transferred from $FADH_2$ and NADH to a series of electron-carrying proteins in the mitochondrial inner membrane in eukaryotes and the cytoplasmic membrane in bacteria and then to the final acceptor, O_2. These proteins are NADH-Q (ubiquinone) reductase, cytochrome reductase, and cytochrome oxidase, and they transfer electrons with the participation of reduced ubiquinone between the first two enzymes and with the participation of cytochrome c between the last two enzymes in an electron transport chain. As electrons are being transported within the membrane, protons are translocated across the membrane to the outside. The protons accumulate in the intermembrane space in mitochondria in eukaryotes, the periplasmic space in Gram-negative bacteria, and the cell wall outside the membrane in Gram-positive bacteria, presumably mediated by the phosphate groups of teichoic acids. The proton gradient across the membrane provides the free energy for the transmembrane enzyme ATP synthase, which mediates the phosphorylation of ADP to form ATP.

Under anaerobic conditions, the final electron acceptor can be a molecule like nitrate, fumarate, and sulfate, resulting in anaerobic respiration. The metabolism of one glucose molecule under aerobic conditions can yield 38 ATP molecules, compared with only two ATP molecules under anaerobic conditions. Aerobic microorganisms in an oxygen-rich environment will multiply more rapidly than aneorobes.

Based on their sources of carbon and energy, bacteria can be classified into the following groups:

- Photoautotrophs use CO_2 as a carbon source. They can "fix" the CO_2 into ribulose bisphosphate, converting it into phosphoglyceric acid via the Calvin-Benson cycle. The phosphoglyceraldehyde that is produced in the cycle can then join central metabolism. Photoautotrophs use light energy via photosynthesis. An example is the anaerobe *Chromatium vinosum*.
- Chemoautotrophs obtain energy by oxidizing inorganic substances such as sulfides and nitrites. An example is the aerobic bacterium *Thiobacillus thiooxidans*.
- Photoheterotophs use organic molecules as a source of carbon and generate energy via photosynthesis. An example is the hydrogen gas–producing *Rhodopseudomonas palustris*, which may be a source of fuel in the future.
- Chemoheterotrophs use chemical oxidation-reduction reactions to generate energy and obtain carbon from organic molecules. Most medically important bacteria are in this group.

Bacteria are also classified according to their optimal growth temperature and the effect of oxygen on their metabolism. Most human pathogens are mesophiles whose optimal growth temperature is 37°C, with a range of 10°C to 45°C. Psychrophiles grow optimally at 20°C and within the range of 0°C to 30°C. An example is *Listeria monocytogenes*, which can grow at 4°C. Thermophiles grow optimally at 50°C to 55°C and can grow in the range of 25°C to 90°C. Resistance of microorganisms to heat is associated with the thermostability of their proteins. Many thermophilic microorganisms are in the domain Archaea.

With respect to the effect of oxygen on growth and metabolism, bacteria can be classified into four groups:

1. Obligate, or strict, aerobes require oxygen for growth, as they depend on oxidative phosphorylation (respiration), with the final electron acceptor being oxygen. Examples of obligate aerobes are *M tuberculosis* and *P aeruginosa*. Microaerophiles are microorganisms that grow at oxygen concentrations below that of air, including *Helicobacter pylori* and *Borrelia burgdorferi*. These microorganisms have low levels of superoxide dismutase and catalase that detoxify reactive oxygen species.
2. Obligate anaerobes cannot grow in the presence of oxygen or are killed by oxygen. They are not able to detoxify the partial reduction products of O_2 produced during respiration, including hydrogen peroxide (H_2O_2) and superoxide radical (O_2^-). Examples of such bacteria are *P gingivalis*, *Bacteroides fragilis*, and *Clostridium tetani*.
3. Facultative aerobes, such as *E coli*, grow in the presence or absence of oxygen. They obtain their energy by fermentation under anaerobic conditions and by oxidative phosphorylation (aerobic respiration) in the presence of oxygen.
4. Aerotolerant anaerobes generally grow fermentatively both in the presence and absence of oxygen and have some ability to remove partial reduction products of oxygen. Many dental-related bacteria, including streptococci, lactobacilli, and *Fusobacterium nucleatum*, are in this group.

RESEARCH

What are the diseases caused by *L monocytogenes, M tuberculosis, P aeruginosa, B burgdorferi, P gingivalis, B fragilis, C tetani, Clostridium perfringens, E coli,* and *F nucleatum*?

RESEARCH

What are the reactions that detoxify oxygen and the enzymes that catalyze them?

Bacterial Genetics

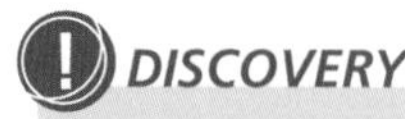

DISCOVERY

Frederick Griffith published his findings on the transforming principle in 1928. He injected mice with a strain of *S pneumoniae* with a rough (R) colony phenotype; the mice did not develop disease (Fig 6-16). When he injected the smooth (S) colony type, however, the mice developed disease and died. If he heat-killed the S strain and injected it, the mice did not develop disease, as expected. Griffith then injected mice with a mixture of the live R strain with the heat-killed S strain (both of which did not cause disease individually). The mice in this case died. Griffith was able to isolate from the mice R forms that had newly acquired the capsular structure.

DISCOVERY

In 1944, Oswald T. Avery, Colin McLeod, and Maclyn McCarty purified the material capable of causing genetic exchange between the different strains of *S pneumoniae* (the transforming principle) and showed it to be DNA.

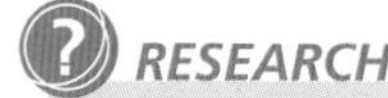

RESEARCH

How did Avery and colleagues figure out that the transforming principle was DNA?

Bacterial genes are located on a single circular loop of DNA, the bacterial chromosome. Each gene is a distinct sequence of DNA that codes for a particular sequence of amino acids in a polypeptide chain. Some genes code for ribosomal RNA (rRNA) and transfer RNA (tRNA). Bacterial genes are haploid. The bacterial genome is composed of exons that are transcribed into messenger RNA (mRNA), unlike eukaryotes that also have introns, noncoding sequences that are interspersed between genes and are spliced out from the RNA transcript as mature mRNA is produced.

DISCOVERY

The flow of genetic information from DNA to mRNA to protein was described as the central dogma of molecular biology by Francis Crick. This concept was modified in 1970 with the discovery of reverse transcriptase in retroviruses by David Baltimore, Howard Temin, and Satoshi Mizutani. This enzyme transcribes RNA into DNA, which is then integrated into the genome of infected cells.

The total genetic potential of DNA is the genotype of the bacterium. The expressed proteins, and hence the structure and function of the organism, is the phenotype. The nucleotides of a gene are arranged in groups of three bases, called codons. During translation, tRNA bound to a specific

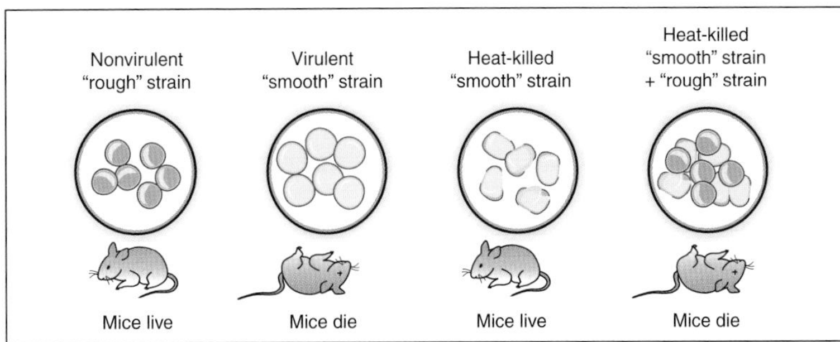

Fig 6-16 The Frederick Griffith experiment.

amino acid recognizes the codon on mRNA via its anticodon that complements the codon sequence.

The function of a gene can be altered or inhibited by genetic mutation. Salvador Luria and Max Delbrück showed the presence of spontaneous mutations in bacteria in 1943. Auxotrophic mutants are defective in the synthesis of an essential metabolite; they cannot proliferate in media that supports the growth of the original wild-type bacteria. The mutagenicity of a chemical is determined readily with the Ames test, developed by Bruce Ames. Strains of *Salmonella* that have lost their ability to synthesize histidine, called *histidine auxotrophs*, are used for this test. When these strains undergo mutations, they can synthesize histidine. If a substance is a mutagen, it will increase the rate at which these organisms revert to histidine synthesizers. To mimic the conversion of various chemicals to mutagens by liver metabolism, rat liver extract is also included in the test.

Silent mutations change the DNA sequence but do not alter the amino acid sequence, since the genetic code is degenerate and several codons code for the same amino acid. A missense mutation causes the insertion of a different amino acid in the protein, usually resulting in the production of a nonfunctional protein.

A nonsense mutation changes the DNA sequence to one coding for a stop codon, causing protein synthesis to be terminated prematurely. In a frameshift mutation, a small deletion or insertion (but not in multiples of three) causes a change in the reading frame, thus altering the amino acid sequence of the protein. Extensive insertion or deletion, or gross rearrangement of chromosome structure, leads to null mutations that completely impair gene function. Mutagens include nucleotide base analogs such as 5-bromouracil, frameshift mutagens such as ethidium bromide that intercalates between bases, and DNA-reactive chemicals like nitrosoguanidine.

Transposons are relatively short pieces of DNA that can move from one place in DNA to another. Enzymes called transposases mediate the cleavage of donor DNA and its insertion into target DNA. Transposition is a rare event, ranging from once every 10^3 to 10^8 bacterial cell divisions. The smaller transposons are about 1,000 base pairs long and may encode only the transposase; these are termed insertion sequence elements. The ends of transposons contain sequences that run in the opposite direction and are called inverted repeats. These sequences are recognized by transposases, which also bind to one another, forming a loop with the transposon DNA. The loop is excised and inserted into the recipient DNA. Composite transposons are formed when certain genes are incorporated between two insertion sequence elements. For example, the transposon Tn5 contains the genes for resistance to kanamycin (Kan^r), bleomycin (Ble^r), and streptomycin (Str^r) flanked by insertion sequences called IS50. Such composite transposons appear to have been assembled in naturally occurring plasmids called R factors. As might be expected, insertion of transposons or insertion sequences into DNA can cause major changes in the genes into which they insert, as well as in adjacent genes.

RESEARCH

What are the molecular targets of the antibiotics kanamycin, bleomycin, and streptomycin?

DISCOVERY

Transposable DNA elements were first observed by Barbara McClintock, who was studying maize genetics in the 1940s and 1950s. She developed a theory by which these movable elements, which she called "controlling elements," regulated genes by selectively inhibiting or modulating their action. These controlling elements could be the answer to the problem of how complex organisms can develop many different kinds of cells and tissues during development when each cell in the organism has the same set of genes. McClintock was awarded the Nobel Prize in 1983 at the age of 81 years.

Regulation of Gene Expression

Bacteria must be capable of adapting quickly to changes in the concentration of certain nutrients in the environment. To minimize the requirement for energy, ideally a particular metabolic system should be operational only when it is needed. Genes encoding enzymes of a particular pathway are grouped together structurally in an operon. The ability to hydrolyze lactose is latent; when the environment changes, β-galactosidase is induced to metabolize lactose (inducible gene) (Fig 6-17). Repressible genes are turned off by the end product of the biosynthetic pathway. For example, histidine is synthesized if the amino acid is not supplied in the medium; but if there is histidine, the genes for the histidine pathway are repressed.

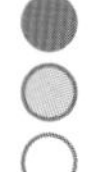

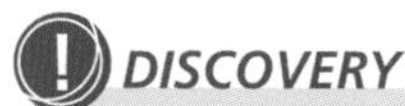

Jacques Monod, in his Nobel Lecture in 1965, described in detail the work that led to the discovery of the *lac* operon and the manner in which it operated (see Fig 6-17). According to François Jacob, one of the other co-discoverers and Nobel laureates, Monod started working on the enzymes that metabolize lactose because they were much simpler to assay than those for maltose. Until World War II, genes in bacteria were not studied; but afterward, Luria and Delbrück analyzed bacterial mutations, and Lederberg and Tatum studied what was then called "adaptation," where bacteria placed from a glucose medium to a lactose medium took some time to generate the enzymes necessary to metabolize lactose. This process was called enzyme "induction." The model that Jacob proposed to Monod was that a gene was making an mRNA and that the control of gene expression was at the level of mRNA production. At first Monod did not like the model, arguing that the enzyme could be produced at different rates, and the model did not explain this. Monod started to make mutants that were unable to metabolize lactose, and he showed that no galactosidase was made in some of these mutants. He and his colleagues also found that there was another gene (permease) adjacent to the first one that facilitated the entry of lactose into the cell.

Plasmids

Plasmids are small genetic elements that replicate independently of the bacterial chromosome (and, as such, are referred to as replicons). They are circular, double-stranded DNA consisting of 1.5 to 400 kilobase pairs (kbp), and they enable bacteria to respond to different environmental challenges. For comparison, the *E coli* chromosome is 4,000 kbp. Plasmids code for resistance to toxins and antibiotics (R plasmids), the fertility factor, and certain adhesiveness or protective-coating properties. Plasmids also code for bacteriocins (colicins in *E coli*) that inhibit the growth of other bacterial strains or related species by destroying DNA, arresting protein synthesis, or increasing membrane permeability to ions.

Gene Exchange

Gene exchange is an important process in bacterial populations that enables the bacteria to acquire new genes, including those that confer antibiotic resistance. Gene exchange between bacteria can occur via three mechanisms: transformation, conjugation, and transduction.

1. Transformation is the introduction of foreign pieces of DNA into bacteria. Mostly done in laboratory experiments, it also occurs naturally in *Haemophilus*, *Neisseria*, *Streptococcus*, and *Bacillus* species. Bacterial species may acquire traits from other species or strains by horizontal gene transfer. In Gram-positive bacteria, a peptidic signal molecule called competence factor is exported outside the cell, and as its concentration increases in a dividing population of bacteria, it binds ComD sensor kinase, which then activates (via a phosphorylation cascade) the operon synthesizing the components of the structure called the translocasome. The translocasome assembled on the membrane binds extracellular DNA and degrades one strand as it imports the other strand into the cell. The DNA can then be incorporated into the bacterial chromosome by recombination. In Gram-negative bacteria, like *Neisseria* and *Haemophilus* species, DNA is imported through the type IV pilus assembly/disassembly system; the disassembling pilus drags the transforming DNA into the periplasm, and a single strand of DNA is translocated through the Rec2/ComF transport system into the cytoplasm. In *Neisseria* and *Haemophilus* species, only specific DNA sequences, primarily species-specific DNA, are taken up. The lung pathogen *Acinetobacter calcoaceticus*, however, can take up DNA from any source.

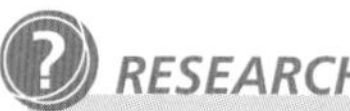

What are the diseases caused by *Neisseria*, *Haemophilus*, and *Acinetobacter* species?

Artificial transformation requires the addition of agents like calcium chloride or the use of high-voltage pulses that induce membrane perturbations that allow DNA to enter cells (electroporation).

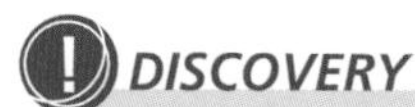

In 1947, when Joshua Lederberg and Edward Tatum mixed different strains of *E coli*, they observed strains that were not genetically similar to either of the original strains. They suspected that the strains exchanged DNA, although the presence of plasmids was not known at the time. They were working, unknowingly, with the fertility (F) plasmid.

2. Bacterial conjugation involves the direct transfer of the DNA of the donor into the recipient bacterium. In fertility factor positive (F^+) donor bacteria such as *E coli*, the sex pilus first attaches to a receptor on fertility factor negative (F^-) bacteria and then contracts, facilitating the formation of a conjugation complex. The fertility factor is located on a plasmid that is transferred with high frequency. The plasmid-encoded helicase/endonuclease makes a site-specific cleavage of the phosphodiester backbone at the *oriT* (origin of transfer) site, and the nick initiates rolling circle replication. The displaced single strand of DNA is directed to the recipient cell via the conjugation complex. The transferred

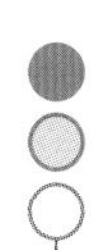

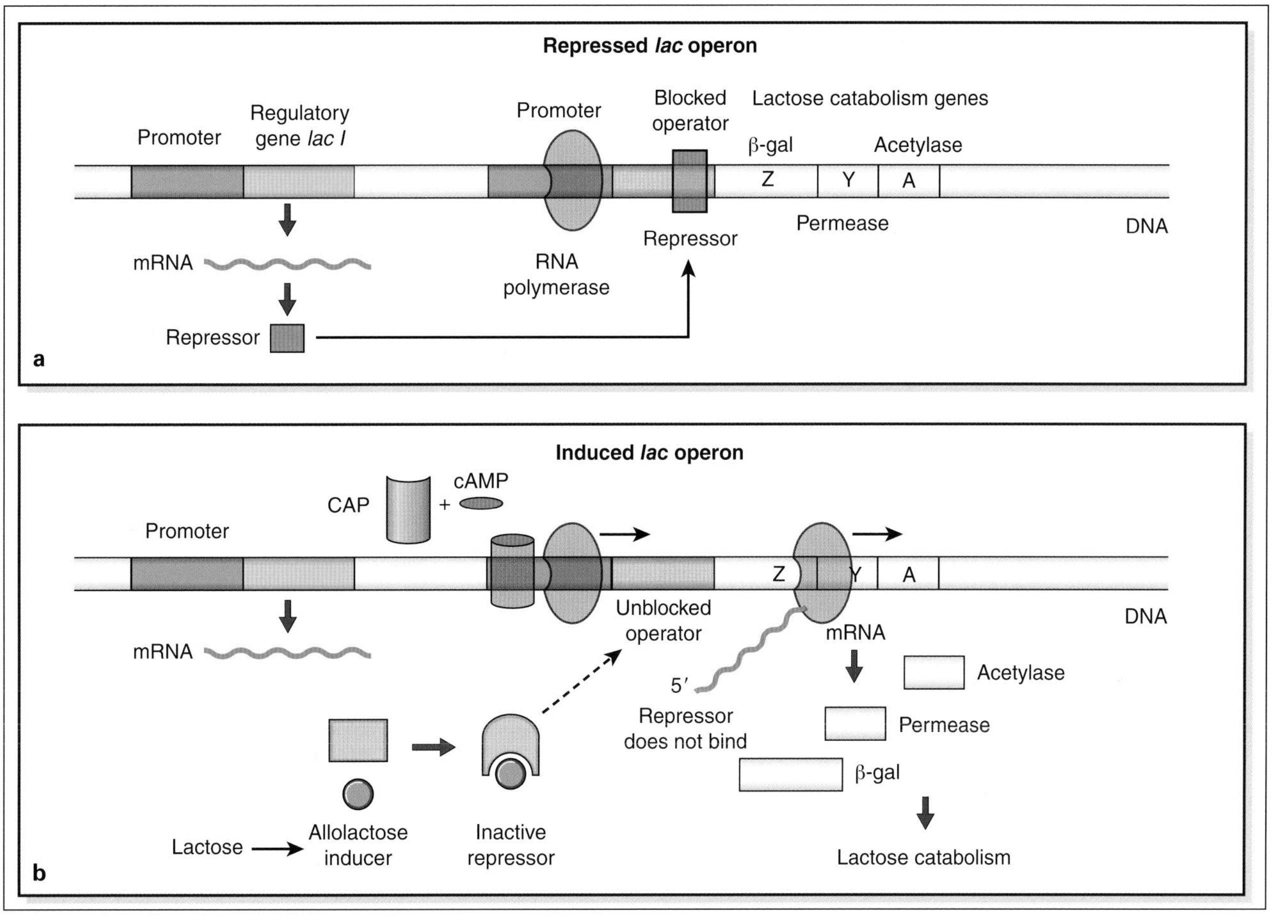

Fig 6-17 The lactose operon. The mRNA encoding the proteins β-galactosidase (β-gal, Z), permease (Y), and acetylase (A) is transcribed from the promoter. The repressor protein is encoded by the *lac I* gene. *(a)* In the absence of lactose, the repressor binds to the operator region of DNA and prevents the RNA polymerase from transcribing the genes. *(b)* In the presence of lactose, an isomer of lactose—allolactose—is produced and binds to the repressor, causing a conformational change in the protein. The modified repressor cannot bind to the operator, and the *lac* operon is transcribed at a low level. If the bacterium is in a poor medium that also contains lactose, the catabolite gene-activator protein (CAP) can be activated by cyclic adenosine monophosphate (cAMP) and binds to the promoter. The promoter is then fully activated and facilitates the transcription of a high level of *lac* mRNA. However, in a poor medium without lactose, although the CAP-cAMP complex can bind to the promoter, the repressor is active because there is no allolactose as an inducer. The *lac* operon therefore will not be activated.

DNA is then circularized, and its complementary strand is synthesized. The recipient cell now becomes F^+.

Sometimes the F^+ plasmid can integrate into the chromosome at sites that have similar DNA sequences in the two pieces of DNA, including insertion elements that may be common in both the plasmid and the chromosome. This bacterial cell is described as high-frequency recombination (Hfr). When conjugation occurs with Hfr bacteria, part of the plasmid sequence starting at *oriT* and a segment of the adjacent bacterial chromosome are transferred to the recipient cell. If the transfer is interrupted at a particular time, only the genes following the *oriT* will be inserted into the recipient chromosome. The further a particular gene is located from the integrated plasmid in the direction of the transfer, the less frequently it is transferred. The DNA advances at a constant rate (approximately 1% of the total DNA per minute at 37°C). Thus, distances on a chromosome can be measured in units of time, the entire genome taking about 100 minutes (compared to 5 minutes for a free F plasmid). The fertility factor can be inserted at different sites along the bacterial chromosome. This leads to different sequences being transferred. These studies have led to the mapping of the genes along the chromosome of *E coli*.

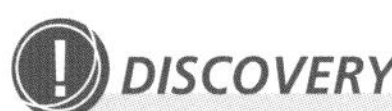

DISCOVERY

In 1952, Joshua Lederberg and Norton Zinder discovered yet another mechanism of gene transfer in *Salmonella*. Transduction is the transfer of bacterial DNA from one cell to another by means of a bacterial virus (bacteriophage) infection.

3. When the phage DNA is introduced into the bacterium, the replication of the bacterial chromosome is disrupted, and components of the phage are produced and assembled. The bacterium lyses, and the phage particles are released. In lysogeny, infection by a temperate bacteriophage does not cause lysis, but the genome of the phage integrates into the bacterial chromosome, and this "prophage" is replicated as part of the chromosome for many generations. Temperate phages may revert to a virulent state that leads to the production of phage particles and bacterial lysis. The new phage may carry with it a part of the bacterial chromosome. This segment of DNA, when delivered to a new host bacterium, may confer a new characteristic to the bacterium, a process called lysogenic conversion. In generalized transduction, any gene from the donor bacterium can be taken and transferred to a recipient bacterium. In restricted or specialized transduction, only a few closely linked genes can be transferred.

The Genetic Code, Genetic Engineering, and Gene Sequencing

The double helical structure of DNA was described by Francis Crick and James Watson in their paper published in *Nature* on April 25, 1953. Experiments by Matt Meselson and Frank Stahl, utilizing an isotope of nitrogen that gets incorporated into DNA as bacteria divide, indicated that DNA replicates in a semiconservative manner, the daughter double helical DNA having one strand from the parent and another synthesized de novo.

The code that dictates which triplet of nucleic acids on an mRNA gives rise to the incorporation of a particular amino acid into the growing polypeptide change during translation in the ribosome was largely worked out by Marshall Nirenberg and Gobind Khorana (Table 6-1). Nirenberg and Khorana were awarded the Nobel Prize in Physiology or Medicine in 1968.

In the 1960s, Werner Arber discovered bacterial enzymes that can cleave DNA at highly specific palindromic sequences. These enzymes, called restriction enzymes, were able to cleave the DNA of bacteriophages, thereby protecting the bacteria. In the early 1970s, Herbert Boyer, who was working on restriction enzymes, and Stanley Cohen, who was an expert on antibiotic resistance plasmids and their transformation into bacteria, collaborated to cut the genes conferring resistance to kanamycin and tetracycline and to place them in the same plasmid. These experiments led to the development of DNA cloning techniques, where a particular DNA segment from a genome could be cleaved using a particular restriction enzyme that would produce "sticky ends" of DNA and "pasted" into a plasmid (a cloning vector) that had been treated with the same restriction enzyme (Fig 6-18).

Table 6-1 The genetic code: The triplet sequences (codons) on mRNA that encode each of the amino acids*

Amino acid	RNA codon
Alanine (Ala)	GCA GCC GCG GCU
Arginine (Arg)	AGA AGG CGA CGC CGG CGU
Asparagine (Asn)	AAC AAU
Aspartic acid (Asp)	GAC GAU
Cysteine (Cys)	UGC UGU
Glutamic acid (Glu)	GAG GAA
Glutamine (Gln)	CAG CAA
Glycine (Gly)	GGG GGA GGC GGU
Histidine (His)	CAC CAU
Isoleucine (Ile)	AUA AUC AUU
Leucine (Leu)	CUG CUA CUC CUU UUG UUA
Lysine (Lys)	AAG AAA
Methionine (Met)	AUG
Phenylalanine (Phe)	UUC UUU
Proline (Pro)	CCG CCU CCA CCC
Serine (Ser)	UCG UCA UCC UCU AGC AGU
Threonine (Thr)	ACG ACA ACC ACU
Tryptophan (Trp)	UGG
Tyrosine (Tyr)	UAC UAU
Valine (Val)	GUG GUA GUC GUU
Stop codons	UAA UAG UGA

*Most of the code is "redundant" in that a number of triplet codons specify a single amino acid. Stop codons indicate the end of the coding segment of the gene. The Met codon also functions as the start codon. (Inspired by Watson.)

The ability to produce large amounts of a certain gene also provided the opportunity to determine the exact sequence of bases in the gene. Fred Sanger developed a method for DNA sequencing that involved the use of the nucleotide analogs, dideoxycytidine, dideoxythymidine, dideoxyadenosine, and dideoxyguanosine. In the more recent of the methods for DNA sequencing, the analogs are labeled with different fluorescent probes and included in small amounts in addition to the normal nucleotides. When the dideoxynucleotide is added to the complementary chain being copied off the template DNA by means of DNA polymerase, the chain is terminated because there is no OH group on the ribose of DNA to which the next phosphate group can bind. This process produces an entire set of DNA molecules (or fragments) of different length, termi-

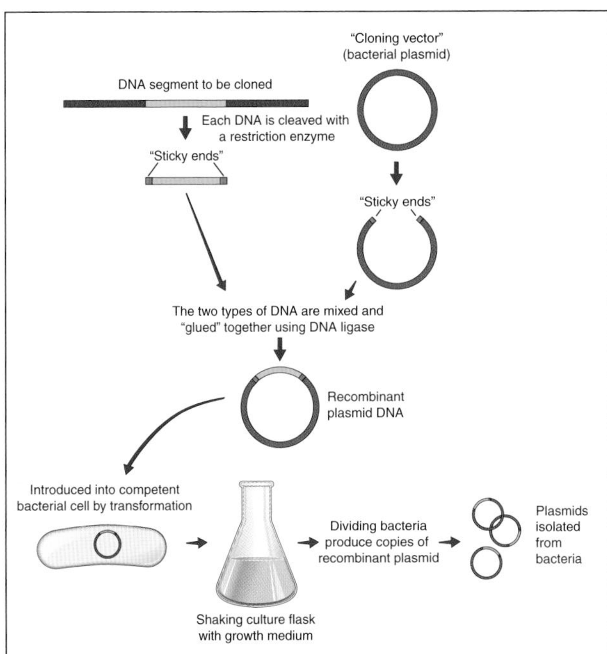

Fig 6-18 Production of recombinant DNA to clone a gene. (Adapted from Watson.)

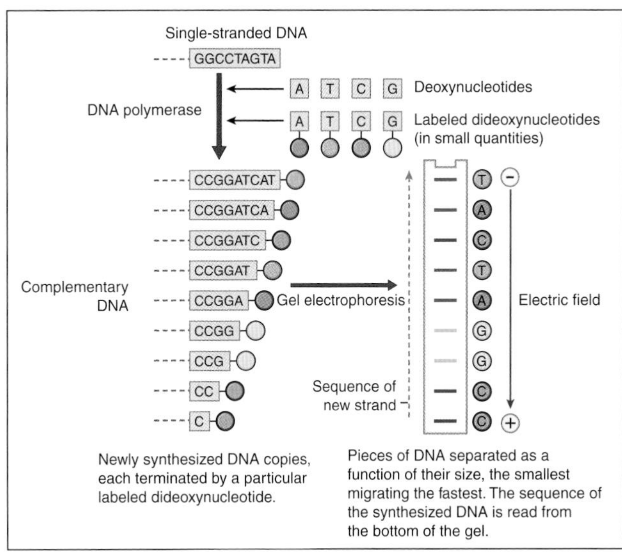

Fig 6-19 The advanced Sanger method of DNA sequencing using the four dideoxynucleotides, each labeled with a different fluorescent probe. (Adapted from Watson.)

nating with a particular dideoxynucleotide. These fragments are separated by gel electrophoresis, where the smallest fragment travels the fastest. The flow of the fragments can be detected by a fluorescence detector, which can essentially "read" the sequence of nucleotides (Fig 6-19). Sanger was awarded the Nobel Prize in Chemistry in 1980 for developing this method.

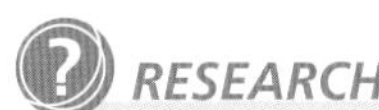

Because eukaryotic genes have introns interspersed between exons that actually encode the final protein product, how can such genes be cloned into bacterial plasmids without the introns present?

Bibliography

The Barbara McClintock Papers. Profiles in Science: National Library of Sciences. http://profiles.nlm.nih.gov/ps/retrieve/Narrative/LL/p-nid/49. Accessed 4 May 2015.

Engleberg NC, DiRita V, Dermody TS. Schaechter's Mechanisms of Microbial Disease, ed 4. Baltimore: Lippincott Williams & Wilkins, 2007.

Fronzes R, Christie PJ, Waksman G. The structural biology of type IV secretion systems. Nat Rev Microbiol 2009;7:703–714.

Greenwood D, Slack R, Peutherer J, Barer M. Medical Microbiology, ed 17. Edinburgh: Churchill Livingstone/Elsevier, 2007.

History of the Microscope. Anton van Leeuwenhoek: A history of the compound microscope. www.history-of-the-microscope.org/anton-van-leeuwenhoek-microscope-history.php. Accessed 4 May 2015.

Ingraham JL, Ingraham CA. Introduction to Microbiology: A Case History Approach. Pacific Grove, CA: Brooks/Cole (Thomson), 2004.

Innovators and Pioneers: Anton van Leeuwenhoek. www.pbs.org/wnet/redgold/printable/p_leeuwenhoek.html. Accessed 4 May 2015.

Meselson M, Stahl F. The replication of DNA in *Escherichia coli*. Proc Natl Acad Sci USA 1958;44:671–682.

Monod J. From enzymatic adaptation to allosterin transitions. In: Nobel Lectures, Physiology or Medicine, 1963–1970. Amsterdam: Elsevier, 1965. www.nobelprize.org/nobel_prizes/medicine/laureates/1965/monod-lecture.pdf. Accessed 4 May 2015.

Murray PR, Rosenthal KS, Pfaller MA. Medical Microbiology, ed 6. Philadelphia: Mosby/Elsevier, 2009.

Pedrotti PW. Antonj van Leeuwenhoek. www.vanleeuwenhoek.com. Accessed 4 May 2015.

Ryan KJ, Ray CG. Sherris Medical Microbiology, ed 5. New York: McGraw-Hill, 2010.

Slonczewski JL, Foster JW. Microbiology: An Evolving Science. New York: Norton, 2009.

Snyder L, Peters JE, Henkin TM, Champness W. Molecular Genetics of Bacteria, ed 4. Washington, DC: ASM Press, 2013.

Watson JD. DNA: The Secret of Life. New York: Knopf, 2003.

Watson JD, Crick FHC. Molecular structure of nucleic acids: A structure for deoxyribose nucleic acid. Nature 1953;171:737–738.

Willett NP, White RR, Rosen S. Essential Dental Microbiology. Norwalk, CT: Appleton & Lange, 1991.

Take-Home Messages

- Bacteria can be classified structurally into Gram-positive and Gram-negative, depending on their staining with a procedure developed by Christian Gram.
- Gram-positive bacteria have a single lipid bilayer membrane surrounded by a thick layer of peptidoglycan.
- Gram-negative bacteria have both a cytoplasmic membrane and an outer membrane with a thin peptidoglycan layer in between. The outer monolayer of the outer membrane is mostly composed of LPS.
- LPS has three structural domains. The lipid A domain has endotoxin activity.
- Peptidoglycan is a mesh of linear polysaccharide co-polymer chains composed of N-acetylglucosamine and N-acetylmuramic acid. The chains are cross-linked by peptides.
- In Gram-positive bacteria, the peptide bridge consists of L-alanine–D-glutamic acid–L-lysine–D-alanine–D-alanine and is attached to N-acetylmuramic acid.
- The peptide sequence of the peptidoglycan in Gram-negative bacteria is L-alanine–D-glutamic acid–mesodiamino-pimelic acid–D-alanine–D-alanine.
- The subunits of peptidoglycan are translocated across the cytoplasmic membrane by the action of bactoprenol-pyrophosphate.
- Transpeptidases, which are penicillin-binding proteins, link the peptides in adjoining polysaccharides.
- Bacteria transport synthesized proteins across their membranes via the general secretory pathway and various secretion systems.
- The external structures of bacteria include the capsule, flagella, and pili.
- The generation time is the time required for cells to divide, doubling the population. Exponential growth is given by the formula $N = 2^n$, where N is the number of cells and n is the number of generations.
- Growth in a closed system with no new nutrients being added to the culture goes through a lag phase, followed by exponential, stationary, and death phases.
- During cell division, the cell wall in the middle of the growing structure invaginates to form a septum, helped by tubulin-like contractile proteins (FtsZ). The actin-like protein MreB controls cell width and length.
- Certain Gram-positive bacteria form spores, especially under adverse environmental conditions.
- Bacteria use the glycolytic (Embden-Meyerhof-Parnas) pathway, the pentose phosphate pathway, and the tricarboxylic acid (Krebs) cycle to metabolize glucose.
- Fermentation takes place under anaerobic conditions and involves the conversion of pyruvate to various end products such as ethanol and lactic acid.
- In oxidative phosphorylation, the energy-rich molecules $FADH_2$ and NADH transfer electrons to electron-carrying proteins in the mitochondrial inner membrane in eukaryotes and the cytoplasmic membrane in bacteria and then to the final acceptor, O_2. This process also generates a proton gradient across the membrane that drives an ATP synthase to form ATP.
- Bacteria can be classified into four groups with respect to the effect of oxygen on growth and metabolism: *(1)* obligate, or strict, aerobes; *(2)* obligate anaerobes; *(3)* facultative anaerobes; and *(4)* aerotolerant anaerobes.
- Bacterial genes are located on a single circular loop of DNA, the bacterial chromosome.
- The function of a gene can be altered or inhibited by genetic mutation.
- Genes encoding enzymes of a particular pathway are grouped together structurally in an operon.
- Gene exchange enables bacteria to acquire new genes, including those that confer antibiotic resistance, and is mediated by transformation, conjugation, or transduction.

7 Bacterial Pathogenesis

The ability of a microorganism to cause disease is related to its pathogenicity. Pathogenesis is both the mechanism by which the microorganism infects the host and the mechanism of disease development. Virulence is a measure of the pathogenicity of an organism and can be measured by the number of organisms necessary to cause disease in an animal model. The lethal dose 50 (LD_{50}) is the number of bacteria that causes death in 50% of an animal population, and the effective dose 50 (ED_{50}) is the number of bacteria causing a particular disease symptom in 50% of the animals.

Infection

Bacterial infections can be classified into several different types. Opportunistic infections are caused by the normal human flora or transient bacteria when intact immunologic or anatomical defenses are compromised (eg, coagulase-negative staphylococci residing on the skin or mucosal surfaces may enter normally sterile anatomical sites or might cause infection if competing bacteria are removed by antibiotic treatment). Primary infections cause clinical disease by invading and multiplying within tissues and causing injury in individuals with intact or impaired immune systems (eg, dysentery caused by *Shigella* or meningitis caused by virulent strains of *Neisseria meningitidis*). Secondary infections are caused by bacterial invasion after a viral infection damages barriers to infection (eg, pneumococcal pneumonia after an influenza infection of the lungs). Acute infections start rapidly, within hours or days of exposure, and have a relatively short duration of days to weeks (eg, strep throat caused by *Streptococcus pyogenes*). Chronic infections continue for a relatively long time, on the order of months or years (eg, leprosy caused by *Mycobacterium leprae*).

Infections can be symptomatic, subclinical, or latent. In a subclinical infection, the microorganism can be isolated or antibody titers can increase, indicating that the immune system has responded to the infection. Subclinical, or inapparent, infections do not have readily detectable clinical symptoms (eg, *Chlamydia* infections in women).

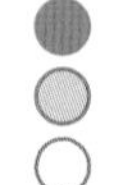

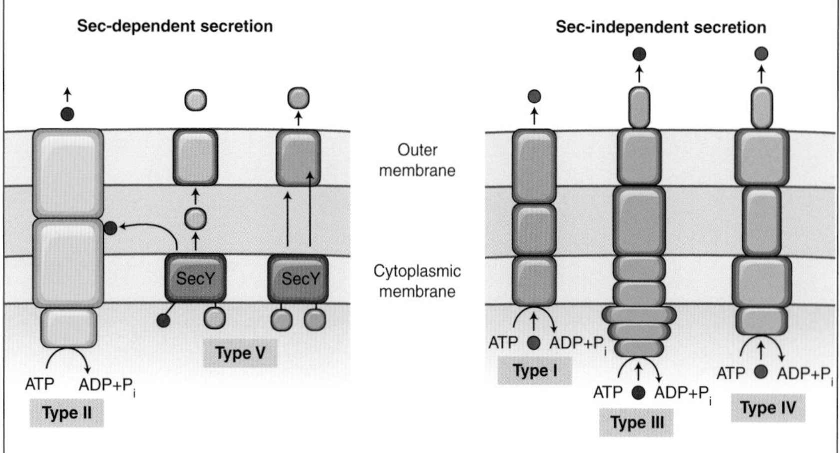

Fig 7-1 Secretion systems in Gram-negative bacteria. (Adapted from Fronzes et al.)

In a latent infection, the microorganism does not cause apparent disease but can be activated later (eg, if the body is under stress or the immune system is compromised). Some infections result in a chronic carrier state in the host, as in the case of *Salmonella* Typhi that survive and multiply in the gall bladder. Chronic carriers can transmit the microorganism to other hosts. Infections can be localized, as in the case of staphylococcal boils, or generalized, when they are spread throughout the body (eg, bacteremia). Pus-forming infections, such as those due to staphylococci or streptococci, are called pyogenic infections. Some infections are mixed or polymicrobial infections. An example is the group of microorganisms that cause periodontal disease.

A microorganism is a pathogen if it is capable of causing a disease. Microbial pathogenicity refers to the structural and biochemical mechanisms by which microorganisms cause disease. Bacteria cause diseases by two major mechanisms: *(1)* Invasion and inflammation. For example, *Mycobacterium tuberculosis* infects and resides in macrophages, the very cells that would normally fight infection. *(2)* Toxin production. For example, *Corynebacterium diphtheriae* releases diphtheria toxin that enters epithelial cells in the throat and inhibits protein synthesis. Exotoxins are polypeptides released by the bacteria. Endotoxin, or lipopolysaccharide (LPS), is an integral part of the outer membrane of Gram-negative bacteria. It induces fever (and is also termed *exogenous pyrogen*) and can cause shock as a result of a drastic reduction in blood pressure.

Protein Secretion

How are exotoxins secreted from bacteria? Both Gram-negative and Gram-positive bacteria utilize the general secretory pathway (GSP) (see Fig 6-9). A signal peptide at the leading end of the protein is guided by "chaperone" proteins (SecB), via proteins with propelling functions (SecA), and through a channel formed by SecY, SecE, and SecG proteins. The signal peptide is removed once the protein goes through the GSP.

In Gram-negative bacteria, there are additional transport systems that enable the export of proteins (Fig 7-1). The type II and type V systems enable proteins that have reached the periplasmic space to be exported outside the bacterium. The type III system not only transports proteins across the two membranes but also injects them into eukaryotic host cells through a syringe-like apparatus. The type IV transport system can export both proteins and DNA into target cells.

Transmission

Most infections are transmitted from external sources and thus are termed exogenous. Other infections are endogenous in origin and are caused by members of the normal flora (eg, uropathogenic *Escherichia coli*). Opportunistic infections are caused by bacteria (or fungi) only when the host is immunocompromised, such as patients with HIV infection or malignancies or those undergoing immunosuppressive therapy.

The most common route of transmission of microorganisms is generally believed to be the respiratory route; (eg, *Bordetella pertussis*, which causes pertussis). Microorganisms like *Clostridium tetani* and *Staphylococcus aureus* are transmitted via breaks in the skin and cause tetanus and abscesses, respectively. Some microorganisms are transmitted via the fecal-oral route (mouth or gastrointestinal tract) and include *Vibrio cholera* and *E coli*. The genital tract is the route of transmission of sexually transmitted diseases, including gonorrhea caused by *Neisseria gonorrhoeae* and syphilis caused by *Treponema pallidum*. Microorganisms can also be transmitted congenitally and include group B streptococci, *Chlamydia trachomatis*, and *Listeria monocytogenes*.

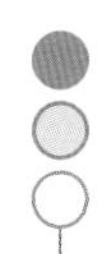

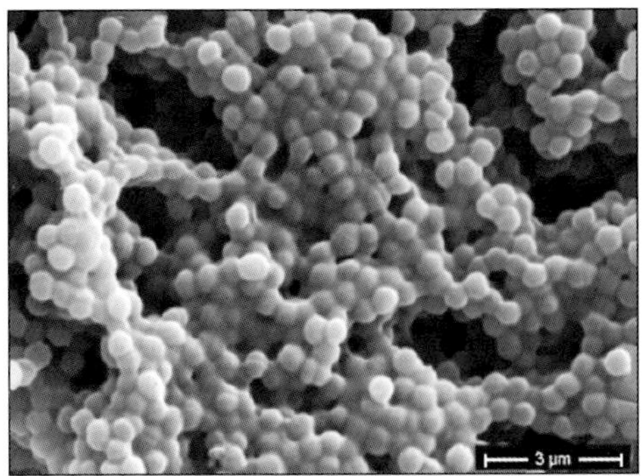

Fig 7-2 Scanning electron micrograph of an *S aureus* biofilm found on the luminal surface of an indwelling catheter. The biofilm is composed of coccoid cells attached to each other and the substrate via polysaccharide polymers. (Photograph by Rodney M. Donlan and Janice Haney Carr, courtesy of the Centers for Disease Control and Prevention.)

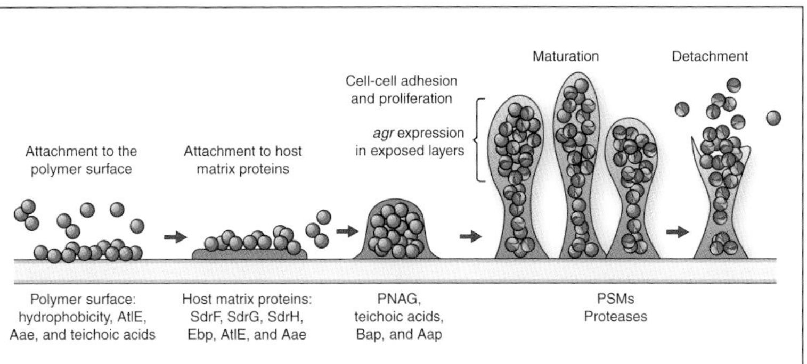

Fig 7-3 Biofilm development by *Staphylococcus epidermidis*. Attachment to an uncoated surface is dependent mainly on the hydrophobicity of the bacterial cell surface. Adhesion to host matrix-covered devices is facilitated by bacterial surface proteins. After adhesion to the surface, exopolysaccharide (eg, poly-*N*-acetylglucosamine [PNAG]), specific proteins like Bap and Aap, and accessory macromolecules such as teichoic acids mediate intercellular aggregation. Biofilm maturation may involve the expression of detergent-like peptides (phenol-soluble modulins [PSMs]) and proteolytic activity induced by "quorum sensing" in exposed layers of the biofilm. PSMs are involved in both biofilm structuring and detachment. The gene-expression profile is significantly different in the biofilm compared with that in the planktonic mode of growth and includes downregulation of basic cell processes. (Adapted from Otto.)

Attachment

Bacteria have specialized structures or produce substances that facilitate their attachment to the surface of host cells or prostheses (eg, dentures, artificial heart valves, catheters). Mutants that lack these mechanisms are usually not pathogenic. *N gonorrhoeae* and *E coli* use adhesin proteins at the tips of their pili to mediate attachment to carbohydrate receptors on the surface of urinary tract epithelium. Thus, adhesins can be termed lectins, which are carbohydrate-binding proteins. The cariogenic bacterium *Streptococcus mutans* uses extracellular polysaccharides such as mutan and glucan to mediate its attachment to the salivary pellicle on tooth surfaces and to other bacteria. Lipoteichoic acid that is part of the cell wall of Gram-positive staphylococci and streptococci mediate the attachment of the bacteria to mucosal cells. The complex of lipoteichoic acid and M protein on Group A streptococci bind to fibronectin on host cell surfaces. *Mycoplasma pneumoniae* binds to sialic acid on lung epithelial cells via its P1 protein.

Bacterial Biofilms

Biofilms are a complex structured community of microbial cells attached strongly to a surface and enclosed in a matrix primarily made of polysaccharides produced by the cells. Microorganisms in biofilms differ from unattached, free, planktonic organisms in terms of the genes that they express. Biofilms may form on living tissues, indwelling catheters, water lines, dentures, and tooth surfaces (dental plaque). The structure of the biofilm and the extracellular matrix protects the biofilm-associated bacteria from host defenses and antibiotics (Figs 7-2 and 7-3).

Invasion

Bacteria can get through mucosal and other tissue barriers by destroying them or by entering the cells that constitute the barrier. Pathogenic bacteria secrete degrading enzymes that enable the spread of the organisms. Collagenase degrades collagen, and hyaluronidase degrades hyaluronic acid, thereby breaking down connective tissue. Coagulase secreted by *S aureus* facilitates the formation of a fibrin clot from fibrinogen to produce a clotlike barrier. Streptococci produce streptolysins S and O, hyaluronidase, deoxyribonucleases, and streptokinases.

Toxin Production

Toxins produced by bacteria can either cause damage to tissues directly (eg, destructive enzymes) or initiate biologic activities that are harmful to the host (eg, LPS). The cytotoxin leukocidin, such as that produced by the periodontopathogen *Aggregatibacter actinomycetemcomitans*, can destroy neutrophils and macrophages. The exotoxin streptolysin produced by *S pyogenes* has a similar function. Preformed toxins produced by *S aureus* and *Bacillus cereus* cause food poisoning, and botulinum toxin produced by *Clostridium botulinum* causes botulism without the need for these bacteria to multiply in the host. Toxin genes can be on plasmids (labile toxins and stable toxins of enterotoxigenic *E coli*) or within the genome of lysogenic phages, such as β-corynephage that carries the *tox* gene encoding diphtheria toxin expressed by pathogenic *C diphtheriae*.

Diphtheria toxin is an example of a dimeric toxin with subunits called A and B. The A subunit is the active component; ie, diphtheria toxin A fragment enzymatically inhibits protein synthesis in target cells and kills them. The B subunit facilitates the entry of the A subunit by binding to a host cell surface receptor; in the case of diphtheria toxin, the receptor is a precursor of the heparin-binding epidermal growth factor receptor. Other A-B type toxins include *Pseudomonas* exotoxin A (receptor: α2-macroglobulin receptor), Shiga toxin (receptor: globotriosyl ceramide, Gb3), tetanus toxin (receptor: polysialogangliosides + 15 kDa glycoprotein), and cholera toxin (receptor: ganglioside, GM1). Shiga toxin (formerly called *Shiga-like toxin* or *verotoxin*) is responsible for the hemolytic uremic syndrome caused by *E coli* O157:H7. It enters endothelial cells in the kidneys a nd in small blood vessels lining the intestines and causes cytotoxicity.

Such exotoxins are considered to be among the most toxic substances known. They are strong immunogens and induce the synthesis of protective antibodies, also known as *antitoxins*. Treatment with formaldehyde, acid, or heat can neutralize exotoxins, and these toxoids are used in vaccines, as they retain their antigenicity. The diphtheria and tetanus vaccines are prepared in this way.

Endotoxin, or LPS, is the main component of the external leaflet of the outer membrane of Gram-negative bacteria. The lipid A segment of LPS is responsible for endotoxin activity, such as the acute-phase response and inflammation. LPS binds to the receptors CD14 and Toll-like receptor 4 (TLR4) on macrophages and other cells. Toll-like receptors recognize pathogen-associated molecular patterns, including LPS, on microorganisms. Stimulation of macrophages by LPS leads to the production of tumor necrosis factor-alpha (TNF-α), interleukin-1 (IL-1), and IL-6, which are acute-phase cytokines. LPS at low concentrations stimulates the immune system and causes fever and vasodilation as part of the normal inflammatory response. In patients with Gram-negative sepsis, LPS levels in blood can be very high, and this can cause the activation of the complement system, with accompanying vasodilation and leakage of capillaries. Together with the action of IL-1 and TNF-α, hypotension and shock can ensue. Activation of the blood-clotting system can result in disseminated intravascular coagulation. *N meningitidis* LPS can cause high fever, capillary leakage (resulting in skin lesions called *petechiae*), and shock because of increased vascular permeability and the inability to maintain blood pressure.

Interference with the Host Immune System

Bacteria express various virulence factors that interfere with the ability of the host immune system to fight infection. *Streptococcus pneumoniae*, *N meningitidis*, *Haemophilus influenzae*, *Klebsiella pneumoniae*, and *S* Typhi have polysaccharide capsules that can inhibit phagocytosis by macrophages and neutrophils. The *S pyogenes* capsule consists of hyaluronic acid, which mimics connective tissue. Biofilms with a matrix of capsular material can evade antibody or complement binding to the bacteria in the biofilm. Proteins that are part of the cell wall of Gram-positive cocci, including the M protein of *S pneumoniae* and *S pyogenes* and protein A of *S aureus* can also inhibit phagocytosis. Protein A can bind to the Fc region of antibodies and thus mask the bacteria as a particle with the Fab regions exposed.

Immunoglobulin A (IgA) is normally found on mucosal surfaces as a protective mechanism against microbial infection. IgA proteases of *N gonorrhoeae*, *H influenzae*, and *S pneumoniae* can degrade IgA and render it ineffective. This, in turn, facilitates the attachment of the bacteria to the mucosal surfaces. *N gonorrhoeae* can undergo antigenic variation, thereby evading the immune system. *Mycobacteria* can grow inside phagosomes of macrophages, the very cells that would normally fight invading microorganisms. They also inhibit the fusion of phagosomes with lysosomes. Some bacteria, including *Salmonella* Typhimurium (*Salmonella enterica* serovar Typhimurium), *Salmonella* Enteritidis, and *M leprae* can resist lysosomal enzymes.

L monocytogenes and *Francisella tularensis* can enter the host cell cytoplasm and replicate there, avoiding exposure to the immune system. The O-antigen of LPS in Gram-negative bacteria can prevent complement access to the bacterial membrane. The coagulase of *S aureus* can form a clotlike barrier, protecting the site of infection from attack by the immune system. The *S pyogenes* streptolysin can lyse phagocytotic cells.

Inflammation

Bacteria can cause pyogenic or granulomatous inflammation. Neutrophils are found predominantly in pyogenic (or pus-producing) inflammation. *S aureus*, *S pyogenes*, and *S pneumoniae* are the most common pyogenic bacteria. For example, pustular impetigo is caused primarily by *S aureus* and to some extent by *S pyogenes*. Macrophages and T cells are the predominant cells in granulomatous (granuloma-forming) inflammation. *M tuberculosis* is an important inducer of granulomatous inflammation.

Koch's Postulates

Robert Koch (1843–1910), the German microbiologist, set forth a set of four rules for establishing the connection between a microbe and a disease:

1. The microbe must be associated with the symptoms of the disease and must be present at the site of infection. Koch showed the presence of *Bacillus anthracis* in anthrax lesions and *M tuberculosis* in people suffering from "consumption."
2. The microbe must be isolated from the lesions of disease and grown as a pure culture. Koch had to develop methods to culture slow-growing microorganisms like *M tuberculosis* as well as solid agar to be able to isolate individual colonies. Some microorganisms cannot be grown alone in culture medium, including *Chlamydophila pneumoniae* and *T pallidum*. These microorganisms can be grown in cultured eukaryotic cells. For example, *T pallidum* can be grown in BHK-21 (baby hamster kidney) cells.
3. A pure culture of the microbe, when inoculated into a susceptible host, must reproduce the disease in the experimental host. Koch used the Guinea pig model of tuberculosis (even though these animals do not succumb to tuberculosis in nature) to show that pure cultures of *M tuberculosis*, when inoculated experimentally, could cause disease pathology and death.
4. The microbe must be re-isolated in pure culture form from the experimentally infected host.

The proposed fifth postulate is that the elimination of the disease-causing microbe from the infected host, or prevention of exposure of the host to the microbe, should eliminate or prevent the disease.

There are modern alternatives to satisfying Koch's postulates. Microbes in diseased tissue can be identified by the polymerase chain reaction or immunohistochemistry. Vaccination can be used to show that the specific disease can be prevented. The disease can be treated with an antibiotic to which the microorganism is susceptible. Disinfection and hygiene measures can be employed to prevent exposure to the microbe.

Bibliography

Baron S (ed). Medical Microbiology, ed 4. Galveston: University of Texas Medical Branch at Galveston, 1996.

Fronzes R, Christie PJ, Waksman G. The structural biology of type IV secretion systems. Nat Rev Microbiol 2009;7:703–714.

Greenwood D, Slack R, Peutherer J, Barer M. Medical Microbiology, ed 17. Edinburgh: Churchill Livingstone/Elsevier, 2007.

Ingraham JL, Ingraham CA. Introduction to Microbiology: A Case History Approach. Pacific Grove, CA: Brooks/Cole (Thomson), 2004.

Murray PR, Rosenthal KS, Pfaller MA. Medical Microbiology, ed 6. Philadelphia: Mosby/Elsevier, 2009.

Otto M. *Staphylococcus epidermidis*—The 'accidental' pathogen. Nat Rev Microbiol 2009;7:555–567.

Ryan KJ, Ray CG. Sherris Medical Microbiology, ed 5. New York: McGraw-Hill, 2010.

Willett NP, White RR, Rosen S. Essential Dental Microbiology. Norwalk, CT: Appleton & Lange, 1991.

Wilson BA, Salyers AA, Whitt DD, Winkler ME. Bacterial Pathogenesis: A Molecular Approach, ed 3. Washington, DC: ASM, 2011.

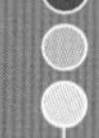

Take-Home Messages

- *Pathogenesis* refers to both the mechanism by which the microorganism infects the host and the mechanism of disease development.
- Bacteria can cause opportunistic, primary, secondary, acute, chronic, subclinical, latent, localized, generalized, pyogenic, and polymicrobial infections.
- Bacteria cause diseases by two major mechanisms: *(1)* invasion and inflammation and *(2)* toxin production.
- Pathogenic bacteria produce a large variety of toxins (eg, leukocidin, streptolysin, botulinum toxin, diphtheria toxin, tetanus toxin, and cholera toxin).
- Exotoxins are secreted from bacteria via the general secretory pathway or through other types of secretion systems. The type III secretion system can inject the toxins directly into eukaryotic host cells.
- Microorganisms can be transmitted via the respiratory route, the fecal-oral route, the skin, and the genital tract.
- Bacteria can attach to host cells or prosthetic surfaces by means of specialized proteins called *adhesins*, polysaccharides, or lipoteichoic acid.
- Microbial cells can form biofilms, which are complex structured communities embedded in a polysaccharide matrix.
- Pathogenic bacteria secrete degrading enzymes that enable the spread of the organisms.

8 Antibacterial Chemotherapy

The most important concept underlying antimicrobial chemotherapy is selective toxicity, which was introduced by Paul Ehrlich.

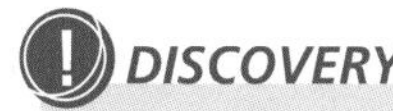

DISCOVERY

In 1908, the Nobel Prize in Physiology or Medicine was awarded jointly to Ilya Ilyich Mechnikov and Paul Ehrlich for their work on immunity. Following his appointment as the director of the Royal Institute of Experimental Therapy in Frankfurt in 1899, Ehrlich focused on chemotherapy, basing his work on the idea that "the chemical constitution of drugs must be studied in relation to their mode of action and their affinity for the cells of the organisms against which they were directed." His aim was "to find chemical substances which have special affinities for pathogenic organisms, to which they would go, as antitoxins go to the toxins to which they are specifically related." Ehrlich and his assistants tested hundreds of chemicals, selected from a larger set that he had collected, against the spirochete that causes syphilis. Among the arsenic-containing drugs already tested for other purposes was one—the 606th of the series tested—that had been abandoned earlier as being ineffective. Ehrlich and visiting scientist Hata tested this compound in an animal model of syphilis and found that it was very effective. The name "Salvarsan" was given to this compound. Further experiments showed that compound 914, "Neosalvarsan," was easier to manufacture and to administer. Ehrlich had to fight much opposition before Salvarsan or Neosalvarsan was accepted for the treatment of syphilis, but eventually he was considered as one of the founders of chemotherapy.

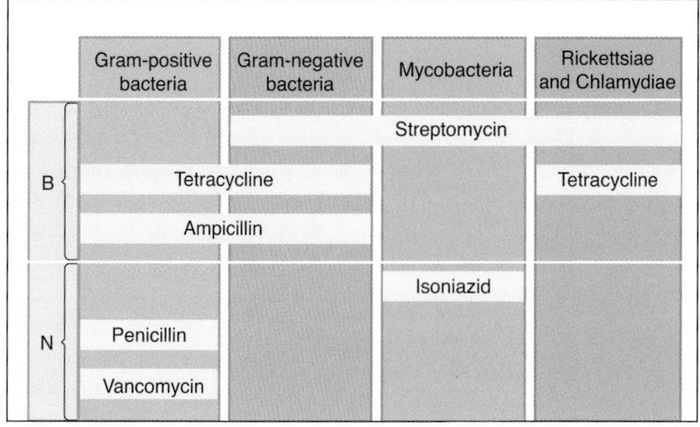

Fig 8-1 The activity of broad-spectrum (B) and narrow-spectrum (N) antibiotics against different types of bacteria. (Adapted from Ingraham and Ingraham.)

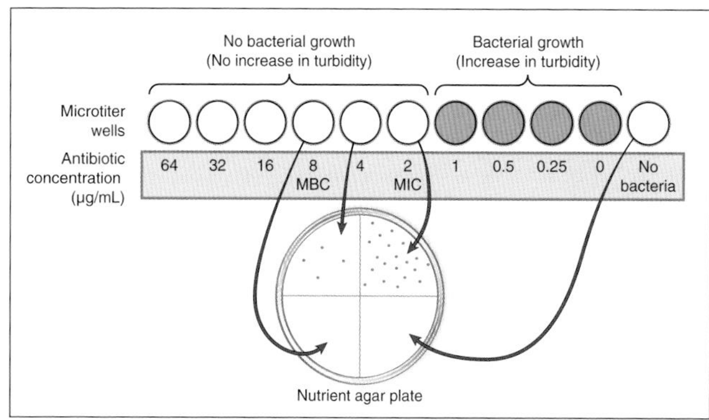

Fig 8-2 Determination of the minimum inhibitory concentration (MIC) and the minimum bactericidal concentration (MBC). The antibiotic to be tested is diluted serially into the wells of a microtiter (96-well) plate (shown) or into tubes. The same concentration of bacterium is added to all the tubes except the control. Following incubation under appropriate conditions to show sufficient turbidity in the "no drug" tube, the growth inhibition is assessed. No growth has occurred at 2 µg/mL or higher drug concentrations. Thus, 2 µg/mL is the MIC. Samples from this well and the wells with higher drug concentrations are plated on a nutrient agar plate. Bacteria from the MIC tube form colonies because they were not killed. When these bacteria are placed in a medium without the antibiotic, they will form colonies. The bacteria treated with 8 µg/mL of the antibiotic do not form any colonies because they were killed by the antibiotic. Therefore, 8 µg/mL can be designated as the MBC. Some microbiologists, however, prefer to designate the MBC as the concentration of antibiotic that causes a 99.9% reduction in the colony-forming units in the initial inoculum (ie, the untreated bacteria). (Adapted from Ingraham and Ingraham.)

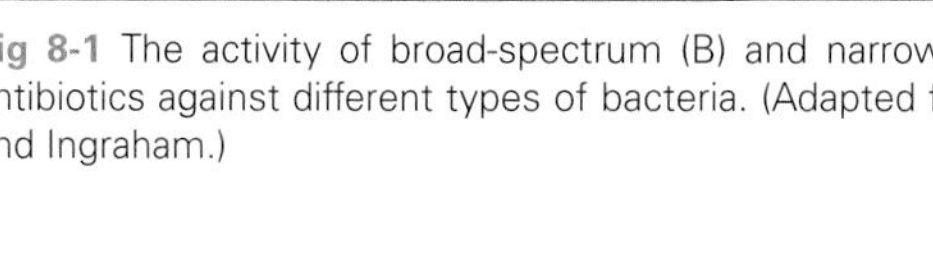

DISCOVERY

The aminoglycoside antibiotic streptomycin was discovered by Albert Schatz, a graduate student in the laboratory of Selman Waksman at Rutgers University, as part of an effort to find a drug against *Mycobacterium tuberculosis*. The antibiotic is produced by certain strains of *Streptomyces griseus*. Although Schatz and Waksman published the discovery together in 1943 and were awarded a patent, only Waksman was awarded the Nobel Prize in 1952.

The antibacterial spectrum of an antibiotic is the range of activity of a drug against bacteria. Broad-spectrum antibiotics can inhibit a large variety of bacteria. For example, tetracyclines are active against many Gram-negative bacilli, chlamydiae, mycoplasmas, and rickettsiae (Fig 8-1). These antibiotics should be reserved for when the etiologic agent of an infection cannot be determined at the time therapy must be initiated or for immunocompromised patients who may be infected with a variety of bacteria. Narrow-spectrum antibiotics are active against one or a few types of bacteria. For example, vancomycin is used against some Gram-positive cocci, such as staphylococci and enterococci (see Fig 8-1).

The antimicrobial activity of a drug against microorganisms may be expressed as the lowest concentration of the drug that inhibits growth of the microorganism. This is designated as the minimum inhibitory concentration (MIC) (Fig 8-2). The bactericidal activity is the ability of a drug to kill a bacterium and is expressed as the minimum bactericidal concentration (MBC). The MBC of a bactericidal antibiotic is close to the MIC, whereas for bacteriostatic antibiotics, the MBC is usually much higher than the MIC, and it may not be safe to administer these high doses.

Bactericidal antibiotics are useful in infections that are life-threatening, in patients whose polymorphonuclear leukocyte (PMN) count is below 500/µL, and in case of endocarditis where phagocytosis is limited by the fibrinous network of bacteria. Penicillin is bactericidal, but it kills cells only when they are growing. Bacteriostatic antibiotics only inhibit bacterial growth, and the immune response is necessary to kill the bacteria (Fig 8-3).

Antibiotic combinations are used to broaden the antibacterial spectrum in possible multiple infections, to prevent the appearance of resistant strains, and to obtain a synergistic effect (Fig 8-4). Antibiotic synergism is obtained if a combination of antibiotics has enhanced bactericidal activity compared with each alone. In antibiotic antagonism, one antibiotic interferes with the bactericidal activity of another. When administering antibiotics, it is important to consider the potential side effects of the treatment. The ratio of the toxic dose of a drug to the effective dose is termed the therapeutic index.

The selectivity of antibiotics for bacteria may result from a number of factors. The aminoglycoside antibiotics are selective for prokaryotic 70S ribosomes and not the 80S ribosomes of eukaryotes. Penicillins inhibit the synthesis of the murein (peptidoglycan) layer of the bacterial cell wall; there is no counterpart of this structure in host cells. While bacteria can concentrate tetracycline, host cells do not. The 50% effective concentration of trimethoprim to inhibit dihydrofolate reductase activity in bacteria is 50,000-fold lower than that in mammalian cells. The toxicity and immunogenicity of antibiotics should also be considered in treatment. For example, penicillin can cause allergies in about 8% of the population. Aminoglycosides can cause nephrotoxicity and ototoxicity. Broad-spectrum antibiotics can upset the balance of bacteria in the intestines, potentially leading to colitis.

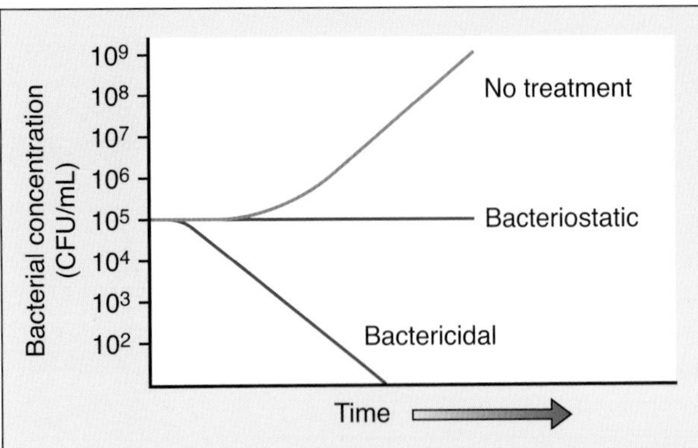

Fig 8-3 Bactericidal versus bacteriostatic activity of antimicrobial agents. A culture is started at 10^5 colony-forming units (CFUs) per mL and incubated at 37°C for various times in the presence of the antibiotics. In the absence of an antimicrobial agent, the CFUs increase. In the presence of a bacteriostatic agent, no growth occurs, but the cells are not killed. With a bactericidal antibiotic, the CFUs decrease by 99.9% during a standardized test period.

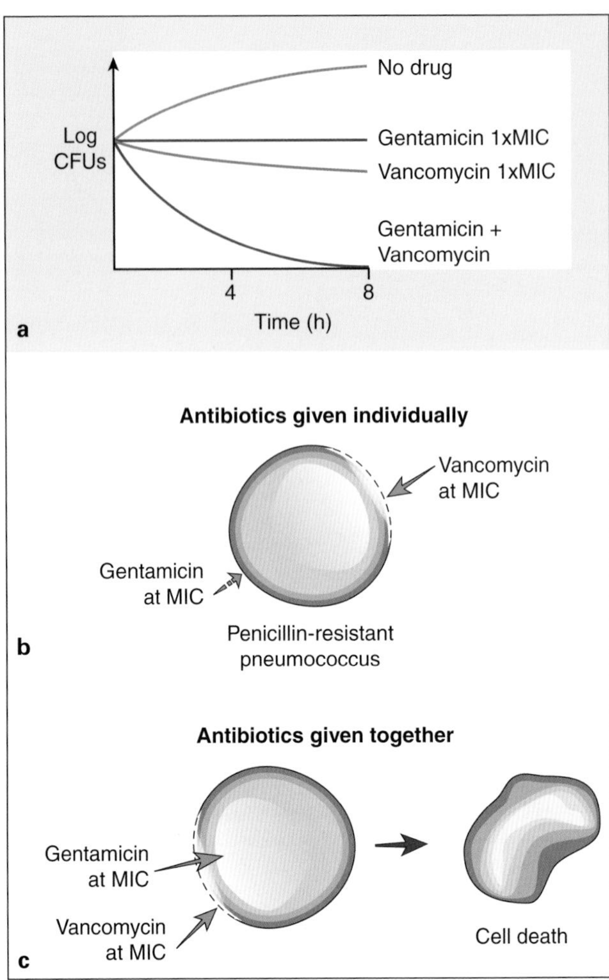

Fig 8-4 *(a to c)* An example of synergy between two antibiotics. *(b)* Vancomycin or gentamicin is given. The growth of the cells is inhibited. *(c)* Vancomycin and gentamicin are given at the same time. Vancomycin opens holes in the cell wall through which aminoglycosides (gentamicin) can enter and reach the ribosomes to halt protein synthesis, resulting in a bactericidal effect. (Adapted from Wecker et al.)

Mechanisms of Antibiotic Action

Inhibition of cell wall synthesis

Enzymes that cross-link precursors of the cell wall during biosynthesis also bind penicillin and are called *penicillin-binding proteins (PBP)*. Penicillin enters through porins and binds PBPs, inhibiting cell wall synthesis and causing the release of autolytic enzymes (lysins or murein hydrolases).

Alteration of cell membranes

Polymyxins disrupt the cytoplasmic membrane of susceptible bacteria with a detergent-like activity. The antibiotics amphotericin B and nystatin have a similar activity on fungal membranes.

Inhibition of protein synthesis

Tetracycline and aminoglycosides inhibit protein synthesis by binding to ribosome subunits after entering through porins. Antibiotic binding results in *(1)* inhibition of the initiation of protein synthesis, *(2)* inhibition of protein elongation, or *(3)* misreading of tRNA and the production of deformed proteins.

Inhibition of nucleic acid synthesis

Rifampin inhibits nucleic acid synthesis by binding to RNA polymerase. Quinolones inhibit DNA gyrase and thus inhibit the relief in the strain of the DNA as the DNA is being unwound by helicase.

Antimetabolic activity

An antimetabolite prevents a cell from performing a metabolic reaction. It may function in two ways: *(1)* by competitive inhibition of enzymes or *(2)* by being incorporated into nucleic acids. Para-aminobenzoic acid (PABA) is required for folic acid synthesis, which is necessary for nucleic acid synthesis. Sulfanilamide, a prescription drug, and PABA are chemically similar. When sulfanilamide is bound to the enzyme that reacts with PABA, the bacterium cannot synthesize folic acid.

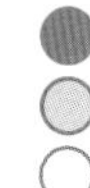

Penicillin G | Penicillin V | Ampicillin | Methicillin

Fig 8-5 Penicillin G and its derivatives. Penicillin V and ampicillin are acid-stable analogs of penicillin G. Methicillin is a β-lactamase–resistant derivative. (From the NIH Open Chemistry Database [pubchem.ncbi.nlm.nih.gov].)

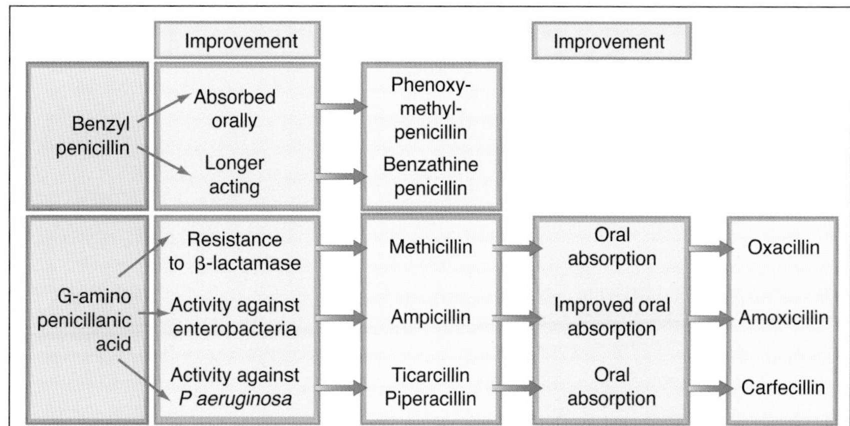

Fig 8-6 Development of penicillins. In this scheme, the term "improvement" indicates a qualitative improvement in the activity or stability of penicillin. (Adapted from Greenwood et al.)

Antibiotics That Inhibit Cell Wall Synthesis

Penicillins

The characteristic structure of penicillin is a β-lactam (cyclic amide) ring (see Fig 8-5). It was originally identified in cultures of the mold *Penicillium chrysogenum* by Alexander Fleming in 1928. Penicillins inhibit the bacterial enzyme transpeptidase, which catalyzes the final cross-linking step in the synthesis of peptidoglycan. They also bind to PBPs, of which there are 6 kinds in *Staphylococcus aureus* and 13 kinds in *Escherichia coli*, and have different activities. These include transglycosylation of the glycan strand, transpeptidation, hydrolysis of the last D-alanine of the peptide (DD-carboxypeptidation), and hydrolysis of the peptide bond connecting two glycan chains (endopeptidation). The inhibitory action of penicillin activates autolytic enzymes, called murein (peptidoglycan) hydrolases. In this respect, penicillins and other β-lactam antibiotics are considered to be bactericidal antibiotics.

Derivatives of penicillin can be produced that are acid stable and thus have increased gastrointestinal absorption (eg, penicillin V, ampicillin); are resistant to penicillinase (β-lactamase; eg, methicillin, nafcillin, oxacillin, cloxacillin); or have a broader spectrum of activity, including against Gram-negative organisms (eg, the aminopenicillins ampicillin and amoxicillin, the carboxypenicillins carbenicillin and ticarcillin, and piperacillin) (Fig 8-5). The development of new penicillins and the improvements in the activity of these antibiotics are described in Fig 8-6.

Penicillin G is inactivated by gastric acid but may be given intravenously against streptococci or gonococcus. Some staphylococci produce penicillinase; penicillinase-resistant penicillins such as nafcillin and cloxacillin can be used against infection by such bacteria. Enhanced spectrum penicillins such as carbenicillin and ticarcillin can be used parenterally against Gram-negative bacteria (eg, *Enterobacter* and *Pseudomonas*). Penicillin G has low toxicity, but up to 8% of the general population is allergic to it. Other adverse effects of penicillin are leukopenia, hepatitis, interstitial nephritis, diarrhea, and platelet dysfunction.

Penicillins can be used in combination with a β-lactamase inhibitor, such as clavulanate. Examples of such combinations are amoxicillin-clavulanate (called Augmentin), ticarcillin-clavulanate, and piperacillin-tazobactam.

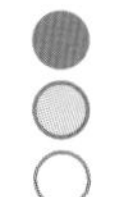

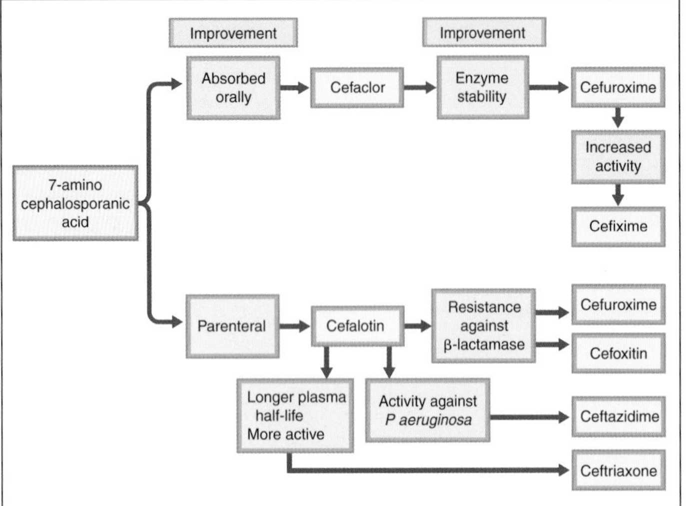

Fig 8-7 Development of cephalosporins. In this scheme, the term "improvement" indicates a qualitative improvement in the activity or stability of cephalosporin. (Adapted from Greenwood et al.)

Cephalosporins

Cephalosporins are β-lactam antibiotics originally isolated from the mold *Cephalosporium*. Their mechanism of action is similar to that of penicillin, but they have a wider spectrum, are resistant to β-lactamases, and have improved pharmacokinetic properties. Cephalosporins have low toxicity but may induce allergic reactions in people allergic to penicillin.

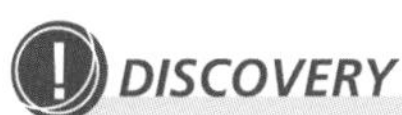

The first cephalosporin was discovered in 1945 by Giuseppe Brotzu, who was the rector of the University of Cagliari in Sardinia, Italy. He was curious why there were no cases of typhoid (which was endemic in Sardinia and acquired while bathing in the sea and eating shellfish obtained from the area) in the vicinity of a sewage outflow pipe near the university. He isolated a filamentous fungus identified as *Cephalosporium acremonium*, which is now renamed *Acremonium chrysogenum*. Cultures of the organism inhibited Gram-positive and Gram-negative pathogens. Brotzu sent a culture of the fungus to the Dunn School of Pathology at Oxford. There, Edward Abraham and Guy Newton discovered the presence of cephalosporin C in culture filtrates while they were working to determine the molecular weight of penicillin N, which was abundant in the filtrates and had been identified earlier. It was resistant to penicillinase and to acid, and most importantly, it was active against *S aureus*, which was widespread in hospitals and difficult to treat.

The first-generation cephalosporins (eg, cephalothin and cephazolin) have activities similar to that of ampicillin. They are narrow-spectrum antibiotics, with activities restricted to *E coli*, *Klebsiella* species, and some Gram-positive cocci.

The second-generation cephalosporins have an expanded spectrum of activity against *Haemophilus influenzae*, a pediatric pathogen (cefaclor and cefuroxime); *Bacteroides fragilis*, an anaerobic pathogen (cefoxitin and cefotetan), and *Enterobacter* and *Citrobacter*. They also have improved stability against enterobacterial β-lactamases.

The third-generation cephalosporins have a broader spectrum of activity that includes almost all Enterobacteriaceae and *Pseudomonas aeruginosa* (cefsulodin, cefoperazone). Extended spectrum fourth-generation antibiotics have increased stability to β-lactamases over that of third-generation cephalosporins. Cefepime and cefpirome are highly effective against Enterobacteriaceae and *P aeruginosa* and are used against nosocomial infections. The development of new cephalosporins and the improvements in the activity of these antibiotics are described in Fig 8-7.

Other β-lactams

The carbapenem antibiotics (imipenem, meropenem) are β-lactam antibiotics that have a broad spectrum. Monobactams have a narrow spectrum, being effective against Gram-negative, aerobic bacteria, and have the advantage that they will not affect the normal bacterial microflora of the patient.

Glycopeptides

Vancomycin is a complex glycopeptide that blocks transpeptidation by interacting with the D-alanine-D-alanine terminal segment of the pentapeptide side chains of peptidoglycan. It was initially isolated from *Streptomyces orientalis*. It is effective in the treatment of gastrointestinal diseases caused by *S aureus* or *Clostridium difficile* because it is not absorbed effectively in the gut. It is used intravenously against methicillin-resistant staphylococci or in patients with penicillin allergy. Teicoplanin is an antibiotic with a similar mechanism of action as vancomycin and was isolated from the actinobacterium *Actinoplanes teichomyceticus*. These antibiotics are ineffective against Gram-negative bacteria because they cannot pass through the outer membranes.

A gene encoding vancomycin resistance located in a transposon that is part of a conjugative plasmid has been transferred from *Enterococcus faecalis* to *S aureus*. The transposon has also been integrated into the multidrug-resistance plasmid of *S aureus*. The potential transfer of this plasmid to other bacteria via conjugation may have serious medical consequences.

Other inhibitors of cell wall synthesis

Bacitracin is a polypeptide antibiotic obtained from *Bacillus licheniformis* and used topically against skin infections caused by *Staphylococcus* and Group A *Streptococcus*. It inhibits the recycling of the lipid carrier that transports peptidoglycan precursors through the cell membrane. It may also damage the cytoplasmic membrane. Isoniazid and ethionamide are inhibitors of mycolic acid synthesis in mycobacteria. Ethambutol inhibits the synthesis of arabinogalactan in mycobacteria. Cycloserine inhibits two enzymes involved in cell wall synthesis.

Antibiotics That Alter Cell Membranes

Polymyxins are cyclic polypeptides that act as cationic detergents and lyse bacterial cell membranes. They are obtained from *Bacillus polymyxa*. Some polymyxins are nephrotoxic, and they are used externally to treat local infections of the ear, eye, and skin. However, some systemic infections by drug-resistant, Gram-negative bacteria can be treated with colistin (polymyxin E).

Daptomycin is a cyclic lipopeptide produced by *Streptomyces roseosporus*; it binds to the bacterial cytoplasmic membrane and disrupts transmembrane ionic gradients. It is effective against drug-resistant streptococci, staphylococci, and enterococci.

Antibiotics That Inhibit Protein Synthesis

Aminoglycosides consist of a six-member aminocyclitol ring connected to amino sugars. They are effective against bacteria that can transport them into the cell by a process involving oxidative phosphorylation. Therefore, they are not active against anaerobic or facultatively anaerobic bacteria that use fermentation for their metabolism. They bind to ribosomes, destabilize them, and block initiation complexes. Streptomycin, which was the first aminoglycoside identified, binds to the 30S ribosomal subunit. It has been used for the treatment of tuberculosis and gentamicin-resistant streptococci and enterococci. The newer aminoglycosides bind to multiple sites on 30S and 50S subunits and are less susceptible to bacterial drug resistance resulting from mutations in the ribosomal binding sites of the antibiotics. Gentamicin and tobramycin are used to treat serious infections of Gram-negative bacilli, including *Pseudomonas*, *Acinetobacter*, and Enterobacteriaceae, and some Gram-positive organisms such as staphylococci. Amikacin and streptomycin are combined with other antibiotics in the treatment of tuberculosis and other mycobacterial diseases. Amikacin is not modified easily by bacteria and thus is used to treat bacteria resistant to other aminoglycosides. Neomycin is used topically in ointments such as Neosporin (Johnson & Johnson); it is toxic when given systemically.

Aminoglycosides are poorly absorbed by the gut; therefore, they are administered intravenously or intramuscularly. The therapeutic levels of aminoglycosides are close to toxic levels; therefore, serum levels must be controlled to avoid nephrotoxicity and ototoxicity.

Tetracyclines are broad-spectrum bacteriostatic antibiotics obtained from *Streptomyces*, and they inhibit protein synthesis by blocking the binding of tRNA to the 30S ribosome subunit. They are used in the treatment of rickettsial disease, brucellosis, *Mycoplasma pneumoniae*, chlamydial urethritis, gonorrhea, and acne.

They are absorbed rapidly through the gastrointestinal tract. Divalent cations in antacids and dairy products bind tetracyclines and prevent absorption. The antibiotic localizes in bones and teeth and causes discoloration and enamel damage. Tetracyclines do not accumulate in the cerebrospinal fluid and thus are ineffective against meningitis. Tigecycline is a recently developed derivative with a broad-spectrum activity, and it is recommended for use in polymicrobial intra-abdominal infections and deep tissue infections.

Chloramphenicol prevents the attachment of amino acids to the peptide chain on the 50S subunit of ribosomes by inhibiting peptidyl transferase. It is used in the treatment of typhoid fever, penicillin-resistant strains of *H influenzae*, meningococcal infections in penicillin-allergic patients, and severe rickettsial infections. It also interferes with protein synthesis in bone marrow cells and can cause aplastic anemia (defective regeneration of blood cells) and inflammation of nerves.

Macrolide antibiotics include erythromycin, azithromycin, and clarithromycin and comprise a macrocyclic lactone ring bound to two saccharide moieties. Erythromycin was initially isolated from cultures of *Streptomyces erythreus*. The macrolides act by binding to the 50S ribosomal subunit and are used to treat pulmonary infections caused by *Legionella*, *Mycoplasma*, *Chlamydophila*, and Gram-positive organisms in patients with penicillin allergy. They are also effective against *Mycobacterium avium-intracellulare*. Telithromycin is a derivative of erythromycin (in a set of antibiotics called ketolides) that is more stable under acidic conditions. It is effective against *Streptococcus pneumoniae*, *H influenzae*, *Legionella pneumophila*, *M pneumoniae*, and *Chlamydophila pneumoniae*.

Clindamycin is active against anaerobic Gram-positive bacteria (*Clostridium perfringens*) and anaerobic Gram-negative bacteria (*B fragilis*). It is a derivative of lincomycin, produced by *Streptomyces lincolnensis*. It binds the 50S ribosomal subunit and inhibits peptidyl transferase by causing the release of peptidyl-tRNA from the ribosome. It is administered orally or intravenously, but oral administration can cause gastrointestinal disturbances such as diarrhea and pseudomembranous colitis. The latter is caused by suppression of the normal flora of the bowel and overgrowth of a drug-resistant strain of *C difficile*.

Linezolid (Zyvox) is a relatively novel antibiotic that inhibits protein synthesis and is administered orally. It is used in the treatment of vancomycin-resistant Enterococcus faecium, which causes skin and blood infections as well as pneumonia.

Synercid (a combination of quinupristin and dalfopristin) is another protein synthesis inhibitor that is effective against streptococci, staphylococci, and vancomycin-resistant *E faecium*. Dalfopristin binds to the 50S ribosomal subunit, inhibits peptide chain elongation, and facilitates the binding of quinupristin to the ribosome. Quinupristin causes the early release of polypeptide chains from the ribosome.

Antibiotics That Inhibit Nucleic Acid Synthesis

Rifampin (also called *rifampicin*) is a derivative of rifamycin B that is produced by *Streptomyces mediterranei* and is used against *M tuberculosis* and aerobic Gram-positive cocci. It inhibits bacterial DNA-dependent RNA polymerase, and because resistance can develop as a result of a mutation in the polymerase β subunit, it is usually combined with other antibiotics. Rifampin is also used in the treatment of methicillin-resistant *S aureus* and *Borrelia burgdorferi* infections. Rifampin can cause hepatotoxicity and upregulate cytochrome P450 enzymes that then increase the metabolism of other drugs in the liver, with a decrease in their effective concentration in the blood. A derivative of rifampin, rifabutin is effective against *M avium*.

Quinolones have two fused six-member rings that may also include fluorine, rendering the group of antibiotics known as fluoroquinolones. They inhibit DNA gyrase (the main target in Gram-negative bacteria and the enzyme that nicks, negatively supercoils, and seals DNA during replication) and topoisomerase type IV (the main target in Gram-positive bacteria) required for DNA replication. The lower frequency of bacterial resistance and the enhanced activity of the newer fluoroquinolones is the result of binding to multiple sites on the topoisomerase, reducing the likelihood of a single mutation causing resistance. They are used against a variety of microorganisms, including enterobacteria, *Haemophilus* species, *Neisseria* species, *Legionella*, and *Bordetella*. The quinolones include ciprofloxacin, levofloxacin, ofloxacin, and the extended-spectrum quinolones moxifloxacin, gatifloxacin, and clinafloxacin. Ciprofloxacin is effective against *P aeruginosa* and ofloxacin against *Chlamydia*. It is recommended that moxifloxacin be used for acute sinusitis, bronchitis, and pneumonia only if other antibiotics have failed or cannot be used.

Metronidazole is a nitroimidazole compound that acts as a prodrug in that it is converted to its active form by the reduction of the nitro group by metabolic pathways linked to the ferredoxin- or flavodoxin-like electron transport components. These pathways are characteristic of anaerobic bacteria or protozoa and are not found in aerobic or microaerophilic bacteria. The reduced drug causes cytotoxicity by damaging bacterial DNA but also acts at other sites in the cell. It is useful in the treatment of anaerobic infections, including periodontal and *B fragilis* infections. To cover anaerobic and facultative bacteria that may also be involved in polymicrobial infections, it is generally used in conjunction with another antibiotic (eg, a β-lactam).

Antibiotics with Antimetabolic Activity

Sulfonamides block a step in folic acid synthesis by competing with p-aminobenzoic acid, because they are structural analogs, and are used primarily for the treatment of urinary tract infections with the Enterobacteriaceae family, particularly *E coli*. They are well absorbed by the oral route and excreted at high concentrations in the urine, so they are well suited for such infections. They are also effective against *Nocardia* and *Chlamydia*. Trimethoprim inhibits dihydrofolate reductase and hence the production of tetrahydrofolate. This in turn inhibits the production of thymidine and some purines as well as methionine and glycine. The combination trimethoprim-sulfamethoxazole inhibits two consecutive steps in the synthesis of folate. It is effective in treating urinary tract and lower respiratory tract infections, otitis media, sinusitis, prostatitis, infectious diarrhea, as well as *Pneumocystis carinii* (*P jirovecii*) infections.

Miscellaneous Antibiotics

Clofazimine is effective against *M tuberculosis*, *Mycobacterium leprae*, and other atypical mycobacteria. It binds to mycobacterial DNA. Its red color can cause skin discoloration. The low pH found in macrophage phagolysosomes enables pyrazinamide to act against phagocytosed *M tuberculosis*. However, the exact mechanism of action of this antibiotic is not known.

Bacterial Resistance to Antibiotics

Microorganisms are considered to be sensitive or susceptible to an antibiotic if their MICs are achievable in the blood, cerebrospinal fluid, or urine at the recommended doses. They are resistant to an antibiotic if their MICs are not achieved or exceeded by the recommended doses.

As new antibiotics are introduced, drug-resistant microorganisms emerge. It appears that the development of

Table 8-1 **The time frame of the regulatory approval of new classes of antibiotics and the development of drug-resistant bacteria**

Antibiotic	Year introduced	Year drug resistance observed	First resistant microorganism
Penicillin	1943	1940*	*Staphylococcus*
Tetracycline	1950	1960	*Shigella*
Erythromycin	1953	1968	*Staphylococcus*
Methicillin	1960	1962	*Staphylococcus*
Gentamicin	1967	1980	*Enterococcus*
Vancomycin	1972	1988†	*Enterococcus*
Ceftazidime	1985	1987	Enterobacteriaceae
Imipenem	1985	1996	Enterobacteriaceae
Levofloxacin	1996	1996	*Streptococcus pneumoniae*
Linezolid	2000	2001	*Staphylococcus*
Daptomycin	2003	2009	*Staphylococcus*
Ceftaroline	2010	2011	*Staphylococcus*

*Resistance to penicillin was discovered before the drug was approved.
†Vancomycin is used as a last resort, which may be why the development of resistance took 16 years.
(Data from Hede.)

resistance is occurring at a faster rate than in years past (Table 8-1). Bacteria may be resistant to certain antibiotics or can develop resistance by a number of different mechanisms (Fig 8-8).

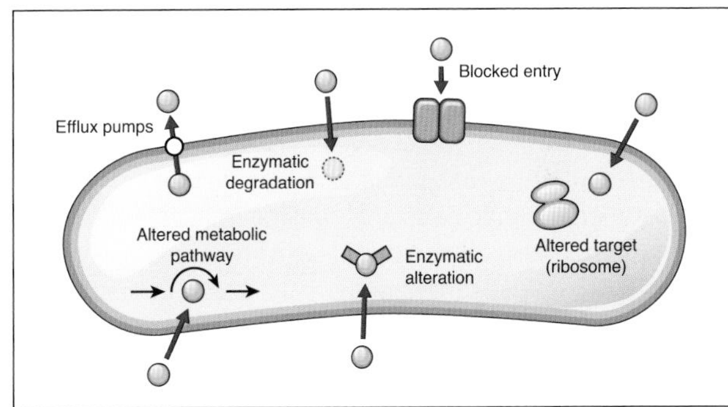

Fig 8-8 The major mechanisms of bacterial resistance to antibiotics.

Impaired permeability of antibiotics

The outer membrane of Gram-negative bacteria constitutes a barrier to antibiotics. The main reason β-lactam antibiotics are less effective against Gram-negative bacteria than Gram-positive bacteria is their inability to permeate the outer membrane. Some antibiotics can penetrate the outer membrane through the porin channels, depending on their molecular structure, hydrophobicity, and charge. Mutations in the porin proteins may prevent the entry of antibiotics that are normally effective against a particular Gram-negative species. Bacteria that do not have the molecular machinery to actively transport aminoglycosides are resistant to the antibiotic (eg, enterococci, streptococci, and anaerobes). Some bacteria have membrane transport systems that pump antibiotics out of the cells, similar to the mammalian P-glycoprotein that pumps anticancer drugs out of the cells. For example, erythromycin may be pumped actively out of the bacterial cell. When *P aeruginosa* loses its outer membrane protein involved in transporting imipenem, it becomes resistant to this antibiotic.

Alteration of the molecular targets of antibiotics

When the 30S ribosomal subunit mutates, this may impair the binding of streptomycin and hence its antibacterial activity. Newer aminoglycosides, such as amikacin, bind to multiple sites on the ribosome, making it more difficult for the bacterium to develop resistance to these drugs. PBPs with transpeptidase activity may also undergo mutations, which may prevent β-lactam antibiotics from binding to and inhibiting the enzyme. The decrease in the susceptibility of a mutated bacterium to penicillin may be gradual and not absolute, such that a higher concentration of the antibiotic may surpass the MIC for the mutated bacterium and thus still be effective. Changes in PBPs are the main reason for the emergence of methicillin-resistant *Staphylococcus aureus* (MRSA) and penicillin-resistant pneumococci.

Vancomycin resistance in enterococci is attributed to the emergence of bacterial enzymes that place ala-lys at the terminus of the peptide segment of peptidoglycan rather than ala-ala, because vancomycin does not bind to the altered dipeptide. Mutations in DNA gyrase may lead to resistance to quinolones. Methylation of the 23S ribosomal RNA prevents the binding of clindamycin to the 50S ribosomal subunit. This alteration also affects erythromycin binding to the ribosome.

Enzymatic inactivation of antibiotics

Some organisms synthesize enzymes that destroy drugs, such as β-lactamase, which cleaves the β-lactam ring of penicillins and cephalosporins (see Fig 8-8). Different β-lactamases have varying activities against antibiotics in the same family. The original penicillinase from staphylococci can degrade ampicillin but not methicillin or cephalosporins. Clavulanic acid can bind some penicillinases but not others. Extended-spectrum β-lactamases (ESBLs) are of medical concern because they can inactivate different cephalosporins. ESBLs are inducible enzymes, so they may be difficult to detect because the conditions in susceptibility tests may not be sufficient to induce them.

Bacteria produce numerous enzymes that can acetylate, phosphorylate, or adenylate hydroxyl or amino groups of aminoglycosides, which can no longer bind to ribosomes. Esterase and phosphotransferase enzymes in bacteria can modify erythromycin, and acetylase can alter chloramphenicol, thus conferring resistance to these antibiotics.

Resistance to antibiotics may be intrinsic, for example the result of constitutive production of β-lactamase, especially in Gram-negative bacteria. A β-lactam antibiotic may activate the chromosomal genes encoding β-lactamase, and the increased production of the enzyme may render the bacterium resistant to additional β-lactam antimicrobials. Acquired resistance may be the result of mutations or the transfer of genetic material from resistant microorganisms, often by plasmids (R plasmid) that also mediate conjugation. R plasmids are found in various Gram-negative bacilli such as *Shigella*, *Salmonella*, *Klebsiella*, *Vibrio*, *Pasteurella*, and *Escherichia*. Some R plasmids can be transferred only to closely related strains, whereas others can be transferred to other species or genera. Resistance genes can be on transposons, which can insert into other plasmids or the chromosome. Although plasmids can undergo recombination, transposition is more likely to carry the entire resistance gene into the target plasmid.

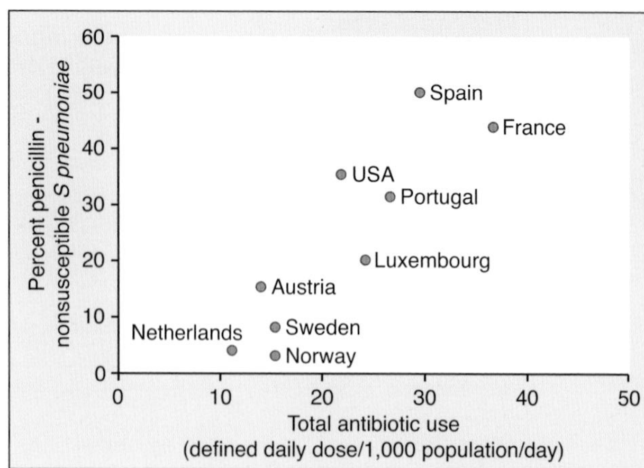

Fig 8-9 The prevalence of penicillin-nonsusceptible *S pneumoniae* strains versus total antibiotic use in the outpatient setting. (Adapted from Albrich et al.)

Drug resistance is a serious problem in the treatment of bacterial infections. Hospital-acquired infections may be particularly difficult to treat because these bacteria have been exposed to a large number of antibiotics over the years and may have developed resistance to the commonly used antibiotics. There is also a correlation between the total antibiotic use in a particular country and the percentage of penicillin-nonsusceptible *S pneumoniae* strains in that country (Fig 8-9).

Another problem is drug resistance in food-borne pathogens, including *Salmonella* and *Campylobacter*. Despite the strong opposition of the Centers for Disease Control and Prevention, the use of ciprofloxacin at farms to treat illnesses, prevent infections, and fatten animals on less feed has resulted in the emergence of quinolone-resistant *Salmonella* and *Campylobacter* species. Vancomycin-resistant enterococci have arisen as a result of the treatment of livestock by an analogous antibiotic (avoparcin). This antibiotic is no longer used in the European Union.

The gene for vancomycin resistance contained within a transposon has been transferred in vivo from *E faecalis* to the *S aureus* multiresistance plasmid. This plasmid now encodes resistance to β-lactams, vancomycin, and aminoglycosides.

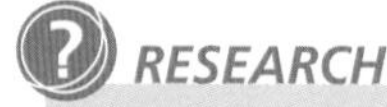

What is the potential danger of an R plasmid in a nonpathogenic bacterium of the normal gut microflora?

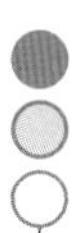

Take-Home Messages

- The antibacterial spectrum of an antibiotic is the range of bacteria against which the drug is effective.
- The lowest concentration of a drug that inhibits growth is the minimum inhibitory concentration (MIC). The ability of a drug to kill a bacterium is expressed as the minimum bactericidal concentration (MBC).
- The ratio of the toxic dose of a drug to the effective dose is the therapeutic index.
- Antibacterial agents may inhibit cell wall synthesis, protein synthesis, metabolic activity, or nucleic acid synthesis or alter cell membranes.
- Penicillins inhibit bacterial transpeptidase that catalyzes the final cross-linking step in the synthesis of peptidoglycan.
- Penicillins can be used in combination with a β-lactamase inhibitor, including clavulanate.
- Cephalosporins act similarly to penicillin, but they have a wider spectrum and are resistant to β-lactamases.
- Vancomycin is a complex glycopeptide that blocks transpeptidation and is used intravenously against methicillin-resistant staphylococci.
- Aminoglycosides bind to ribosomes, destabilize them, and block initiation complexes. They are effective against bacteria that can transport them into the cell by a process involving oxidative phosphorylation.
- Tetracyclines are broad-spectrum bacteriostatic antibiotics that inhibit protein synthesis by blocking the binding of tRNA to the 30S ribosome subunit.
- The macrolide antibiotics bind to the 50S ribosomal subunit and are used to treat pulmonary infections caused by *Legionella*, *Mycoplasma*, and *Chlamydophila*.
- Rifampin inhibits bacterial DNA-dependent RNA polymerase and is used against *M tuberculosis* and aerobic Gram-positive cocci.
- Quinolones inhibit DNA gyrase in Gram-negative bacteria and topoisomerase type IV in Gram-positive bacteria.
- Sulfonamides block a step in folic acid synthesis by competing with p-aminobenzoic acid, and trimethoprim inhibits dihydrofolate reductase and hence the production of tetrahydrofolate.
- Resistance to antibiotics can develop by bacteria limiting their permeability, altering the molecular targets of the antibiotics, or inactivating the antibiotics.
- Drug resistance is a serious problem in the treatment of bacterial infections, especially in hospitals.

Bibliography

Albrich WC, Monnet DL, Harbarth S. Antibiotic selection pressure and resistance in *Streptococcus pneumoniae* and *Streptococcus pyogenes*. Emerg Infect Dis 2004;10:514–517.

Cottagnoud P, Cottagnoud M, Täuber MG. Vancomycin acts synergistically with gentamicin against penicillin-resistant pneumococci by increasing the intracellular penetration of gentamicin. Antimicrob Agents Chemother 2003;47:144–147.

eMedExpert. Cephalosporins (Cephems). www.emedexpert.com/compare/cephalosporins.shtml. Accessed 11 May 2015.

Engleberg NC, DiRita V, Dermody TS. Schaechter's Mechanisms of Microbial Disease, ed 4. Baltimore: Lippincott Williams & Wilkins, 2007.

Greenwood D, Slack R, Peutherer J, Barer M. Medical Microbiology, ed 17. Edinburgh: Churchill Livingstone/Elsevier, 2007.

Hamilton-Miller JMT. The cephalosporins and Sir Edward Abraham: Recollections about a great scientist and his part in the discovery of these antibiotics. J Antibiotics 2000;53:1003–1007.

Hede K. Antibiotic resistance: An infectious arms race. Nature 2014;509(7498, suppl):S2–S3.

Ingraham JL, Ingraham CA. Introduction to Microbiology: A Case History Approach. Pacific Grove, CA: Brooks/Cole (Thomson), 2004.

Murray PR, Rosenthal KS, Pfaller MA. Medical Microbiology, ed 6. Philadelphia: Mosby/Elsevier, 2009.

Nobelprize.org. "Paul Ehrlich - Biographical." Nobel Media AB 2013. http://www.nobelprize.org/nobel_prizes/medicine/laureates/1908/ehrlich-bio.html. Accessed 11 May 2015.

Sauvage E, Kerff E, Terrak M, Ayala JA, Charlier P. The penicillin-binding proteins: Structure and role in peptidoglycan biosynthesis. FEMS Microbiol Rev 2008;32:234–258.

Soares GM, Figueiredo LC, Faveri M, Cortelli SC, Duarte PM, Feres M. Mechanisms of action of systemic antibiotics used in periodontal treatment and mechanisms of bacterial resistance to these drugs. J Appl Oral Sci 2012;20:295–309.

Wecker L, Crespo L, Dunaway G, Faingold C, Watts S. Brody's Human Pharmacology, ed 5. New York: Mosby/Elsevier, 2009.

Sterilization, Disinfection, and Antisepsis

9

Sterilization

The total destruction of all microbes, including bacterial spores, mycobacteria, naked capsid viruses, and fungi is termed *sterilization*, which is achieved by dry or wet heat, certain gases, and certain chemicals. Moist (autoclave) and dry heat are used to sterilize most materials, except heat-sensitive, toxic, or volatile chemicals. Ultraviolet or ionizing radiation can also be used. Instruments that cannot be autoclaved can be sterilized with ethylene oxide gas, but the instrumentation has to be strictly monitored because the gas is flammable and carcinogenic. Hydrogen peroxide vapors can be used for the sterilization of instruments. In plasma gas sterilization, hydrogen peroxide is vaporized, and microwave-frequency or radio-frequency energy is used to produce free radicals. Peracetic acid (CH_3CO_3H) is an oxidizing agent that has sterilizing activity and has the advantage that the end products—acetic acid and oxygen—are nontoxic. Glutaraldehyde is also a sterilizing agent, but it must be handled with care.

Autoclaving involves the exposure of suitable materials to moist heat under a pressure of 15 lb/in^2 at 121°C to 132°C for at least 15 minutes. The high temperature results in protein denaturation. The rate of killing organisms is affected by a number of factors, including the size of the autoclave, the temperature and time, the steam flow rate, the location of the material in the chamber, and the density and size of the load. Air pockets in the load inhibit penetration of the steam, and thus must be avoided. The functionality of the autoclave should be checked routinely by including a commercially available ampule of *Bacillus stearothermophilus* spores in the middle of the load and incubating it after the autoclaving at 37°C in a supplied medium. If there is an error in the sterilization process, the spores germinate and grow, producing a turbid suspension. If sterilization is successful, the incubation medium is clear.

Dry heat treatment for sterilization of heat-resistant instruments involves exposure to 160°C for 2 hours or 171°C for 1 hour. Ultraviolet radiation sterilizes by damaging DNA, and ionizing radiation sterilizes by knocking off electrons from biomolecules.

Table 9-1 Antimicrobial properties of disinfectants and antiseptic agents

Agent(s)	Bacteria	Myco-bacteria	Bacterial spores	Fungi	Viruses
Disinfectants					
Alcohol	+	+	–	+	+/–
Hydrogen peroxide	+	+	+/–	+	+
Formaldehyde	+	+	+	+	+
Phenolics	+	+	–	+	+/–
Chlorine	+	+	+/–	+	+
Iodophors	+	+/–	–	+	+
Glutaraldehyde	+	+	+	+	+
Quaternary ammonium	+/–	–	–	+/–	+/–
Antiseptics					
Alcohol	+	+	–	+	+
Iodophors	+	+	–	+	+
Chlorhexidine	+	+	–	+	+
Parachlorometaxylenol	+/–	+/–	–	+	+/–
Triclosan	+	+/–	–	+/–	+

(Adapted from Murray et al.)

Disinfection

Disinfection is the use of physical or chemical methods to destroy most microorganisms. Bacterial spores and some resistant organisms like mycobacteria and viruses may survive disinfection procedures. High-level disinfection can usually emulate the efficiency of sterilization. In intermediate-level disinfection, bacterial spores can survive. Low-level disinfection kills most vegetative bacteria and lipid-enveloped viruses. Many factors influence the efficiency of disinfection, including the type and concentration of the disinfectant, the number and nature of the organisms, the amount of organic material present that can inactivate the disinfectant, the time of exposure to the agent, and the temperature.

Certain surgical instruments or endoscopes that cannot be sterilized by autoclaving can be treated with high-level disinfectants after cleaning the instruments to remove any organic matter. High-level disinfectants include glutaraldehyde, peracetic acid, chlorine compounds, and hydrogen peroxide (Table 9-1).

Intermediate-level disinfectants kill all microbial pathogens except bacterial spores and include phenolic compounds, alcohols, and iodophor compounds. These compounds are used to clean surfaces or instruments under conditions where contamination with bacterial spores is not likely. Such instruments include flexible fiberoptic endoscopes and anesthesia breathing circuits.

Quaternary ammonium compounds provide low-level disinfection and can be used to disinfect noncritical instruments, including stethoscopes.

Appropriate disinfectants must be chosen to clean surfaces that present a risk of cross infection. A high-level disinfectant is appropriate for decontaminating an instrument exposed to blood or a surface contaminated with *Clostridium difficile* or *Pseudomonas aeruginosa*, which can be involved in nosocomial infections.

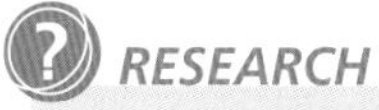

What are the diseases caused by *C difficile* and *P aeruginosa*? What makes them nosocomial pathogens?

Antisepsis

Antisepsis is the use of chemical agents (antiseptics) on living tissue to inhibit or eliminate microbes (see Table 9-1). These compounds are selected for their safety and efficacy. Ethyl and isopropyl alcohol at concentrations in the range 70%–90% are active against all groups of organisms, but

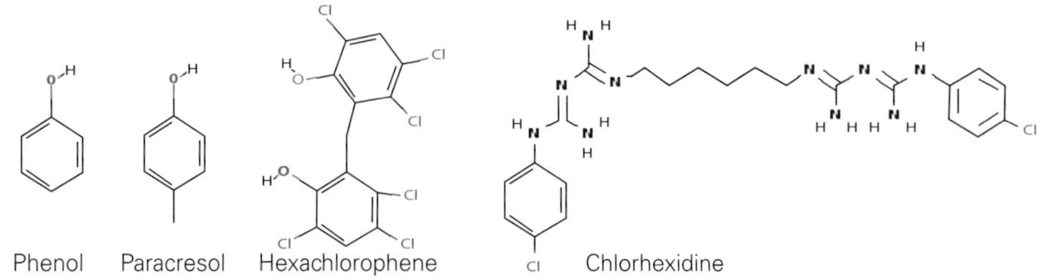

Phenol Paracresol Hexachlorophene Chlorhexidine

Fig 9-1 Phenol and phenolics.

not spores. Iodophors at 1 to 2 mg free iodine/liter are effective antiseptic agents on the skin, having a range of activity similar to that of alcohols. Chlorhexidine kills organisms at a much slower rate than alcohol, but its activity persists on tissues. Parachlorometaxylenol has limited activity against Gram-positive bacteria and is included in liquid soaps because it is nontoxic and persistent. Triclosan is active against bacteria and is used in deodorant soaps and some toothpastes. Extensive use of antimicrobial soaps and toothpastes with triclosan can result in the accumulation of the antiseptic and its byproducts in groundwater. Ultraviolet radiation can convert triclosan into polychlorinated dibenzodioxin, which has many toxic effects in humans.

Classes of Germicides and Mechanisms of Action

Phenols and phenolics

Phenol was the original antiseptic used by Joseph Lister to treat wound infections in the 19th century (Fig 9-1). Phenols denature proteins and disrupt lipidic membranes. Paracresol was the original Lysol disinfectant. Phenol is not effective against spores at room temperature and has poor activity against naked capsid viruses. Phenolic compounds are active against mycobacteria, presumably because these bacteria have a cell wall rich in lipids and waxes. The addition of chlorine to phenolics enhances their activity. Two phenol compounds can be linked together to form bisphenols, whose activity can be increased by the addition of chlorine. An example is hexachlorophene, which is active against Gram-positive bacteria. This antiseptic is available by prescription only because of its potential neurotoxicity.

RESEARCH

Explore Joseph Lister's first case in which he used phenol as an antiseptic.

Chlorhexidine is used instead of hexachlorophene as a hand and skin antiseptic and is often prescribed as an antiseptic in dentistry. It has a broad spectrum of action, and because it binds to tissues, it has persistent antibacterial activity. It reduces gingival inflammation, plaque, and bleeding. It may be used as an alternative to mechanical oral hygiene after an oral surgical procedure or as a preoperative rinse. Chlorhexidine inhibits a number of bacterial processes: *(1)* sugar transport in streptococci; *(2)* amino acid uptake and catabolism in *Streptococcus sanguinis*; *(3) Porphyromonas gingivalis* protease; *(4)* membrane functions, including adenosine triphosphate (ATP) synthase and maintenance of ion gradients in streptococci; and *(5)* binding of plaque-forming bacteria. Mutans streptococci are especially susceptible to the activity of chlorhexidine. Because it is positively charged, it is neutralized by anionic detergents and soaps.

Alkylating agents

Alkylating agents inactivate proteins by attaching short chains of carbons (alkyl groups) (Fig 9-2). Formaldehyde and glutaraldehyde are used as sterilizing agents or high-level disinfectants. Formaldehyde gas dissolved in water at a final concentration of 37% is termed formalin, to which stabilizers like methanol are added. Formaldehyde can be toxic to the skin or mucous membranes. The microbicidal activity of formaldehyde can be enhanced by combining it with alcohol (eg, 20% formalin in a 70% alcohol solution). Glutaraldehyde becomes polymerized in solution and interacts with amino acids in proteins or peptidoglycan, thereby inactivating them. It is used in disinfecting instruments with lenses or apparatuses for respiratory therapy that cannot be autoclaved. Because glutaraldehyde is inactivated by organic material, items to be disinfected must be cleaned first. Glutaraldehyde is less toxic than formaldehyde, but it can damage skin or mucous membranes.

Ethylene oxide is a colorless, flammable, and potentially explosive gas used to sterilize heat-sensitive items. It inactivates microorganisms by replacing hydrogen atoms on hydroxyl, sulfhydryl, and carboxyl groups in biomolecules, particularly adenine and guanine. It is also a mutagen. Sterilizers using ethylene oxide use 10% of the gas mixed with carbon dioxide at 50°C to 60°C for 4 to 6 hours, with an optimal relative humidity of about 30%. Ethylene oxide is toxic; therefore, the chamber must be aerated for 16 hours or longer to prevent any absorbed gas on the material from damaging tissues or skin. Artificial heart valves are sterilized with ethylene oxide because they are damaged by the heat of the autoclave.

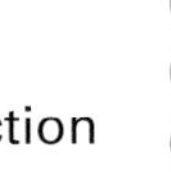

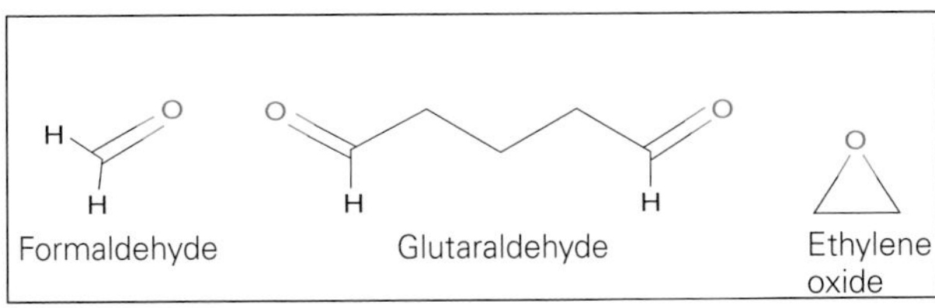

Fig 9-2 Alkylating agents.

Dimethyldodecylbenzyl-ammonium chloride

Fig 9-3 A quaternary ammonium salt.

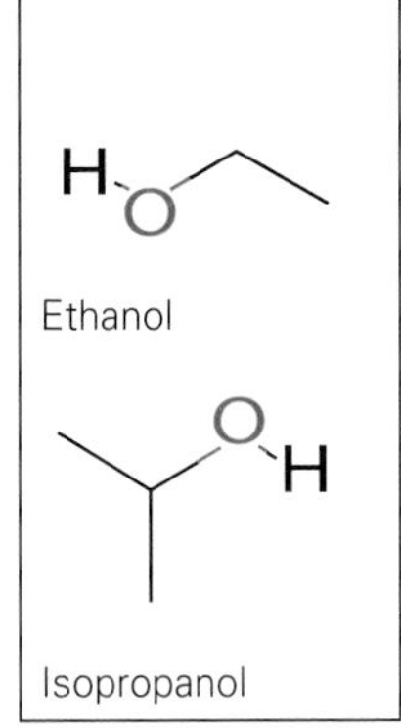

Fig 9-4 Alcohols.

Oxidizing agents

Oxidizing agents, including ozone, halogens, and hydrogen peroxide, oxidize functional groups on proteins and thereby inactivate them. Compounds containing iodine or chlorine are used extensively as disinfectants and antiseptics. The highly reactive halogen iodine can precipitate proteins and oxidize enzymes and has strong microbicidal activity. It was originally used as a 2% solution in 50% alcohol, which sometimes caused hypersensitivity reactions. Elemental iodine can be complexed with a carrier compound such as polyvinylpyrrolidone (povidone iodine), and such a complex is termed an *iodophor*, "iodo" referring to iodine and "phor" to carrier.

Aqueous solutions of chlorine are bactericidal. Chlorine in water may be found as hypochlorous acid (HOCl), hypochlorite ion (ClO^-), or elemental chlorine. Chlorine can oxidize irreversibly sulfhydryl groups of proteins. Hypochlorite ions form toxic *N*-chloro compounds in the cytoplasm, thereby interfering with metabolism. Chlorine has greater activity under acidic conditions, indicating that hypochlorous acid is the more active substance compared with hypochlorite ion. Spore-forming organisms are up to three orders of magnitude more resistant to chlorine than vegetative microorganisms. Organic matter and alkaline detergents can decrease the efficacy of chlorine compounds.

Hydrogen peroxide as a 3% solution in water acts as an antiseptic. In the range 3% to 6%, it can kill most bacteria, and in the range 10% to 25%, it can destroy spores. It attacks membrane lipids and other cellular components. It can be used to disinfect surgical prostheses, plastic implants, and contact lenses. Hydrogen peroxide is thermodynamically unstable and is broken down to water and oxygen. It is most stable in dilute, acidic solutions kept in cold temperatures. When applied to skin, bubbling occurs as a result of the production of oxygen through the action of catalase ($2H_2O_2 \rightarrow 2H_2O + O_2$). The active form of hydrogen peroxide is the free hydroxyl radical ($^{\cdot}OH$) formed by the decomposition of hydrogen peroxide.

Surfactants

Surfactant molecules have hydrophobic and hydrophilic parts and can penetrate the cytoplasmic membrane of bacteria, altering the surface properties of the membrane and causing the leakage of intracellular ions and compounds. Quaternary ammonium salts ("quats") consist of four organic groups, including a long hydrocarbon chain, linked covalently to a charged nitrogen atom. The most effective of these compounds are those with hydrocarbon chains of 8 to 18 carbons. The cationic detergents benzalkonium chloride (Fig 9-3) and cetylpyridinium chloride are examples of quaternary ammonium salts. They are neutralized by anionic compounds, such as soaps, and by organic matter. They are safe to use on skin at concentrations of 0.1%. *Pseudomonas*, *Mycobacterium*, *Trichophyton*, bacterial spores, and many viruses are resistant to quats. Some *Pseudomonas* strains survive and grow in quaternary ammonium solutions.

Alcohols

Alcohols can disrupt the membrane lipids of microorganisms and denature proteins. Ethanol and isopropanol (Fig 9-4) are the two most commonly used alcohols and have bactericidal activity against vegetative bacteria, mycobacteria, certain fungi, and lipid-containing viruses. They are not effective against bacterial spores, and they are not very effective against some fungi and naked capsid viruses. Alcohol activity is greater in the presence of water; thus, 70% alcohol is more active than 95% alcohol, because proteins are denatured more efficiently in the presence of water. The most effective concentration range is 60% to 90% volume in water. Alcohol followed by an iodophor is used as an antiseptic for the skin before surgical procedures.

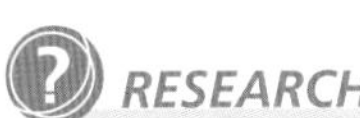

RESEARCH

How long does it take for ethanol solutions to kill microorganisms like *P aeruginosa*, *Mycobacterium tuberculosis*, and *Staphylococcus aureus*?

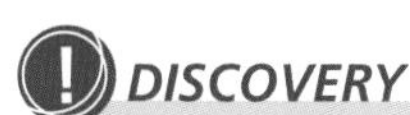

DISCOVERY

"Childbed fever," also called *puerperal endometritis,* was a major problem at the Vienna General Hospital in the 1840s, causing 600 to 800 maternal deaths per year. Ignaz Semmelweis, an assistant obstetrician at the hospital, examined the hospital statistics over several years and discovered that the death rate in Division I of the hospital was 10 times higher than that in Division II. Both obstetricians and students delivered the babies in Division I, which was the teaching unit. All deliveries in Division II were by midwives. The mortality rate was also very low for deliveries at home, and there was no epidemic elsewhere in Vienna. Semmelweis hypothesized that the main difference between the two divisions was that the obstetricians and students performed autopsies, sometimes on women who had died of childbed fever or other infections. These "health care" personnel did not use good hand-washing practices and, according to Semmelweis, carried "invisible cadaver particles" to the pregnant women. Starting in 1847, Semmelweis required thorough hand washing with a chlorine solution. The mortality rate in Division I was reduced from 11.4% in 1846 to 1.3% in 1848 (the first full year of chlorine hand washing), and that in Division II was also reduced from 2.7% to 1.3%. Childbed fever is now known to have been caused primarily by Group A streptococci.

Bibliography

Centers for Disease Control. Guideline for Disinfection and Sterilization in Healthcare Facilities, 2008. www.cdc.gov/hicpac/Disinfection_Sterilization/6_0disinfection.html. Accessed 8 May 2015.

Ingraham JL, Ingraham CA. Introduction to Microbiology: A Case History Approach. Pacific Grove, CA: Brooks/Cole (Thomson), 2004.

Marsh PD, Martin MV. Oral Microbiology, ed 5. Edinburgh: Churchill/Livingstone, 2009.

Murray PR, Rosenthal KS, Pfaller MA. Medical Microbiology, ed 7. Philadelphia: Saunders, 2013.

Ryan KJ, Ray CG. Sherris Medical Microbiology, ed 5. New York: McGraw-Hill, 2010.

Varoni E, Tarce M, Lodi G, Carrassi A. Chlorhexidine (CHX) in dentistry: State of the art. Minerva Stomatol 2012;61:399–419.

Take-Home Messages

- Sterilization is the total destruction of all microbes, including bacterial spores, mycobacteria, naked capsid viruses, and fungi.
- Autoclaving involves the exposure of suitable materials to moist heat under a pressure of 15 lb/in^2 at 121°C to 132°C for at least 15 minutes.
- Disinfection is the use of physical or chemical methods to destroy most microorganisms.
- Antisepsis is the use of chemical agents (antiseptics) on living tissue to inhibit or eliminate microbes.
- Phenolic compounds denature proteins and disrupt lipid membranes. Paracresol was the original Lysol disinfectant.
- Chlorhexidine is prescribed often as an antiseptic in dentistry. It has a broad spectrum of action, and it has persistent antibacterial activity because it binds to tissues. It reduces gingival inflammation, plaque, and bleeding.
- Alkylating agents inactivate proteins by attaching short chains of carbons (alkyl groups).
- Ethylene oxide inactivates microorganisms by replacing hydrogen atoms on hydroxyl, sulfhydryl, and carboxyl groups in biomolecules, particularly adenine and guanine. It is a flammable and potentially explosive gas used to sterilize heat-sensitive surgical items.
- Oxidizing agents, including ozone, halogens, and hydrogen peroxide, oxidize functional groups on proteins and inactivate them.
- Iodine can precipitate proteins and oxidize enzymes and has strong microbicidal activity.
- Hydrogen peroxide as a 3% solution in water acts as an antiseptic, and it can kill most bacteria in the concentration range of 3% to 6%.
- Surfactant molecules have hydrophobic and hydrophilic parts and can penetrate the cytoplasmic membrane of bacteria, alter the surface properties of the membrane, and cause the leakage of intracellular ions and compounds.
- Alcohols can disrupt the membrane lipids of microorganisms and denature proteins.

Microbial Identification and Molecular Diagnostics

10

Microbial Identification

Microscopic methods

In bright-field light microscopy, the specimen to be identified is observed by light passing through the condenser to the specimen (see Fig 6-3). The image is magnified by the objective lens and the ocular lens, the total magnification being the product of the magnifications of the two lenses. The low power (10×) lens is used to get a general appearance of the specimen. The 40× objective lens enables the visualization of parasites and filamentous fungi. The 100× oil immersion lens is used to examine yeasts and bacteria as well as the details of eukaryotic cells. The resolving power, *d*, of a microscope is the distance between two points that can just be distinguished as being separate:

$$d = \lambda/2NA$$

where λ is the wavelength of light and *NA* is the numerical aperture of the objective lens. NA reflects the ability of the lens to gather light and resolve specimen detail at a fixed object distance. Higher values of numerical aperture allow increasingly oblique rays to enter the objective lens, producing a more highly resolved image. The use of immersion oil with the 100× lens reduces the dispersion of light, enhancing the resolving power. The resolving power of the best bright-field microscopes is about 0.2 μm. Because the refractive indices of microorganisms and background are similar, it is difficult to distinguish the microorganisms without using stains.

In dark-field microscopy, a condenser prevents transmitted light from directly illuminating the specimen but enables scattered light to reach the specimen and illuminate it against a black background. The resolving power of dark-field microscopy is significantly better than that of bright-field microscopy. This method is used to detect spirochetes such as *Treponema pallidum*, *Treponema denticola*, and *Leptospira* species.

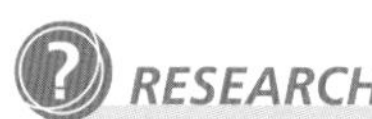

RESEARCH

What are the diseases caused by *T pallidum, T denticola,* and *Leptospira* species?

Light waves travel at different speeds through materials that have different refractive indices. Therefore, light rays that go through the microbial specimen are out of phase to varying degrees with the light rays that go outside the specimen. In phase-contrast microscopy, peaks of light waves that arrive at different times interfere with each other and reduce the intensity of the light. That is, the light rays moving through the more dense material are retarded more than those going through the medium. The rays arriving at the same time augment each other. This creates a three-dimensional image of the microorganism and permits more detailed analysis of the internal structures.

Fluorescent compounds absorb light at a particular wavelength and emit light at a higher visible wavelength. In fluorescence microscopy, microorganisms are stained with fluorescent dyes and then observed in a fluorescence microscope. Microorganisms stained with fluorescent compounds are brightly "lit" against a dark background. Microorganisms can be identified by immunofluorescence microscopy, where fluorescence-labeled antibodies specific for antigens on the microorganism are added to the sample and unbound antibodies are washed off.

The simplest method for examining microbial samples is to place them on a microscope slide in an aqueous medium. This method is called a wet mount. The medium may contain potassium hydroxide to eliminate debris and a contrasting dye that stains the microorganisms. The capsule of certain microorganisms, such as *Pseudomonas aeruginosa*, may be visualized by staining the background with India ink in a procedure called negative staining.

Differential stains can distinguish different types of microorganisms. The Gram stain delineates two major types of bacteria. Fungi also stain positively with this method. *Plasmodium* species can be stained with the Wright-Giemsa stain. The acid-fast staining methods can identify mycobacteria that retain stain after an acidic decolorizing agent. The specimen needs to be heated for the Ziehl-Neelsen stain but not for the Kinyoun and auramine-rhodamine fluorescent stains.

Fluorescent dyes can be used to distinguish live and dead bacteria or eukaryotic cells. For example, the SYTO 9 dye labels all bacterial DNA green, whereas propidium iodide penetrates bacteria with damaged membranes and labels them red. Antibodies labeled with fluorescent dyes can detect specific antigens on microorganisms that can be used to identify them in the direct fluorescent antibody test.

Culture

The colony characteristics on nutrient agar can help with initial diagnosis. The shape, elevation, color, and translucency of the colonies as well as their ability to grow under aerobic or anaerobic conditions or in the presence of carbon dioxide all help with identifying particular microorganisms.

Culturing certain microorganisms requires particular media. For example, some strains of *Neisseria* grow best on chocolate agar, which is a modified (heated) form of blood agar. Blood agar contains the basal medium, which may be tryptic soy agar, and (usually) sheep blood. This medium is useful in the identification of β-hemolytic bacteria such as *Streptococcus pyogenes*. *Legionella* grows on buffered charcoal yeast extract (BCYE) and requires iron and L-cysteine in the medium. The addition of certain antibiotics to BCYE renders this a selective medium for the isolation of *Brucella*. Mueller-Hinton agar is used for the antibiotic susceptibility testing of bacteria. Thioglycolate broth is an enrichment broth that facilitates the recovery of low numbers of bacteria. Sabouraud dextrose agar is useful in the isolation and growth of fungi. The addition of antibacterial agents and the use of low pH renders this agar selective for fungi.

Selective media are used to recover particular microorganisms from a mixed sample. MacConkey agar is selective for Gram-negative bacteria (as the crystal violet and bile salts in the agar inhibit Gram-positive bacteria) and can differentiate between lactose fermenters, which produce acid and turn an indicator dye red, and nonfermenters. Xylose lysine deoxycholate agar can differentiate between *Salmonella* and *Shigella* species. Mycobacteria can be isolated by the use of Löwenstein-Jensen medium and Middlebrook agar. Mannitol salt agar is used for isolating staphylococci, which grow in the presence of high salt. In this medium, *Staphylococcus aureus* ferments mannitol and turns the phenol red yellow. CandiSelect 4 agar and CHROMagar can be used for the identification of various *Candida* species.

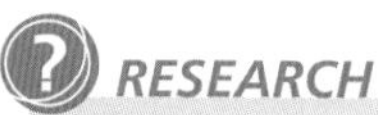

RESEARCH

What are the mechanisms by which xylose lysine deoxycholate agar works?

Certain microorganisms such as *Chlamydia* and *Treponema* can only be grown in cultured eukaryotic cells. Likewise, animal viruses need eukaryotic cells in which to replicate. The cytopathic effect of certain viruses in particular cell types can help with identification.

Biochemistry

Microorganisms can be identified based on their ability to produce acidic or gaseous end products after feeding on a particular carbohydrate, such as glucose or mannitol. Enzymatic activities, including cytochrome oxidase, catalase, lecithinase, or urease, may also help in identification. Metabolic products or fatty acids of microorganisms may be analyzed by automated systems and compared with databases to identify a particular microorganism.

Molecular Diagnostics

Molecular diagnostic techniques are highly sensitive and specific. They are also safe to use, because the infectious agent does not need to be isolated or grown in culture and chemically inactivated samples can be analyzed. Very small samples of the DNA of the microorganism can be identified. Molecular diagnostic techniques can identify mutations in the genetic material of different strains. Drug-resistant human immunodeficiency virus (HIV) strains can be identified that can help with the development of alternative antiviral drugs.

DNA probe analysis

DNA probes are synthetic oligonucleotides that can hybridize with specific DNA sequences of the microorganism to be detected in tissues or cells. The sample to be tested is heated to dissociate the Watson and Crick DNA strands, the probe is added, and the sample is cooled to allow for hybridization of complementary sequences. The DNA probe is labeled with a fluorescent probe or biotin. The fluorescent DNA can be visualized directly under a fluorescence microscope. In the case of the biotin-labeled probe, avidin labeled with either horseradish peroxidase or a fluorescent probe is added to the sample. Avidin binds biotin with high affinity and specificity and thus reveals whether the probe has bound to the DNA in the cell or tissue.

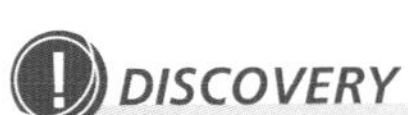

DISCOVERY

Kary Mullis developed the polymerase chain reaction technique in 1985 at the Cetus Corporation, one of the first biotechnology firms in Emeryville, California. He placed a small amount of the DNA containing the gene of interest into a test tube, together with all four nucleotides necessary to produce complementary sequences. Mullis synthesized short DNA "primers" that were complementary to sequences on each side of the desired gene. He also added DNA polymerase. He heated the test tube to separate the two original strands of DNA. When the temperature was lowered, the primers bound to their complementary sequences of the DNA sample. The polymerase recognized the primers and started to copy the template DNA. At the end of the reaction, there were two double helices. Mullis repeated the heating and cooling, each time doubling the number of DNA copies.

Because the technique was labor-intensive, scientists at Cetus worked on automating the procedure. Fresh DNA polymerase had to be added to each cycle. To address this part of the technique, Cetus engineers developed the first thermocycling machine, called "Mr Cycle." After the introduction of the thermostable polymerase from *Thermus aquaticus* (Taq), the DNA thermal cycler was developed to more rapidly cycle between the different temperatures.

The polymerase chain reaction (PCR) is used to copy particular segments of DNA in an exponential manner to generate about a million copies. Short DNA oligonucleotides, called *primers*, that are complementary to sequences on each side of the desired gene are used to initiate the generation of complementary copies using a polymerase, in the presence of dNTPs (deoxynucleoside triphosphates). The two original strands of DNA are separated by heating, and as the temperature is lowered, the primers bind to their complementary sequences of the DNA sample. A heat-resistant DNA polymerase, usually from the thermophilic microorganism *T aquaticus*, copies the DNA strands starting at the primers. The heating and cooling steps are repeated many times, and thus the original DNA is replicated at every cycle, producing a very large number of copies.

PCR can be used to detect chromosome-integrated or episomal DNA from retroviruses and herpesviruses. Species-specific oligonucleotides can be used to amplify the 16S rRNA to identify oral bacteria. Alternatively, the gene for leukotoxin from *Aggregatibacter actinomycetemcomitans*, the fimbrillin gene of *Porphyromonas gingivalis*, and the glucosyltransferase gene of *Streptococcus sanguinis*, *Streptococcus mutans*, and *Streptococcus sobrinus* can be used to detect these microorganisms (Fig 10-1).

In multiplex PCR, more than one gene is amplified in the same reaction, necessitating the use of multiple primers. This method has been used for the simultaneous detection of *A actinomycetemcomitans* and *P gingivalis* in periodontal samples and *Dialister pneumosintes*, *Prevotella intermedia*, and *Porphyromonas endodontalis* from endodontic samples (see Fig 10-1).

The reverse transcription polymerase chain reaction (RT-PCR) uses the reverse transcriptase enzyme to copy viral genomic RNA or mRNA to DNA, followed by the regular PCR procedure. This method is useful in the identification of emerging viruses that may have sequence homology to known viruses.

Real-time PCR can be used to determine the amount of DNA or RNA (by RT-PCR) in a sample by measuring how fast new DNA is made through the increase in fluorescence of a reporter molecule (eg, SYBR green) or a sequence-specific molecular beacon as it binds the DNA (see Fig 10-1). The HIV viral load in plasma can be readily determined with this method.

Oligonucleotide probes, which are 15 to 30 nucleotides long, can hybridize with specific sequences in target DNA. When tagged with fluorescent probes, they are used in fluorescence in situ hybridization to detect particular gene sequences in cultured mammalian cells or in bacteria, such as 16S rRNA (see Fig 10-1).

In another technique utilizing hybridization, the genomic DNA of a particular microorganism is labeled with digoxigenin, which is a steroid isolated from the plant *Digitalis purpurea* (foxglove). DNA is extracted from samples to be tested and spotted on a nylon membrane. The known DNAs are then hybridized to the samples, detected by using anti-

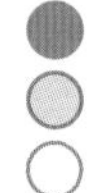

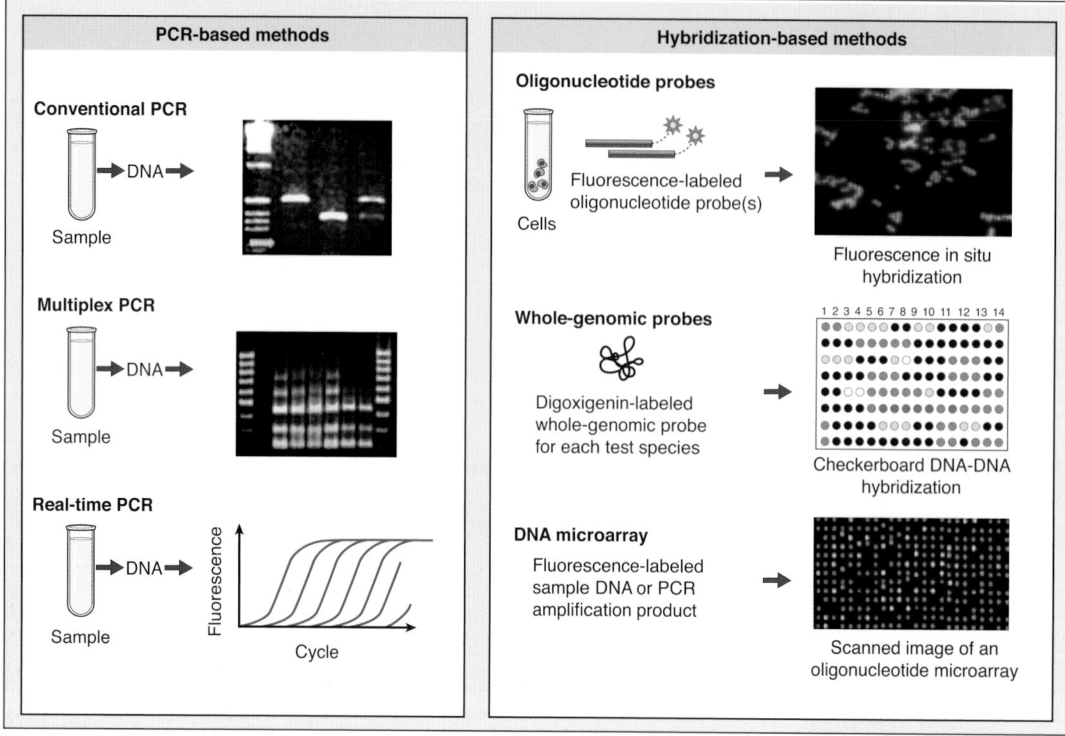

Fig 10-1 Molecular techniques used in the detection and identification of oral microflora. (Adapted with permission from Asikainen and Karched.)

digoxin antibodies conjugated to alkaline phosphatase, and incubated with a chemiluminescent substrate for the enzyme (see Fig 10-1). This method, called **whole genomic checkerboard DNA-DNA hybridization**, has been used to monitor the presence of selected oral bacteria in plaque, saliva, and mucosal surfaces.

In **DNA microarray analysis**, the expression of bacterial (or eukaryotic) genes under different conditions (eg, when the bacteria are sporulating) can be measured. First, a microarray is created by microspotting each gene of a bacterial species on a glass slide. The RNA expressed under two different conditions is extracted and reverse transcribed to cDNA, and the DNA is labeled with a fluorescent label, green for one condition and red for the other condition. The labeled DNA is layered over the microarray. If a gene has been expressed, the labeled DNA corresponding to that RNA will bind to the spot (or set of spots) corresponding to that gene (see Fig 10-1). The relative amounts of the green and red DNA at the spot can be measured and indicate the relative expression of that gene under the different conditions (eg, sporulation).

DNA sequencing can be used to determine the sequence of the 16S RNA gene to identify bacterial species. Viral genomes can be sequenced to identify viruses and their mutants.

In the **dot blot**, clinical samples can be analyzed for the presence of specific nucleic acid sequences by placing a small aliquot on a nitrocellulose filter, followed by the addition of a labeled DNA probe. Pieces of DNA produced by restriction enzyme cleavage of specific palindromic sequences in genomic DNA are separated by electrophoresis, and the pieces are transferred onto a nitrocellulose filter, retaining the same pattern on the electrophoresis gel. The DNA on the filter can then be visualized by hybridizing with a sequence-specific, labeled DNA in a **Southern blot**. This is the basis of restriction endonuclease typing or restriction fragment length polymorphism. In a Northern blot, pieces of RNA (eg, mRNA from a cell or tissue) are electrophoresed, transferred to a nitrocellulose filter, and detected by hybridization with labeled DNA.

Immune detection

Enzyme-linked immunosorbent assay (ELISA) is used to detect either *(1)* antibodies by using antigen-coated wells of a 96-well plastic plate or *(2)* antigens by using antibody-coated wells and detecting the bound antigen by a secondary antibody (Fig 10-2).

Immunofluorescence detection of antigens in or on cell or tissue samples involves the use of fluorescently labeled antibodies specific for the antigen. When the antigen-recognizing antibody is labeled, the procedure is called **direct immunofluorescence** (Fig 10-3). When the antigen-recognizing (specific) "primary" antibody is not labeled, a

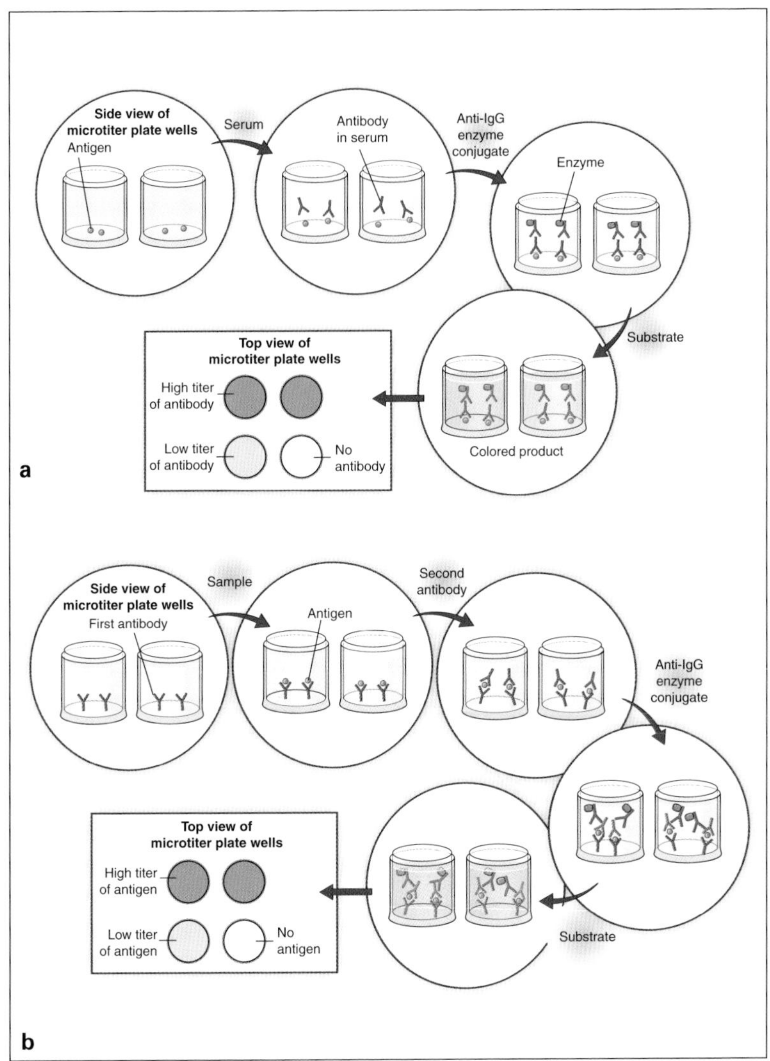

Fig 10-2 Enzyme immunoassays for quantitation of antibody or antigen. *(a)* Antibody detection by antigen-coated wells. *(b)* Antigen capture by antibody-coated wells and detection by secondary antibody.

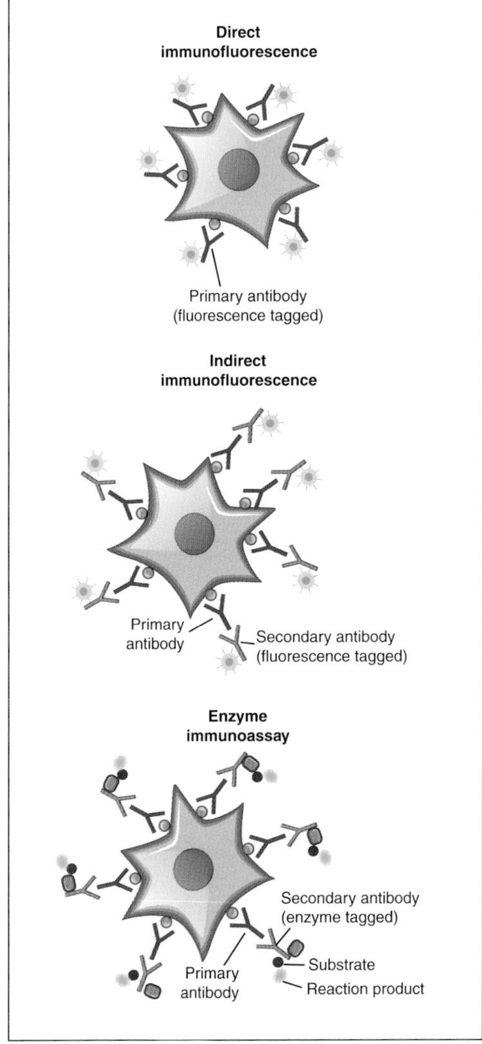

Fig 10-3 Immunofluorescence and enzyme immunoassay for antigen localization in cells.

fluorescently labeled secondary antibody that recognizes the first antibody is used. For example, if the first antibody is a mouse monoclonal antibody, the second antibody may be a rabbit anti-mouse antibody that recognizes the Fc region of the first antibody. This procedure is known as indirect immunofluorescence. The indicator on the antibody can be an enzyme like horseradish peroxidase or alkaline phosphatase, in which case the addition of the substrate will produce a colored product that stains the recognized cells. The enzyme may be on the primary or secondary antibody. This procedure is known as enzyme immunoassay.

Flow cytometry is used to measure the immunofluorescence of cells in suspension labeled with a fluorescent antibody to cell surface antigens. The fluorescence is activated by a laser incident on individual cells as they flow rapidly through the path of the laser. Thus, the fluorescence intensity of each cell can be measured. The intensity data are usually presented as a histogram of the number of cells (y-axis) at each channel of fluorescence intensity (x-axis). For immunologic studies on lymphocytes, the relative amounts of CD4 and CD8 cells can be determined.

Western blotting can be used to identify proteins that have been separated by gel electrophoresis or to detect if patient sera have antibodies against a set of antigens (eg, that of HIV). The proteins are first transferred onto a nitrocellulose filter. The filter is then incubated with an antibody that is specific for the protein of interest or with patient sera. The specific antibody or antibodies in patient sera bind to the target protein or proteins. The bound specific antibody is detected by an enzyme-conjugated antibody against it. The bound patient antibodies can be recognized by an enzyme-conjugated antihuman secondary antibody. Western blot analysis can be used to determine if a patient has antibodies against a number of HIV antigens.

Take-Home Messages

- The resolving power, *d*, of a microscope is the distance between two points that can just be distinguished as being separate. $d = \lambda/2NA$, where λ is the wavelength of light and *NA* is the numerical aperture of the objective lens.
- In phase-contrast microscopy, peaks of light waves that arrive at different times interfere with each other and reduce the intensity of the light. The light rays moving through more dense material are retarded more than those going through the medium, creating a three-dimensional image.
- In fluorescence microscopy, microorganisms are stained with fluorescent dyes (eg, on a specific antibody) and then observed in a fluorescence microscope. Fluorescent compounds absorb light at a particular wavelength and emit light at a higher visible wavelength.
- Differential stains can distinguish different types of microorganisms. The Gram stain delineates two major types of bacteria.
- Culture media should include components that are essential for the growth of certain types of bacteria. Blood agar is useful in the identification of β-hemolytic bacteria. BCYE with iron and L-cysteine is essential for the growth of *Legionella*. Sabouraud dextrose agar is useful in the isolation and growth of fungi.
- Selective media are used to recover particular microorganisms from a mixed sample. MacConkey agar is selective for Gram-negative bacteria. Mannitol salt agar is used to isolate staphylococci, which grow in the presence of high salt.
- DNA probes are synthetic oligonucleotides that can hybridize with specific DNA sequences of the microorganism to be detected in tissues or cells.
- PCR is used to copy particular segments of DNA in an exponential manner to generate about a million copies.
- Real-time PCR can be used to determine the amount of DNA or RNA (by reverse transcription PCR) in a sample by measuring how fast new DNA is made through the increase in fluorescence of a reporter molecule.
- Whole-genomic checkerboard DNA-DNA hybridization is used to detect the presence of certain oral bacteria in plaque, saliva, and mucosal surfaces.
- In DNA microarray analysis, the expression of bacterial (or eukaryotic) genes under different conditions can be measured.
- ELISA is used to detect antibodies or antigens in samples from patient serum or other sources.
- Immunofluorescence detection of antigens in or on cell or tissue samples involves the use of fluorescently labeled antibodies specific for the antigen or fluorescent "secondary" antibodies that bind to the specific "primary" antibodies.
- Flow cytometry is used to measure the immunofluorescence of cells in suspension labeled with a fluorescent antibody to cell surface antigens.

Bibliography

Asikainen S, Karched M. Molecular techniques in oral microbial taxonomy, identification and typing. In: Rogers AH (ed). Molecular Oral Microbiology. Norfolk, UK: Caister Academic, 2008.

Greenwood D, Barer M, Slack R, Irving W. Medical Microbiology, ed 18. Edinburgh: Churchill Livingstone/Elsevier, 2012.

Ingraham JL, Ingraham CA. Introduction to Microbiology: A Case History Approach. Pacific Grove, CA: Brooks/Cole (Thomson), 2004.

Levinson W. Review of Medical Microbiology and Immunology, ed 11. New York: McGraw-Hill, 2010.

Mullis KB, Faloona FA. Specific synthesis of DNA in vitro via a polymerase-catalyzed chain reaction. Methods Enzymol 1987; 155:335–350.

Murray PR, Rosenthal KS, Pfaller MA. Medical Microbiology, ed 7. Philadelphia: WB Saunders, 2013.

Ryan KJ, Ray CG. Sherris Medical Microbiology, ed 5. New York: McGraw-Hill, 2010.

Smithsonian Institution Archives. The History of PCR. siarchives.si.edu/research/videohistory_catalog9577.html. Accessed 8 May 2015.

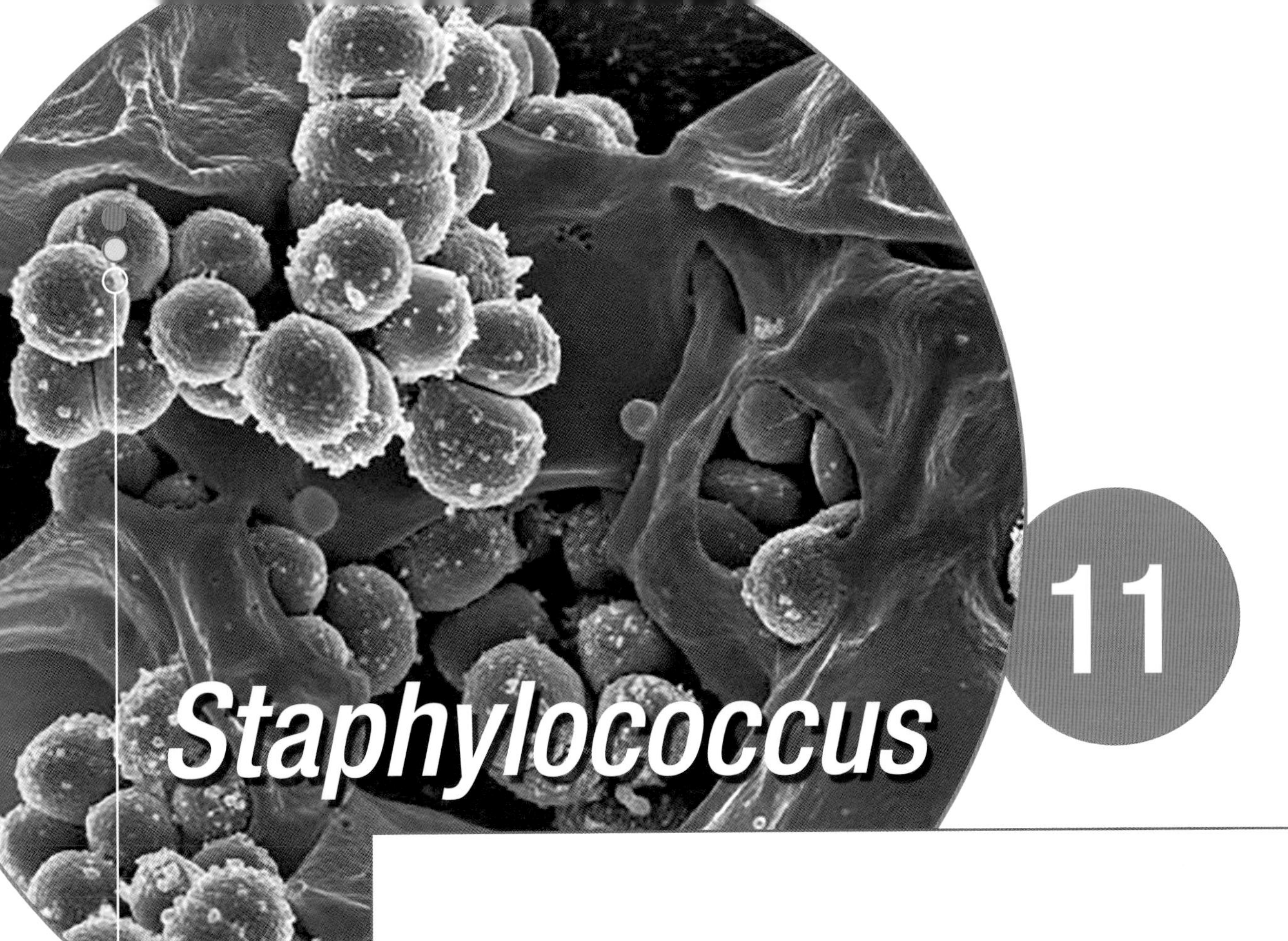

Staphylococci are spherical, facultatively anaerobic, catalase-positive Gram-positive cocci usually arranged in irregular grapelike clusters (Fig 11-1). They are found on the skin and mucous membranes. Staphylococci cause diseases ranging from food poisoning to toxic shock syndrome, wound infections, bacteremia, pneumonia, endocarditis, meningitis, and urinary tract infections. *Staphylococcus aureus*, *Staphylococcus epidermidis*, *Staphylococcus haemolyticus*, *Staphylococcus lugdunensis*, and *Staphylococcus saprophyticus* are the species most commonly associated with disease. *S aureus* is the most virulent and best-known member of the genus. It forms golden colonies because of a carotenoid pigment it produces. It also synthesizes coagulase that binds to a factor in serum, thus mediating the conversion of fibrinogen to fibrin, which polymerizes to form a blood clot. The other species in the genus are generally identified as coagulase-negative cocci.

S aureus

Clinical syndromes and diagnosis

Diseases caused by staphylococcal toxins

S aureus causes a wide range of diseases. Staphylococcal scalded skin syndrome, also called *Ritter disease*, primarily affects newborns and young children and starts with inflammation around the mouth that spreads to the rest of the body. Blisters appear on the skin, followed by peeling of the epithelial cells (desquamation), and the skin looks scalded. The blisters do not contain bacteria or leukocytes, suggesting that that the pathology is caused by a toxin. In bullous impetigo, skin blisters are localized and are infected with the organism. Toxic shock syndrome, caused by toxic shock syndrome toxin-1 (TSST-1)–producing strains of *S aureus*, became a national concern in the United States in 1980 when it was reported that menstruating women using highly absorbent tampons developed this disease (Fig 11-2). The disease is

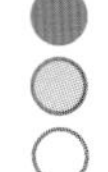

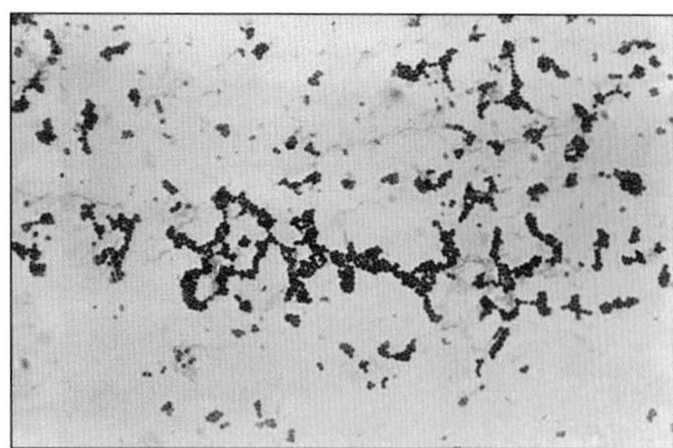

Fig 11-1 Gram stain of *Staphylococcus aureus*. (Public Health Image Library image 2296, courtesy of Dr Richard Facklam.)

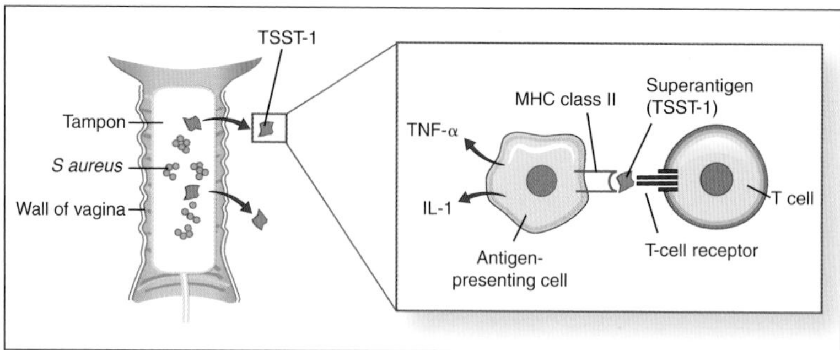

Fig 11-2 Pathogenesis of staphylococcal toxic shock syndrome. IL, interleukin; MHC, major histocompatibility complex; TNF, tumor necrosis factor. (Adapted from Ryan and Ray.)

characterized by fever, low blood pressure, a widespread rash, and involvement of multiple organs. TSST-1 acts as a superantigen and causes the release of multiple cytokines, including tumor necrosis factor.

Staphylococcal food poisoning is caused by heat-stable enterotoxins (thus, heating the food will kill the bacteria but not inactivate the toxin) that contaminate food from an infected food-preparer. About half the carriers are asymptomatic, and colonization is mainly in the nasopharynx. The onset of disease is abrupt after ingestion of contaminated food, with symptoms of vomiting, diarrhea, abdominal pain, and nausea.

Diseases caused by primary infection

S aureus causes a number of cutaneous infections. Impetigo starts as a small reddening of the skin (macule) and progresses to a pustule and additional vesicles with pus. In some cases, Group A streptococci are also associated with this condition. The pyogenic infection of hair follicles results in folliculitis; when folliculitis occurs at the base of the eyelid, it is termed a stye. Furuncles, or boils, are superficial skin infections in hair follicles, sweat glands, or sebaceous glands. Infection can spread from a furuncle into adjacent tissue and form abscesses, forming a carbuncle. This is observed most often on the back of the neck. Carbuncles can result in the spread of the bacteria to other tissues, with concomitant fever and chills.

Bones, joints, deep organs, and surgical wounds can be infected by *S aureus*, which can form abscesses and also lead to bacteremia and endocarditis. More than half of *S aureus* bacteremia cases are the result of surgical procedures or contaminated catheters. *S aureus* endocarditis cases have a mortality rate around 50%. Inhalation of oral secretions containing *S aureus* can result in aspiration pneumonia, especially in the elderly, in young children, and in cystic fibrosis or influenza patients. Necrotizing pneumonia is caused by community-acquired methicillin-resistant *S aureus* (MRSA) and can result in coughing up of blood (hemoptysis), septic shock, and death. *S aureus* can also cause osteomyelitis (localized or generalized infection of bone and bone marrow) and septic arthritis.

Community-acquired MRSA infections in the United States are associated mostly with the USA300 strain, which is highly virulent and contagious and causes epidemic outbreaks of mostly skin and soft tissue infections. Community-acquired MRSA is now the most frequent cause of death by a single infectious agent in the United States. A study in 2008 indicated that MRSA infections account for more deaths each year than AIDS.

S aureus can be diagnosed by Gram staining of clinical specimens taken from the base of an abscess, by nucleic acid amplification tests, and by culturing on blood agar or mannitol salt agar (only *S aureus*, not other staphylococci). The microorganism can also be identified by fluorescence in situ hybridization of DNA probes specific for *S aureus* DNA.

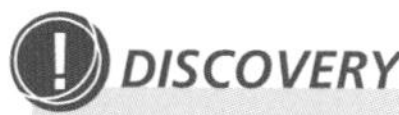

DISCOVERY

S aureus was discovered in 1880 by Sir Alexander Ogston, a Scottish surgeon. He described it as "beautiful tangles, tufts, and chains of round organisms in great numbers which stood out clear and distinct among the pus cells and debris." He was examining pus in the laboratory he had built at the back of his house in Aberdeen.

Pathogenesis and epidemiology

S aureus has a large number of virulence factors that facilitate disease. The polysaccharide capsule inhibits chemotaxis and phagocytosis by leukocytes and mediates attachment to catheters and other synthetic materials. The peptidoglycan has endotoxin-like activity, attracts polymorphonuclear leukocytes, and activates complement. Lysozyme, which is present in mucosal secretions such as tears and saliva, breaks the bond between the two saccharide components of peptidoglycan and thus acts as a natural barrier to staphylococcal infections. Protein A is the main protein in the cell wall of *S aureus* and prevents the antibody-mediated immune response by binding to the Fc portion of immunoglobulin G (IgG). Protein A bound to chromatography gels is also used in the biochemical purification of IgG. Phosphate-containing polymers in the cell wall called teichoic acids can bind to the extracellular matrix component fibronectin and mediate the attachment of staphylococci to mucosal surfaces. The bacteria also express surface-bound coagulase, called clumping factor, that binds fibrinogen.

S aureus expresses and secretes a number of exotoxins that can defend it against the immune system and that cause tissue damage. These include cytotoxins that damage cell membranes or act as hemolysins, causing the leakage of hemoglobin from erythrocytes. Alpha toxin can lyse red blood cells, leukocytes, and other types of cells by forming a pore in the membrane. Beta toxin is a sphingomyelinase C that lyses red blood cells, leukocytes, and fibroblasts. Gamma toxin is a leukocidin and also lyses red blood cells. Panton-Valentine leukocidin is found in all strains of community-acquired MRSA but only in 5% of hospital-acquired strains. Delta toxin acts as a detergent. Phenol-soluble modulins not only lyse host cells but also have antimicrobial activity against other bacteria. *S aureus* also secretes molecules that inhibit neutrophil function, including chemotaxis inhibitory protein of *S aureus* (CHIPS) and extracellular adherence protein (Eap). The golden carotenoid pigment and superoxide dismutase of *S aureus* inhibit the killing activity of neutrophils mediated by reactive oxygen species.

Exfoliative toxin has serine protease activity that can degrade a component of desmosomes that bind cells together. It facilitates staphylococcal scalded skin syndrome. TSST-1 can go through mucosal barriers and acts as a superantigen and thus causes the release of cytokines. This can result in hypovolemic shock. Enterotoxins are associated with food poisoning, are resistant to hydrolysis by gastrointestinal enzymes, and are heat-stable (100°C for 30 min). *S aureus* produces cell-bound and free coagulase that converts fibrinogen to insoluble fibrin.

Staphylococci produce catalase that converts H_2O_2 into H_2O and O_2 as well as hyaluronidase that hydrolyzes the acidic mucopolysaccharide of connective tissue and facilitates the spread of the microorganism in tissues. Fibrinolysin (staphylokinase) can dissolve fibrin clots, also mediating the spread of the infection. *S aureus* and about a third of the strains of staphylococcus produce lipases that degrade the lipids of cell membranes and help with the invasion of cutaneous and subcutaneous tissues.

Staphylococci are found on the skin and in the nasopharynx; moist skin folds can be transiently colonized with *S aureus*. About one-third of healthy adults are persistent carriers of nasopharyngeal *S aureus*. It can be transmitted via respiratory droplets or via contaminated clothing or bed linen. The incidence is higher in hospitalized patients, medical personnel, and individuals who use needles regularly. A large number of nosocomial (hospital-acquired) infections are reported per year. The estimated number of hospitalizations for *S aureus* infection was 478,000 in 2005, according to the Centers for Disease Control and Prevention. Of these, about 278,000 were related to MRSA. Thorough hand washing and aseptic management of lesions can reduce the spread of staphylococci.

Treatment and prevention

In the United States, more than 90% of *S aureus* strains are resistant to penicillin. Semisynthetic penicillins have been developed that are resistant to β-lactamase, including methicillin, nafcillin, and oxacillin. Nevertheless, MRSA strains have become common (30% to 50% of isolates). Vancomycin is effective against MRSA, but vancomycin-resistant strains emerged in 1997.

Linezolid (Zyvox, Pfizer) was approved by the US Food and Drug Administration in 2000 and can be used against vancomycin-resistant strains. Daptomycin (Cubicin, Cubist Pharmaceuticals) was approved in 2003 for the treatment of complicated skin and skin structure infections. Tigecycline (Tygacil, Pfizer) was approved in 2005 for adults with complicated skin and skin structure infections caused by *S aureus* as well as other infections.

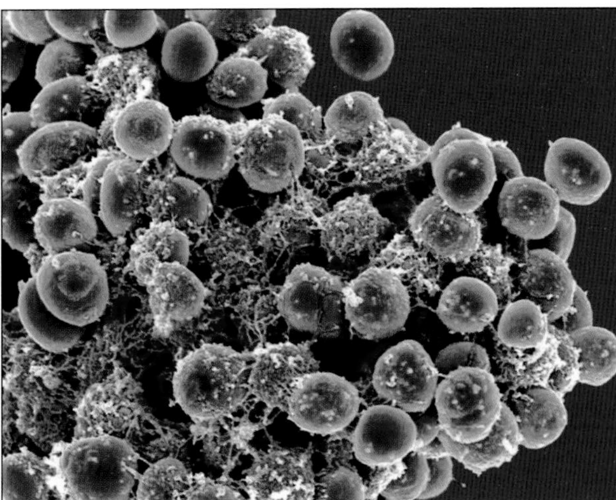

Fig 11-3 *S epidermidis* embedded in an extracellular matrix material. The bacterium is a commensal found on skin and mucosal surfaces. The use of catheters and implants can cause infection in patients. (Public Health Image Library image 18135, courtesy of the National Institute of Allergy and Infectious Diseases.)

S epidermidis, S lugdunensis, and *S saprophyticus*

These are coagulase-negative staphylococci. *S epidermidis* is part of the normal human flora on the skin and mucous membranes and can cause infections of intravenous catheters and heart valves. It may adhere to medical devices through the production of a polysaccharide slime.

S lugdunensis, which is named after Lugdunum (the Latin name for Lyon, France, where it was first isolated), is also a skin commensal, but it is not as frequent a pathogen as *S aureus* and *S epidermidis*. Infections are more similar to those caused by *S aureus*. These staphylococci can form biofilms (Fig 11-3) and can cause highly destructive native valve endocarditis, requiring both antimicrobial therapy and surgical intervention. *S lugdunensis* can also cause urinary tract, wound, intravascular catheter, and implanted medical device infections, as well as bacteremia.

S saprophyticus is associated with urinary tract infections, particularly in sexually active young women. It is the second most prevalent cause of community-acquired urinary tract infections in this population, the most common infection being caused by *Escherichia coli*.

Endocarditis due to coagulase-negative staphylococci is treated with vancomycin or ampicillin/sulbactam and an aminoglycoside. *S epidermidis* is susceptible to linezolid, streptogramins, tigecycline, and daptomycin and has intermediate resistance to vancomycin.

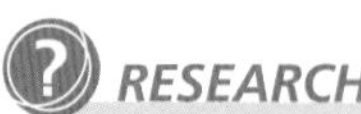

How did *S aureus* become methicillin resistant?

Bibliography

Ala Aldeen D. *Staphylococcus aureus*: Molecular and Clinical Aspects. Chichester, IL: Harwood, 2004.

Centers for Disease Control and Prevention. Methicillin-resistant *Staphylococcus aureus* (MRSA). http://www.cdc.gov/mrsa/-index.html. Accessed 21 May 2015.

Centers for Disease Control and Prevention. Public Health Image Library. phil.cdc.gov. Accessed 4 August 2015.

Frank KL, Del Pozo JL, Patel R. From clinical microbiology to infection pathogenesis: How daring to be different works for *Staphylococcus lugdunensis*. Clin Microbiol Rev 2008;21:111–133.

Greenwood D, Slack R, Peutherer J, Barer M. Medical Microbiology, ed 17. Edinburgh: Churchill Livingstone/Elsevier, 2007.

Krishna S, Miller LS. Host-pathogen interactions between the skin and *Staphylococcus aureus*. Curr Opin Microbiol 2012;15:28–35.

Murray PR, Rosenthal KS, Pfaller MA. Medical Microbiology, ed 6. Philadelphia: Mosby/Elsevier, 2009.

Otto M. Looking toward basic science for potential drug discovery targets against community acquired MRSA. Med Res Rev 2010;30:1–22.

Ryan KJ, Ray CG. Sherris Medical Microbiology, ed 5. New York: McGraw-Hill, 2010.

Take-Home Messages

- Staphylococci are spherical, facultatively anaerobic, catalase-positive Gram-positive cocci usually arranged in irregular grapelike clusters.
- *S aureus* infection can cause staphylococcal scalded skin syndrome, bullous impetigo, toxic shock syndrome, and food poisoning.
- TSST-1 acts as a superantigen and stimulates the immune system to release multiple cytokines.
- *S aureus* infection can also result in bacteremia, endocarditis, aspiration pneumonia, necrotizing pneumonia, osteomyelitis, and septic arthritis.
- The virulence factors of *S aureus* include the capsule, the peptidoglycan, protein A, teichoic acids, clumping factor, alpha toxin, beta toxin, gamma toxin, CHIPS, Eap, exfoliative toxin, TSST-1, enterotoxins, catalase, hyaluronidase, fibrinolysin, and lipases.
- In the United States, more than 90% of *S aureus* strains are resistant to penicillin. Vancomycin, linezolid, daptomycin, and tigecycline can be used for specific manifestations of the infection.
- *S epidermidis* is part of the normal human flora on the skin and mucous membranes.
- *S epidermidis* can cause infections of intravenous catheters and heart valves.
- *S saprophyticus* is the second most prevalent cause of community-acquired urinary tract infections in sexually active women.

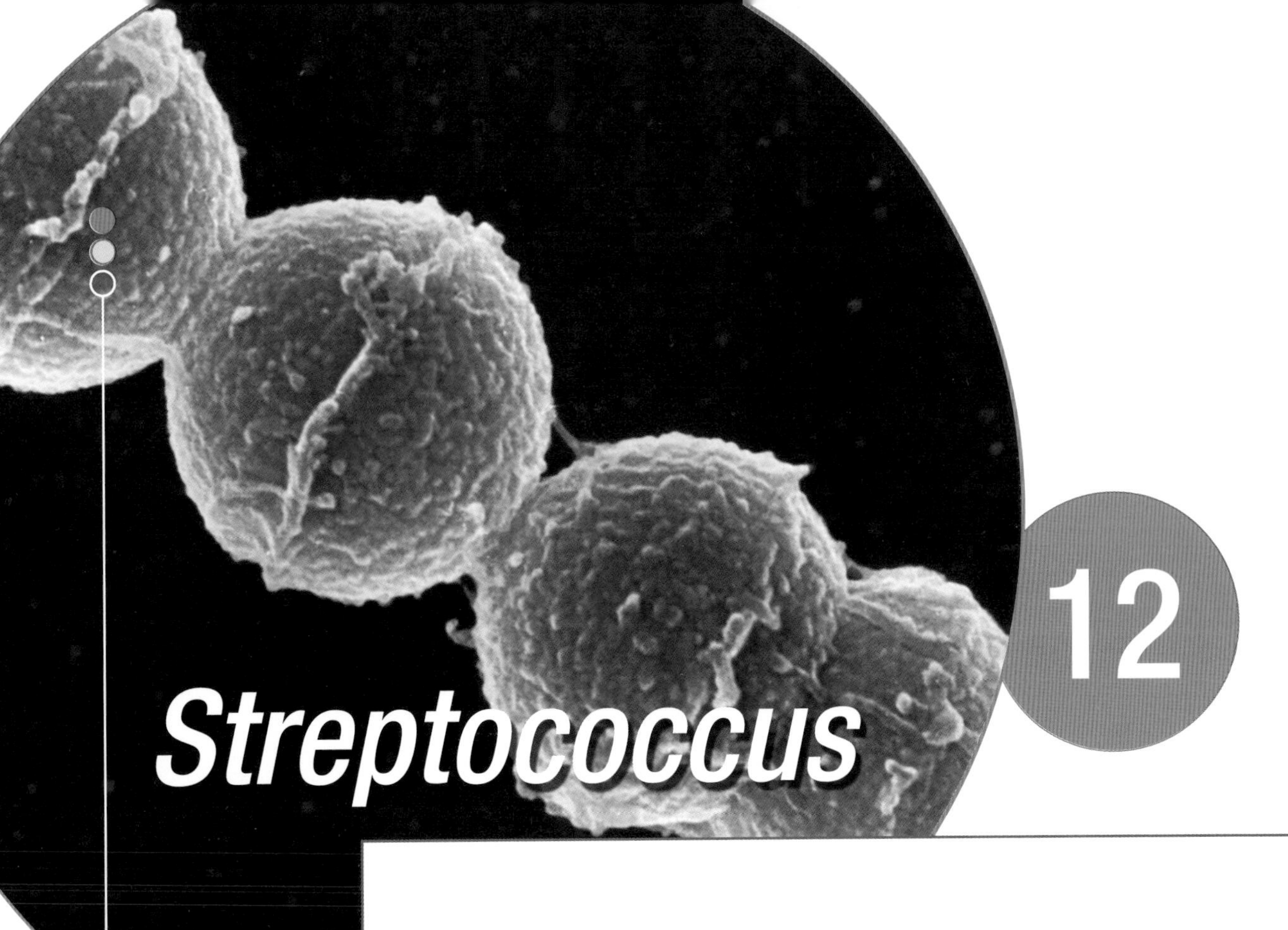

12 Streptococcus

Streptococci are Gram-positive cocci arranged in pairs and chains and are part of the normal microflora of humans and animals. They are facultatively anaerobic (ie, they can grow both aerobically and anaerobically), except for some species that grow under a CO_2-enhanced atmosphere (which are called *capnophilic*). They are catalase-negative and ferment carbohydrates, resulting in the production of lactic acid. Streptococci have been classified into groups by the microbiologist Rebecca Lancefield based on the cell surface carbohydrates, and thus the groups are named after her (eg, Lancefield Group A). Group A streptococci include *Streptococcus pyogenes*, which causes "strep throat" and scarlet fever (Fig 12-1). Group B streptococci include *Streptococcus agalactiae*, which is associated with neonatal diseases. Viridans streptococci include the oral microorganisms *Streptococcus mutans* and *Streptococcus mitis*. *Streptococcus pneumoniae* is the most common cause of pneumonia (Fig 12-2). Group D streptococci include *Enterococcus faecium*.

Groups A and B cause a particular type of hemolysis called β-hemolysis when grown on sheep blood agar plates (Fig 12-3). This is characterized by a yellow ring around the colony, indicative of the release of hemoglobin from erythrocytes. Viridans streptococci and *S pneumonia* cause α-hemolysis, which produces a greenish color around the colonies when grown on blood agar. γ-hemolysis is somewhat of a misnomer, referring to the absence of hemolysis.

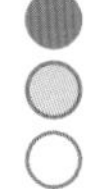

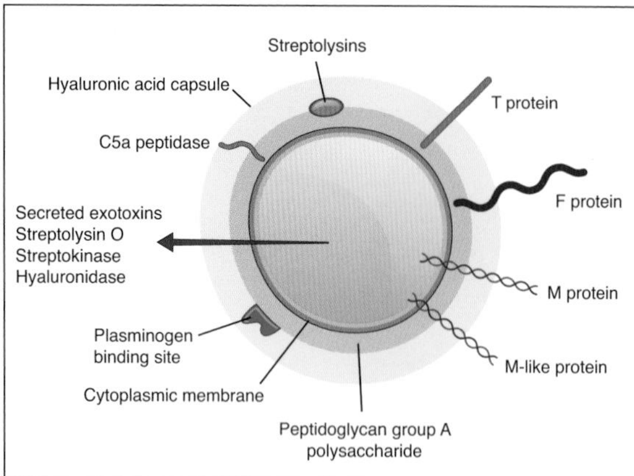

Fig 12-1 Schematic diagram of the location of virulence-associated molecules of *S pyogenes*. (Adapted from Greenwood et al.)

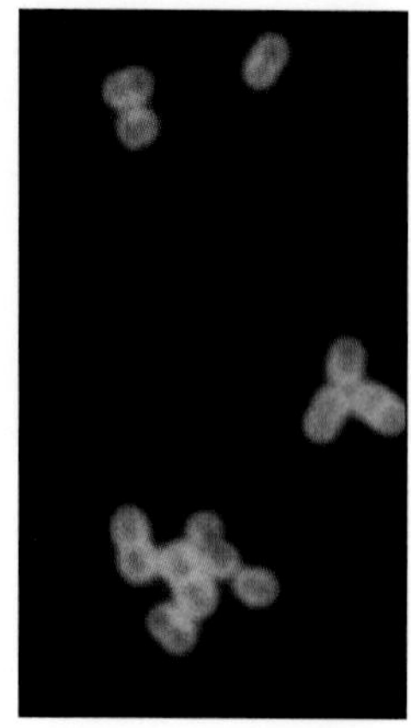

Fig 12-2 *S pneumoniae*. (Public Health Image Library image 1003, courtesy of Dr M. S. Mitchell.)

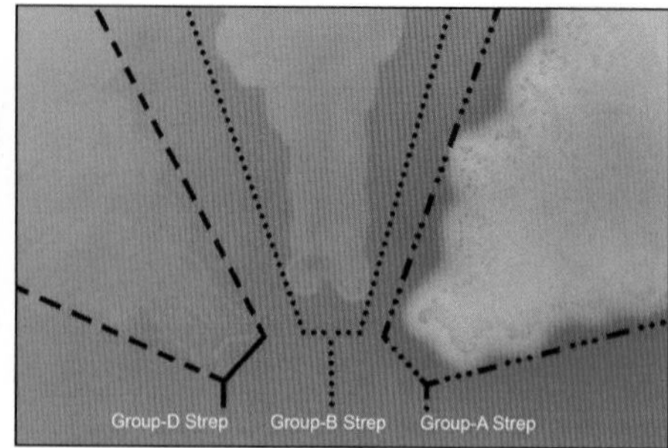

Fig 12-3 Hemolytic reactivity of streptococci on a blood agar plate. (Public Health Image Library image 10862, courtesy of Dr Richard Facklam.)

S pyogenes (Group A *Streptococcus*)

Clinical syndromes and diagnosis

Group A *Streptococcus* (*S pyogenes*) may cause suppurative (pus-forming) or nonsuppurative diseases. The suppurative diseases include pharyngitis (generally known as strep throat) (Fig 12-4); scarlet fever, which is a complication of streptococcal pharyngitis; erysipelas, an acute infection of the skin; and other skin infections called pyoderma or impetigo. The two very severe diseases caused by *S pyogenes* are invasive fasciitis (commonly known as *flesh-eating disease*), and streptococcal toxic shock syndrome caused by pyrogenic exotoxins of the bacterium. The nonsuppurative diseases include acute rheumatic fever and acute glomerulonephritis.

An oral manifestation of scarlet fever is "strawberry tongue," characterized by a red surface that is seen after an initial yellowish-white coating on the tongue is shed (Fig 12-5). Pharyngitis caused by *S pyogenes* can be recognized by the erythematous appearance of the pharynx, together with an exudate.

The microorganism can be identified by microscopy, antigen detection, and culture. The Signify Strep A Dipstick kit detects carbohydrate antigens of Group A streptococci collected on a throat swab.

Pathogenesis and epidemiology

The diseases caused by *S pyogenes* are mediated by the virulence factors of the bacterium. The capsule comprises hyaluronic acid identical to that found in the connective tissue of the host and hence does not elicit an immune response. It also inhibits the phagocytosis of the bacterium by phagocytes. The M protein is located at the end of the fimbriae and is also involved in inhibiting phagocytosis.

M-like proteins on *S pyogenes* bind the Fc portion of immunoglobulin (Ig) G and IgM, thereby preventing the recognition of antibody-bound bacteria by Fc receptors on phagocytes. The F protein binds fibronectin, which is part of the extracellular matrix and in turn binds cell surface integrin; this interaction mediates bacterial attachment to epithelial cells of the pharynx and the skin.

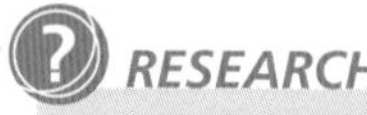

RESEARCH

What is the potential role of autophagy in fighting intracellular Group A *Streptococcus* infections?

Pyrogenic exotoxins are produced by lysogenic strains of streptococci and induce fever, act as superantigens, and are responsible for the red rash observed in scarlet fever. Superantigens can interact with both major histocompatibility complex class II (MHC II) molecules and T-cell receptors, thereby stimulating the T cell to proliferate and release cytokines in an uncontrolled manner. The excessive amount of cytokines cause damage to epithelial and endothelial cells, leading to the leakage of capillaries and hypotension. Streptococcal superantigens include the pyrogenic exotoxins A, C, and G through J. Superantigens are thought to be involved in toxic shock syndrome, scarlet fever, and food poisoning.

Streptolysin S is a nonimmunogenic, cell-bound hemolysin that can lyse erythrocytes, leukocytes, and platelets and can facilitate the autolysis of phagocytes. Streptolysin O is immunogenic and can kill leukocytes by autolysis. The antistreptolysin O diagnostic test is used to determine a recent infection and to evaluate whether it may have caused rheumatic fever or glomerulonephritis. Streptokinase (fibrinolysin) catalyzes the conversion of plasminogen to plasmin, which then degrades fibrin in blood clots,

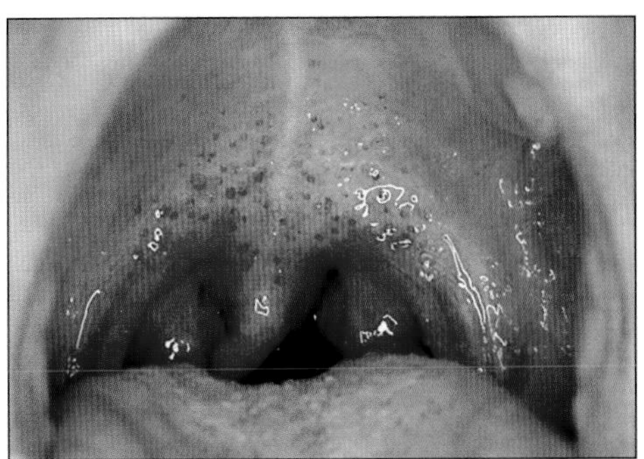

Fig 12-4 Strep throat, caused by Group A *Streptococcus*, characterized by inflammation of the oropharynx and small red spots (petechiae) on the soft palate. The bacteria are spread via direct contact with mucus from the nose or throat of infected individuals or by contact with infected skin wounds. (Public Health Image Library image 3185, courtesy of Dr Heinz F. Eichenwald.)

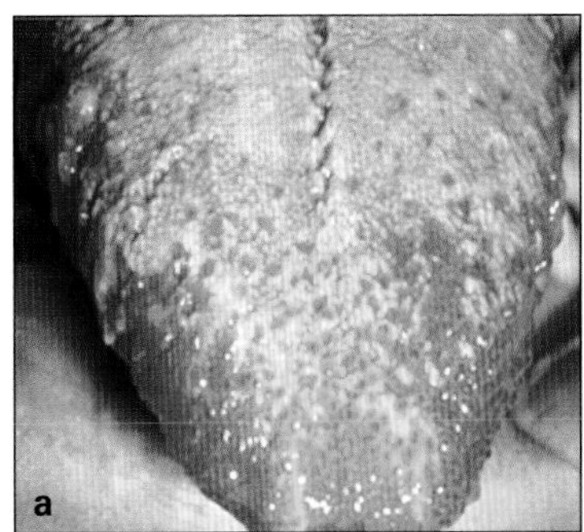

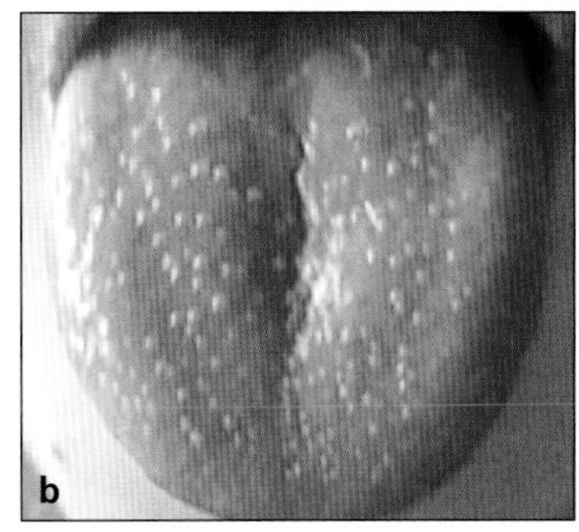

Fig 12-5 White strawberry tongue with prominent papillae *(a)* and red strawberry tongue of scarlet fever with edematous papillae *(b)*. (Reprinted with permission from Neville et al.)

thereby causing the disintegration of the blood clot. This is a mechanism by which the microorganism can invade the host beyond the protective blood clot around the lesion. DNase degrades DNA present in pus, thereby reducing its viscosity and facilitating the spread of the microorganism. Hyaluronidase, also called *spreading factor*, degrades hyaluronic acid, which is part of connective tissue in the host.

S pyogenes is spread by airborne droplets and by contact. It is present as a commensal in the pharynx of healthy children and young adults. Disease is caused by strains that are acquired soon before the onset of the disease and that are capable of infection of the pharynx or skin before the immune system can generate antibodies. Lack of competition from other organisms is also a factor.

Treatment and prevention

The bacterium is very sensitive to penicillin. Erythromycin can be used for patients with penicillin allergies. Azithromycin can be substituted if erythromycin causes gastrointestinal disturbances, like vomiting. Antibiotic prophylaxis is used for patients with a history of rheumatic fever to prevent the recurrence of the disease. Antibiotic prophylaxis is also useful before procedures that can induce transient bacteremia (eg, dental procedures).

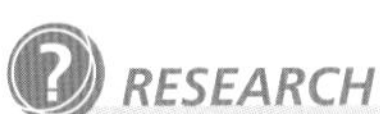

RESEARCH

Can streptococcal pili be utilized in vaccines?

S agalactiae (Group B *Streptococcus*)

Clinical syndromes and diagnosis

Group B *Streptococcus* is part of the normal flora of the female genital tract and is a significant cause of septicemia, pneumonia, and meningitis in newborn children. It can cause early-onset neonatal disease during the first 7 days of life, with bacteremia, pneumonia, and meningitis. Symptoms include fever, lethargy, and difficulty feeding. With early diagnosis and supportive care, the mortality rate is below 5%. Some survivors of meningitis will have neurologic complications, including blindness and deafness. Late-onset neonatal disease is caused by infection from an exogenous source and is characterized by bacteremia and meningitis. The disease causes coughing, congestion, fever, lethargy, and difficulty feeding. Although the survival rate is high, neurologic complications are seen in 25% to 50% of the patients who develop meningitis. *S agalactiae* can cause urinary tract and wound infections and postpartum endometritis in pregnant women.

S agalactiae can be diagnosed by a polymerase chain reaction test, culturing in a selective medium (that inhibits the growth of other microorganisms), and the CAMP test (where a heat-stable protein produced by the bacterium enhances the β-hemolysis caused by *Staphylococcus aureus*).

Pathogenesis and epidemiology

The virulence factors for *S agalactiae* include hemolysins, the capsule, C5a peptidase, hyaluronidase, IgA-binding proteins, and adhesins. The microorganism tends to infect neonates lacking maternal antibodies to it or those with low levels of complement. Antibodies that develop against the type-specific capsular antigens are protective against infection. In some strains, the polysaccharides that constitute the capsule have terminal sialic acid (neuraminic acid) residues that can inhibit the alternate complement pathway. *S agalactiae* is found in the genitourinary tract and the lower gastrointestinal tract. Infection can occur in utero, at the time of birth, or during the first few months of life.

Treatment and prevention

Although the minimum inhibitory concentration (MIC) of penicillin G for *S agalactiae* is about 10 times greater than it is with *S pyogenes*, it is the preferred drug. Patients who have serious infections are treated with a combination of penicillin and an aminoglycoside, and those with penicillin allergy are given vancomycin. Pregnant women should be screened for *S agalactiae*, and those who are infected or have high risk factors should be given intravenous penicillin G 4 hours before birth.

S pneumoniae

S pneumoniae are oval or lancet-shaped Gram-positive cocci that appear either as diplococci (arranged in pairs) or as short chains. They are part of the mitis group of viridans streptococci (see later section). They form α-hemolytic colonies on blood agar; the green color results from the degradation of hemoglobin by pneumolysin (see Fig 12-3). The C polysaccharide of the bacterium is a teichoic acid that is exposed on the surface, even protruding through the capsule. It interacts with a serum protein called C-reactive protein, which is elevated under acute inflammatory conditions and can be used to monitor inflammation. The F-antigen is a lipoteichoic acid anchored in the bacterial membrane. Phosphocholine is a component of these teichoic acids and is necessary for the action of the bacterial autolysin that hydrolyzes the cell wall during cell division.

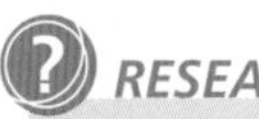

What is the structure of teichoic acid?

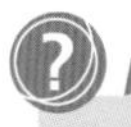

RESEARCH

Why are bacterial autolysins important during bacterial cell division?

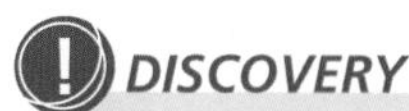

In 1928, while working at the Ministry of Health of the United Kingdom, Frederick Griffith used smooth (S, capsulated) and rough (R, noncapsulated) colonies of *S pneumoniae* in mice and interpreted his results with the transforming principle (see Fig 6-16). The pathogenic S forms caused the death of mice, whereas the R forms were nonpathogenic. Although heat-killed S forms did not cause death if administered alone, they resulted in death of the mice when given together with R forms, and live S forms were isolated from the animals. Griffith concluded that the R forms were transformed by a "transforming principle" from the dead S forms. In 1944, while working at the Rockefeller Institute for Medical Research, Oswald Avery, Colin MacLeod, and Maclyn McCarty identified the transforming agent as DNA.

Clinical syndromes and diagnosis

S pneumoniae can cause pneumonia as a result of the aspiration of an endogenous oral organism that then infects the lower lobes of the lungs, hence the name lobar pneumonia. The symptoms include fever between 39°C and 41°C, severe shaking chills, productive cough with bloody sputum, and chest pain. Patients who have splenic dysfunction cannot efficiently clear the bacteria from blood and can suffer severe pneumonia. Sinusitis and otitis media caused by *S pneumoniae* are usually preceded by a viral infection of the upper respiratory tract. Otitis is usually seen in children.

Meningitis is caused by *S pneumoniae* that has spread into the central nervous system following bacteremia or ear and sinus infections. It is the cause of most pneumococcal meningitis cases in children and adults. Septicemia (bacteremia) is observed in about a quarter of patients with pneumonia and in about 80% of patients with meningitis.

Diagnosis can be done by Gram staining of sputum, which reveals lancet-shaped diplococci. The Quellung (swelling) reaction, in which antibodies to the bacteria are added and cause an increase in the refractiveness next to the bacteria, can be used to confirm the staining test. The C polysaccharide of the bacterium can be detected in the urine of patients with bacteremia or in the cerebrospinal fluid in patients with meningitis using an immunoassay. In the bile solubility test, colonies of *S pneumoniae* disintegrate after exposure to bile. The microorganism can also be identified by its sensitivity to the chemical optochin while growing on blood agar plates.

Pathogenesis and epidemiology

S pneumoniae binds epithelial cells of the oropharynx via its adhesin proteins. The bacteria produce secretory IgA protease that interferes with entrapment in mucin that is normally mediated by secretory IgA. They also secrete pneumolysin that creates pores in ciliary epithelial cells and phagocytes. One of the pathogenic mechanisms of *S pneumoniae* is to elicit a strong inflammatory response via the activation of the alternative complement pathway by teichoic acid and fragments of peptidoglycan. The classical complement pathway is activated by pneumolysin, and this results in the production of proinflammatory cytokines such as interleukin-1 (IL-1) and tumor necrosis factor-alpha (TNF-α), which in turn cause leukocyte migration, tissue destruction, and fever. Bacterial phosphocholine facilitates binding to platelet-activating factor receptors on cells in the lungs and meninges as well as to leukocytes and platelets. Binding may be followed by cell entry, which may facilitate the spreading of the bacterium into the blood and the central nervous system. The capsule of *S pneumoniae* prevents phagocytosis and destruction and is found on strains that cause disease.

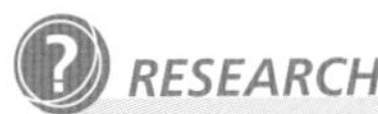

RESEARCH

What is the difference between the alternative and classical complement pathways?

S pneumoniae is commensal in the throat and nasopharynx of healthy individuals and is transmitted via respiratory droplets. Disease occurs when the bacteria spread to the lungs, causing pneumonia, or to the sinuses, ears, and meninges, causing sinusitis, otitis media, and meningitis, respectively. Bacterial pneumonia is usually preceded by a viral respiratory infection and is related to other conditions that interfere with defense against bacteria, such as chronic pulmonary disease, diabetes, congestive heart failure, or dysfunction of the spleen.

Treatment and prevention

Penicillin is the drug of choice. Penicillin-resistant strains arose in 1977, and now 15% to 30% of strains worldwide are multidrug resistant (ie, resistant to three or more classes of drugs). In the case of severe infections, vancomycin with ceftriaxone or a fluoroquinolone is used.

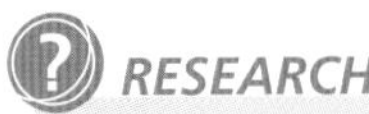

RESEARCH

What are the mechanisms of action of vancomycin, ceftriaxone, and fluoroquinolones?

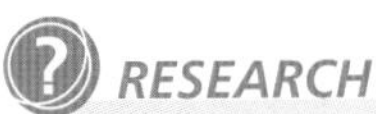

RESEARCH

How might *S pneumoniae* acquire the ability to become antibiotic resistant?

A vaccine that includes antigens from 23 different serotypes (Pneumovax [Merck] and Pnu-Imune [Wyeth]) protects against most strains and is long lasting. However, it is not highly effective in people especially at risk for pneumococcal disease (eg, renal transplant patients, young children, and the elderly). The pneumococcal conjugate vaccine (PCV13) protects against 13 strains of *S pneumoniae* and is recommended for infants and toddlers. In this vaccine, the polysaccharide antigens are conjugated to proteins to elicit helper T cell responses. The 23-valent polysaccharide vaccine stimulates mature B cells, and this response is not well developed in very young children.

RESEARCH

Can infection by noncapsulated pneumococci be protective against capsulated pneumococci?

Viridans Streptococci

Viridans streptococci are characterized by their α-hemolytic properties in blood agar, characterized by the production of a green border around the colonies (see Fig 12-3). The name comes from *viridis*, which is Latin for "green." Most viridans streptococci are commensals in the oropharynx and in the gastrointestinal and genital tracts. They have been placed in four groups, based on 16S rRNA sequence analysis:

1. Salivarius group (*Streptococcus salivarius, Streptococcus thermophilus, Streptococcus vestibularis*)
2. Mitis group (*Streptococcus oralis, Streptococcus gordonii, Streptococcus sanguinis, Streptococcus parasanguinis, S pneumoniae, Streptococcus cristatus, S mitis*)
3. Anginosus group (*Streptococcus constellatus, Streptococcus intermedius, Streptococcus anginosus*)
4. Mutans group (*Streptococcus sobrinus, S mutans*)

The anginosus group is associated with head and neck, brain, lung, and abdominal infections as well as abscess formation, and these streptococci have β-hemolytic activity. The salivarius group can cause bacteremia and endocarditis. The mitis group is associated with subacute endocarditis, pneumonia, and meningitis, and the mutans group initiates dental caries and can cause bacteremia. Although viridans streptococci are very sensitive to penicillin, with MICs less than 0.1 μg/mL, the bacteria in the mitis group have developed moderate (MIC in the range of 0.2 to 2 μg/mL) and high (MIC greater than 2 μg/mL) resistance.

Take-Home Messages

- Streptococci are Gram-positive cocci arranged in pairs and chains and are one of the normal microflora of humans and animals.
- They are catalase-negative and ferment carbohydrates, with the production of lactic acid.
- *Streptococcus* Groups A and B cause a particular type of hemolysis called *β-hemolysis* when grown on sheep blood agar plates.
- *S pyogenes* infections can cause pharyngitis, scarlet fever, erysipelas, and pyoderma and impetigo.
- The virulence factors of *S pyogenes* include the capsule, M protein, F protein, pyrogenic exotoxins, streptolysin S, streptolysin O, streptokinase, DNase, and hyaluronidase.
- *S agalactiae* is part of the normal flora of the female genital tract and can cause septicemia, pneumonia, and meningitis in newborns.
- In some strains of *S agalactiae*, capsular polysaccharides have terminal sialic acid residues that can inhibit the alternative complement pathway.
- Patients with a serious infection are treated with a combination of penicillin and an aminoglycoside.
- *S pneumoniae* can cause pneumonia, following aspiration of an endogenous oral organism that infects the lower lobes of the lungs, as well as meningitis and septicemia.
- The virulence factors of *S pneumoniae* are secretory IgA protease, pneumolysin, phosphocholine, and the capsule.
- A vaccine comprising antigens from 23 different serotypes of *S pneumoniae* protects against most strains. The pneumococcal conjugate vaccine protects against 13 strains of the bacterium.
- Most viridans streptococci are commensals in the oropharynx and in the gastrointestinal and genital tracts. They are divided into four groups: salivarius, mitis, anginosus, and mutans.

Bibliography

Centers for Disease Control and Prevention. Pneumococcal Vaccination. http://www.cdc.gov/vaccines/vpd-vac/pneumo/default.htm#-vacc. Accessed 29 May 2015.

Centers for Disease Control and Prevention. Public Health Image Library. phil.cdc.gov. Accessed 4 August 2015.

Dockrell DH, Whyte MK, Mitchell TJ. Pneumococcal pneumonia: Mechanisms of infection and resolution. Chest 2012;142:482–491.

Greenwood D, Slack R, Peutherer J, Barer M. Medical Microbiology, ed 17. Edinburgh: Churchill Livingstone/Elsevier, 2007.

Maeda Y, Goldsmith CE, Coulter WA, et al. The viridans group streptococci. Rev Med Microbiol 2010;21(4):69–79.

Murray PR, Rosenthal KS, Pfaller MA. Medical Microbiology, ed 6. Philadelphia: Mosby/Elsevier, 2009.

Musser JM, DeLeo FR. Toward a genome-wide systems biology analysis of host-pathogen interactions in group A *Streptococcus*. Am J Pathol 2005;167:1461–1472.

Neville BW, Damm DD, Allen CM, Bouquot JE. Oral and Maxillofacial Pathology, ed 3. St Louis: Saunders, 2009.

Ofek I, Hasty DL, Doyle RJ. Bacterial Adhesion to Animal Cells and Tissue. Washington, DC: ASM, 2003.

Rajagopal L. Understanding the regulation of Group B Streptococcal virulence factors. Future Microbiol 2009;4:201–221.

Ryan KJ, Ray CG. Sherris Medical Microbiology, ed 5. New York: McGraw-Hill, 2010.

Miscellaneous Gram-Positive Bacilli

13

This chapter focuses on numerous species of Gram-positive bacilli. These include the aerobic or facultatively anaerobic spore-forming bacilli *Bacillus anthracis* and *Bacillus cereus*, the aerobic or facultatively anaerobic non–spore-forming bacilli *Corynebacterium diphtheriae* and *Listeria monocytogenes*, the facultatively anaerobic or strictly anaerobic *Actinomyces*, and the aerobic *Nocardia* species.

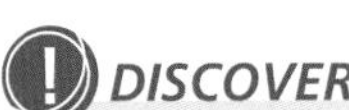

In 1863, the French parasitologist Casimir Davaine reported that anthrax can be transmitted by the injection of blood from diseased animals to healthy ones and that rod-shaped microscopic bodies could be found in blood from these animals. Because the animals did not get sick in the absence of these rod-shaped bodies, Davaine proposed that the disease is caused by these microorganisms. In 1877, Robert Koch was able to culture these organisms using pure culture techniques and observed their filamentous structure, together with translucent bodies (spores) inside them. Koch demonstrated that the dry spores could survive in the environment, explaining how the disease could be transmitted to animals (eg, sheep) from fields that had not been used for grazing for long periods. Koch defined the criteria, now known as *Koch's postulates*, that need to be met to prove that a particular microorganism causes a particular disease. Louis Pasteur developed an attenuated *B anthracis* vaccine and field-tested it with sheep, goats, and cows that were protected from the disease; grateful local farmers cheered and carried Pasteur on their shoulders.

B anthracis

These rod-shaped bacteria generate spores aerobically and form filamentous structures (Fig 13-1). They have a prominent polypeptide capsule composed of D-glutamate, which can be visualized by "negative staining" with India ink (Fig 13-2). Antibodies against the capsule are not protective. The bacteria form mucoid-type colonies as a result of their capsule.

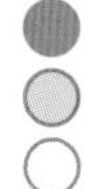

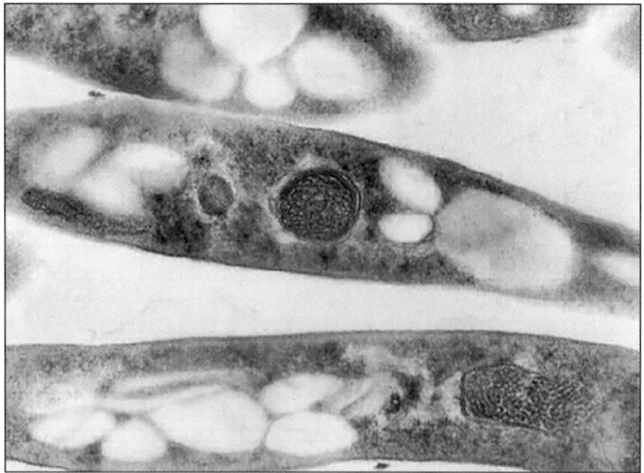

Fig 13-1 Transmission electron micrograph of *B anthracis*. (Public Health Image Library image 1824, courtesy of Dr Sherif Zaki and Elizabeth White.)

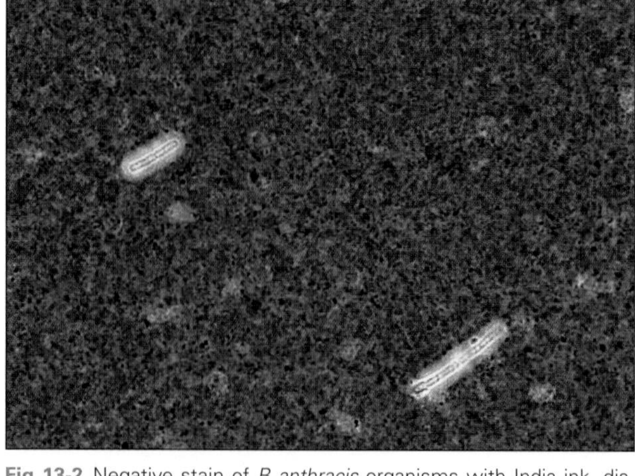

Fig 13-2 Negative stain of *B anthracis* organisms with India ink, displaying the extensive capsule that resists staining. (Public Health Image Library image 1882, courtesy of Larry Stauffer, Oregon State Public Health Laboratory.)

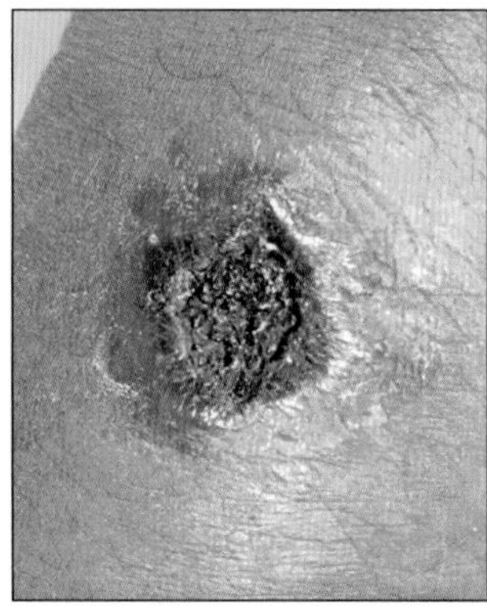

Fig 13-3 Anthrax lesion on the skin of the forearm caused by the bacterium *B anthracis*. The disease has manifested itself as a cutaneous ulceration, which has begun to turn black, hence the origin of the name *anthrax*, after the Greek word for coal. (Public Health Image Library image 2033, courtesy of Dr James H. Steele.)

Clinical syndromes and diagnosis

Anthrax is primarily a disease of livestock, but it can infect people in close contact with these animals. Cutaneous anthrax is caused by *B anthracis* spores entering abrasions in the skin. After the spores germinate, edema develops at the site, which then transforms into a papule, a vesicle, a malignant pustule, and a necrotic ulcer with a black scab, termed an eschar (Fig 13-3). The infection may spread from this ulcer and cause sepsis, leading to death in about 20% of patients if untreated.

Inhalation anthrax is also called *pulmonary anthrax* and "woolsorter's disease." It can have a long incubation period (1 to 43 days) in the nasal passages, or the spores can be engulfed by macrophages and transported to mediastinal lymph nodes. The disease appears initially like a viral respiratory illness, with fever, myalgias, malaise, and a nonproductive cough; it can then progress to respiratory failure, sepsis, and shock. The mortality rate is greater than 95% if untreated.

B anthracis can be identified by Gram staining of infected blood samples, visualization of the capsule by negative staining or direct fluorescence antibody against a capsular antigen test, and the polymerase chain reaction.

Pathogenesis and epidemiology

The virulence factors of *B anthracis* are the poly-D-glutamic acid capsule and anthrax toxin. Anthrax toxin consists of three proteins: *(1)* protective antigen (PA), *(2)* lethal factor (LF), and *(3)* edema factor (EF). PA facilitates the cellular entry of the other two toxins. After binding to its receptor on the cell surface, PA is cleaved by cellular proteases and forms a heptameric prepore. LF, which is a zinc metalloprotease, inhibits cell growth. EF is an adenylate cyclase that causes an increase in the intracellular concentration of cyclic adenosine monophosphate (cAMP). LF and EF bind to the heptamer and are endocytosed. In the acidified endosome, the prepore transforms into a pore, releasing the factors into the cell.

B anthracis spores are transmitted through exposed skin or mucous membranes from contaminated soil or infected animal products or by contact with sick animals to cause cutaneous anthrax. Inhalation anthrax is rare in humans and more common in herbivores. Nevertheless, specially prepared anthrax spores are a biological and bioterrorism weapon.

Treatment and prevention

Treatment requires early antibiotic treatment. Ciprofloxacin or doxycycline treatment for 60 days is recommended for adults. Amoxicillin should be prescribed for children and pregnant women.

Vaccination of animal herds and people in endemic areas is necessary for adequate protection. Animals that die of anthrax are usually incinerated or buried. The current vaccine, known as AVA (Anthrax Vaccine Adsorbed) and BioThrax (Emergent BioSolutions), is produced from the cell-free filtrates of a toxigenic strain of *B anthracis* and contains PA as well as aluminum hydroxide as an adjuvant.

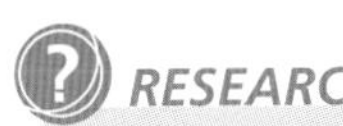

RESEARCH

What did the outbreaks of anthrax in 1979 in Sverdlovsk, Russia (currently Ekaterinburg) and in 2001 in the United States teach us about the disease?

B cereus

B cereus resembles *B anthracis* but lacks the capsule. It is a saprophyte found in soil, water, and vegetation. It is found in most raw foods.

Clinical syndromes and diagnosis

B cereus causes food poisoning, gastroenteritis, ocular infections, and intravenous catheter-mediated sepsis. The emetic (vomiting) form is caused by contaminated rice, in which heat-resistant spores survive and germinate, and occurs within 6 hours of ingestion. The infection results in nausea, vomiting, and abdominal cramps, similar to enteritis caused by *Escherichia coli* or *Salmonella enterica*. The diarrheal form is transmitted via contaminated meat or vegetables and occurs within 8 to 24 hours of ingestion.

Diagnosis is based on culturing samples from the suspected food. *B cereus* forms large, gray, irregular "anthracoid" colonies after incubation on blood agar.

Pathogenesis and epidemiology

Spores of *B cereus* can survive in soil. The heat-stable enterotoxin (vomiting toxin) acts as a superantigen and causes gastroenteritis with vomiting. The heat-labile enterotoxin (diarrheal toxin) ADP-ribosylates a cell surface G protein, resulting in the stimulation of adenylate cyclase, the production of cAMP, fluid loss, and diarrhea.

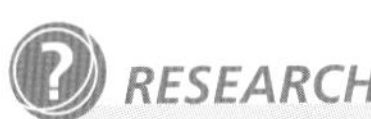

RESEARCH

What is the prevalence of *B cereus* in rice samples obtained from retail food stores?

Treatment and prevention

Treatment is symptomatic. Proper refrigeration of food is essential. Cooked rice should not be kept warm for long periods.

Bacillus stearothermophilus and Bacillus subtilis

These species are used in sterilization monitoring. *B stearothermophilus* spores in a culture medium are placed in autoclaves and exposed to moist 121°C to 132°C heat for 15 minutes. They are then placed in medium at 37°C to grow. If growth is observed, it indicates that the autoclave is malfunctioning. Similarly, *B subtilis* spores are utilized to monitor sterilization by dry heat (171°C for 1 hour or 160°C for 2 hours). Killing of these species following these treatments ensures that the sterilization devices would be able to eliminate other less resistant microorganisms.

C diphtheriae

C diphtheriae are aerobic or facultatively anaerobic, Gram-positive, non–spore-forming, club-shaped rods, which are wider at one end. They form short chains or clumps and cause respiratory and cutaneous diphtheria. Other species that cause disease are *Corynebacterium ulcerans* (pharyngitis and pharyngeal ulcers) and *Corynebacterium jeikeium* (bacteremia and intravenous catheter colonization). *Corynebacteria* have a complex cell wall architecture. Beyond the plasma membrane and the peptidoglycan layer is an arabinogalactan layer and an "outer membrane" of mycolic acids with acyl chains in the range of 22 to 36 carbon atoms. The latter membrane corresponds to the outer membrane of Gram-negative bacteria and is similar to the overall architecture of *Mycobacteria*. In addition, there is a layer of free polysaccharides, glycolipids, and proteins.

Clinical syndromes and diagnosis

C diphtheriae can cause respiratory or cutaneous diphtheria. The respiratory disease can be classified into anterior nasal diphtheria, pharyngeal and tonsillar diphtheria, and laryngeal diphtheria. The symptoms of respiratory diphtheria develop within approximately 2 to 5 days of exposure and include malaise, low-grade fever, sore throat, exudative pharyngitis, and the formation of a thick "pseudomembrane" comprising bacteria, lymphocytes, plasma cells, fibrin, and dead cells. The pseudomembrane may cause airway obstruction, and hence the disease has to be treated expeditiously. Cultures may not always reveal the organism; polymerase chain reaction of the exotoxin gene can provide a definitive diagnosis. Myocarditis may develop and lead to congestive heart failure, cardiac arrhythmias, and even death. Neuropathy can develop in the soft palate and pharynx and lead to oculomotor and ciliary paralysis, as well as peripheral neuritis.

Cutaneous diphtheria is caused by the entry of the bacterium into subcutaneous tissue through breaks in the skin. The infection causes a papule that evolves into a nonhealing ulcer, sometimes covered with a grayish membrane.

Pathogenesis and epidemiology

The main virulence factor of *C diphtheriae* is the exotoxin secreted by the bacterium. The B subunit of the toxin binds to cell surface receptors through its receptor-binding domain. The membrane-translocation domain of the protein facilitates the entry of the A subunit into the cytoplasm. The A subunit adenosine diphosphate (ADP)-ribosylates elongation factor 2 (EF-2)

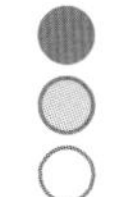

by transferring ADP-ribose from nicotinamide adenine dinucleotide, resulting in the inhibition of protein synthesis. A single molecule of A subunit can kill the target cell by acting enzymatically on all EF-2s.

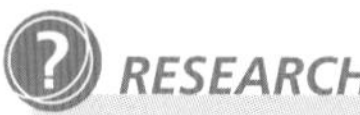

RESEARCH

What is the function of elongation factor?

C diphtheriae is transmitted by inhalation of airborne droplets or skin contact at the site of a preexisting lesion. Humans are the only natural host. Some patients can harbor the bacteria for weeks or months and become convalescent pharyngeal or nasal carriers. *C ulcerans* can infect animals.

In 1921, there were 206,000 cases of diphtheria in the United States, causing 15,520 deaths. After the 1920s, diphtheria rates began to decline following the introduction of vaccination. There were no reported cases in the United States between 2004 and 2008. In 2011, 4,887 cases were reported worldwide to the World Health Organization.

Treatment and prevention

Treatment involves early administration of diphtheria antitoxin and penicillin G or erythromycin to eliminate the organism and terminate toxin production. Active immunization is achieved with diphtheria toxoid during childhood (as part of the DTaP vaccine) and with booster shots every 10 years (Tdap).

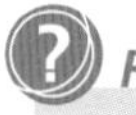

RESEARCH

What do "T" and "aP" represent in the DTaP and Tdap vaccines? What is the difference between DTaP and Tdap?

L monocytogenes

L monocytogenes is a non–spore-forming, facultatively anaerobic bacillus measuring 0.4 μm by 1.0 to 1.5 μm. It is found in water, soil, food, and the gastrointestinal tracts of humans and animals and causes listeriosis, manifesting as meningitis and bacteremia. Listeriosis is seen primarily in neonates, pregnant women, immunocompromised patients with defective cell-mediated immunity, and the elderly. However, the disease can also develop in healthy individuals.

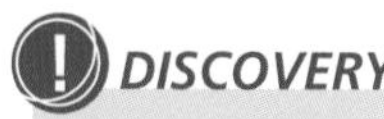

DISCOVERY

Everitt Murray was Lecturer in Pathology at Cambridge University when in 1926 he and his colleagues isolated a bacterium that was infecting and killing laboratory rabbits. They first named it *Bacterium monocytogenes*; the name was later changed to *Listerella monocytogenes* and finally to *Listeria monocytogenes* in honor of Joseph Lister, the Scottish surgeon who introduced the use of antiseptics in the treatment of wounds.

Clinical syndromes and diagnosis

Early-onset neonatal disease is acquired transplacentally in utero and results in disseminated abscesses and granulomas. Late-onset disease occurs soon after birth and causes meningitis or meningoencephalitis with septicemia. In healthy adults, *L monocytogenes* causes mild, influenza-like illness. In immunocompromised patients, it causes severe illness, including meningitis, bacteremia, and high-grade fever. Listeriosis should be suspected in organ-transplant patients, patients with cancer, or pregnant women developing meningitis.

The microorganism may be identified by culturing blood or cerebrospinal fluid samples on blood agar. Cold enrichment may be used to distinguish *Listeria* from rapidly growing bacteria. Biochemical and serologic tests are used for definitive identification.

Pathogenesis and epidemiology

L monocytogenes can grow in macrophages and epithelial cells. Pathogenic strains can exit the phagocytotic vacuole, multiply in the cytoplasm, recruit actin from the cytoplasm to induce motility, and then infect neighboring cells, where they start this cycle again. Thus, listeriae can spread in host tissues protected from humoral immunity. Virulent strains produce listeriolysin O and two different phospholipase C enzymes, both acting as hemolysins, and proteins that mediate attachment to cells, called internalins. The ActA protein mediates the polymerization of actin and the motility of *Listeria* in the host cell.

Organisms can cross the intestines and are carried by the lymph or blood to mesenteric lymph nodes, the spleen, and the liver. Kupffer cells in the liver destroy many of the organisms and initiate the immune response involving T-cell proliferation and cytokine induction.

L monocytogenes is transmitted via contaminated food, such as milk, soft cheese, undercooked meat, processed meats, unwashed raw vegetables, cabbage, and cantaloupes. It can replicate at 4°C to 8°C. It can reach the fetus in pregnant women who are bacteremic. The incidence of disease in AIDS patients is 100-fold greater than the normal population. The mortality rate in the United States is about 16% to 18%.

RESEARCH

What is the molecular target of phospholipase C? What is the result of this activity?

Treatment and prevention

The treatment of choice is gentamicin with either penicillin or ampicillin. Trimethoprim-sulfamethoxazole has bactericidal activity against *L monocytogenes* and is thus useful in treatment. Raw or partially cooked foods of animal origin, soft cheeses, and unwashed raw vegetables should be avoided, especially for individuals at risk.

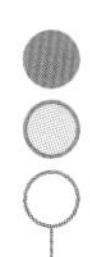

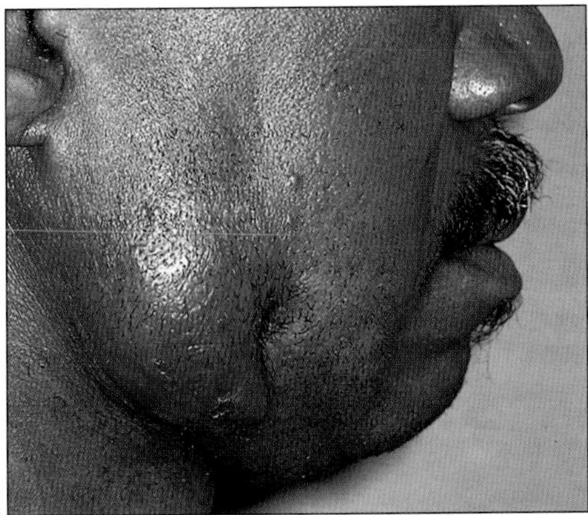

Fig 13-4 Cervicofacial actinomycosis manifested as a "lumpy jaw" with abscess and fibrosis. (Reprinted with permission from Marx and Stern.)

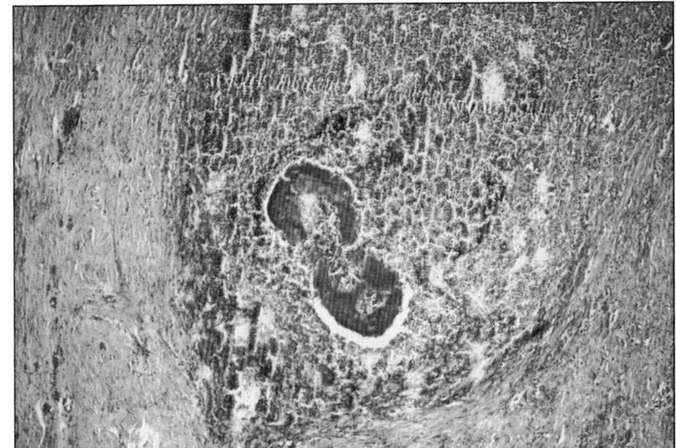

Fig 13-5 A colony of *Actinomyces*, or sulfur granule, surrounded by a ring of necrosis and then by fibrosis. The surrounding structures may explain the resistance of *Actinomyces* to the immune system and antibiotics. (Reprinted with permission from Marx and Stern.)

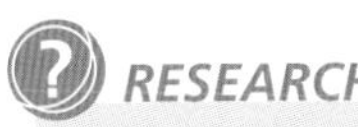

RESEARCH

How could *L monocytogenes* be used in immunotherapy against cancer?

Actinomyces

Actinomyces is one of the genera of Actinomycetes, the others being *Nocardia* and *Streptomyces*. The name *Actinomyces* is derived from the Greek for "ray fungus." These bacteria are facultatively anaerobic or strict anaerobic Gram-positive bacilli and form long branching filaments reminiscent of *Mycobacteria*, but they are not acid-fast. They cause slowly developing, chronic infections. Most human infections by this genus are caused by the species *Actinomyces israelii*. *Actinomyces* form sulfur granules in the sinus tract of the infected patient; the granules are a conglomeration of filamentous microorganisms bound by calcium phosphate.

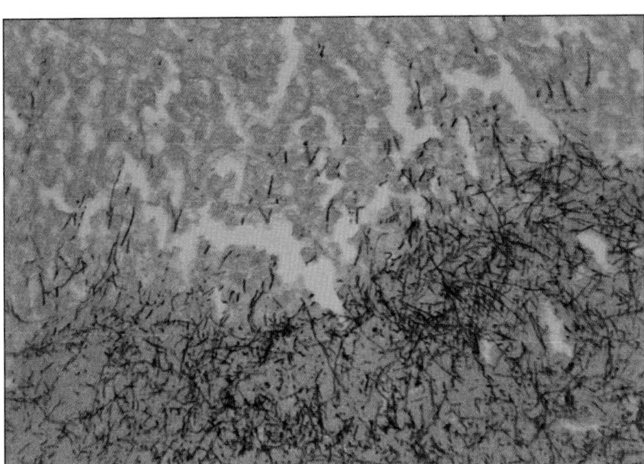

Fig 13-6 Gram staining of a sulfur granule showing the filamentous and sometimes coccoid *Actinomyces* microorganisms. (Reprinted with permission from Marx and Stern.)

Clinical syndromes and diagnosis

Actinomyces species cause opportunistic infections of the upper respiratory tract, the gastrointestinal tract, and the female genital tract when normal mucosal barriers are disrupted. Actinomycosis is characterized by multiple abscesses connected by sinus tracts. Cervicofacial actinomycosis may occur after dental procedures, and the dentist may be the first to diagnose the swelling resulting from this condition (Fig 13-4). Thoracic actinomycosis is established via inhalation or via the bloodstream. Abdominal infections are caused usually by surgery or trauma. Pelvic infections may result from abdominal infections or the use of intrauterine devices. Central nervous system infections are caused by *Actinomyces* spread from other locations.

For diagnosis, specimens are obtained from the lesion by biopsy, needle aspiration, or fiber-optic bronchoscopy. The sulfur granules are crushed between glass slides and stained with the Gram and Ziehl-Neelsen methods, revealing Gram-positive mycelia. The microorganisms can also be visualized in tissue sections by the direct fluorescent antibody test.

Pathogenesis and epidemiology

The characteristic feature of actinomycosis is chronic granulomatous lesions that form abscesses connected by sinus tracts. Colonies of *Actinomyces* can be observed in the abscesses and sinus tracts, presenting as sulfur granules, circumscribed by an area of necrosis, which in turn is surrounded by fibrosis (Figs 13-5 and 13-6). Most actinomycosis infections are endodontic, odontogenic, or implant-

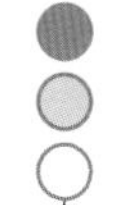

associated infections. Invasive dental procedures, trauma to the oral cavity, and poor oral hygiene are risk factors for the development of actinomycosis.

Treatment and prevention

Treatment of *Actinomyces* infections involves surgical debridement and long-term administration of penicillin, macrolides, carbapenems, or clindamycin. An undrained focus must be suspected if infections do not respond to prolonged therapy. Good oral hygiene is necessary for prevention.

Nocardia

Nocardia is another genus of Actinomycetes. They are strictly aerobic, Gram-positive bacilli that form branched hyphae. Their cell wall contains mycolic acids that are also found in *Mycobacteria*. In contrast to *Actinomyces*, they are acid-fast when stained with the Ziehl-Neelsen dye. *Nocardia asteroides* causes bronchopulmonary disease that can spread to the skin, and central nervous system *Nocardia brasiliensis* causes cutaneous disease.

Clinical syndromes and diagnosis

In the United States, *Nocardia* primarily causes pulmonary and central nervous system infections. Symptoms of bronchopulmonary infections include dyspnea (difficulty in breathing), fever, and cough. In the central nervous system, *Nocardia* infections may cause single or multiple brain abscesses. Cutaneous infections result in cellulitis (inflammation of the soft or connective tissue), pyoderma (purulent skin disease), chronic ulcerative lesions, and subcutaneous abscesses. Lymphocutaneous infections involve the local lymph nodes. *Nocardia* can cause a chronic granulomatous disease, termed mycetoma, particularly in the foot. It may spread to the bone, connective tissue, and muscle. The foot gets enlarged, with multiple draining sinus tracts.

Pathogenesis and epidemiology

Nocardia is found worldwide in organic-rich soil and causes exogenous infections; ie, the bacteria are not among the normal human flora. It colonizes the oropharynx. The lower airways may be infected by aspiration of oral secretions. It can survive in phagocytes and causes necrosis and abscess formation. Patients with impaired cell-mediated immunity and immunocompetent patients with chronic pulmonary disease, such as bronchitis and emphysema, are at risk for *N asteroides* infection. *N brasiliensis* can cause skin infections in immunocompetent persons.

Treatment and prevention

Treatment involves proper wound care and trimethoprim-sulfamethoxazole (Bactrim, Roche) treatment for 6 weeks or more. The prognosis is poor for immunocompromised patients with disseminated disease.

Bibliography

American Society for Microbiology. Significant Events in Microbiology 1861–1999. http://www.asm.org/index.php/choma3/71-membership/archives/7852-significant-events-in-microbiology-since-1861. Acessed 9 July 2015.

Burkovski A. Cell envelope of corynebacteria: Structure and influence on pathogenicity. ISRN Microbiol 2013;2013:935736.

Centers for Disease Control and Prevention. Diphtheria. www.cdc.gov/diphtheria/clinicians.html. Accessed 1 June 2015.

Centers for Disease Control and Prevention. Public Health Image Library. phil.cdc.gov. Accessed 4 August 2015.

DiSalvo A. Actinomycetes. Microbiology and Immunology On-line. University of South Carolina School of Medicine. http://www.microbiologybook.org/mycology/mycology-2.htm. Accessed 1 June 2015.

Engleberg NC, DiRita V, Dermody TS. Schaechter's Mechanisms of Microbial Disease, ed 4. Baltimore and Philadelphia: Lippincott Williams & Wilkins, 2007.

Greenwood D, Slack R, Peutherer J, Barer M. Medical Microbiology, ed 17. Edinburgh: Churchill Livingstone/Elsevier, 2007.

Marx RE, Stern D. Oral and Maxillofacial Pathology: A Rationale for Diagnosis and Treatment, ed 2. Chicago: Quintessence, 2012.

Murray PR, Rosenthal KS, Pfaller MA. Medical Microbiology, ed 6. Philadelphia: Mosby/Elsevier, 2009.

Ryan KJ, Ray CG. Sherris Medical Microbiology, ed 5. New York: McGraw-Hill, 2010.

Society for General Microbiology. Obituary notice: E.G.D. Murray, 1890–1964. J Gen Microbiol 1967;46:1–21.

Stevenson LG. Robert Koch. Encyclopedia Britannica Online. www.britannica.com/EBchecked/topic/ 320834/Robert-Koch. Accessed 1 June 2015.

Todar K. *Bacillus anthracis* and anthrax. Todar's Online Textbook of Bacteriology. www.textbookofbacteriology.net/Anthrax_3.html. Accessed 1 June 2015.

Vázquez-Boland JA, Kuhn M, Berche P, et al. *Listeria* pathogenesis and molecular virulence determinants. Clin Microbiol Rev 2001;14:584–640.

Wright JG, Quinn CP, Shadomy S, Messonnier N. Use of anthrax vaccine in the United States. MMWR Morb Mort Wkly Rep 2010;59:1–30.

Take-Home Messages

- *B anthracis* and *B cereus* are spore-forming bacilli. *C diphtheriae*, *L monocytogenes*, and *Actinomyces* are non–spore-forming bacilli.
- The virulence factors of *B anthracis* are the capsule and anthrax toxin.
- *B anthracis* causes cutaneous and inhalation anthrax. Early antibiotic treatment with ciprofloxacin or doxycycline is essential.
- *B cereus* causes food poisoning. Contaminated rice causes the emetic form of the disease. Treatment is symptomatic.
- *B stearothermophilus* and *B subtilis* are used for sterilization monitoring.
- *C diphtheriae* causes respiratory and cutaneous diphtheria. The respiratory infection results in the formation of a pseudomembrane in the throat that may cause airway obstruction; thus, the disease must be treated expeditiously.
- The *C diphtheriae* exotoxin inhibits protein synthesis.
- Diphtheria antitoxin and penicillin G or erythromycin are administered to treat infections by *C diphtheriae*.
- *L monocytogenes* causes granulomas and meningitis in neonates and bacteremia and fever in immunocompromised adults.
- The bacterium produces listeriolysin O and two phospholipase C enzymes (both acting as hemolysins) and internalins that mediate attachment to cells.
- *Actinomyces* species cause opportunistic infections and multiple abscesses connected via sinus tracts.
- Cervicofacial actinomycosis may occur after dental procedures.
- *Nocardia* primarily causes pulmonary and central nervous system infections.

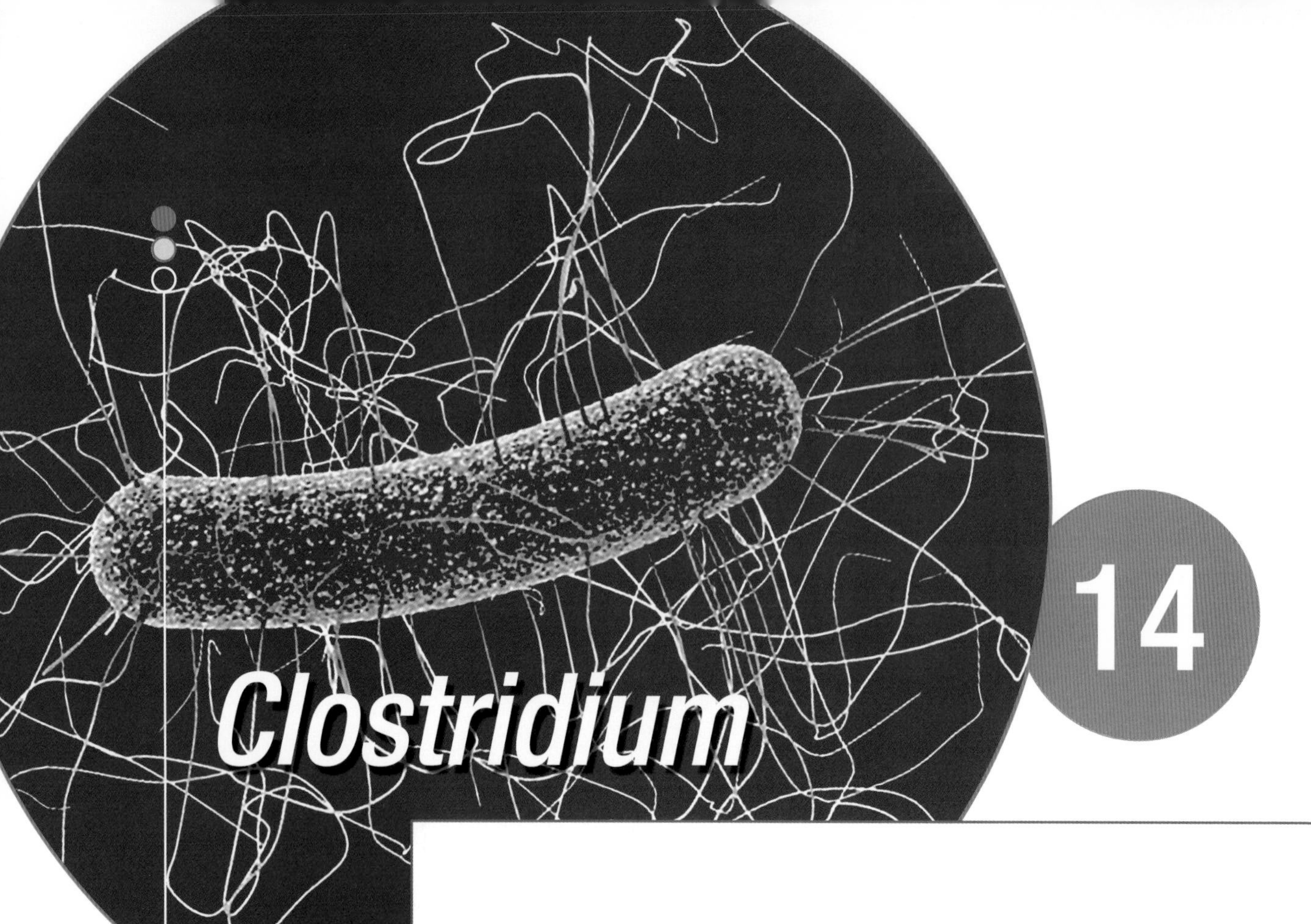

Clostridia are Gram-positive, strictly anaerobic, spore-forming bacilli. The genus includes *Clostridium perfringens, Clostridium tetani, Clostridium botulinum, Clostridium difficile*, and *Clostridium septicum*.

C perfringens

Clinical syndromes and diagnosis

C perfringens causes a range of dangerous diseases. Myonecrosis (gas gangrene) is a life-threatening disease resulting in muscle necrosis, shock, renal failure, and death, usually within 2 days of onset. The typically observed gas in the infected tissues is the hydrogen and carbon dioxide generated by the metabolic activity of the bacteria. In some infections, soft tissues can develop erythema and edema accompanied by gas formation, a condition termed cellulitis; however, unlike gas gangrene, there is no pain, swelling, or toxicity.

C perfringens can also infect the endometrium, particularly when necrotic tissue is retained in the uterus (eg, following abortions performed with nonsterile instruments). Suppurative myositis can ensue when pus accumulates in the planes of muscle.

C perfringens can cause food poisoning, with abdominal cramps and watery diarrhea and without nausea or vomiting. Type C microorganisms secrete beta toxin and cause necrotizing enteritis, characterized by bloody diarrhea and peritonitis.

Pathogenesis and epidemiology

C perfringens forms spores that enable the microorganism to survive adverse environmental conditions in water, soil, and sewage. It is also a normal resident of the gastrointestinal tract. Exposure to exogenous *C perfringens* is more common than the spread of the endogenous bacteria. Infection is initiated in damaged tissue with an impaired blood supply and reduced oxygen tension, extravasated fluid, foreign

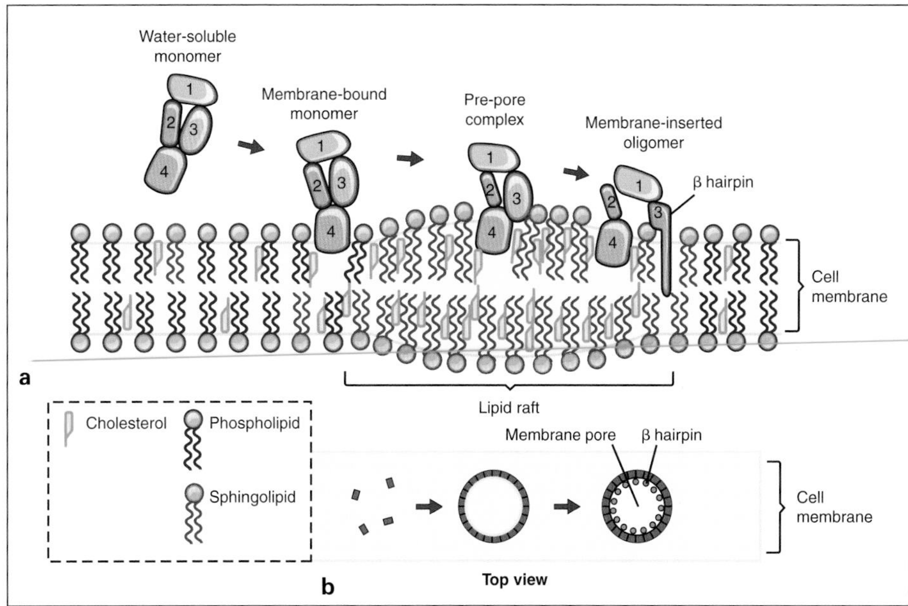

Fig 14-1 Perfringolysin O. *(a)* Insertion of monomers into membranes containing cholesterol. *(b)* Schematic structure of the perfringolysin O oligomeric membrane pore complex.

bodies, and a coincident pus-producing infection. The bacteria produce a large number of toxins and enzymes that damage adjacent healthy tissue, rendering the environment more anaerobic and hence favorable for multiplication. Hyaluronidase breaks down the extracellular matrix and mediates the spread of the bacterium. Collagenase and other proteinases degrade connective tissue and muscle. Alpha toxin is a phospholipase C that hydrolyzes phosphatidylcholine and sphingomyelin, leading to the lysis of erythrocytes, leukocytes, and platelets. It also causes increased vascular permeability and bleeding. Beta toxin creates pores in cell membranes and causes the loss of mucosa, leading to necrotizing enteritis.

Perfringolysin O forms transmembrane pores in cholesterol-containing membranes (Fig 14-1). Epsilon toxin increases the vascular permeability of the gastrointestinal wall. The enzymatic component of iota toxin adenosine diphosphate (ADP) ribosylates actin, causing the rounding and death of cells, and thus contributes to the necrotic activity of type E *C perfringens*. Enterotoxin, which is produced by type A strains that are involved in food poisoning as well as gas gangrene and soft tissue infections, binds to the brush border membrane in the small intestine and causes ion and fluid loss.

Treatment and prevention

Because infection can lead to deterioration of tissue as well as death, rapid treatment is essential. The necrotic tissue needs to be removed by surgical debridement, and high-dose penicillin G therapy should be initiated. Broad-spectrum cephalosporins are also added to the treatment, because nonclostridial anaerobes and Enterobacteriaceae also infect the wound site. Patients can be placed in hyperbaric oxygen chambers to increase the tissue levels of oxygen to slow the spread of the disease.

To prevent infections, skin and deep tissue wounds should be cleaned thoroughly, foreign bodies and dead tissue should be removed, and hematomas should be drained. Prophylactic antibiotics should also be given. Prevention of food poisoning by *C perfringens* can be avoided by proper cooking and refrigeration.

C tetani

C tetani, which is a motile spore-forming bacillus, causes tetanus, also known as trismus (or lockjaw). It frequently stains Gram-negative, and the spore at one end of the bacterium gives the appearance of a drumstick.

Clinical syndromes and diagnosis

C tetani infections cause generalized or localized tetanus. Generalized tetanus often affects the masseter muscles initially, which results in the inability to open the mouth, or trismus. Contraction of the facial muscles leads to the characteristic *risus sardonicus*, the apparent "smile." In severe cases, back muscles contract to deform the body backward. When the autonomic nervous system is affected, the disease leads to cardiac arrhythmias, blood pressure fluctuations, dehydration, and hyperthermia. Untreated generalized tetanus has a mortality rate ranging from 15% to greater than 60%.

Localized tetanus involves only the muscles in the area of primary injury; the prognosis is favorable for this condition. Cephalic tetanus results when the cranial nerves are affected and has a very poor prognosis.

Neonatal tetanus is caused by the infection of the umbilical cord when it is severed under nonsterile conditions, and it has a very poor prognosis when the mother is not immunized against tetanus.

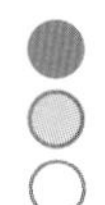

Pathogenesis and epidemiology

The neurotoxic effects of *C tetani* are mediated by tetanospasmin, or tetanus toxin. It is synthesized as an A-B toxin, where the B chain binds to a receptor on neuronal membranes, and the A chain, a zinc endopeptidase, degrades a protein involved in neurotransmitter release via vesicles in presynaptic nerve terminals of inhibitory synapses. The inhibition of the inhibitory neurotransmitters glycine and γ-aminobutyric acid causes the excitatory synaptic activity to be unregulated, leading to spastic paralysis. Tetanus toxin affects peripheral motor end plates, the spinal cord, the brain, and the sympathetic nervous system.

Spores of *C tetani* are found in fertile soil and the gastrointestinal tract of many animals and humans. The disease follows minor trauma to the skin with a spore-contaminated splinter or nail. Spore germination occurs preferably in necrotic tissue and tissue with a poor blood supply. It is estimated that there are more than 1 million cases worldwide, with a mortality rate between 20% and 50%. In the United States, there have been an average of 29 reported cases per year in the period 1996 to 2009.

Treatment and prevention

Treatment should begin with debridement of the primary wound and immediate administration of metronidazole and human tetanus immunoglobulin, followed by vaccination with tetanus toxoid. For preventive vaccination, three doses of the DTaP vaccine are given at 2, 4, and 6 months and again at 15 through 18 months of age. A DTaP booster is recommended for children ages 4 through 6 years. Because immunity to tetanus decreases over time, older children need to get the Tdap vaccine. This vaccine contains a full dose of tetanus and lower doses of diphtheria and pertussis and should also be administered every 10 years as a booster, since it contains inactivated tetanus and diphtheria toxins, which are not as immunogenic as vaccines with live attenuated microorganisms.

C botulinum

Clinical syndromes and diagnosis

C botulinum can cause food-borne botulism, particularly following the ingestion of home-canned foods. The symptoms include weakness and dizziness a few days later, dry mouth, blurred vision, abdominal pain, and constipation. The progressive disease caused by *C botulinum* is characterized by weakening of peripheral muscles and flaccid paralysis. This can lead to respiratory paralysis. Complete recovery may take months to years as the paralyzed nerve endings regenerate. Infant botulism is caused by the ingestion of spores in food, such as honey. The initial symptoms include failure to thrive, constipation, and a weak cry.

Pathogenesis and epidemiology

Botulinum toxin inhibits cholinergic synaptic transmission, thereby blocking the excitation of muscle, leading to flaccid paralysis. The toxin is an A-B toxin, where the A subunit has zinc-endopeptidase activity. The B subunit binds to sialic acid and glycoproteins on motor neurons, is endocytosed, and facilitates the cytoplasmic release of the A fragment when the endosome lumen becomes acidified.

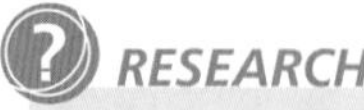

RESEARCH

What are the clinical applications of botulinum toxin?

Treatment and prevention

Because *C botulinum* infection can lead to respiratory paralysis, ventilatory support is very important. Gastric lavage and metronidazole or penicillin therapy is used to eliminate the microorganism from the gastrointestinal tract. Botulinum antitoxin against toxins from strains A, B, and E can neutralize the preformed toxin.

Prevention involves keeping foods in acid pH and at or below 4°C to inhibit the germination of spores and heating to 60° to 100°C for 10 minutes to denature preformed toxin molecules. Honey should not be given to children younger than 1 year, since infant botulism is related to the ingestion of spore-contaminated honey.

C difficile

C difficile can cause antibiotic-associated gastrointestinal diseases, including life-threatening pseudomembranous colitis. It is found among the intestinal microflora of some healthy people and of hospitalized patients, and spores of *C difficile* have been found in hospital rooms of patients infected with the microorganism.

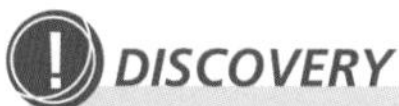

DISCOVERY

The first report of a pseudomembranous lesion of the intestine came from J. M. T. Finney at Johns Hopkins Hospital in 1893. Although the lesion was in the small intestine of a 22-year-old woman who had undergone surgery for the resection of a tumor in the gastric pylorus, it was described as a "diphtheritic membrane." Reports of pseudomembranous enterocolitis became more common after the introduction of antibiotics. In 1974, F. J. Tedesco and colleagues described patients with severe diarrhea attributed to clindamycin, which had become the drug of choice for anaerobic infections. Tedesco undertook a prospective study involving 200 patients who were receiving clindamycin. Those who developed diarrhea underwent colonoscopy to detect pseudomembranous colitis; 21% percent of the patients had diarrhea, and 10% had pseudomembranous colitis. This was a potentially life-threatening complication of a commonly prescribed antibiotic.

Clinical syndromes and diagnosis

C difficile infections cause diarrhea and are associated with the formation of pseudomembranes, which are yellow-white plaques, on the colonic mucosa. In addition to the clinical symptoms, infection with *C difficile* is confirmed by immunoassays for the enterotoxin and cytotoxin. The mere detection of these toxins, for example in young children, does not indicate disease. Stool samples can be tested for the presence of the microorganism; however, positive cultures do not necessarily indicate disease but rather show colonization.

Pathogenesis and epidemiology

Antibiotics such as clindamycin, cephalosporins, and fluoroquinolones can alter the normal gastrointestinal microflora and enable the overgrowth of *C difficile*, which is relatively resistant to these antibiotics (Fig 14-2). Disease develops if the organism overgrows in the colon and produces toxins. The microorganism produces two toxins: enterotoxin and cytotoxin. Enterotoxin (toxin A) damages the tight junctions between intestinal epithelial cells and causes hemorrhagic necrosis and watery diarrhea. It also induces neutrophil chemotaxis. Cytotoxin (toxin B) causes actin depolymerization, thus damaging the colonic mucosa and leading to pseudomembrane formation.

C difficile is found in the gastrointestinal tract of about 3% of the general population and up to 30% of hospitalized patients. It is the most common nosocomial cause of diarrhea. Spores can be a major source of nosocomial outbreaks. In 2004, a new epidemic strain of *C difficile* emerged and caused hospital outbreaks. It produces higher amounts of enterotoxin and cytotoxin and is more resistant to fluoroquinolones.

Treatment and prevention

Treatment is initiated by the discontinuation of the implicated antibiotic and administration of metronidazole or vancomycin. Some strains appear to be resistant to metronidazole, although antibiotic susceptibility tests in the laboratory do not indicate such resistance. Patients should be monitored carefully to ascertain that they are responding to therapy.

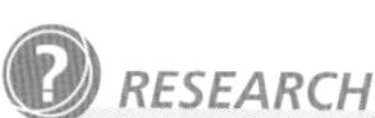

RESEARCH

Why should dentists be concerned about *C difficile* infection in their patients?

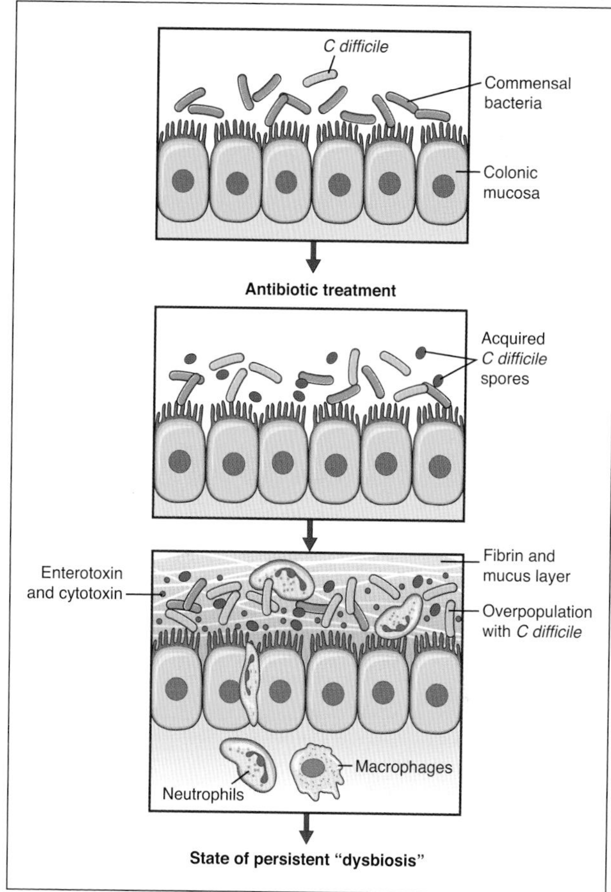

Fig 14-2 Changes in the colonic epithelium following antibiotic treatment and overpopulation by *C difficile*.

C septicum

C septicum causes atraumatic gas gangrene and necrotizing enterocolitis. *C septicum* infections are mostly seen in cases of colon cancer, leukemia, diabetes, and rarely Crohn's disease. The microorganism can spread into tissues if the structure of the gastrointestinal mucosa is compromised, destroying the tissue and producing gas. The mortality rate is 50% or more.

C septicum has four different toxins that cause tissue necrosis, disseminated intravascular coagulation, intravascular thrombosis, and hemolysis. Infections can be treated with penicillin, metronidazole, or imipenem.

Take-Home Messages

- Clostridia are Gram-positive, strictly anaerobic, spore-forming bacilli.
- *C perfringens* causes myonecrosis, or gas gangrene, a life-threatening disease resulting in muscle necrosis, shock, renal failure, and death. Other clinical manifestations are cellulitis, suppurative myositis, endometriosis, and food poisoning.
- Tissue damage is mediated by hyaluronidase, collagenase, alpha toxin, beta toxin, perfringolysin O, epsilon toxin, iota toxin, and enterotoxin.
- Rapid treatment is essential. The necrotic tissue should be removed by surgical debridement, and high-dose penicillin G therapy should be started.
- *C tetani* infections cause generalized or localized tetanus. Generalized tetanus often affects the masseter muscles initially, which results in the inability to open the mouth (trismus).
- Neonatal tetanus is caused by the infection of the umbilical cord when it is severed under nonsterile conditions.
- Tetanus toxin is a zinc endopeptidase that degrades a protein involved in neurotransmitter release in presynaptic nerve terminals of inhibitory synapses. The inhibition of inhibitory neurotransmitters causes the excitatory synaptic activity to be unregulated and leads to spastic paralysis.
- Treatment begins with debridement of the primary wound and administration of metronidazole and human tetanus immunoglobulin, followed by vaccination with tetanus toxoid.
- *C botulinum* causes food-borne botulism, characterized by weakness, dizziness, dry mouth, blurred vision, abdominal pain, and constipation. The progressive disease caused by *C botulinum* causes weakening of peripheral muscles and flaccid paralysis.
- Botulinum toxin has zinc-endopeptidase activity and inhibits cholinergic synaptic transmission, thus blocking the excitation of muscle and leading to flaccid paralysis.
- Ventilatory support is used to counter flaccid paralysis. Gastric lavage and metronidazole or penicillin therapy are used to eliminate the microorganism.
- *C difficile* can cause antibiotic-associated gastrointestinal diseases, including life-threatening pseudomembranous colitis.
- It produces enterotoxin (toxin A) and cytotoxin (toxin B), leading to hemorrhagic necrosis and pseudomembrane formation.
- Treatment is initiated by discontinuation of the causative antibiotic and administration of metronidazole or vancomycin.
- *C septicum* causes atraumatic gas gangrene and necrotizing enterocolitis, seen mostly in cases of colon cancer, leukemia, and diabetes.

Bibliography

Bartlett JG. *Clostridium difficile* infection: Historic review. Anaerobe 2009;15:227–229.

Centers for Disease Control and Prevention. Information about the Current Strain of *Clostridium difficile*. www.cdc.gov/HAI/organisms/cdiff/Cdiff-current-strain.html. Accessed 12 June 2015.

Centers for Disease Control and Prevention. Tetanus. www.cdc.gov/features/tetanus. Accessed 12 June 2015.

Greenwood D, Slack R, Peutherer J, Barer M. Medical Microbiology, ed 17. Edinburgh: Churchill Livingstone/Elsevier, 2007.

Heibl C, Knoflach P. *Clostridium septicum* causing sepsis with severe disseminated intravascular coagulation in a patient with Crohn's disease. Am J Gastroenterol 2011;106:170–171.

Moe PC, Heuck AP. Phospholipid hydrolysis caused by *Clostridium perfringens* α-toxin facilitates the targeting of perfringolysin O to membrane bilayers. Biochemistry 2010;49:9498–9507.

Murray PR, Rosenthal KS, Pfaller MA. Medical Microbiology, ed 6. Philadelphia: Mosby/Elsevier, 2009.

Ryan KJ, Ray CG. Sherris Medical Microbiology, ed 5. New York: McGraw-Hill, 2010.

Bordetella, *Legionella*, and Miscellaneous Gram-Negative Bacilli

15

Bordetella pertussis

Bordetella are small, strictly aerobic bacilli. *B pertussis* is transmitted by airborne droplets and causes pertussis, or whooping cough. The organism attaches to ciliated epithelial cells via its filamentous hemagglutinin and pertussis toxin, proliferates, and causes tissue damage.

Clinical syndromes and diagnosis

B pertussis is spread from patients with clinically apparent pertussis or mild unrecognized disease. The first stage of the disease (7–10 days after infection) is the catarrhal stage, which resembles a common cold. This stage poses the highest risk for transmission of the disease, because production of bacteria is at a peak and the disease is not recognized as pertussis. The paroxysmal stage (characterized by convulsions or seizures) begins 1 to 2 weeks after the onset of the catarrhal stage, with repetitive coughs followed by an inspiratory whoop. These paroxysms end with vomiting and exhaustion. About 2 to 8 weeks later, the convalescent stage begins, in which the paroxysmal cough is reduced in severity and frequency. The rate of convalescence depends on the rate at which damaged respiratory epithelial cells regenerate. However, secondary complications, such as pneumonia and encephalopathy, can occur. In patients with partial immunity, the disease may not follow these classic symptoms. *B pertussis* constitutes a potential health hazard to pediatricians and dental professionals treating children.

Cultures must be immediately transferred to special medium (Regan-Lowe medium) because the organism is sensitive to drying. Cotton swabs must be avoided because they are toxic. Specimens can be identified by direct fluorescent antibody or by the polymerase chain reaction. Culture methods are not always reliable.

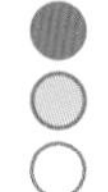

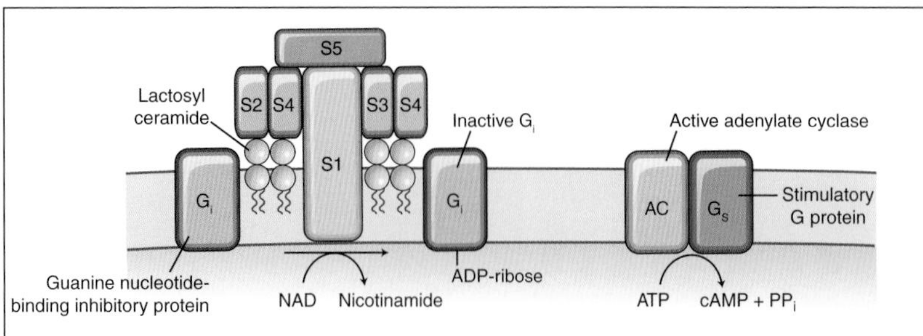

Fig 15-1 Schematic diagram of the mechanism of action of pertussis toxin. NAD, nicotinamide adenine dinucleotide; ATP, adenosine triphosphate; cAMP, cyclic adenosine monophosphate.

Pathogenesis and epidemiology

The bacterium is spread from person to person through airborne droplets. It is estimated that 30 to 50 million people are infected globally every year, and about 300,000 deaths occur every year as a result. In the United States, there were 48,277 cases and 20 deaths reported to the Centers for Disease Control and Prevention in 2012. The highest incidence was in infants less than 1 year old (126.7 per 100,000), followed by children 7 to 10 years old (58.5 per 100,000). Many cases are undiagnosed or unreported.

B pertussis has a number of virulence factors. Pertussis toxin is secreted by the type IV secretion system, adenosine diphosphate (ADP)-ribosylates guanine nucleotide-binding proteins at the cell membrane (Fig 15-1), and interferes with signal transduction by chemokine receptors, resulting in the inability of lymphocytes to enter lymphoid tissue. This results in an increase in the number of lymphocytes in the blood (lymphocytosis). Inactivation of the inhibitory G protien causes uncontrolled adenylate cyclase activity and an increase in cyclic adenosine monophosphate (cAMP) concentration. This results in an increase in respiratory secretions and mucus production. A domain of the toxin mediates binding of the toxin to glycosylated molecules on respiratory epithelial cells. The toxin has an active subunit (A) and a pentameric cell-binding subunit (B) that is similar to the B pentamer of cholera toxin.

Adenylate cyclase toxin causes an increase in cAMP levels in cells and inhibits *(1)* leukocyte chemotaxis, phagocytosis, and killing; *(2)* oxidative activity of alveolar macrophages; and *(3)* cell lysis by natural cytotoxic cells. Tracheal cytotoxin inhibits ciliary movement in epithelial cells (ciliostasis). It inhibits DNA synthesis, impairing the regeneration of damaged cells. Filamentous hemagglutinin and the 69 kD pertactin (P69 protein) mediate the attachment of the bacterium to ciliated cells.

Treatment and prevention

Treatment is supportive; antibiotics do not lessen the clinical course. Macrolides (erythromycin, azithromycin, clarithromycin) can be used to eradicate the organism, but this has limited value because the disease is contagious while still unrecognized. They are useful, however, in prevention of disease in exposed, unimmunized individuals. They should also be given to immunized children younger than 4 years who have been exposed, because vaccine-induced immunity is not fully protective.

The acellular pertussis vaccine is given in combination with diphtheria and tetanus toxoids and is composed of inactivated pertussis toxin, filamentous hemagglutinin, and pertactin. Pertussis toxin used for this vaccine is inactivated genetically by introducing two amino acid changes that eliminate its ADP-ribosylating activity but maintain its antigenicity. This DTaP vaccine is given at 2, 4, 6, and 15 to 18 months as well as at 4 to 6 years. The "adult vaccine" (Tdap) is given at 11 to 12 years and again between 19 and 65 years. The pertussis component of this vaccine contains five components: inactivated pertussis toxin, filamentous hemagglutinin, pertactin, and fimbria 2 and 3.

Francisella tularensis

Francisella tularensis is a small aerobic coccobacillus in the gamma-proteobacteria group (which also includes *Legionella* and *Pseudomonas*), named after Edward Francis. It causes tularemia, also known as *glandular fever, rabbit fever,* or *tick fever.*

Clinical syndromes and diagnosis

The clinical symptoms include abrupt onset of fever, chills, malaise, and fatigue. The most common type of tularemia is ulceroglandular, with skin ulcers and lymphadenopathy. Oculoglandular infections, resulting from contamination of the eye and presenting with swollen cervical lymph nodes, and oropharyngeal tularemia are also observed.

F tularensis can be diagnosed by staining with fluorescence-labeled antibodies following preliminary identification by Gram staining, which is very light. Cysteine-containing culture media are essential for growth. The laboratory performing the analysis should be informed of the suspicion of *F tularensis* because it is highly infectious and can penetrate through unbroken skin.

Pathogenesis and epidemiology

The bacteria can survive for long periods in macrophages of the reticuloendothelial system by inhibiting phagosome-lysosome fusion. Pathogenic strains have a capsule that can inhibit phagocytosis. Because it is intracellular, it is not affected by humoral immunity.

The disease spreads via tick bites, contact with an infected animal, consumption of infected meat or water, and inhalation of infected aerosols. The most common in the United States is tick-borne tularemia from a rabbit reservoir. Exposure to 10 organisms by a tick bite or to 50 by aerosol can cause disease; ie, *F tularensis* is highly infectious.

Treatment and prevention

Gentamicin is the treatment of choice. Reservoirs of infection, including rabbits and ticks, should be avoided. Live attenuated vaccines are not completely protective but can be used by persons at high risk of exposure.

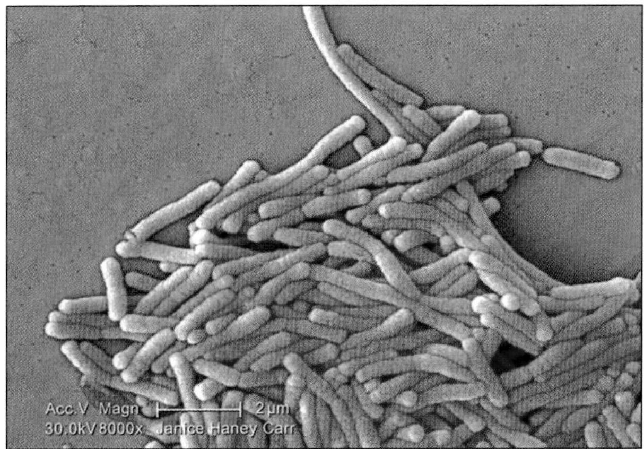

Fig 15-2 Scanning electron micrograph of *L pneumophila* grown on buffered charcoal yeast extract. (Public Health Image Library image 11149, courtesy of Janice Haney Carr.)

Brucella

Brucella are small, nonmotile, non-encapsulated Gram-negative coccobacilli. Four species of *Brucella* can cause human brucellosis or undulant fever. The microorganisms were first isolated and described by David Bruce and Bernhard Bang. Thus, the disease is also called Bang's disease. The worldwide incidence is greater than 500,000 per year, while the number of cases in the United States was only 115 in 2010.

Clinical syndromes and diagnosis

Brucella melitensis is the most common cause of severe brucellosis with serious complications. The initial manifestations are malaise, chills, myalgias, arthralgias, and nonproductive cough. Fever is common and undulant (intermittent). Granulomas can form in the liver, spleen, and bone marrow and result in enlargement of the liver, spleen, and lymph nodes. *Brucella suis* can form destructive lesions.

Prolonged incubation on enriched blood agars is necessary. *Brucella* can be identified by its microscopic and colony morphology and reactivity with specific antibodies.

Pathogenesis and epidemiology

Brucella organisms reside in the macrophages of the liver sinusoids, bone marrow, and spleen and secrete proteins that induce granuloma formation. They inhibit phagosome-lysosome fusion and the myeloperoxidase system. They inactivate hydrogen peroxide by their catalase and superoxide by superoxide dismutase. They also inhibit apoptosis, thereby prolonging the life of infected cells. Bacteria are released intermittently into the bloodstream from the granulomas, causing the recurrent fever and chills characteristic of the disease.

Disease is transmitted to humans who have direct contact with animals or who consume unpasteurized milk or cheese.

Treatment and prevention

Doxycycline plus an aminoglycoside is the preferred treatment. Ciprofloxacin, trimethoprim-sulfamethoxazole, and rifampin can also be used as combination therapy. Prevention involves minimizing exposure to the source of infection and pasteurizing dairy products. Animals are vaccinated with an attenuated strain of *Brucella abortus*.

Legionella

Legionella pneumophila was recognized as the species responsible for the deaths of many attendees of the American Legion convention in a Philadelphia hotel in 1976. The organism had not been detected before 1976 because it does not stain well and does not grow on conventional media. These aerobic organisms appear as coccobacilli in tissues but acquire filamentous structures in culture (Fig 15-2).

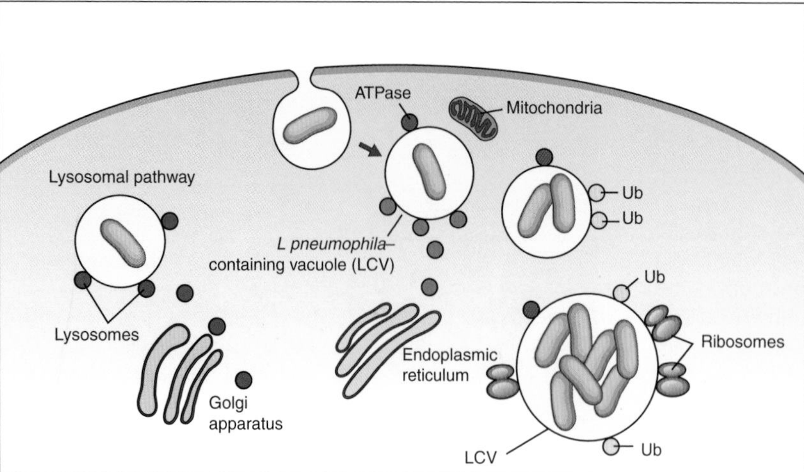

Fig 15-3 Intracellular life cycle of *L pneumophila*. The *L pneumophila*–containing vacuole (LCV) bypasses the common endocytotic trafficking pathway that normally delivers the contents to the lysosomal compartments (left side of the cell). The LCV avoids phagosome-lysosome fusion by employing materials carried in vesicles *(blue)* from the endoplasmic reticulum. The LCV also attracts mitochondria and ribosomes as the infection progresses. The phagosome containing the bacteria is transformed into a specialized compartment that provides an environment where the bacteria multiply. Ubiquitinated proteins (Ub) and vacuolar adenosine triphosphatases (ATPases) are also localized on the LCV membrane. (Adapted from Xu and Luo.)

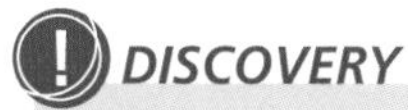
DISCOVERY

Following the American Legion convention in July 1976, there were a total of 182 cases and 29 deaths from acute pneumonia. Epidemiologic studies led by David Fraser of the US Centers for Disease Control and Prevention linked the deaths to the Bellevue Stratford Hotel and concluded that the disease was most probably spread by the airborne route. Joseph McDade, a rickettsiologist, was assigned to investigate whether legionnaires disease was caused by *Coxiella burnetii*, the agent of Q fever. He inoculated guinea pigs with human lung homogenates and passaged potentially infected material in embryonated eggs, but he could not demonstrate an infectious agent, although the guinea pigs fell ill. He stained guinea pig tissues with the Gimenez stain, which stains rickettsia and other bacteria, but only saw an occasional bacillus. Upon re-examination of guinea pig tissue slides, however, he found clusters of rods. When he repeated the inoculation of eggs without adding the standard antimicrobials used for rickettsial isolation, he recovered a microorganism from the embryos. McDade also showed that patients with legionnaires disease had antibodies to the bacterial isolate, thus discovering the etiology of legionnaires disease.

The Gimenez stain contains carbol fuchsin, which intensely stains Gram-negative rods as well as rickettsia. Conventional stains used to detect bacteria in tissues could not detect *L pneumophila* in the lungs of patients with the disease, despite the very large number of bacteria in the lungs of fatal cases. The Gimenez stain effectively detects the bacterium in culture, in infected macrophages, and in infected fresh and formalin-fixed lungs. However, it does not stain the bacteria in paraffin-embedded lungs, making it unlikely that pathologists using the stain would have detected the microorganism.

Clinical syndromes and diagnosis

L pneumophila causes Pontiac fever and legionnaires disease. Pontiac fever is the mild, flu-like form of *Legionella* infection that does not result in pneumonia. The symptoms include fever, chills, myalgia, malaise, and headache developing in 12 hours and persisting for 2–5 days. Legionnaires disease is apparent after 2 to 10 days of incubation and starts with an abrupt onset of fever, chills, headache, and nonproductive cough. It is a multiorgan disease, with abnormalities in the gastrointestinal tract, central nervous system, liver, and kidneys. Pulmonary function deteriorates if not treated.

The most sensitive test for microscopic determination of *Legionella* is the direct fluorescent antibody test. Cultures can be stained with Gimenez or Dieterle silver stains. *Legionella* requires cysteine for growth, and iron enhances growth. The most common medium for *Legionella* is buffered charcoal yeast extract (BCYE) agar. If the organism grows on BCYE with cysteine, but does not grow without cysteine, there is a good chance that it is *Legionella*.

Pathogenesis and epidemiology

The C3b component of complement binds the bacterial porin and facilitates uptake into alveolar macrophages through the CR3 complement receptor.

Legionella multiply in the macrophages and inhibit phagosome-lysosome fusion (Fig 15-3). This inhibition is facilitated by a type IV secretion system (Dot/Icm) that spans the two bacterial membranes and the phagosome membrane and transports into the cytoplasm proteins that affect vesicle traffic in the host cell. Tissue destruction may be the result of the production of proteolytic and other degrading enzymes. Nevertheless, protease-deficient mutants of *L pneumophila* are also virulent. All species have a low potential for causing disease, which is seen most of-

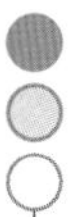

ten in individuals with compromised immune systems or pulmonary function. Macrophages need to be activated by interferon gamma, produced by sensitized helper T cells, to be able to kill the intracellular pathogen.

The microorganisms are present in lakes, streams, air-conditioning cooling towers, and potable water systems (including dental unit waterlines). In nature, they infect and grow in amoebae. Infection occurs via exposure to aerosols containing *Legionella* from humidifiers, showers, respiratory therapy equipment, and water fountains.

Treatment and prevention

The macrolides azithromycin and clarithromycin and the fluoroquinolones ciprofloxacin and levofloxacin are the antibiotics of choice. (Macrolides are also effective against pulmonary infections caused by *Mycoplasma pneumoniae* and *Streptococcus pneumoniae*). β-lactam antibiotics are generally ineffective because most strains produce β-lactamases. Aminoglycosides, penicillins, and cephalosporins cannot enter macrophages where the microorganisms reside.

Prevention requires reducing the microbial burden in the environmental source, such as hyperchlorination or elevated temperatures, but this has only been moderately successful.

Bacteroides

Bacteroides are obligate anaerobic, non–spore-forming, Gram-negative bacilli that colonize the oropharynx, gastrointestinal tract, and genital tract. The *Bacteroides fragilis* group is pleomorphic in size and shape, biochemically related, antibiotic resistant, and grows rapidly in culture.

A major component of the cell wall structure is lipopolysaccharide, but it has no endotoxin activity because it lacks the phosphate groups on the glucosamines and the number of fatty acids is less than that in normal lipopolysaccharide. The capsule of *B fragilis* contains three polysaccharides—PS A, PS B, and PS C. The extent of the capsule observed in electron micrographs may be a function of the staining technique used to visualize the capsular material.

Bacteroides melaninogenicus subspecies *asaccharolyticus* has been reclassified and includes *Porphyromonas gingivalis* (prominent in patients with periodontal disease) and *Porphyromonas endodontalis* (isolated from infected root canals in humans).

Clinical syndromes and diagnosis

Patients presenting with abdominal pain and who have a history of appendicitis and diverticulitis may have intra-abdominal abscesses. *B fragilis* is the most common cause of intra-abdominal infections such as sepsis, peritonitis, and abscesses. Although there are a very large number of species in the gastrointestinal tract and *B fragilis* comprises only about 1% to 2% of the microflora, it is the bacterium most commonly found in these infections. *B fragilis* can form abscesses in gynecologic infections and cause significant disease if it is introduced via contamination of a traumatized surface into skin and soft tissue. *Bacteroides*, *Fusobacterium*, and *Peptostreptococcus* can cause necrotizing fasciitis in the neck (Fig 15-4). *B fragilis* can also cause bacteremia, and enterotoxin-producing strains can result in a self-limited gastroenteritis.

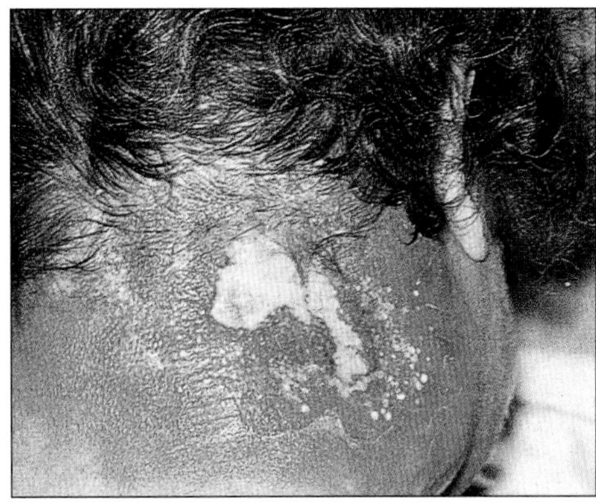

Fig 15-4 Necrotizing fasciitis of the neck, with a central area of necrosis and a large area of rapidly advancing erythema. *Bacteroides*, *Fusobacterium*, and *Peptostreptococcus* species account for 50% to 60% of cases. (Reprinted with permission from Marx and Stern.)

Specimens for culture should be transported to the laboratory in an oxygen-free system (degassed, stoppered collection tubes) and incubated in an anaerobic environment. Selective media containing bile, esculin (a glycosidic substrate), and gentamicin enables the growth of *B fragilis*. Thus, colony morphology, resistance to several antibiotics, and growth in bile provide a preliminary identification. Definitive identification can be made with 16S ribosomal RNA gene sequencing and biochemical assays.

Pathogenesis and epidemiology

Although *Bacteroides distasonis* and *Bacteroides thetaiotamicron* are the predominant species of *Bacteroides* found in the gastrointestinal tract, *B fragilis* is the major cause of intra-abdominal infections. The primary reason for this is the virulence of the bacterium. The oxygen-susceptible and avirulent organisms are cleared by the immune system, while the virulent microorganisms proliferate. The capsule of *B fragilis* and *B melaninogenicus* prevents phagocytosis, mediates adhesion to peritoneal surfaces, and promotes abscess formation. *Bacteroides* can adhere to epithelial cells and extracellular molecules like fibrinogen and fibronectin by means of its fimbriae. The lipopolysaccharide stimulates leukocyte chemotaxis by activating the alternate pathway of complement, via the production of the chemoattractant C5a. Anaerobes that cause disease are generally able to tolerate oxygen. Catalase inactivates hydrogen peroxide, and superoxide dismutase inactivates superoxide free radicals.

Abscess formation is related to the ability of the zwitterionic motif (with both positive and negative charges) on the PS A polysaccharide to activate $CD4^+$ T cells. Abscess formation is also thought to require synergy between facultative and strict anaerobic bacteria, for example by the former depleting residual oxygen, enabling the strict anaerobes to take over.

Enterotoxigenic strains of *B fragilis* that cause diarrheal disease produce a zinc metalloprotease that causes F-actin rearrangement in intestinal epithelial cells. This results in chloride secretion and fluid loss.

During infection, the endogenous bacterial population spreads by trauma or disease from normally colonized mucosal surfaces to sterile tissues or fluids. Diagnostic or surgical procedures that disrupt barriers surrounding mucosal surfaces can introduce these organisms into normally sterile sites. The *B melaninogenicus* group is common in pleuropulmonary and central nervous system infections.

Treatment and prevention

Antibiotics with the best activity against Gram-negative anaerobic bacilli are metronidazole (Flagyl, Pfizer), carbapenems (eg, imipenem), and β-lactam plus β-lactam inhibitor combinations (eg, piperacillin-tazobactam). Resistance to clindamycin and tetracycline has developed in *B fragilis* and is mediated by transferable plasmids.

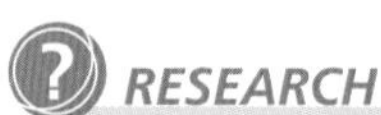

B fragilis exposed to low concentrations of piperacillin-tazobactam undergo phenotypic changes, such as the expression levels of certain proteins. Which techniques can be used to identify such proteins?

Fusobacterium

This bacterium has a fusiform shape (spindle-shaped). Its lipopolysaccharide is similar to that of other Gram-negative bacilli and stimulates leukocyte chemotaxis by activating the alternate pathway of complement (via C5a).

Fusobacteria are slow-growing anaerobes and are often found in association with other bacteria (such as the fusospirochetal complex). They are present in the oropharynx and the gastrointestinal and genitourinary tracts of healthy individuals and can spread by bacteremia to other sites or may be aspirated into the lungs. *Fusobacterium nucleatum* is often seen in periodontal disease. It produces butyric acid (a tissue irritant) and proteases. Agglutinins on *F nucleatum* cause adherence to erythrocytes and epithelial surfaces as well as co-agglutination with other bacteria. *Fusobacterium necrophorum* may cause necrotizing tonsillitis and septicemia, leading to development of abscesses in the lung and brain. Fusobacteria in blood can cause thromboembolic metastasis, especially in the lungs. Butyric acid and other metabolic products produce a foul smell that is seen in all fusobacterial infections. *Wolinella* is a fusobacterium that populates the oropharynx. Fusobacterial infections can be treated with metronidazole.

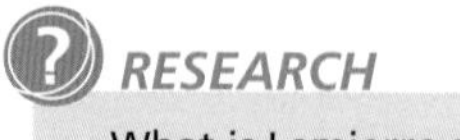

What is Lemierre syndrome?

Cardiobacterium

Cardiobacterium hominis is a facultatively anaerobic, small bacillus that can be found in the respiratory tract of about 70% of healthy individuals. Most patients who develop *C hominis* endocarditis have a history of oral disease or dental procedures before clinical symptoms developed as well as preexisting heart disease. This bacterium enters the bloodstream from the oropharynx, adheres to the damaged heart tissue, and multiplies. The disease progresses slowly, and complete recovery ensues following appropriate antibiotic therapy (penicillin or ampicillin for 2 to 6 weeks). Maintenance of good oral hygiene and prophylactic antibiotics at the time of dental manipulations for persons with certain heart conditions must be considered. These conditions include artificial heart valves, a history of infective endocarditis, and a transplanted heart with a problem with a valve.

Eikenella

Eikenella corrodens, named after Eiken, who observed the ability of the organism to "corrode" or form pits in agar, is a nonmotile, non–spore-forming, facultatively anaerobic bacillus. It is a normal resident of the upper respiratory tract. It is an opportunistic pathogen that causes infections in immunocompromised patients and in patients with diseases or trauma in the oral cavity. Clinically, it presents as sinusitis, meningitis, brain abscesses, pneumonia, lung abscesses, and endocarditis. It has been associated with human bites and fistfight injuries. Amoxicillin-clavulanate and moxifloxacin are recommended for treatment.

Capnocytophaga

This filamentous, fusiform bacterium can grow aerobically or anaerobically in the presence of carbon dioxide. The DF-1 group colonizes the oropharynx and is associated with periodontal disease and septicemia. The DF-2 strains are found in the oral cavities of cats and dogs and can cause bite-wound infections. Amoxicillin-clavulanate is recommended for treatment.

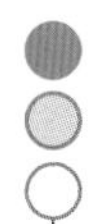

Pasteurellaceae

The family Pasteurellaceae are facultatively anaerobic and include the species *Haemophilus influenzae*, *Haemophilus parainfluenzae*, *Aggregatibacter actinomycetemcomitans*, and *Pasteurella multocida*.

H influenzae

Haemophilus species are facultatively anaerobic rods that colonize human mucous membranes. Encapsulated strains of *H influenzae* can cause meningitis, epiglottitis, otitis, and sinusitis. Non-encapsulated *H influenzae* strains cause primarily pediatric ear and sinus infections. *H parainfluenzae* is associated with dental plaque and periodontal disease. The majority of facultatively anaerobic Gram-negative bacilli (rods) in the oral cavity belong to the genus *Haemophilus*.

Clinical syndromes and diagnosis

H influenzae can cause meningitis, epiglottitis, cellulitis, otitis, sinusitis, and arthritis. Type b *H influenzae* was the major cause of meningitis in children before the use of the conjugated vaccine. In nonimmune children who develop meningitis and are treated promptly, the mortality rate is less than 10%. Epiglottitis involves cellulitis and swelling of the local tissues and is therefore life-threatening. Cellulitis presents as reddish-blue patches on the cheeks and around the eyes. Other clinical syndromes of *H influenzae* include ear and sinus infections in children and infections of the lower respiratory tract (particularly in the elderly). *H influenzae* and *S pneumoniae* are the two most common causes of otitis and sinusitis. *H parainfluenzae* as well as *Haemophilus segnis* and *Haemophilus aphrophilus* are found in dental plaque.

Haemophilus species can be identified in cerebrospinal fluid in patients with meningitis using microscopy (Gram-negative coccobacilli to long pleomorphic filaments) and detection of capsular polyribitol phosphate (PRP) antigen (using latex agglutination). The bacterium can be cultured in chocolate agar (in which inhibitors of V factor are heat inactivated).

Pathogenesis and epidemiology

Most species of *Haemophilus* (Greek for "blood loving") require hemin ("X factor") and nicotinamide adenine dinucleotide (NAD, "V factor") for growth. Most strains of *H influenzae* have a polysaccharide capsule composed of PRP, with six antigenic serotypes (a to f). The b serotype was responsible for the great majority of infections before the introduction of the vaccine (Hib) against this serotype. Most infections are now caused by non-encapsulated strains. In the United States in 2012, there were 10 cases of serotype b and 701 total cases per 100,000 population, according to the Centers for Disease Control and Prevention. Nevertheless, the vaccine is not distributed adequately in many countries, and it is estimated that there are about 8.1 million cases and 370,000 fatalities worldwide each year.

Lipid A may be responsible for meningeal inflammation. Immunoglobulin A1 proteases produced by the bacteria degrade mucosal IgA and facilitate the colonization of mucosal surfaces.

Treatment and prevention

Without antimicrobial therapy, the mortality rate in patients with meningitis and epiglottitis is almost 100%. For the treatment of children under 7 years of age, the Infectious Disease Society of America recommends a combination of vancomycin and a broad-spectrum cephalosporin such as ceftriaxone or cefotaxime. Less severe infections, including sinusitis or otitis media, can be treated with ampicillin (in non–β-lactamase–producing strains) or amoxicilin-clavulanate.

Vaccination against *H influenzae* has been highly successful. The Hib vaccine contains the capsular PRP antigen covalently attached to proteins like tetanus toxoid or diphtheria toxoid. It is administered three times to children before the age of 6 years.

Actinobacillus

Actinobacilli are small, facultatively anaerobic bacilli that are part of the normal oropharyngeal population. They are associated with rare bite-wound infections and opportunistic infections such as bacteremia and pneumonia.

Aggregatibacter

Bacteria formerly known as *Haemophilus aphrophilus* and *Actinobacillus actinomycetemcomitans* have been classified into a new genus, *Aggregatibacter*. These microorganisms populate the oral cavity and can enter the bloodstream following dental procedures or in patients with periodontitis, where they can attach to a damaged heart valve, causing endocarditis. Infection can be treated with ceftriaxone.

Pasteurella

Pasteurella are facultatively anaerobic, small coccobacilli. The natural reservoir for *P multocida* and *Pasteurella canis* is the oropharynx of animals. After an animal bite or scratch, localized cellulitis and lymphadenitis is observed. Chronic respiratory disease in patients can be exacerbated by the aspiration of infected oral secretions. *Pasteurella* species can cause systemic infection in people who are immunocompromised.

The antibiotic of choice is penicillin G. Expanded-spectrum cephalosporins, tetracyclines, macrolides, and fluoroquinolones can also be used.

Take-Home Messages

- *Bordetella* are small, strictly aerobic bacilli. *B pertussis* is transmitted by airborne droplets and causes pertussis, or whooping cough.
- The catarrhal stage poses the highest risk for transmission of the disease.
- Pertussis toxin ADP-ribosylates guanine nucleotide-binding proteins in the host cell membrane and interferes with signal transduction by chemokine receptors; this results in the inability of lymphocytes to enter lymphoid tissue.
- The acellular pertussis vaccine, DTaP, is given in combination with diphtheria and tetanus toxoids and contains inactivated pertussis toxin, filamentous hemagglutinin, and pertactin.
- *F tularensis* is an aerobic coccobacillus that causes tularemia, or glandular fever.
- Four species of *Brucella* can cause human brucellosis, or undulant fever.
- *L pneumophila* multiplies in alveolar macrophages and inhibits phagosome-lysosome fusion. It causes legionnaires disease, a multiorgan disease involving pneumonia and abnormalities in the gastrointestinal tract, central nervous system, liver, and kidneys.
- *Bacteroides* are obligate anaerobic, non–spore-forming, Gram-negative bacilli that colonize the oropharynx, gastrointestinal tract, and genital tract. *B fragilis* is the major cause of intra-abdominal infections.
- Fusobacteria are slow-growing anaerobes and are often found in association with other bacteria, as in the fusospirochetal complex in dental plaque. They are present in the oropharynx and other mucosal surfaces but can spread by bacteremia to other sites.
- Most patients who develop *C hominis* endocarditis have a history of oral disease or dental procedures as well as preexisting heart disease.
- Encapsulated strains of *H influenzae* can cause meningitis, epiglottitis, otitis, and sinusitis. Non-encapsulated *H influenzae* strains cause pediatric ear and sinus infections.

Bibliography

Carbonetti NH. Pertussis toxin and adenylate cyclase toxin: Key virulence factors of *Bordetella pertussis* and cell biology tools. Future Microbiol 2010;5:455–469.

Centers for Disease Control and Prevention. Brucellosis. www.cdc.gov/brucellosis/index.html. Accessed 16 June 2015.

Centers for Disease Control and Prevention. Pertussis (Whooping Cough). www.cdc.gov/pertussis/surv-reporting.html. Accessed 16 June 2015.

Centers for Disease Control and Prevention. Public Health Image Library. phil.cdc.gov. Accessed 4 August 2015.

Edelstein PH. Legionnaires disease: History and clinical findings. In: Heuner K, Swanson M (eds). *Legionella*: Molecular Biology. Poole, UK: Caister Academic, 2008. www.open-access-biology.com/legionella/edelstein.html. Accessed 16 June 2015.

Engleberg NC, DiRita V, Dermody TS. Schaechter's Mechanisms of Microbial Disease. Baltimore and Philadelphia: Lippincott Williams & Wilkins, 2007.

Marx RE, Stern D. Oral and Maxillofacial Pathology: A Rationale for Diagnosis and Treatment, ed 2. Chicago: Quintessence, 2012.

Mosby's Dictionary of Medicine, Nursing and Health Professions, ed 9. Philadelphia: Mosby/Elsevier, 2012.

Murray PR, Rosenthal KS, Pfaller MA. Medical Microbiology, ed 6. Philadelphia: Mosby/Elsevier, 2009.

Pumbwe L, Skilbeck CA, Wexler HM. The *Bacteroides fragilis* cell envelope: Quarterback, linebacker, coach—Or all three? Anaerobe 2006;12:211–220.

Roberts GL. Fusobacterial infections: An underestimated threat. Br J Biomed Sci 2000;57:156–162.

Ryan KJ, Ray CG. Sherris Medical Microbiology, ed 5. New York: McGraw-Hill, 2010.

Stefanopoulos PK, Tarantzopoulou AD. Facial bite wounds: Management update. Int J Oral Maxillofac Surg 2005;34:464–472.

Xu L, Luo ZQ. Cell biology of infection by *Legionella pneumophila*. Microbes Infections 2012;15:157–167.

Neisseria and Neisseriaceae

16

Neisseria are aerobic, Gram-negative diplococci, which makes the presumptive identification of these bacteria relatively straightforward. The genus includes *Neisseria gonorrhoeae*, *Neisseria meningitidis*, *Neisseria sicca*, *Neisseria mucosa*, and *Neisseria lactamica*. *N gonorrhoeae* causes sexually transmitted infections. *N meningitidis* colonizes the upper respiratory tract and causes meningitis, septicemia, pneumonia, arthritis, and urethritis. *N sicca*, *N mucosa*, and *N lactamica* are commensals in the oropharynyx and nasopharynx. There have been isolated cases of meningitis, osteomyelitis, endocarditis, respiratory infections, acute otitis media, and acute sinusitis caused by these *Neisseria* species.

Other members of the Neisseriaceae family include *Eikenella corrodens*, *Kingella kingae*, and *Moraxella catarrhalis*, organisms that colonize the oropharynx and can cause opportunistic infections.

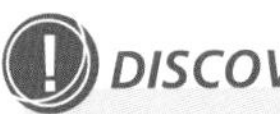

DISCOVERY

The genus *Neisseria* is named after the German physician Albert Ludwig Neisser. Admission statistics at the Breslau Hospital were begun in 1886, when gonorrhea accounted for about 9% of venereal disease admissions. With the microscopic examination of secretions that Neisser introduced, 54% of these admissions were diagnosed as gonorrhea. In 1900, Neisser called gonorrhea "a social danger for the people" that requires "the most careful attention from the authorities who are responsible for the public health."

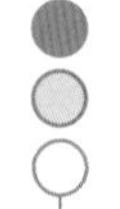

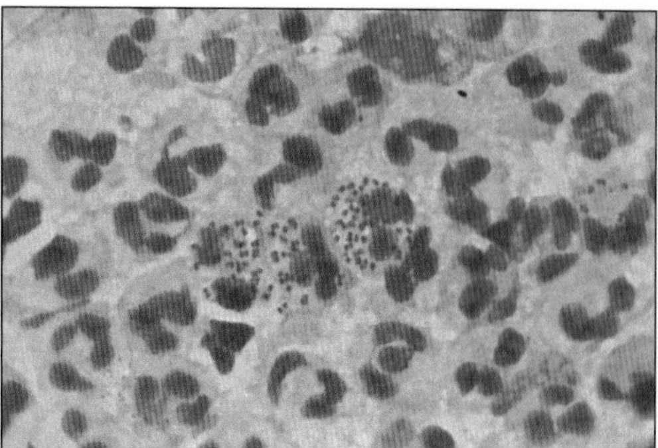

Fig 16-1 Gram-negative diplococcal *N gonorrhoeae* in neutrophils. (Public Health Image Library image 15018, courtesy of Bill Schwartz.)

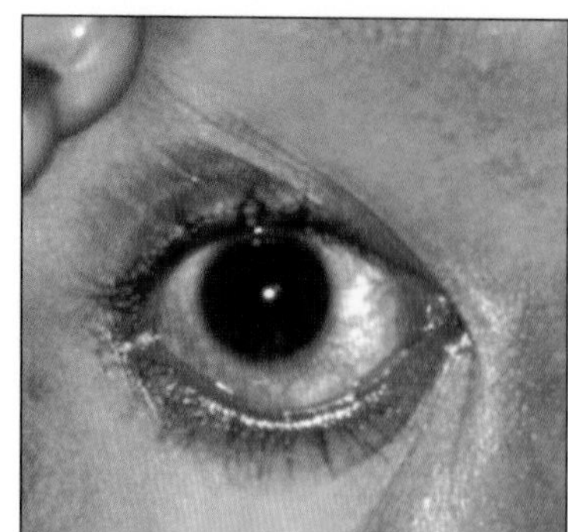

Fig 16-2 A patient presenting with gonococcal conjunctivitis in the right eye, following the dissemination of gonococcal urethritis. Rash and joint pain are additional manifestations of disseminated *N gonorrhoeae*. (Public Health Image Library image 6784, courtesy of Joe Miller.)

N gonorrhoeae

N gonorrhoeae (also called *gonococci*) are Gram-negative diplococci with pili. They are nonmotile, and they metabolize glucose oxidatively (Fig 16-1).

Clinical syndromes and diagnosis

In men, the infection manifests itself as acute urethritis, dysuria (painful, burning urination), the presence of a purulent urethral discharge, and rare complications such as epididymitis (acute or chronic inflammation of the epididymis) and prostatitis. In women, the bacterium causes infection of endocervical columnar epithelial cells, purulent vaginal discharge, intermenstrual bleeding, dysuria, and abdominal pain. In 10% to 20% of female patients, ascending genital infections are observed, including salpingitis (inflammation or infection of the fallopian tube) and pelvic inflammatory disease. These infections can cause ectopic pregnancy and sterility.

In some patients, infection results in septicemia, with a pustular rash on the skin, suppurative arthritis in the joints, and conjunctivitis (Fig 16-2). Other clinical manifestations include perihepatitis (Fitz-Hugh–Curtis syndrome), anorectal gonorrhea in homosexual men, and purulent conjuctivitis in newborns infected during delivery (ophthalmia neonatorum).

Diagnosis includes the observation of Gram-stained diplococci in neutrophils, nucleic acid–based assays, and culture in both nonselective and selective media. Culturing is particularly important in identifying antibiotic susceptibility. The oxidase reaction also helps in identifying *Neisseria* species, as they are oxidase-positive and contain cytochrome c.

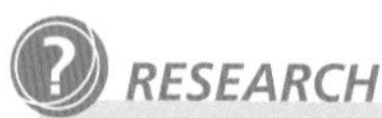

RESEARCH

What does the oxidase test actually measure?

Pathogenesis and epidemiology

The pili constitute one of the virulence factors of the bacterium. They mediate attachment to mucosal cell surfaces and are antiphagocytotic. Strains of bacteria that do not have pili are not virulent. There are more than 100 serotypes of pilin proteins that make up the pili; these different proteins cause antigenic variations of the bacteria. PorB (protein I) prevents phagosome-lysosome fusion in neutrophils, facilitates invasion of epithelial cells, and confers resistance to complement-mediated killing of the bacterium. Opa (protein II) mediates attachment to epithelial cells. Tbp1 and Tbp2 are transferrin-binding proteins and facilitate the acquisition of iron, which is essential for enzymes that are involved in the synthesis of nucleic acids. Lbp is a lactoferrin-binding protein that also helps in the acquisition of iron for the bacterium.

The lipooligosaccharide lacks the O-antigen but has endotoxin activity that induces the production of inflammatory cytokines, including tumor necrosis factor-alpha (TNF-α) production, by the host. The bacterium releases outer membrane blebs containing the lipooligosaccharide that enhance endotoxin activity and membrane proteins that can act as decoys by binding antibodies directed against the microorganism. The bacterial immunoglobulin A (IgA) protease degrades secretory IgA found on mucous surfaces, and the plasmid-encoded penicillinase breaks down β-lactam antibiotics.

The disease occurs only in humans. The bacterium is transmitted by sexual contact, and the risk of transmission is 50% in women and 20% for men. The major reservoirs of the bacterium are asymptomatic carriers.

Treatment and prevention

Penicillin G is not recommended because of the more than 200-fold increase in the required therapeutic dose since 1945. Resistance to penicillin is the result of a β-lactamase (penicillinase) encoded by a transmissible plasmid. The bacteria also have chromosomally mediated resistance to tetracyclines, erythromycin, and aminoglycosides because of changes of the cell surface that prevent antibiotic binding and penetration. The Centers for Disease Control and Prevention recommends the following treatment regimen:

- For uncomplicated cases, a single dose of ceftriaxone (Rosephin [Roche]; injectable) plus a single dose of azithromycin (or doxycycline twice daily for 7 days)
- If ceftriaxone cannot be given (eg, because of allergy), 2 g of azithromycin should be given.
- If ceftriaxone is not available, cefixim (Suprax [Lupin]; oral) plus a single dose of azithromycin (or doxycycline twice daily for 7 days).

Because sexually promiscuous individuals can get multiple infections, it appears that there is a lack of protective immunity. This may be the result of the variability in the immunodominant portion of the pilin protein. Thus, vaccines have not been effective. Chemoprophylaxis is used only in newborns to prevent gonococcal eye infections, and this therapy involves the use of a 1% silver nitrate solution, 1% tetracycline, or 0.5% erythromycin eye ointments. Prevention of the spread of gonorrhea involves education and the identification of infected individuals and their sexual partners.

N meningitidis

N meningitidis has about 90% DNA homology to *N gonorrhoeae*. However, it differs in that it has a capsule and that infection of the bloodstream causes a life-threatening disease.

Clinical syndromes and diagnosis

N meningitidis causes an abrupt and intense headache, stiff neck, vomiting, coma, and fever. Between 2,500 and 3,000 cases of the infection are reported per year in the United States. It is 100% lethal without antibiotic intervention and still less than 10% lethal with antibiotics. Meningococcemia (septicemia) causes disseminated intravascular coagulation, with accompanying shock, fever, and skin manifestations such as petechiae (purple or red spots on the skin resulting from hemorrhage in the dermal or submucosal layers) (Fig 16-3). These are manifestations of the induction of cytokines, including TNF-α and interleukin-1, by endotoxin.

N meningitidis is diagnosed from blood or cerebrospinal fluid samples as an oxidase-positive, Gram-negative diplococcus that grows on chocolate agar. The virulence of disseminated microorganisms pose a safety risk to laboratory personnel. Agglutination tests and polymerase chain reaction can also be used to confirm the species.

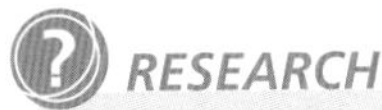

RESEARCH

What are other oxidase-positive microorganisms?

Pathogenesis and epidemiology

Meningococcal disease starts with the colonization of the nasopharynx mediated by pili. Because of the protection by the polysaccharide capsule, the bacterium can spread systemically without antibody-mediated phagocytosis. The toxic effects are caused by the endotoxin activity of the lipooligosaccharide.

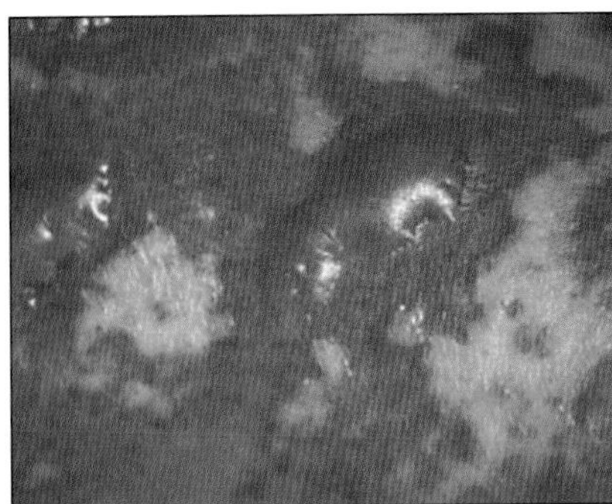

Fig 16-3 Skin lesions in a patient with meningococcemia, with petechial lesions and hemorrhagic bullae. (Reprinted with permission from Murray et al.)

Meningococcal disease is one of the most feared of all infections because of its rapid progression. The microorganism is part of the nasopharyngeal flora of about 10% of healthy individuals and is spread by respiratory droplets. Close, prolonged contact promotes the spread of the bacterium. The disease is most common in children under 1 year and young adults between 15 and 19 years of age.

Maternal antibodies are protective soon after birth, but this passive immunity decreases before acquired immunity develops.

Treatment and prevention

Penicillin and ampicillin are the antibiotics of choice, but rare resistance to penicillin is observed. Ceftriaxone and oily chloramphenicol are the drugs of choice in epidemics, because a single dose is effective in clearing the infection.

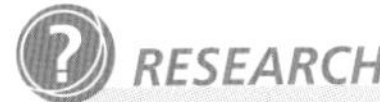

RESEARCH

How can bacterial meningitis be eliminated?

There are three quadrivalent meningococcal vaccines that target *N meningitidis* serogroups A, C, W-135, and Y available in the United States:

1. Menomune (MPSV-4; a polysaccharide vaccine) was cleared by the Food and Drug Administration in 1981 and is used for people aged 9 months to 55 years as well as for older people at risk.
2. Menactra (MCV-4; a diphtheria toxoid conjugate vaccine) was cleared by the FDA in January 2005.
3. Menveo (CRM197 conjugate vaccine) was cleared by the FDA in 2010.

The latter two vaccines are licensed for use in people ages 2 to 55 years. There are no vaccines available against serogroup B *N meningitidis* (MenB) disease, which is responsible for 32% of meningococcal disease in the United States and 45% to greater than 80% in Europe.

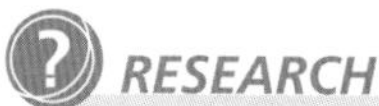

RESEARCH

Why is there no vaccine against serogroup B?

MCV-4 is now recommended for all children and teens aged 11 through 18 years. This vaccine is also used to control an outbreak of disease with a serogroup present in the vaccine, for travelers to hyperendemic areas (such as the meningitis belt in Africa), or for individuals at increased risk such as patients with complement deficiency.

E corrodens

E corrodens are Gram-negative rods and thus differ from the *Neisseria* species in this family. Infections are associated with human bite wounds, resulting in the introduction of oral microflora into deep tissues as well as subacute endocarditis, with a gradual onset of low fever, chills, and night sweats. The bacterium was initially described by M. Eiken as a *Bacteroides* species in 1958, and in 1972 it was classified as *E corrodens* because of its corrosion of the agar medium.

M catarrhalis

M catarrhalis is a Gram-negative diplococcus that can cause otitis media and sinusitis as well as life-threatening infections such as endocarditis and meningitis. It can also cause lower respiratory tract infections in elderly patients with chronic obstructive pulmonary diseases. Chronic bronchitis and pneumonia can also result from *M catarrhalis* infections. It can be treated with amoxicillin–clavulanic acid, cephalosporins, macrolides, and fluoroquinolones.

Bibliography

Centers for Disease Control and Prevention. *Moraxella catarrhalis.* www.cdc.gov/std/gonorrhea/lab/Mcat.htm. Accessed 17 June 2015.

Centers for Disease Control and Prevention. Public Health Image Library. phil.cdc.gov. Accessed 4 August 2015.

Centers for Disease Control and Prevention. Update to CDC's *Sexually Transmitted Diseases Treatment Guidelines, 2010*: Oral cephalosporins no longer a recommended treatment for gonococcal infections. Morb Mort Wkly Rep MMWR 2012;61:590–594.

Engleberg NC, DiRita V, Dermody TS. Schaechter's Mechanisms of Microbial Disease, ed 4. Baltimore and Philadelphia: Lippincott Williams & Wilkins, 2007.

Kirkcaldy RD. New Treatment Guidelines for Gonorrhea: Antibiotic Change. www.medscape.com/viewarticle/768883. Accessed 17 June 2015.

Murray PR, Rosenthal KS, Pfaller MA. Medical Microbiology, ed 6. Philadelphia: Mosby/Elsevier, 2009.

Ryan KJ, Ray CG. Sherris Medical Microbiology, ed 5. New York: McGraw-Hill, 2010.

World Health Organization. Meningococcal meningitis. www.who.int/mediacentre/factsheets/fs141/en/. Accessed 17 June 2015.

Take-Home Messages

- *Neisseria* are aerobic, Gram-negative diplococci.
- In men, *N gonorrhoeae* infection causes acute urethritis, dysuria (painful, burning urination), and a purulent urethral discharge.
- In women, *N gonorrhoeae* infects endocervical columnar epithelial cells and causes purulent vaginal discharge, intermenstrual bleeding, dysuria, and abdominal pain.
- The pili mediate attachment to mucosal cell surfaces and are antiphagocytotic.
- The bacterium releases outer membrane blebs containing the lipooligosaccharide that enhances endotoxin activity.
- For uncomplicated cases, a single dose of ceftriaxone plus a single dose of azithromycin is administered.
- *N meningitidis* has a capsule, and infection of the bloodstream causes a life-threatening disease.
- *N meningitidis* causes an abrupt and intense headache, stiff neck, vomiting, coma, and fever.
- Penicillin and ampicillin are the antibiotics of choice.
- There are three quadrivalent meningococcal vaccines that target *N meningitidis* serogroups A, C, W-135, and Y. No vaccine is available against serogroup B.
- *E corrodens* infections are associated with human bite wounds, resulting in the introduction of oral microflora into deep tissues as well as subacute endocarditis.

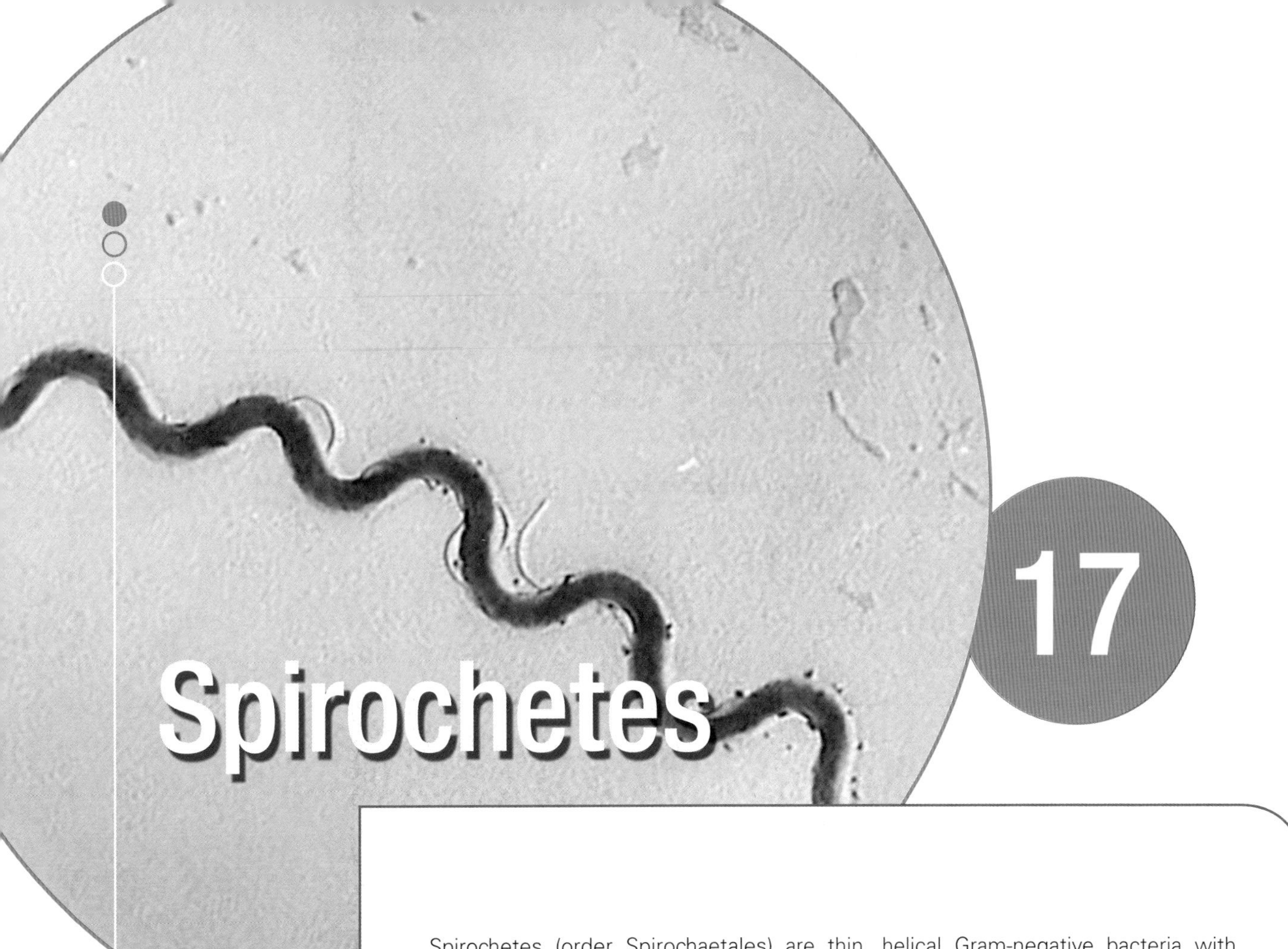

17 Spirochetes

Spirochetes (order Spirochaetales) are thin, helical Gram-negative bacteria with flagellum-like filaments ("axial filaments") in the periplasmic space that run along the length of the spirochete. They were once thought to be strict anaerobes, but it is now known that they can use glucose oxidatively. They can be aerobic, facultatively anaerobic, or anaerobic.

Treponema pallidum subspecies *pallidum*

Treponema pallidum subspecies *pallidum* causes syphilis. It is a thin, coiled spirochete that cannot be grown in cell-free culture but can be grown in Sf1Ep rabbit epithelial cells. Surprisingly, the bacteria can also grow on the surface of the cells. The bacteria are very labile and cannot survive exposure to drying or disinfectants.

Clinical syndromes and diagnosis

The clinical syndromes are observed in three phases. In the primary phase, skin lesions or ulcers called chancres occur at the site of infection (Fig 17-1). The lesion involves the inflammation of arteries, displaying endarteritis and periarteritis, with infiltrating neutrophils and macrophages. The microorganisms frequently survive ingestion by phagocytes. Infection spreads through the lymphatics and the bloodstream. The ulcer usually heals within 2 months (see Fig 17-2).

Disseminated disease is observed during the secondary phase, with skin lesions over the entire body. A flulike syndrome, lymphadenopathy, and a highly infectious mucocutaneous rash are observed. Spontaneous remission may occur in some cases, or the third phase follows.

During the tertiary or late phase, the disease disseminates and causes the destruction of any organ or tissue. The immune response to treponemal antigens causes vasculitis and chronic inflammation. Gummas, or soft masses of inflammatory

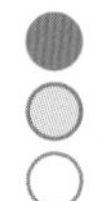

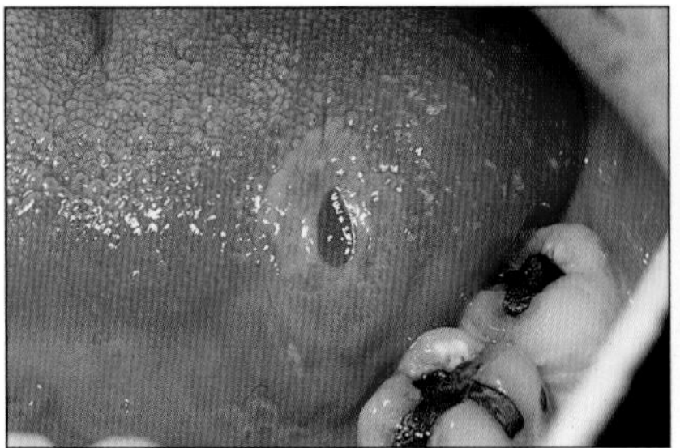

Fig 17-1 Oral manifestation of primary syphilis, in the form of a painless chancre, with elevated margins. (Reprinted with permission from Marx and Stern.)

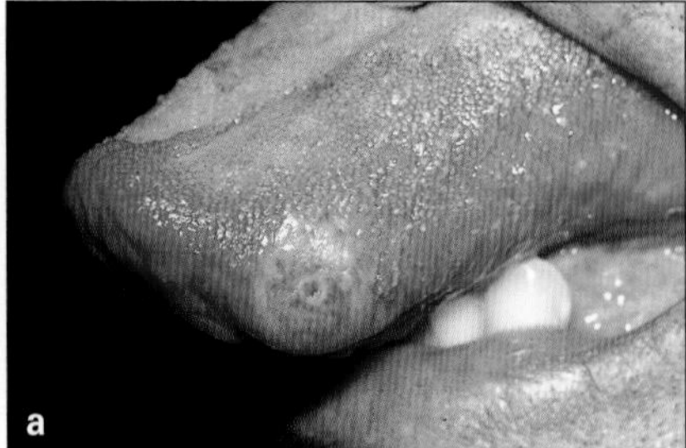

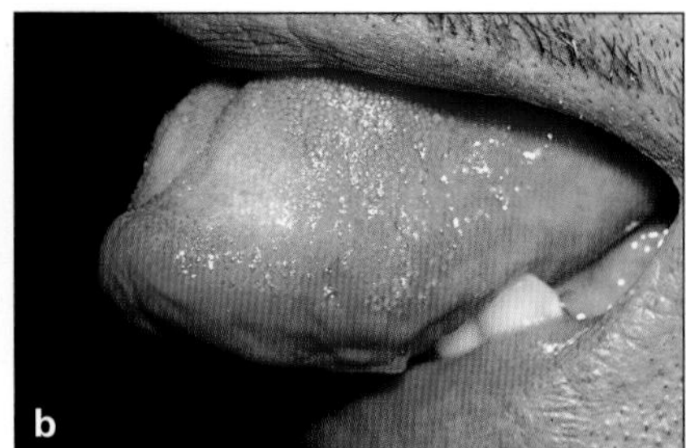

Fig 17-2 *(a)* The oral chancre in Fig 17-1, 1 week after receiving treatment with benzathine penicillin. *(b)* The resolution of the chancre 4 weeks after the administration of benzathine penicillin. (Reprinted with permission from Marx and Stern.)

cells and a few microorganisms, may result in bone and tissue destruction. The disease nomenclature is based on the organ of primary involvement, such as neurosyphilis or cardiovascular syphilis. Advanced disease results in bone destruction and cardiovascular syphilis. At this stage, infection can lead to fatal disease with multiorgan malformations. Neurosyphilis, with symptoms of meningitis, can also develop during the early phases of the disease.

Congenital syphilis is caused by treponemes crossing the placental barrier and can result in premature birth, multiple organ failure, and intrauterine growth retardation. The most common manifestations of congenital syphilis are facial and tooth deformities (Hutchinson incisors and mulberry molars) and, less commonly, deafness and arthritis.

Motile forms of the spirochete can be visualized by darkfield microscopy or by fluorescent antibodies. Nontreponemal tests measure immunoglobulin (Ig) G or IgM (called "reagin" antibodies) against lipids released from damaged cells and present in the cell membrane of treponemes (venereal disease research laboratory [VDRL] test; rapid plasma reagin [RPR] test). These tests examine the flocculation of cardiolipin (known as Wassermann antigen) by the patient's serum. False-positive tests may be obtained in the case of patients with viral infections, rheumatoid arthritis, systemic lupus erythematosus, or liver infections. Treponemal tests utilize the bacterium as the antigen and give fewer false-positive results. The fluorescent treponemal antibody absorption test detects IgG and IgM specific for the bacterium.

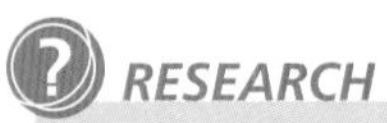

RESEARCH

Which membranes in the human body contain cardiolipin? What is the function of cardiolipin?

Pathogenesis and epidemiology

Virulent spirochetes produce hyaluronidase, which may facilitate perivascular infiltration. Outer membrane proteins promote adherence to host cells. Coating of the microorganism by fibronectin (a glycoprotein of the extracellular matrix and also found in blood) protects the microorganism against phagocytosis. Tissue destruction and lesions of syphilis are believed to be the result of the immune response to infection. When exposed to the bacteria, human cells express intercellular adhesion molecules that can facilitate the adhesion of immune cells and thus enhance local inflammation.

Syphilis is the third most common sexually transmitted disease in the United States after *Neisseria gonorrhoeae* (gonorrhea) and *Chlamydia trachomatis* (chlamydia) infections. It spreads via sexual contact, sometimes congenitally, and rarely via transfusion of contaminated blood. *T pallidum* subsp *pallidum* is transmitted primarily during the early stages of the disease. Syphilis cases reported to the Centers for Disease Control and Prevention (CDC) have increased from 13,970 in 2011 to 15,667 in 2012 (an increase of 12.1%).

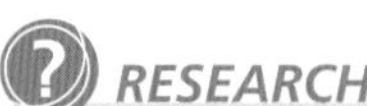

RESEARCH

***T pallidum* can be kept alive in culture only for a few cell divisions. How can the expression of treponemal proteins in *Escherichia coli* help in the identification of virulence factors of *T pallidum*?**

Treatment and prevention

Benzathine penicillin is used for the early stages of the disease (Fig 17-2), and penicillin G is prescribed for congenital or late syphilis. For patients who are allergic to penicillin, tetracycline and doxycycline can be prescribed. Neurosyphilis can only by treated with penicillin; thus, patients with penicillin allergies must be treated first to overcome the allergy. No vaccine is available. Safe sex and treatment of partners is essential. Prenatal care is very important for the prevention of congenital syphilis, since the disease can be prevented by penicillin treatment.

Penicillin treatment of patients with secondary syphilis can result in fever, chills, and myalgias a few hours after receiving the antibiotic. This response is called the Jarisch-Herxheimer reaction and is attributed to the release of endotoxin-like substances from the bacterium. Tumor necrosis factor-alpha (TNF-α) is an important mediator of this reaction, because passive immunization with anti-TNF antibody can prevent the symptoms.

Oral treponemes

Treponema denticola, *Treponema macrodentium*, and *Treponema orale* are part of the normal oral flora. The number of spirochetes increases with the onset of gingival inflammation and periodontal disease. They penetrate intact tissue next to inflamed tissue in acute necrotizing ulcerative gingivitis.

Borrelia

Borrelia species cause relapsing fever and Lyme disease. Borreliae are weakly staining Gram-negative bacilli that are larger than other spirochetes (3 to 30 μm in length). In smears of blood from patients with relapsing fever, the spirochetes stain with the Giemsa stain. Lyme disease is a tick-borne disease that can cause dermatologic, rheumatologic, neurologic, and cardiologic abnormalities. It is caused by numerous *Borrelia* species, primarily *Borrelia burgdorferi* in the United States. W. Burgdorfer discovered the spirochete responsible for Lyme disease.

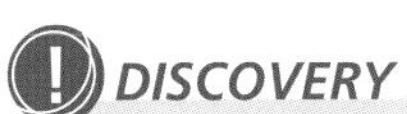

DISCOVERY

In the mid-1970s, an exceptionally large number of cases of juvenile rheumatoid arthritis were noted in Lyme, Connecticut, and two neighboring towns. Scientists first considered exposure to airborne and waterborne microbes but then focused on deer ticks, since most of these children lived and played near wooded areas. The first symptoms were noted during summer, the high season for ticks. Some of the patients noted a skin rash before the onset of arthritis and remembered being bitten by a tick at the rash site. Allen Steere at the Yale University School of Medicine was investigating "Lyme disease" cases in 1977 and contacted Willy Burgdorfer, a zoologist and microbiologist at the Rocky Mountain Laboratories in Montana, to discuss methods of dissecting and preserving tick tissues. Steere mentioned the deer tick as the potential carrier for Lyme disease.

Burgdorfer had studied relapsing fever 30 years earlier and had noted the transmission of spirochetes from soft-bodied ticks to the host. In 1981, while testing numerous deer ticks that Jorge Benach of the New York State Health Department supplied him, Burgdorfer noticed coiled microorganisms and recalled a 1949 conference where the hard ticks were described as spreading spirochetes and causing a European skin disorder called *erythema migrans*. He and his colleagues also found that serum from recovering Lyme disease patients had antibodies that reacted to spirochetes they had found in the deer ticks. Their studies were published in *Science* in 1982. The Lyme disease–causing spirochete was named after Burgdorfer for his role in identifying it.

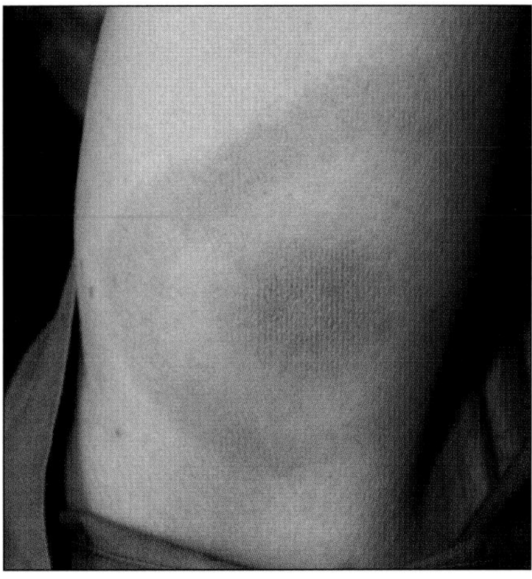

Fig 17-3 Erythema migrans, the characteristic Lyme disease rash, following a tick bite on the posterior upper right arm of a patient. (Public Health Image Library image 9875, courtesy of James Gathany.)

Clinical syndromes and diagnosis

Two forms of relapsing fever are recognized: epidemic louse-borne relapsing fever and endemic tick-borne relapsing fever. Relapsing fever has episodes of fever for several days, followed by a period without fever, and then another episode of fever, recurring from one to four times. The symptoms include fever, body aches, muscle and joint pain, nausea, vomiting, anorexia, headache, dry cough, rash, neck pain, eye pain, confusion, and dizziness. In epidemic relapsing fever, a single relapse is characteristic, but the disease is more severe.

Lyme disease is characterized by a skin lesion at the site of infection 3 to 30 days after the bite, starting as a small macule (a small flat discoloration at the same level as the rest of the skin) and then enlarging to cause erythema migrans in 70% to 80% of patients (Fig 17-3). The diameter of the erythema can range from 5 cm to greater than 50 cm. The lesion has a flat red border and a central clearing. Lyme disease causes malaise, severe fatigue, fever, chills, headache, muscle and joint pains, and swollen lymph nodes (lymphadenopathy), lasting for about 4 weeks. If untreated, the infection can spread to other parts of the body and cause erythema migrans, loss of muscle tone in the face (Bell's palsy), severe headaches, stiff neck due to meningitis, pain and swelling in the knees, heart palpitations, and dizziness resulting from a change in heartbeat. These symptoms will resolve over weeks to months, but if untreated they may lead to the late disseminated stage in about 60% of patients. Arthritis, most likely due to immunologic cross-reactivity, occurs at this stage, with severe joint pain and swelling. Some patients (up to 5%) may develop severe neurologic symptoms, including numbness or tingling in the extremities, shooting pains, and short-term memory loss.

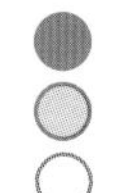

Even some patients who are treated with antibiotics for Lyme disease (10% to 20%) can develop posttreatment Lyme disease syndrome, characterized by muscle and joint pains, fatigue, cognitive defect, and sleep disturbance. It is thought that this stage of the disease is the result of autoimmune responses, and antibiotic treatment is contraindicated.

Giemsa- or Wright-stained preparations of blood from 70% of patients can reveal borreliae that cause relapsing fever. For the detection of Lyme disease, an enzyme-linked immunosorbent assay (ELISA) is used to detect antibodies, but not *B burgdorferi* itself. A positive ELISA is followed by a Western blot assay testing IgG against 10 different *B burgdorferi* proteins. These assays are important confirmatory tests for patients suspected of having Lyme disease; this method, however, is not useful at early stages of the disease, because no antibodies are formed at this time. The absence of antibodies at this early stage can result in a false-negative result for persons with very early Lyme disease. This in turn may cause a delay in treatment.

Pathogenesis and epidemiology

Borreliae are spread via blood following exposure to infected arthropods. The organism is present in low numbers in skin during erythema chronicum migrans, the characteristic skin lesion.

Relapsing fever is caused by *Borrelia recurrentis* as well as a number of other species and is transmitted by the human body louse. The periodic febrile and afebrile cycles of relapsing fever arise from the ability of the borreliae to undergo antigenic variation, periodically changing the molecules on their outer surface as a result of DNA rearrangement. This process enables the microorganism to evade the immune system. The three species that cause relapsing fever in the United States are *Borrelia hermsii*, *Borrelia parkerii*, and *Borrelia turicatae*. The clinical manifestations of relapsing fever are in part a response to the release of endotoxin.

Lyme disease is the major vector-borne disease in the United States. Hard ticks are the major vectors. The major reservoir hosts are the white-footed mouse and white-tailed deer. Ninety percent of infections are caused by ticks at the nymph stage, which is the size of a poppyseed. Hence, many patients do not remember having a tick bite. The pathogenesis of Lyme disease is thought to be the result of autoimmune reactions to the infections. Until recently, the CDC has estimated that there are 30,000 cases of Lyme disease per year in the United States. However, several new preliminary studies from the CDC have indicated that the actual incidence may be greater than 300,000 per year.

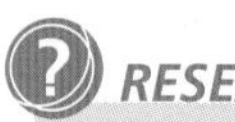

RESEARCH

Is the treatment of chronic Lyme disease (or post-Lyme disease) with antibiotics appropriate? How is the disease related to the ability of *B burgdorferi* to evade the immune system and survive antibiotic therapy?

Treatment and prevention

Relapsing fever has been treated most effectively with tetracycline or erythromycin. The early manifestations of Lyme disease are managed with doxycycline, amoxicillin, or cefuroxime. Despite this intervention, Lyme disease–related arthritis and other complications can occur in a small percentage of patients. Treatment can result in shock-like syndrome (increase in temperature, decrease in blood pressure, and leukopenia) resulting from the rapid killing of bacteria and the possible release of toxic substances (Jarisch-Herxheimer reaction).

Leptospira interrogans

Leptospira interrogans are coiled, thin, Gram-negative aerobic bacilli with a hook at one or both ends of the microorganism. Their motility is conferred by the two periplasmic flagellae.

Clinical syndromes and diagnosis

Initial symptoms of the disease are flulike, and the fever and myalgia may resolve after a week. The severe systemic disease is called Weil's disease and results in renal and hepatic failure, meningitis, vascular collapse, hemorrhage, thrombocytopenia (reduction in the number of platelets), myocarditis, and death.

Microscopic detection of the organism is difficult, even with Gram or silver staining. The spirochete may be cultured in a specific medium and then observed by dark-field microscopy. Antibodies in patient sera can be detected via the microscopic agglutination test, which detects the ability of antibodies to agglutinate (precipitate) different strains of live *Leptospira*.

Pathogenesis and epidemiology

The organism can penetrate into mucous membranes or skin through small cuts, spreads to all tissues, and damages the endothelium of small vessels. Immune complexes with the bacterial antigens can cause glomerulonephritis (renal disease). Infectious strains of *Leptospira* adhere to extracellular matrix components, including collagen, laminin, and fibronectin, via their Lsa24, Lsa21, LigA, and LigB proteins. The bacterium is transmitted from wild animals (most commonly rodents) and domestic animals that harbor the spirochete in their renal tubules. Streams, standing water, and moist soil can be infected with the urine from animals. Humans are considered an end-stage host. Although the incidence in the United States is thought to be low, there are no reporting requirements, which makes it impossible to know the actual incidence of the disease.

Treatment and prevention

Patients with severe disease should be treated with intravenous penicillin G or doxycycline. Vaccination of pets and livestock as well as rodent control have been useful in controlling the disease.

Bibliography

Centers for Disease Control and Prevention. Lyme Disease. www.cdc.gov/lyme/. Accessed 17 June 2015.

Centers for Disease Control and Prevention. Lyme Disease: Two-step Laboratory Testing Process. www.cdc.gov/lyme/diagnosistesting/LabTest/TwoStep/. Accessed 17 June 2015.

Centers for Disease Control and Prevention. Public Health Image Library. phil.cdc.gov. Accessed 4 August 2015.

Centers for Disease Control and Prevention. 2012 Sexually Transmitted Diseases Surveillance: Syphilis. www.cdc.gov/std/stats12/syphilis.htm. Accessed 17 June 2015.

Cinco M. New insights into the pathogenicity of leptospires: Evasion of host defences. New Microbiol 2010;33:283–292.

Engleberg NC, DiRita V, Dermody TS. Schaechter's Mechanisms of Microbial Disease, ed 4. Baltimore and Philadelphia: Lippincott Williams & Wilkins, 2007.

Marx RE, Stern D. Oral and Maxillofacial Pathology: A Rationale for Diagnosis and Treatment, ed 2. Chicago: Quintessence, 2012.

Murray PR, Rosenthal KS, Pfaller MA. Medical Microbiology, ed 6. Philadelphia: Mosby/Elsevier, 2009.

National Institute of Allergy and Infectious Diseases. Diagnostic Research. www.niaid.nih.gov/topics/lymedisease/research/Pages/diagnostics.aspx. Accessed 17 June 2015.

National Institute of Allergy and Infectious Diseases. Finding the Cause of Lyme Disease. www.niaid.nih.gov/topics/lymeDisease/research/Pages/cause.aspx. Accessed 17 June 2015.

Stricker RB, Johnson L. Lyme disease: Call for a "Manhattan Project" to combat the epidemic. PLoS Pathogens 2014;10:e1003796.

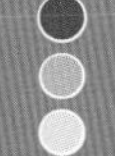

Take-Home Messages

- *T pallidum* subsp *pallidum* causes syphilis.
- In the primary phase of syphilis, skin lesions or ulcers called *chancres* occur at the site of infection.
- In the secondary phase, a flulike syndrome, lymphadenopathy, and a highly infectious mucocutaneous rash are observed.
- In the tertiary phase, the disease disseminates and causes the destruction of organs or tissues. The immune response to treponemal antigens causes vasculitis and chronic inflammation.
- The most common manifestations of congenital syphilis are facial and tooth deformities.
- Syphilis is the third most common sexually transmitted disease in the United States after *N gonorrhoeae* and *C trachomatis* infections.
- The number of *Treponema* in periodontal pockets increases with the onset of gingival inflammation and periodontal disease.
- *Borrelia* species cause relapsing fever and Lyme disease.
- Lyme disease is a tick-borne disease that can cause dermatologic, rheumatologic, neurologic, and cardiologic abnormalities. It is caused by numerous *Borrelia* species, primarily *B burgdorferi* in the United States.
- Relapsing fever is caused primarily by *B recurrentis* and is transmitted by the human body louse. The periodic febrile and afebrile cycles of relapsing fever arise from the ability of the borreliae to undergo antigenic variation.
- *L interrogans* can cause severe systemic disease known as *Weil's disease*, which is characterized by renal and hepatic failure, meningitis, vascular collapse, hemorrhage, thrombocytopenia, myocarditis, and death.

18 Enterobacteria, *Campylobacter*, and *Helicobacter*

The family Enterobacteriaceae are Gram-negative, aerobic and facultatively anaerobic bacilli, including the medically important genera *Escherichia*, *Salmonella*, *Shigella*, *Yersinia*, *Klebsiella*, *Proteus*, *Enterobacter*, *Citrobacter*, *Serratia*, and *Providencia*. The family includes the largest and most heterogeneous collection of pathogenic Gram-negative bacilli. Some bacteria are among the normal flora of the gastrointestinal tract of humans and animals. They are found in soil, water, and vegetation, following excretion from the gastrointestinal tract. They are responsible for about one-third of all septicemias, many intestinal infections, and more than 70% of urinary tract infections.

Shigella, *Salmonella* serotype Typhi, and *Yersinia pestis* are always associated with disease and are not found as normal flora in humans. *Escherichia coli*, *Proteus mirabilis*, and *Klebsiella pneumoniae* are commensals that can cause opportunistic infections.

Enterobacteria ferment glucose and reduce nitrate. They are catalase positive and oxidase negative. Some members of the family (eg, *Klebsiella*) have a polysaccharide capsule that defines the "K antigen." The O antigen refers to the outer polysaccharide portion of lipopolysaccharide (LPS), and the H antigen refers to the flagellar proteins.

The virulence factors of enterobacteria include endotoxin (LPS), the capsule, antigenic phase variation—which is the alternative expression of capsular (K) and flagellar (H) antigens to evade antibody responses—exotoxins, expression of adhesion factors (fimbriae), sequestration of growth factors via hemolysins and iron by siderophores, and the type III secretion system that enables the microinjection of virulence factors into the host cell. Their ability to survive and multiply intracellularly, resistance to complement-mediated killing, and resistance to antimicrobial agents are additional virulence factors.

E coli

Clinical syndromes and diagnosis

E coli (Fig 18-1) causes more than 90% of the approximately 7 million cases of bladder and lower urinary tract infections (cystitis) and a quarter million cases of kidney and upper urinary tract infections (pyelonephritis) annually in the United States. Urinary tract infections mostly originate from the patient's own intestinal flora. Septicemia can be initiated by the spread of bacteria that infect the urinary tract or the gastrointestinal tract. *E coli* and Group B streptococci (ie, *Streptococcus agalactiae*) are the most common causes of neonatal meningitis.

E coli strains that cause intestinal infections are classified according to their virulence and the type of gastroenteritis they cause: enterotoxigenic *E coli* (ETEC), enteroinvasive *E coli* (EIEC), enteropathogenic *E coli* (EPEC), enterohemorrhagic *E coli* (EHEC), and enteroaggregative *E coli* (EAEC).

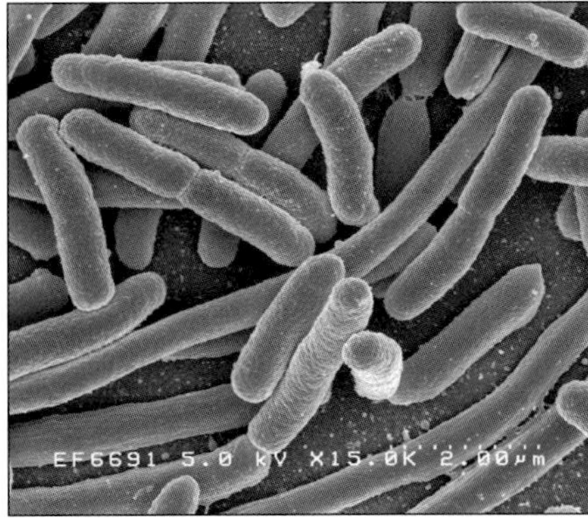

Fig 18-1 Scanning electron micrograph of *E coli*. The flagella and fimbriae are not visible in this type of electron microscopy. (Public Health Image Library image 18160, courtesy of the National Institute of Allergy and Infectious Diseases.)

Enterotoxigenic E coli

ETEC causes diarrhea following an incubation period of 1 to 2 days and persists for 3 to 4 days with cramps, nausea, vomiting, and watery diarrhea. It is the most important cause of traveler's diarrhea in visitors to developing countries, where it is also the leading cause of morbidity and mortality due to diarrhea in the first 2 years of life. It is transmitted by the consumption of contaminated food and water.

ETEC strains produce labile toxin (LT) and stable toxin (ST). LT inactivates part of the G protein in enterocytes, resulting in the accumulation of cyclic adenosine monophosphate and secretion of chloride, electrolytes, and water. ST activates guanylate cyclase, which results in the generation of cyclic guanosine monophosphate; however, the mechanism by which secretion is enhanced is not fully understood. The bacteria do not invade the tissue, and there is no apparent inflammation. Adherence of the bacteria to intestinal microvilli is mediated by fimbriae expressing the colonizing factor (CF) or the coli surface (CS) antigen. The genes for LT, ST, and CF are usually found on a single plasmid in ETEC. Natural immunity develops in the form of secretory immunoglobulin A (sIgA) against the toxins and can be passed on to breast-fed newborns.

LT-producing strains of *E coli* can be diagnosed by polymerase chain reaction (PCR) and enzyme-linked immunosorbent assay.

Enteroinvasive E coli

The pathogenesis of EIEC strains is similar to that of *Shigella* but milder. Ingested bacteria are resistant to gastric acid and bile and multiply in the large intestine. They penetrate the mucous layer, bind to the epithelial cells, and are endocytosed. The endocytotic vesicle lyses, thereby releasing the bacteria into the cytoplasm. The host cells are killed, and the bacterium spreads to neighboring cells with the help of an actin network, causing tissue destruction and inflammation. The initial symptom is watery diarrhea. Some patients develop dysentery, including cramping, fever, and blood and leukocytes in the stool.

Laboratory diagnosis is achieved with molecular techniques that detect genes that encode the invasion plasmid antigen (*ipaH*) and aerobactin (*iuc*).

Enteropathogenic E coli

EPEC is a major cause of pediatric diarrhea in communities with poor hygiene. Rare outbreaks occur in daycare nurseries in developed countries. Sometimes severe and protracted watery diarrhea is characteristic of EPEC infections. The microorganisms attach to epithelial cells of the small intestine and destroy the microvilli. The bacteria aggregate and form colonies on the surface of the epithelial cells with the aid of bundle-forming pili (BFP). The bacteria inject proteins into the enterocytes by the type III secretion system. The bacterial translocated intimin receptor (Tir) is inserted into the host cell membrane and acts as a receptor for the bacterial adhesion protein intimin. Cytoskeletal proteins accumulate below the intimin receptor, and the cell begins to deteriorate.

EPEC can be identified by lactose fermentation on MacConkey agar, followed by PCR detection of the intimin-encoding *aea* gene.

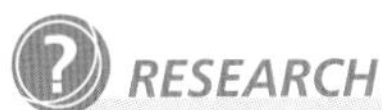

RESEARCH

What are the properties of MacConkey agar?

Enterohemorrhagic E coli

This strain of *E coli* is also identified as verocytotoxigenic E coli (VTEC) and is associated with hemorrhagic colitis and hemolytic uremic syndrome. EHEC produces verocytotoxin (VT), which is similar to Shiga toxin, but its genes are carried in a lambda-like bacteriophage, whereas Shiga toxin is encod-

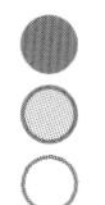

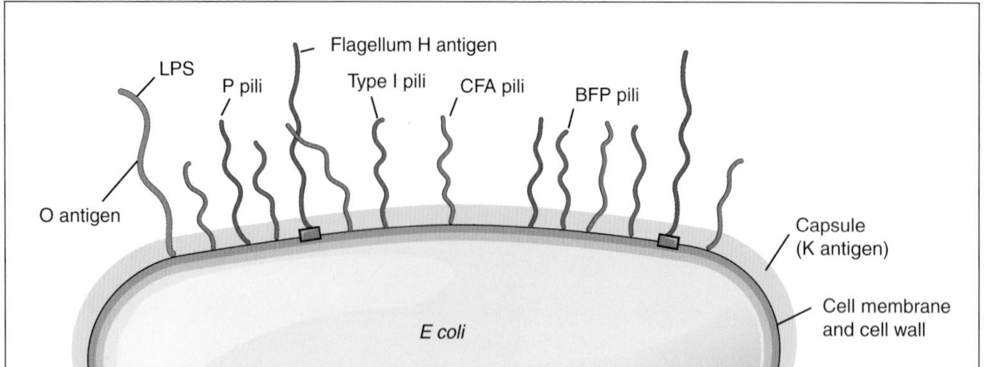

Fig 18-2 Antigenic structure of *E coli*. LPS contains the O antigen. The H antigen and K antigen are the flagellar protein and polysaccharide, respectively. The type I (common) pili are found in most *E coli* strains. Specialized P pili, colonization factor antigens (CFA) pili, and BFP are found in some *E coli* strains in addition to the type I pili.

ed by a chromosomal gene in *Shigella dysenteriae* type 1. The B component of the toxin binds to the glycolipid globotriosylceramide (GB_3), which is found on the villi of intestinal epithelial cells and on kidney endothelial cells. Inflammation resulting from EHEC infection increases the production of GB_3, further exacerbating the disease. The A component of the toxin binds to the 28S rRNA, inactivates 60S ribosomal subunits, and inhibits protein synthesis.

EHEC causes disease ranging from uncomplicated diarrhea to acute bloody diarrhea with abdominal cramps, thrombocytopenia, acute kidney failure, and hemolytic anemia. Outbreaks of these diseases were first recognized in 1982 in the United States, and the strain O157:H7 was identified as the major cause of these syndromes. Strains O145 and O104:H4 also cause disease. Hemolytic uremic syndrome is seen in approximately 8% of infections, results in kidney failure, and requires dialysis and transfusions. Some patients may develop chronic kidney failure, seizures, or stroke. There are an estimated 110,000 infections and 61 deaths each year in the United States resulting from infection with EHEC. The mortality rate is between 3% and 5%. Serious complications of the disease are more likely in children younger than 5 years and the elderly.

While the first cases of O157:H7 infection were reported in the 1980s, an outbreak occurred in 1991 resulting from the consumption of cider pressed from apples that had been contaminated with manure. In 1999, outbreaks occurred at county fairs as a result of cow manure contaminating water. A multistate outbreak of *E coli* O145 infections in 2010 was linked to shredded romaine lettuce from a single processing facility. In 2011, *E coli* O104:H4 infections occurred in a number of European countries as well as in the United States.

Infection is initiated by the consumption of contaminated and improperly cooked ground beef, unpasteurized milk and juice, and contaminated fruits and vegetables as well as contact with cattle. The bacterium can also be acquired through swimming in contaminated lakes or pools or drinking inadequately chlorinated water. It is transmitted readily from person to person, and the spread of the disease has been difficult to control in daycare centers.

Direct culture identification of EHEC may be difficult because the percentage of this bacterium in stool samples may be less than 1%. The bacterium can be concentrated by adherence to magnetic beads coated with O157-specific capture antibodies. The *vtx* genes encoding the two types of VT (VT1 and VT2) may be detected by DNA hybridization or PCR.

Enteroaggregative E coli

These microorganisms adhere to cells in an aggregated pattern that resembles stacked bricks, and they were first recognized in 1987 in an outbreak in Chile. EAEC is associated with chronic diarrhea and growth retardation in children, particularly in countries with poor hygiene conditions. It is rare in industrialized countries.

Some strains produce a Shiga toxin–like toxin, while others express hemolysins and aerobactin (a siderophore). The genes encoding the aggregative phenotype may be transferred to commensal and potentially pathogenic strains of *E coli*. The microorganism can be identified by the pattern of aggregation on human epithelial type 2 cells attached to glass slides and by DNA probes or PCR of the aggregative adhesion genes.

Pathogenesis and epidemiology

The O and K polysaccharides prevent phagocytosis and the attachment of complement. When antibodies to these antigens are present, however, the bacteria may be opsonized. Hemolysin enables accessibility to ferric ions bound to hemoglobin. Enterobactin and aerobactin are siderophores that can extract iron from transferrin and lactoferrin. Strains of *E coli* that cause septicemia, urinary tract infection, and pyelonephritis express aerobactin.

Urinary tract infections by uropathic *E coli* strains are facilitated by the type 1 (common) pili that mediate attachment to the epithelial cells in the bladder (Fig 18-2). The P pili bind to Gal-Gal receptors on uroepithelial cells in the upper urinary tract and are expressed in a majority of pyelonephritis isolates. Once the infection is established, the production of cytotoxic necrotizing factor (CNF) and α-hemolysin leads to the death of host cells. The bacteria can spread to the bloodstream and cause LPS-induced septic shock.

Treatment and prevention

The administration of fluid and electrolytes is most important in the treatment of *E coli* enteritis, as in other diarrheal diseases. The administration of antibiotics may enhance the production of verocytotoxin, however, and thus may be contraindicated. Preventive measures for ETEC involve the availability of safe water and effective hygienic practices in handling food, especially that given to young children. Travelers in countries where *E coli* infections are endemic should consume only hot foods or drinks and avoid salads. Infantile enteritis in hospitals and nurseries is spread from person to person, and thus hand hygiene and prevention of food contamination are essential. EHEC infections can be prevented by thorough cooking of meat and by avoiding contamination with uncooked meats.

Salmonella

Salmonellae are facultatively anaerobic, oxidase-negative, Gram-negative bacilli. The LPS molecules show extensive variability in the saccharide composition and the degree of polysaccharide branching. There are more than 2,000 antigenic types of *Salmonella*, the heterogeneity being attributable to the different LPS structures. The bacteria also express numerous flagella, the protein subunits of which are the basis of the H antigen serotyping (Fig 18-3). The strains that are pathogenic to humans are serotypes of *Salmonella enterica*. The different serotypes were originally designated as different species. The species formerly called *Salmonella enteritidis* is now designated as *S enterica* subsp *enterica* serotype Enteritidis. For convenience, this name is abbreviated as *S* Enteritidis. *S* Typhi has a polysaccharide capsule that may mask the LPS antigens and render identification with antibodies difficult.

Clinical syndromes and diagnosis

Salmonella infection can cause gastroenteritis, septicemia, enteric fever (typhoid fever), and asymptomatic colonization. Noninvasive *Salmonella* serotypes can cause gastroenteritis, with diarrhea, nausea, headache, and malaise. Severe cases manifest as watery, green stools with abdominal pain, fever, shivering, dehydration, hypotension, and renal failure. All *Salmonella* serovars, but especially *S* Typhi, *Salmonella* Paratyphi, and *Salmonella* Choleraesuis, can cause septicemia. Enteric fever is caused by *S* Typhi (typhoid fever), *S* Paratyphi A, and two other strains (paratyphoid fever). The bacteria penetrate the intestinal lining, are phagocytosed by macrophages, and are transported to the liver, bone marrow, and spleen. The symptoms include increasing fever, myalgia, headache, anorexia, and malaise. The intestines are reinfected through the gallbladder, and the disease can continue for a month. These strains can also cause chronic colonization in 1% to 5% of patients. These persistent carriers must register with local public health departments, and as long as they carry *Salmonella* they are barred from occupations involving food and children. They can be treated with antibiotics, or their gallbladders may be removed. The case of Typhoid Mary is an illustration of a chronic carrier who had to be confined to a hospital in New York after being linked to 1,300 cases of typhoid fever.

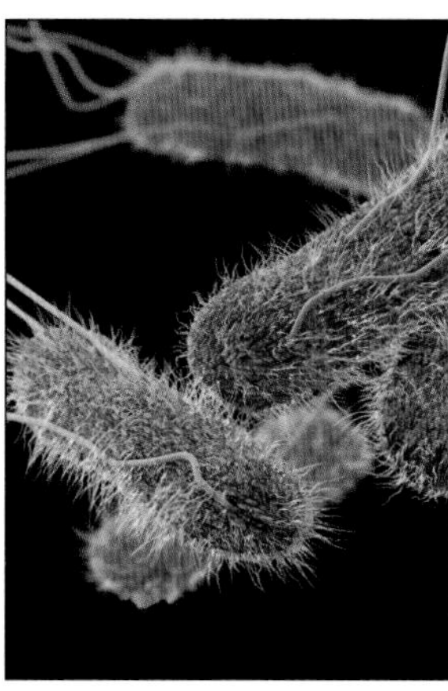

Fig 18-3 Computer-generated image of multidrug-resistant *Salmonella* serotype Typhi, showing the flagella that express the H antigen as well as the short fimbriae. (Public Health Image Library image 16877, courtesy of Melissa Brower.)

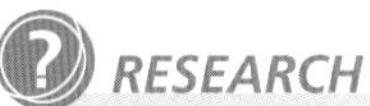

RESEARCH

How are Dr George A. Soper and Typhoid Mary connected?

Salmonella from fecal samples can be identified by growth on selective media such as deoxycholate-citrate agar or xylose-lysine-deoxycholate agar. The O antigen can be identified by slide agglutination, and bacterial samples can be transferred to peptone water for the identification of the flagellar H antigen. The bacteria can also be identified by PCR, but as with all PCR assays, the numbers of bacteria and the amount of DNA must be at sufficient levels that enable successful amplification. The most reliable method of diagnosis for enteric fever is bone marrow or blood culture.

Pathogenesis and epidemiology

Salmonella pathogenesis is initiated by its ability to cross host barriers by invading phagocytotic and nonphagocytotic cells. Entry of *Salmonella* into host cells was thought until recently to require only the type III secretion system (T3SS). However, *Salmonella* can infect cells without T3SS. The outer membrane proteins Rck and PagN are now known to act as invasins. Rck mediates a zipper-like entry mechanism where the cell membrane wraps around the bacterium as a result of the tight adhesion, and actin is polymerized at the site. However, Rck-independent zipper-like entry has also been observed. *Salmonella* binds to and invades both enterocytes and M (microfold) cells in the intestines. The T3SS induces the formation of ruffles on M cells that result from the rearrangement of filamentous actin. This is followed by the uptake of the bacteria by the M cells.

The *Salmonella* pathogenicity island 1 (SPI-1), a cluster of virulence genes in the bacterial chromosome, mediates invasion, replication, and biofilm formation and affects host responses. The T3SS is encoded by genes in the *Salmonella* pathogenicity island 2 (SPI-2). Intracellular replication occurs in a specialized membrane-bound compartment, the *Salmonella*-containing vacuole, and involves

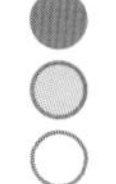

the translocation of approximately 30 effector proteins via the SPI-2 T3SS into the host's intracellular membrane system and the cytoplasm. These proteins maintain the integrity of the vacuole and its localization near the nucleus and interfere with the host cytoskeleton and signaling to the immune system.

Salmonella are found in many animals, including poultry, livestock, rodents, domestic animals, and birds, as well as in humans. *S* Typhi and *S* Paratyphi are highly adapted to man and do not cause disease in nonhuman hosts. Other *Salmonella* strains are adapted to animals, and they can cause severe disease when they infect humans (*S* Choleraesuis). The disease is spread via contaminated water or food products, such as poultry, eggs, and dairy products. It can be transmitted directly by the fecal-oral route in children.

Treatment and prevention

In the late 1940s, the introduction of chloramphenicol decreased the mortality rate of enteric fever from above 20% to less than 2%. However, bone marrow toxicity of this antibiotic led to the use of amoxicillin and co-trimoxazole. The development of resistance to these antibiotics has resulted in the use of ciprofloxacin, ceftriaxone, and cefixime. Antibiotics are not useful in the treatment of gastroenteritis. Patients at risk for developing bacteremia, such as infants under 3 months of age and immunosuppressed individuals, may be treated with antibiotics. *Salmonella* bacteremia requires aggressive treatment with antibiotics.

Proper sanitation, such as the disposal of human excreta and the availability of pure drinking water, is an important control measure. Raw foods of animal origin must not have any contact with cooked foods. Cooked foods should be consumed right after cooking, and any leftovers should be cooled rapidly and refrigerated. Health education of food handlers is a very important prevention method. Two typhoid vaccines are currently available for use in the United States: an oral, live attenuated vaccine (Vivotif Berna [Crucell]) and a Vi capsular polysaccharide vaccine (ViCPS) (Typhim Vi [Aventis Pasteur]) for intramuscular use. These vaccines are 50% to 80% effective.

Shigella

Shigella species are Gram-negative, facultatively anaerobic, oxidase-negative bacilli that cause bacillary dysentery. Dysentery is characterized by the frequent passage of blood-stained, mucopurulent stools and is classified as bacillary or amoebic dysentery. *Shigella* causes about 150 million cases of infectious diarrhea worldwide and 600,000 deaths per year.

Shigella is closely related to enteroinvasive serotypes of *E coli*. DNA analysis has indicated that this genus can be classified as a biogroup within *E coli*. However, they lack flagella and the accompanying H antigen. The genus is subdivided into four species: *(1) Shigella dysenteriae* type 1 produces Shiga toxin and is responsible for the most serious forms of shigellosis. *(2) Shigella sonnei* is responsible for most infections in the United States, and *(3) Shigella flexneri* causes disease in developing countries. *(4) Shigella boydii* is rare.

DISCOVERY

In 1892, Kiyoshi Shiga entered the Tokyo Imperial University School of Medicine, where he was influenced by Dr Shibasaburo Kitasato, a protégé of Robert Koch and discoverer of tetanus antitoxin. After graduation, Shiga started to work with Kitasato. Dysentery epidemics in Japan caused high mortality among the tens of thousands of infected people, and Shiga described the disease as "the most dreaded disease of children from its fulminating course and high mortality." The 1897 epidemic affected more than 91,000 people, with a mortality rate greater than 20%. In the medical literature, the term *dysentery* had been used to describe violent diarrhea of almost any cause. Interestingly, the Japanese term *sekiri* is derived from Chinese characters that indicate "red diarrhea," which is closer to the current definition of dysentery.

Shiga employed simple but precise methods based on Koch's postulates to identify the organism that caused dysentery. He isolated a Gram-negative bacillus from the stools of patients with dysentery and showed that the organism caused diarrhea in experimental dogs. Crucial for his discovery was his observation that the organism agglutinated when exposed to the serum of convalescent dysentery patients. He published his findings in 1898 in German. The organism was initially termed *Bacillus dysenteriae*. Shiga described the production of toxic factors by the organism, one of which is currently called *Shiga toxin*. The genus name was changed to *Shigella* in the 1930 edition of Bergey's *Manual of Determinative Bacteriology*.

Clinical syndromes and diagnosis

Infection causes abdominal cramps, diarrhea, fever, and bloody stools. Symptoms are apparent 1 to 3 days after the bacilli are ingested. The symptoms usually resolve in 5 to 7 days. In children less than 2 years old, severe infection with high fever may result in seizures. In some cases, infected individuals may have no symptoms yet transmit the microorganism to others.

The presence of *Shigella* in stool samples can be detected by selective media such as Hektoen enteric agar, which also contains indicators that reveal specific biochemical reactions. Slide agglutination tests with O group–specific antisera can confirm the particular *Shigella* species.

Pathogenesis and epidemiology

Shigella invades and destroys the intestinal epithelium, causing an intense inflammatory response characterized by mucosal ulceration and abscess formation. The pathway of the microorganism during this invasion is quite intriguing. The bacteria are transcytosed through M cells, are phagocytosed by underlying macrophages, and enter the cytoplasm by penetrating through the phagosome membrane. They induce apoptosis of the macrophages, exit the cell, and invade the enterocytes from the basolateral side by first microinjecting the invasion plasmid antigens IpaA–IpaD through the T3SS. These proteins mediate cytoskeletal reorganization and actin polymerization that facilitate the internalization of the bacteria by endocytosis. Following the escape of the bacteria into the cytoplasm, actin tails form at one end of the bacteria, propel them toward the lateral cell membrane, and push them into the neighboring cell, whose membrane invaginates to accommodate the membrane-*Shigella* complex protruding from the first cell. The bacteria then lyse both membranes and enter the cytoplasm. This process damages the enterocytes and causes ulcers and hemorrhage, enabling the bacteria to reach the lamina propia and causing an acute inflammatory response. The diarrhea caused by the inflammation contains white blood cells, red blood cells, and bacteria. The Shiga toxin of *S dysenteriae* type 1 may cause systemic effects, such as hemolytic uremic syndrome, similar to that caused by EHEC.

Shigella is spread primarily via the fecal-oral route and contaminated hands, making it a "disease of dirty hands." The infectious dose is very low, estimated in some studies to be just 10 bacilli. It is also spread by water or food contaminated by humans. It has no animal reservoirs; the only reservoir is the human intestine. It is largely a pediatric disease in developed countries. It is more widespread in countries with poor sanitary infrastructure. Outbreaks can occur in refugee camps.

About 7,700 cases of shigellosis were reported in the United States in 2012. Because milder cases may not be recognized and reported, the actual number of cases is estimated to be 20 times higher.

Treatment and prevention

Infection is usually self-limited. Antibiotic treatment is recommended to reduce the risk of secondary spread to family members and also to reduce the duration of the disease. If susceptible, the bacteria can be treated with ampicillin. Otherwise, trimethoprim-sulfamethoxazole, ceftriaxone, fluoroquinolones, nalidixic acid, and azithromycin can also be used if the strains are susceptible.

Sewage disposal, water chlorination, hand washing, and proper cooking of food are very effective preventive measures. Nevertheless, hand washing will only reduce the number of bacteria. There are no effective vaccines. Research is focused on live attenuated vaccines that proceed through some of the multistage infection to elicit an immune response.

Yersinia

Yersinia are Gram-negative, facultatively anaerobic, oxidase-negative coccobacilli that cause bubonic plague, pneumonic plague, and gastroenteritis. They are primarily animal pathogens and are occasionally transmitted to humans. The species that cause disease in humans are *Y pestis*, *Yersinia pseudotuberculosis*, and *Yersinia enterocolitica*.

Clinical syndromes and diagnosis

The first clinical manifestations of *Y pestis* infection, occurring within 2 to 7 days of a flea bite, are fever and painful, extensively swollen lymph nodes, most often in the groin ("bubo" from the Greek *boubon* for groin). The mortality rate is 75% in untreated patients. Patients with pneumonic plague experience fever, malaise, and pulmonary symptoms. If untreated, 90% of patients will die.

Y enterocolitica infection results in fever, diarrhea, and abdominal pain for 1 to 2 weeks. Because the infection involves the terminal ileum, it can present symptoms of appendicitis in case of mesenteric lymphadenopathy. The bacterium can also cause transfusion-related bacteremia following the storage of infected, nutritionally rich blood products at 4°C, because it can grow to high concentrations at this temperature.

Diagnosis involves Gram staining of aspirates from a bubo, revealing bipolar-staining Gram-negative bacteria, as well as immunofluorescence for immediate identification of smears or cultures. It is important to notify laboratories regarding suspected *Y pestis* infection to both expedite diagnosis and warn personnel against infection.

Pathogenesis and epidemiology

Y pestis produces different virulence factors in the flea and in the human host. The F1 gene encodes a gel-like protein capsule that inhibits phagocytosis. The plasminogen activator Pla degrades complement components C3a, thereby preventing opsonization, and C5a, thus inhibiting chemotaxis of phagocytes. It also degrades fibrin, enabling the bacteria to spread in tissue. *Yersinia* outer membrane proteins (Yop) can either enzymatically digest host cells or be injected into the host cell through the T3SS. YopH dephosphorylates proteins needed for phagocytosis, YopE disrupts actin filaments, and YopJ/P induces apoptosis of macrophages.

The bacteria spread to the local lymph nodes and cause a suppurative, hemorrhagic lymphadenitis that manifests itself as the bubo. They then enter the bloodstream and cause systemic toxicity via their endotoxin and proteases. In the lungs, the infection produces a necrotizing hemorrhagic pneumonia, hence the term pneumonic plague.

Y enterocolitica virulence factors include invasin that binds host cell integrins and Yop proteins either on the bacterial surface or injected by the T3SS into host cell, where they disrupt biochemical pathways and the actin cytoskel-

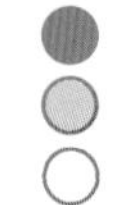

eton. The end result is the paralysis of phagocytes. Thus, the bacterium can populate the reticuloendothelial system.

Plague is a disease of rodents transmitted to humans via the bite of a rat flea. It occurs in two epidemiologic states: sylvatic, referring to plague in wildlife, and urban. Bubonic plague develops following the transmission of the microorganism to humans. Bacteremic spread to the lungs leads to pneumonic plague, which is readily transmitted from person to person, especially in crowded, unsanitary conditions. *Y pestis* caused the Black Death of the Middle Ages in Europe, killing 25 million people between 1346 and 1350, out of an estimated population of 105 million people. Pandemics of plague continued through the end of the 19th and early 20th centuries.

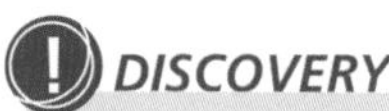

DISCOVERY

The Swiss-French physician Alexandre Yersin, working in Hong Kong in 1894, identified the etiologic agent of the plague and named it *Pasteurella pestis*. The bacterium was renamed in his honor in 1967 as *Yersinia pestis*.

Although urban plague has been eliminated by public health measures, sylvatic plague is still observed in Southeast Asia and even in the southwestern and western United States.

Y enterocolitica is spread by the consumption of contaminated food, such as raw or undercooked pork products, milk, and water. The incidence of culture-confirmed enterocolitis due to this bacterium is 1 in 100,000 each year. *Y pseudotuberculosis* is most likely transmitted to humans from animals, with highest rates reported in Scandinavian and other European countries.

Treatment and prevention

Bubonic or pneumonic plague can be treated with streptomycin or gentamicin. However, timely treatment is essential. Alternative antibiotics are ciprofloxacin, doxycycline, and chloramphenicol. *Y enterocolitica* infections are usually self-limiting; the bacteria are resistant to penicillins and cephalosporins because of the production of β-lactamase. Aminoglycosides, tetracyclines, fluoroquinolones, and ampicillin are effective against *Y pseudotuberculosis*.

Klebsiella

Klebsiella are Gram-negative, facultatively anaerobic, capsulated rods. They primarily cause urinary tract infections but also cause wound and soft tissue infections, endocarditis, and severe bronchopneumonia with multiple abscesses. *K pneumoniae* and *Klebsiella oxytoca* can cause community-acquired or hospital-acquired lobar pneumonia.

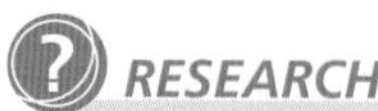

RESEARCH

What are the characteristics of lobar pneumonia, and how are they different from other types of pneumonia?

The polysaccharide capsule is a significant virulence factor, preventing opsonization and complement binding. Type 1 fimbriae and nonfimbrial adhesins (CF29K and CS31A) facilitate binding to host cells.

Klebsiella infections can be treated with combinations of amoxicillin or ampicillin with the β-lactamase inhibitor clavulanic acid and with the β-lactamase–stable cephalosporins cefuroxime and cefotaxime. Pneumonia requires aggressive treatment with an aminoglycoside or a cephalosporin.

Proteus

P mirabilis has a characteristic "swarming growth" when placed at the center of blood agar plates, interspersed with a stationary period. It causes urinary tract infections in children as well as bacteremia in newborns or in patients with other underlying conditions. Some strains produce hemolysins and IgA protease. It produces urease, which hydrolyses urea into CO_2 and NH_3. This raises the pH of urine, causing the precipitation of Ca^{2+} and Mg^{2+} and the formation of kidney stones. The raised pH is also toxic to the epithelial cells lining the urinary tract.

The microorganism is sensitive to ampicillin and other β-lactam antibiotics. All strains are resistant to tetracycline.

Enterobacter

Enterobacter species are similar to *Klebsiella* except that most species are motile with the aid of peritrichous flagella. Hospital outbreaks of *Enterobacter* infection have been traced to contaminated parenteral fluids. It is associated with hospital-acquired infections in patients with a compromised immune system. Gentamicin, fluoroquinolones, carbapenems, and co-trimoxazole are effective against *Enterobacter*.

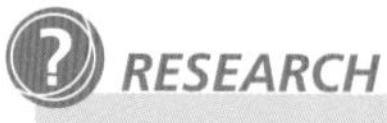

RESEARCH

What are distinguishing features of peritrichous, monotrichous, amphitrichous, and lophotrichous flagella?

Citrobacter

Citrobacter may be found in the normal intestinal flora and may cause opportunistic infections such as bacteremia. *Citrobacter koseri* may cause neonatal meningitis with cerebral abscesses and a high mortality rate. The choice of treatment should be based on in vitro antibiotic susceptibility testing.

Campylobacter

Campylobacter, together with *Helicobacter*, are classified as Epsilonproteobacteria. They are included in this chapter because they cause gastrointestinal diseases. *Campylobacter* are Gram-negative, oxidase-positive, motile rods (Fig 18-4). The capsular polysaccharide can be used in serotyping different strains. *Campylobacter jejuni* and *Campylobacter coli* are some of the most common causes of infectious diarrhea. Thus, it is surprising that they were not recognized as a pathogen until 1973.

Clinical syndromes and diagnosis

Symptoms appear 1 to 7 days after ingestion of *C jejuni* and include fever and lower abdominal pain that may sometimes mimic appendicitis. Within hours, dysenteric stools with pus and blood are observed. The disease usually resolves after 3 to 5 days but sometimes extends to 1 to 2 weeks. A rare complication is the development of Guillain-Barré syndrome in about 1 in 1,000 diagnosed infections. A late, immune-related complication is the development of reactive arthritis, with painful swelling of the joints.

Other *Campylobacter* species, such as *Campylobacter concisus* and *Campylobacter rectus* are involved in periodontal disease.

The bacterium can be diagnosed by the use of a selective medium that inhibits normal flora and incubation under microaerophilic conditions.

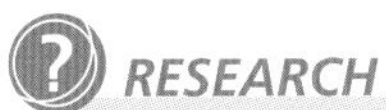

RESEARCH

When was Guillain-Barré syndrome first described? What are its clinical manifestations? Why do some infections by *C jejuni* lead to this syndrome?

Pathogenesis and epidemiology

Following ingestion, *C jejuni* and *C coli* colonize the jejunum and ileum and invade the epithelial cells (Fig 18-5). They produce cytolethal distending toxin that blocks the cell cycle and also express a type VI secretion system (T6SS) that facilitates invasion and colonization. The integrity of the mucosal cell layer is thereby disrupted. This leads to the infiltration of the lamina propia with neutrophils, mononuclear cells, and eosinophils and to the inhibition of the absorptive function, leading to net fluid loss and diarrhea.

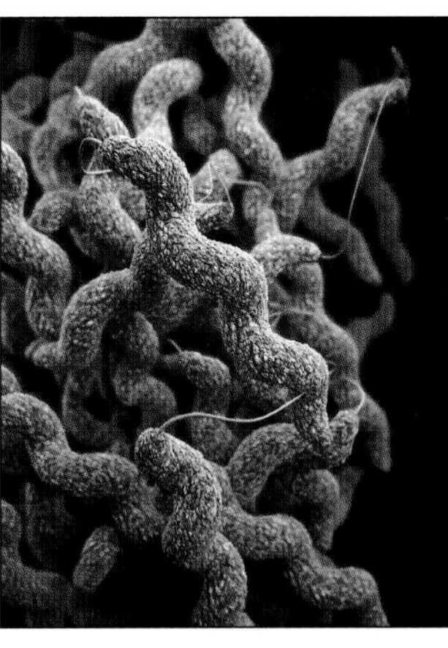

Fig 18-4 Computer-generated image of *Campylobacter jejuni* with bipolar flagella. (Public Health Image Library image 16870, courtesy of Melissa Brower.)

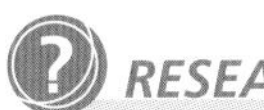

RESEARCH

How can you show that the T6SS is important in invasion and colonization by *C jejuni*?

Infection results in the production primarily of IgG, but repeated exposure increases the levels of IgA, which confers protection. *Campylobacter fetus* can spread from the intestines to the blood and distant tissues, possibly because it is resistant to killing by complement and antibody opsonization in serum. The heat-stable, capsule-like S protein inhibits C3b binding to the bacteria.

Poultry, cattle, and sheep are reservoirs for *C jejuni*. It is transmitted via contaminated food and water. Cats and dogs are reservoirs for *Campylobacter upsaliensis*, which can be transmitted to humans via contact with infected animals. The Foodborne Diseases Active Surveillance Network has estimated that the incidence of *Campylobacter* infections is 14.3 cases per 100,000 population in the United States. It is estimated that there are 76 fatal cases per year.

Treatment and prevention

Campylobacter infections are usually self-limiting and are managed by replacing fluids and electrolytes. Erythromycin and azithromycin are used in cases of severe infection or septicemia. Tetracycline and fluoroquinolones can be employed as secondary antibiotics. However, the use of fluoroquinolone antibiotics, particularly enrofloxacin, in poultry flocks, which was cleared by the Food and Drug Administration (FDA) in 1995, led to an increase in resistance to these antibiotics in human *Campylobacter* infections. The percentage of human *Campylobacter* isolates that were resistant to ciprofloxacin increased from 12% in 1997 to 24% in 2011. In 2005, the FDA rescinded the clearance for the use of fluoroquinolones in poultry.

Prevention measures include reducing the contamination of poultry meat, preventing the consumption of raw milk, and consumer education.

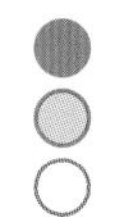

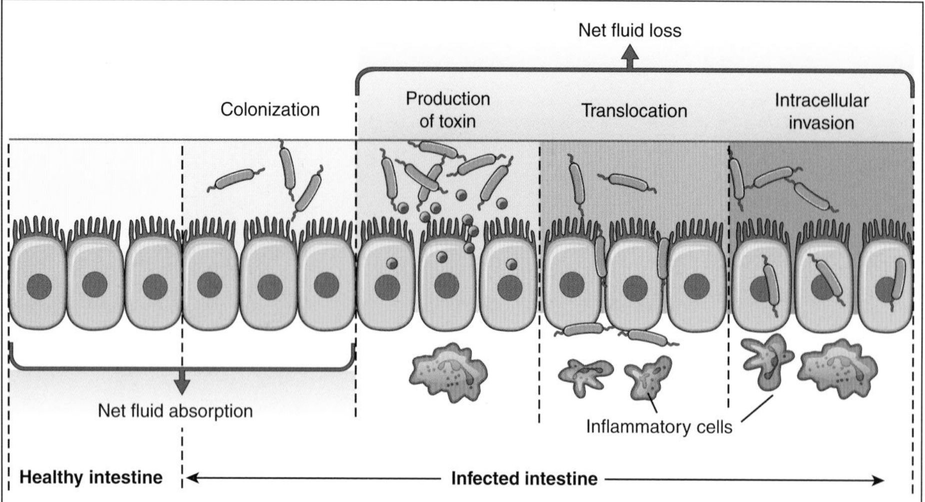

Fig 18-5 Pathogenesis of *C jejuni* and *C coli*. In the undamaged ileal and colonic epithelium, there is net fluid absorption. Following infection, the bacteria reach the mucous layer and the epithelial cell surface, helped by their chemotactic mobility. They then produce cytolethal distending toxin that blocks the cell cycle and synthesize a type VI secretion system (T6SS) that facilitates invasion and colonization. The integrity of the mucosal cell layer is disrupted, and this leads to an inflammatory response as well as to the inhibition of the absorptive function, resulting in net fluid loss and diarrhea. (Adapted from Greenwood et al.)

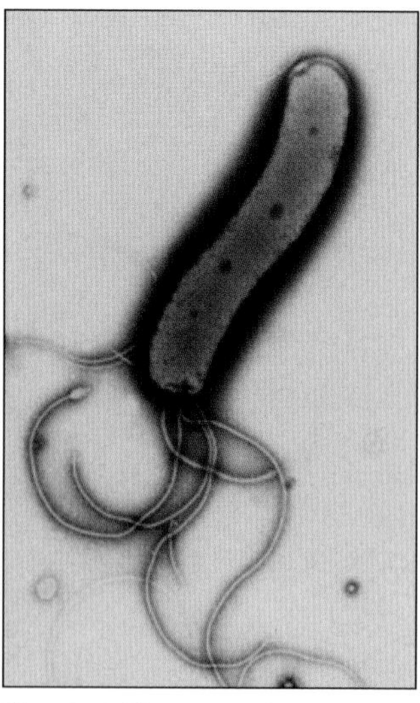

Fig 18-6 Electron micrograph of *Helicobacter pylori* with multiple sheathed, unipolar flagella. (Courtesy of Dr David J. Kelly, University of Sheffield.)

Helicobacter

Helicobacter are Gram-negative, curved bacilli that sometimes appear as coccobacilli in older cultures or under adverse conditions. They have unipolar, sheathed flagella (Fig 18-6), are microaerophilic, and require CO_2. *Helicobacter* is a pathogen that colonizes the human stomach. It is highly motile, utilizing its flagella in a corkscrew-patterned motility. Infection is acquired during childhood and persists if not eradicated. It is estimated that 50% of the world's human population is infected chronically. *Helicobacter pylori* causes chronic gastritis and increases the risk of peptic ulcer disease and gastric cancer.

Clinical syndromes and diagnosis

H pylori infection leads to gastritis, characterized histologically by the infiltration of mononuclear cells and neutrophils into the mucosa. Clinically, the patient experiences nausea, vomiting, abdominal pain, flatulence, and a feeling of being full. The acute phase may develop into chronic gastritis, with some patients (10% to 15%) developing peptic ulcers. Gastric ulcers develop at the junction of the corpus and the antrum, and duodenal ulcers develop at the proximal duodenum.

A manifestation of chronic gastritis is the proliferation of epithelial cells similar to those in the intestines in place of the gastric epithelial cells and the resulting 100-fold increase in the risk of gastric cancer, which is also affected by the strain of *H pylori* and the host immune response to it. Chronic antigen stimulation of B lymphocytes may result in gastric lymphoma.

Biopsy and culture of gastric mucosa is the most sensitive diagnostic method. Urease activity can be detected rapidly in the samples. Culturing is also the most sensitive method to determine the success of therapy. *H pylori*–specific serum IgG and IgA are diagnostic for previous or current exposure.

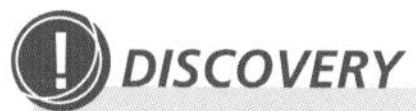

DISCOVERY

The young Australian internist Barry Marshall, who was working with Robin Warren, the discoverer of *H pylori*, hypothesized that gastric and duodenal ulcers are caused by bacteria and not by stress (as was the prevailing dogma). Consistent with Koch's first and second postulates, Marshall and Warren initially showed that *H pylori* could be isolated from ulcer lesions. To satisfy Koch's third postulate, a pure culture of the organism would have to be shown to cause the disease. However, no successful animal models were available. Experimenting on human volunteers would have required approval by the local institutional review board, which would most likely reject the project. Marshall therefore had his stomach examined endoscopically to ensure that it had a healthy mucosa. He then drank a culture of *H pylori*, and within a week he became nauseated and vomited. He also felt unusually hungry and tired. His stomach was again examined near the end of the second week; a region of the lining had an inflamed appearance, and bacteria were found in the mucin layer over this area. The infection eventually healed. As a result of their establishing *H pylori* as the causative agent of stomach ulcers, Marshall and Warren were awarded the Nobel Prize in Physiology or Medicine in 2005.

Pathogenesis and epidemiology

The motility of the bacteria enable them to localize in the less acidic microenvironment in the gastric mucus. The bacteria also produce large amounts of urease that generates ammonia and thus a less acidic medium. Outer membrane proteins mediate adhesion to the gastric epithelial cells. The site most favored by *H pylori* in the stomach is the gastric antrum; however, other parts of the stomach can be colonized when the patient is taking an acid-lowering medication. Mucinase, phospholipase, and vacuolating cytotoxin cause localized tissue destruction, the latter by mediating the vacuolation of the endosomal compartments. *H pylori* infection of the mucosa leads to mild to extensive inflammation, the latter involving lymphocytes, neutrophils, and microabscesses.

The cytotoxin-associated gene (*cagA*) encodes a protein that induces actin depolymerization. It sits on a pathogenicity island (*cag* PAI) of a 40 kb DNA insertion element that comprises about 32 genes. The *cag* PAI encodes a bacterial type IV secretion system (T4SS) and is found in 60% to 70% of Western *H pylori* strains and 100% of East Asian strains. Strains that have the *cag* PAI increase the risk for severe gastritis, dysplasia, gastric adenocarcinoma, and atrophy relative to strains without *cag* PAI. The T4SS facilitates the delivery of bacterial effector proteins into gastric epithelial cells. The CagA protein is phosphorylated in the host cell by the Abl and Src family of kinases, leading to the activation of host signaling pathways that promote epithelial responses with carcinogenic potential.

CagA from certain *H pylori* strains can induce interleukin-8 (IL-8) expression in epithelial cells. The peptidoglycan of *H pylori* is also delivered into host cells by the T4SS. They are then detected by the nucleotide-binding oligomerization domain 1, which is a pattern-recognition molecule. This stimulates the synthesis of the proinflammatory cytokines IL-8, macrophage inflammatory protein-2, and β-defensin by inducing host cell signaling molecules, including nuclear factor kappa B (NF-κB) and Erk.

A large percentage of patients with gastritis, gastric ulcers, and duodenal ulcers are infected with *H pylori*. Transmission from person to person is thought to be via the fecal-oral route.

Treatment and prevention

Treatment involves the use of a proton pump inhibitor, a macrolide, and a β-lactam. Resistance to clarithromycin can lead to treatment failure. Antibiotic susceptibility testing is important if initial treatment is not successful.

H pylori infection is disappearing in countries that have high hygiene standards, clean water, and good living conditions. Studies in an animal model of the disease have indicated that a vaccine that induces a helper T (T_h2) cell response can eradicate the infection, whereas one that induces T_h1 cells enhances inflammation.

Bibliography

Centers for Disease Control and Prevention. *Campylobacter.* http://www.cdc.gov/nczved/divisions/dfbmd/diseases/campylobacter/. Accessed 18 June 2015.

Centers for Disease Control and Prevention. Enterohemorrhagic *Escherichia coli.* http://www.cdc.gov/ncidod/dbmd/diseaseinfo/enterohemecoli_t.htm. Accessed 18 June 2015.

Centers for Disease Control and Prevention. Public Health Image Library. phil.cdc.gov. Accessed 4 August 2015.

Centers for Disease Control and Prevention. Shigellosis. http://www.cdc.gov/shigella/index.html. Accessed 18 June 2015.

Centers for Disease Control and Prevention. *Yersinia.* http://www.cdc.gov/nczved/divisions/dfbmd/diseases/yersinia/. Accessed 18 June 2015.

Figueira R, Holden DW. Functions of the *Salmonella* pathogenicity island 2 (SPI-2) type III secretion system effectors. Microbiology 2012;158:1147–1161.

Greenwood D, Barer M, Slack R, Irving W. Medical Microbiology, ed 18. Edinburgh: Churchill Livingstone/Elsevier, 2012.

Ingraham JL, Ingraham CA. Introduction to Microbiology: A Case History Approach. Pacific Grove, CA: Brooks/Cole (Thomson), 2004.

Lucas MI. Diarrhoeal disease through enterocyte secretion: A doctrine untroubled by proof. Exp Physiol 2010;95:479–484.

Murray PR, Rosenthal KS, Pfaller MA. Medical Microbiology, ed 6. Philadelphia: Mosby/Elsevier, 2009.

Noto JM, Peek RM Jr. The *Helicobacter pylori cag* pathogenicity island. Methods Mol Biol 2012;921:41–50.

Que F, Wu S, Huang R. *Salmonella* pathogenicity island 1(SPI-1) at work. Curr Microbiol 2013;66:582–587.

Ryan KJ, Ray CG. Sherris Medical Microbiology, ed 5. New York: McGraw-Hill, 2010.

Trofa AF, Ueno-Olsen H, Oiwa R, Yoshikawa M. Dr. Kiyoshi Shiga: Discoverer of the dysentery bacillus. Clin Infect Dis 1999;29:1303–1306.

Velge P, Wiedemann A, Rosselin M, et al. Multiplicity of *Salmonella* entry mechanisms, a new paradigm for *Salmonella* pathogenesis. MicrobiologyOpen 2012;1:243–258.

Take-Home Messages

- *Shigella*, *S* Typhi, and *Y pestis* are always associated with disease and are not found as normal flora in humans, whereas *E coli*, *P mirabilis*, and *K pneumoniae* are commensals that can cause opportunistic infections.
- *E coli* causes more than 90% of the approximately 7 million cases of bladder and lower urinary tract infections and a quarter-million cases of kidney and upper urinary tract infections in the United States each year.
- Enterotoxigenic *E coli* causes watery diarrhea with cramps, nausea, and vomiting. It is the leading cause of traveler's diarrhea in visitors to developing countries, where it is also the leading cause of morbidity and mortality due to diarrhea in the first 2 years of life.
- Enteroinvasive *E coli* causes tissue destruction and inflammation in the intestines, accompanied by diarrhea and sometimes dysentery.
- Enteropathogenic *E coli* is a major cause of pediatric diarrhea in communities with poor hygiene.
- Enterohemorrhagic *E coli* is associated with hemorrhagic colitis and hemolytic uremic syndrome. The strain O157:H7 has been identified as the major cause of these syndromes.
- There are more than 2,000 antigenic types of *Salmonella*. This heterogeneity is attributable to the different LPS structures.
- The species formerly called *S enteritidis* is currently designated *S enterica* subsp *enterica* serotype Enteritidis, and it is abbreviated as *S* Enteritidis.
- *Salmonella* infection can cause gastroenteritis, septicemia, and typhoid fever. *Salmonella* binds to and invades both enterocytes and M (microfold) cells in the intestines.
- *Shigella* species are Gram-negative, facultatively anaerobic bacilli that cause bacillary dysentery, characterized by the frequent passage of bloodstained, mucopurulent stools.
- *S dysenteriae* type 1 produces Shiga toxin and is responsible for the most serious forms of shigellosis. *Shigella* causes about 150 million cases of infectious diarrhea worldwide and 600,000 deaths per year.
- *Yersinia* are Gram-negative, facultatively anaerobic coccobacilli that cause bubonic plague, pneumonic plague, and gastroenteritis.
- *Y pestis* caused the Black Death of the Middle Ages in Europe, killing 25 million people between 1346 and 1350 out of an estimated population of 105 million people.
- *Klebsiella* are Gram-negative, facultatively anaerobic, capsulated rods. They primarily cause urinary tract infections but also cause wound and soft tissue infections, endocarditis, and severe bronchopneumonia with multiple abscesses.
- *Citrobacter* may be found in the normal intestinal flora and may cause opportunistic infections including bacteremia.
- *C jejuni* and *C coli* are some of the most common causes of infectious diarrhea. *C concisus* and *C rectus* are involved in periodontal disease.
- *H pylori* are Gram-negative, curved bacilli that cause chronic gastritis and increase the risk of peptic ulcer disease and gastric cancer. It is estimated that 50% of the world's human population is infected chronically.

19 *Mycoplasma* and *Ureaplasma*

Mycoplasmas (class Mollicutes) are the smallest free-living bacteria, with diameters in the range of 0.2 to 0.8 µm. They are unique among bacteria in that they do not have a cell wall. They only have a plasma membrane, but the membrane contains sterols, which confer stability to the membrane. Mycoplasmas require sterols for growth. They are resistant to penicillins and cephalosporins. Most Mycoplasmas are facultatively anaerobic, but *Mycoplasma pneumoniae* ("Eaton's agent"), which causes respiratory disease, is a strict aerobe. *Ureaplasma* organisms produce urease and need acid pH in the growth medium. *Mycoplasma genitalium* has the smallest genome (0.58 Mb) of a self-replicating organism.

Clinical Syndromes and Diagnosis

M pneumoniae causes mild upper respiratory tract disease. The symptoms include low-grade fever, malaise, headache, and a dry, nonproductive cough. Tracheobronchitis can occur where the bronchial passages are infiltrated with lymphocytes and plasma cells. Primary atypical pneumonia or walking pneumonia can also develop, with patchy bronchopneumonia seen on chest radiographs.

M pneumoniae may cause skin rashes and ulcerations of both the oral and vaginal mucosa, appearing as maculopapular, vesicular, or erythematous eruptions. When oral ulceration is associated with the skin rash and conjunctivitis, it is called Stevens-Johnson syndrome.

M genitalium and *Ureaplasma urealyticum* can cause nongonococcal urethritis. *M genitalium* infection may result in pelvic inflammatory disease. *Mycoplasma hominis* has been implicated in pyelonephritis and postpartum fever.

Mycoplasmas stain poorly because they do not have a peptidoglycan layer. The bacteria can be cultured on media with serum and yeast extract for cholesterol and nucleic acid precursors and with penicillin to prevent the growth of other bacteria. Inhibition of growth by specific antisera may aid in the diagnosis. Complement fixation is the

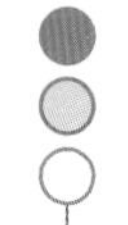

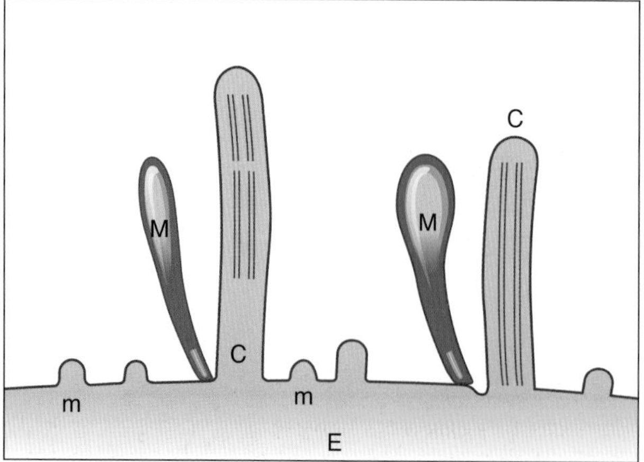

Fig 19-1 Schematic diagram of *M pneumoniae* infection of a tracheal organ culture. E, epithelial cell; C, cilium; m, microvillus; M, mycoplasma attaching to the base of a cilium.

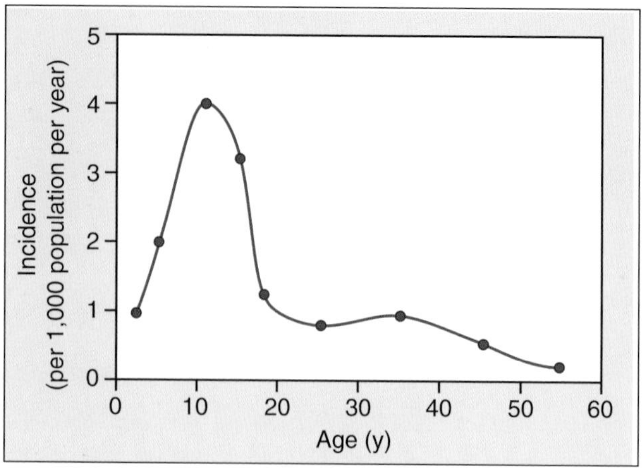

Fig 19-2 Incidence of *M pneumoniae* per 1,000 population per year in different age groups.

most commonly used serologic method to detect *M pneumoniae.* More than two-thirds of patients presenting with *M pneumoniae* developed high titers of cold hemagglutinin. Detection of cold hemagglutinins, however, is not specific, because adenovirus and Epstein-Barr virus infections can also result in the production of these antibodies. Although polymerase chain reaction–based assays are sensitive, they are not necessarily specific and are not widely available.

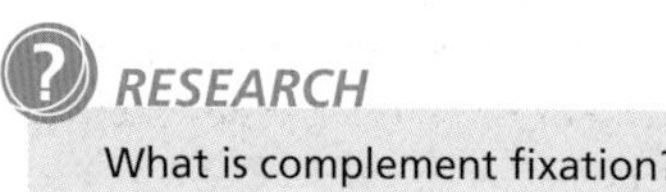

RESEARCH

What is complement fixation?

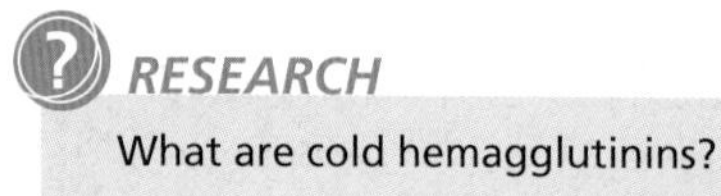

RESEARCH

What are cold hemagglutinins?

Pathogenesis and Epidemiology

Mycoplasmas have evolved mechanisms of mimicry of host antigens, survival within host cells, and phenotypic plasticity. A virulence mechanism of *M pneumoniae* and *M genitalium* is adherence to host cells. *M pneumoniae* adheres to respiratory epithelium by a 168-kD terminal protein attachment factor, P1, which interacts specifically with glycoprotein receptors at the base of the cilia on the epithelial cell surface (Fig 19-1). This results in ciliostasis and destruction of epithelial cells. *M pneumoniae* also interacts with lung surfactant protein D via its membrane glycolipids. It produces a toxin called community acquired respiratory distress syndrome (CARDS) toxin, which most likely helps with colonization, leading to inflammation. Although *M pneumoniae* primarily resides on the surface of respiratory epithelial cells, it can also be endocytosed and can reside inside the host cell.

Infections due to *M pneumoniae* occur more often during the summer, because pneumonia caused by other infectious agents (eg, *Streptococcus pneumoniae* and viruses) is more common during the cold months. *M pneumoniae* is the most common cause of pneumonia in children aged 5 to 15 years (Fig 19-2).

Genital mycoplasma infections of *M hominis, M genitalium,* and *U urealyticum* can occur at birth or as a result of sexual activity.

Oral Mycoplasmas

Mycoplasmas have been isolated from saliva, oral mucosa, and dental plaque, but their significance is not known. *Mycoplasma orale, Mycoplasma salivarium, M hominis,* and *U urealyticum* have been isolated from saliva and have been shown to have proteolytic activity against serum proteins.

Treatment and Prevention

Erythromycin, azithromycin, tetracycline (or doxycycline), and newer fluoroquinolones (gatifloxacin, moxifloxacin) are equally effective in treating *M pneumoniae* infections. Erythromycin is used to treat *Ureaplasma* infections, because these organisms are resistant to doxycycline. *M hominis* is resistant to erythromycin and can be treated with clindamycin. Transmission of *M pneumoniae* via dental aerosols is possible, and thus the use of universal precautions is essential. Patients with *M pneumoniae* are infectious for long periods, even if they are being treated with antibiotics. The sexually transmitted *M hominis, M genitalium,* and *Ureaplasma* infections may be prevented by avoiding sexual contact or by using appropriate barriers.

Take-Home Messages

- Mycoplasmas are the smallest free-living bacteria. They do not have a cell wall, and the cell membrane contains sterols.
- *M pneumoniae* causes mild upper respiratory tract disease, which can develop into primary atypical pneumonia or walking pneumonia, with patchy bronchopneumonia seen on chest radiographs.
- Stevens-Johnson syndrome refers to the oral ulceration that is associated with a skin rash and conjunctivitis.
- *M genitalium* infection may cause pelvic inflammatory disease. *M hominis* has been implicated in pyelonephritis and postpartum fever.
- Mycoplasmas have been isolated from saliva, oral mucosa, and dental plaque.

Bibliography

Centers for Disease Control and Prevention. *Mycoplasma pneumoniae* Infection. www.cdc.gov/pneumonia/atypical/mycoplasma/hcp/index.html. Accessed 18 June 2015.

Haggerty CL, Taylor BD. *Mycoplasma genitalium*: An emerging cause of pelvic inflammatory disease. Infect Dis Obstet Gynecol 2011;2011:959816.

Murray PR, Rosenthal KS, Pfaller MA. Medical Microbiology, ed 6. Philadelphia: Mosby/Elsevier, 2009.

Rottem S. Interaction of mycoplasmas with host cells. Physiol Rev 2003;83:417–432.

Ryan KJ, Ray CG. Sherris Medical Microbiology, ed 5. New York: McGraw-Hill, 2010.

Saraya T, Kurai D, Nakagaki K, et al. Novel aspects on the pathogenesis of *Mycoplasma pneumoniae* pneumonia and therapeutic implications. Front Microbiol 2014;5:410.

Taylor-Robinson D, Jensen JS. *Mycoplasma genitalium*: From chrysalis to multicolored butterfly. Clin Microbiol Rev 2011;24:498–514.

Waites KB, Katz B, Schelonka RL. Mycoplasmas and ureaplasmas as neonatal pathogens. Clin Microbiol Rev 2005;18:757–789.

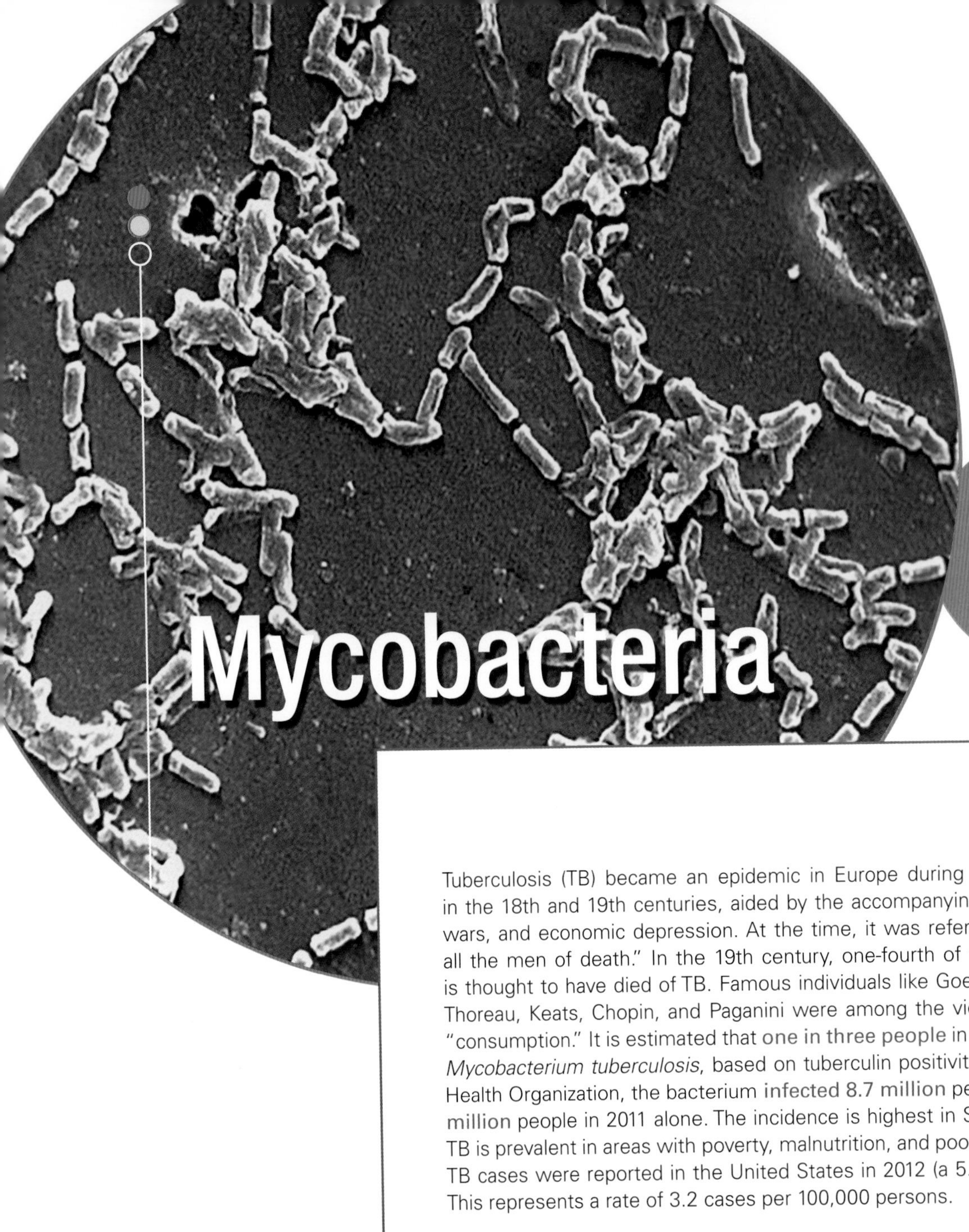

20

Mycobacteria

Tuberculosis (TB) became an epidemic in Europe during the Industrial Revolution in the 18th and 19th centuries, aided by the accompanying urbanization, crowding, wars, and economic depression. At the time, it was referred to as "the captain of all the men of death." In the 19th century, one-fourth of the population of Europe is thought to have died of TB. Famous individuals like Goethe, Rousseau, Chekhov, Thoreau, Keats, Chopin, and Paganini were among the victims of what was called "consumption." It is estimated that one in three people in the world is infected with *Mycobacterium tuberculosis*, based on tuberculin positivity. According to the World Health Organization, the bacterium infected 8.7 million people and killed about 1.4 million people in 2011 alone. The incidence is highest in Southeast Asia and Africa. TB is prevalent in areas with poverty, malnutrition, and poor housing. A total of 9,945 TB cases were reported in the United States in 2012 (a 5.4% decrease from 2011). This represents a rate of 3.2 cases per 100,000 persons.

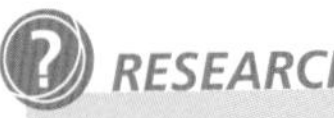

RESEARCH

What is tuberculin positivity?

Mycobacteria are aerobic bacilli 0.2 to 0.6 µm in diameter and 1 to 10 µm in length. The surface of the microorganism is hydrophobic, resulting from the long-chain lipids. This property renders the mycobacteria resistant to many disinfectants and to Gram and Giemsa stains. Once they are stained, the mycobacteria are resistant to decolorization with ethanol–hydrochloric acid solutions; therefore, they are considered acid-fast bacteria (Fig 20-1). They grow very slowly, dividing every 12 to 24 hours. *Mycobacterium leprae*, the etiologic agent of leprosy, cannot be grown in cell-free cultures.

M tuberculosis (MTB) and *Mycobacterium avium-intracellulare* complex (MAC) can cause overwhelming, disseminated disease in immunocompromised patients. MTB is still a significant cause of morbidity and mortality in countries with limited medical resources. Most human mycobacterial infections are caused by MTB, MAC, *Mycobacterium kansasii*, *Mycobacterium fortuitum*, *Mycobacterium chelonae*, and *M leprae*.

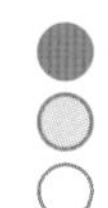

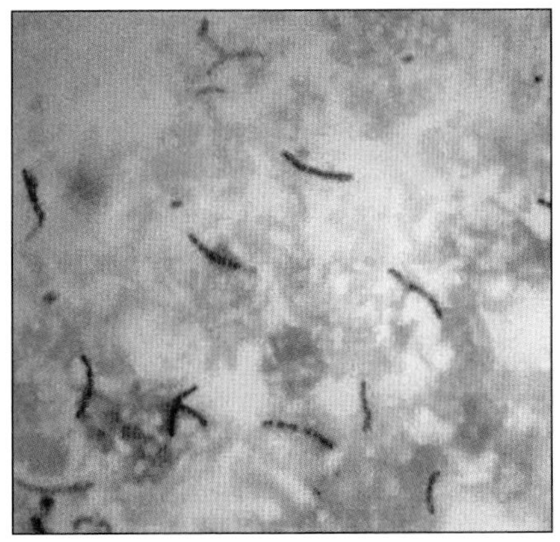

Fig 20-1 Mycobacteria stained with the Ziehl-Neelsen stain. (Public Health Image Library image 5789, courtesy of Dr George P. Kubica.)

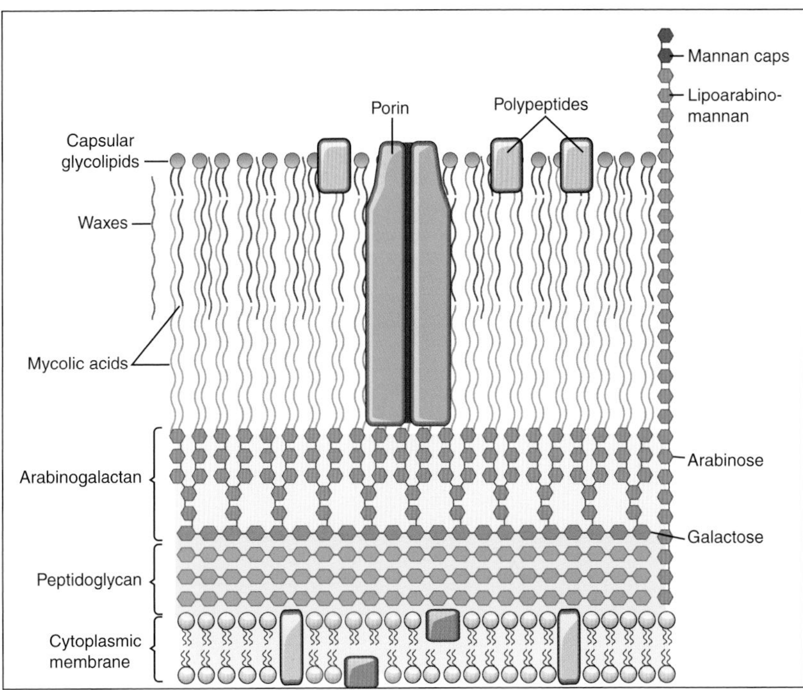

Fig 20-2 The complex cell wall architecture of mycobacteria.

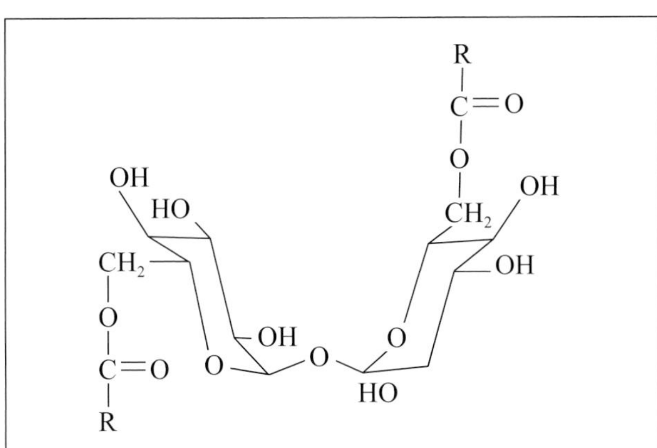

Fig 20-3 Cord factor, 6,6′-dimycolate of trehalose, is a mycoside, which is a complex saturated glycolipid. Cord factor inhibits neutrophil migration and is thought to mediate granuloma formation. The R residues represent very long-chain lipids.

Mycobacteria have a complex cell wall composed of the peptidoglycan layer linked with arabinose-galactose-mycolic acid (arabinogalactan mycolate) (Fig 20-2). Long-chain (C_{70}–C_{90}) mycolic acids are the major lipids in the mycobacterial cell wall. Free lipids are located on the outer layers: waxes (wax D, one of the major components of Freund's adjuvant), mycosides (complex saturated glycolipids), and cord factor (6,6′-dimycolate of trehalose) (Fig 20-3).

The microorganism is relatively resistant to acids and alkalis. Sodium hydroxide (NaOH) is used to concentrate clinical specimens; it destroys unwanted bacteria, human cells, and mucus but not MTB. Mycobacteria grow slowly and form nonpigmented colonies. They have been classified by Runyon into groups according to the rate of growth and pigmentation (yellow-pigmented carotinoids). Organisms that produce pigments after exposure to light are called photochromogens, whereas those producing pigments in both the light and the dark are called scotochromogens.

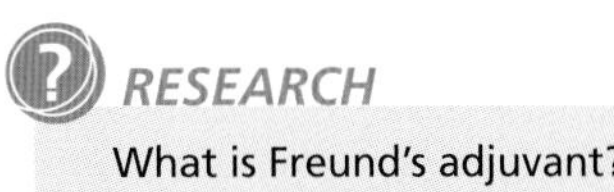

RESEARCH

What is Freund's adjuvant?

M tuberculosis

Clinical syndromes and diagnosis

Primary TB is usually mild and asymptomatic, and in 90% of cases it does not proceed further. Clinical disease develops in the remaining 10% of cases.

The onset is insidious, with complaints of malaise, weight loss, productive cough, and night sweats. Sputum production may be scant or bloody (hemoptysis) and purulent (containing or forming pus). Necrosis may erode blood vessels, which can rupture and cause death through hemorrhage.

Once organisms have made their way into the lung, they have four potential fates:

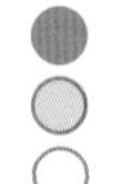

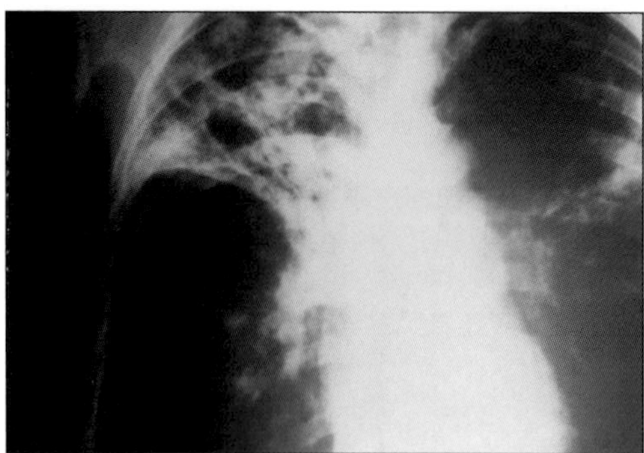

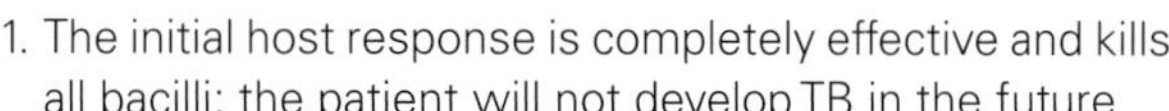

Fig 20-4 A chest radiograph of a TB patient with far-advanced TB, showing bilateral infiltrates and "caving formation" in the right apical region *(top left)*. (Public Health Image Library image 14805, courtesy of the Centers for Disease Control and Prevention.)

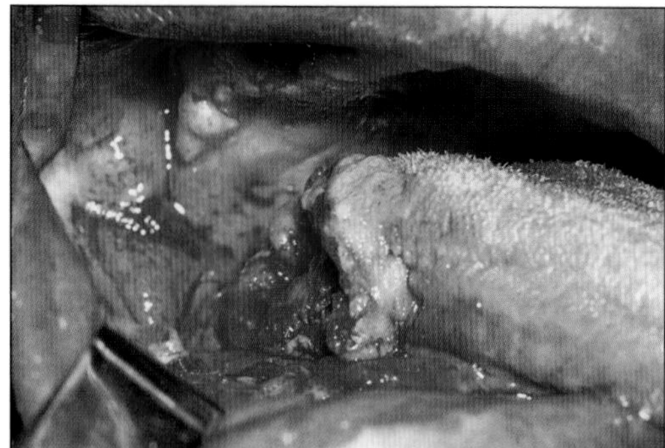

Fig 20-5 Deep, ragged, and painful tuberculous ulcer of the tongue. (Reprinted with permission from Marx and Stern.)

1. The initial host response is completely effective and kills all bacilli; the patient will not develop TB in the future.
2. The organisms multiply immediately after infection and cause clinical disease (primary TB).
3. The bacilli become dormant and never cause disease; the patient has "latent infection," evident only by a positive tuberculin skin test.
4. The latent organisms eventually grow, with resultant clinical disease termed reactivation TB.

TB is primarily a disease of the lungs (Fig 20-4) but may spread to other sites and proceed to a generalized infection ("miliary" TB). TB may also have severe oral manifestations, including painful, ragged ulcers, mainly on the posterior aspect of the tongue or palate (Fig 20-5). These lesions are most commonly secondary to active TB, which can infect the oral site via coughed-up sputum. Confirmation of the disease is achieved by radiographic evidence of pulmonary disease, a positive skin test, and laboratory diagnosis of mycobacteria.

Most infections are restricted to the lungs, but the disease can disseminate to other parts of the body, including the lymph nodes, pleura, the liver, the genitourinary tract, and the meninges.

Infection in an individual can be determined via the skin test, using either "old tuberculin" or purified protein derivative (PPD), which is the recommended method. The antigens are introduced to the intradermal layer of the skin. Forty-eight hours later, an induration (a region of firm or hard tissue) of 10 mm or more indicates that the patient has been exposed to MTB.

For identification by microscopy, the clinical specimen (eg, sputum) is stained with carbolfuchsin (Ziehl-Neelsen and Kinyoun stains) or fluorochrome dyes (Truant auramine-rhodamine), decolorized with acid-alcohol solution, and counterstained. For identification by culture, specimens are treated briefly with a decontaminating reagent (2% NaOH) that will kill rapidly growing bacteria and spare the mycobacteria. MTB is grown on Löwenstein-Jensen (egg-based) medium or Middlebrook (agar-based) medium, but it takes 3 weeks or more to grow. Specially formulated broth cultures measure the metabolism of ^{14}C-palmitic acid by its conversion to $^{14}CO_2$ using the BACTEC instrument, which aspirates the gas above the culture medium in sealed vials and counts the radioactivity. Biochemical tests evaluate the production of niacin and nitrate reductase activity, which is particular for MTB. Nucleic acid amplification of both DNA and ribosomal RNA sequences is highly specific for MTB, but the sensitivity of the technique is no better than culture identification. Moreover, live cultures are necessary for evaluating antibiotic sensitivity.

Pathogenesis and epidemiology

The route of infection for TB is inhalation of infectious aerosols. MTB replicates freely in alveolar macrophages and destroys the cells. Infected macrophages migrate to the local (tracheobronchial) lymph nodes, the bloodstream, and other tissues (bone marrow, spleen, kidneys, central nervous system). Two types of lesions occur: *(1)* The exudative lesion is the result of an acute inflammatory response at the initial site of infection, usually the lungs. *(2)* The granulomatous lesion, the tubercle, consists of a central area of alveolar macrophages, epithelioid (epithelium-like) cells, and Langhans cells, which are fused epithelioid cells (Fig 20-6). The histologic marker for MTB infection is granulomatous inflammation. This tissue destruction and dissemination continues until cell-mediated immunity arrests the infection. A positive skin test indicates the development of immunity.

In extensive, active disease, a caseous (cheese-like) necrosis and cavitation are seen, resulting from the cellular immune responses, enzymes, lipids, and reactive oxygen intermediates from dying macrophages (see Fig 20-6). Tissue destruction is caused by the patient's immune response. MTB can manipulate the immune response to bring about an effective $CD4^+$ T-cell response that controls the disease, but it also facilitates the formation of increasingly destructive lesions in the lung. Tubercles may heal spontaneously, become fibrotic or calcified, and persist as such for a lifetime in people who are otherwise healthy. Latent bacilli can be reactivated years later when the patient's immune system is weakened.

Cord factor is a virulence factor that mediates the parallel alignment of mycobacteria and inhibits neutrophil migration. The waxy coat allows the microorganism to withstand drying and thus to survive for long periods of time in air and household

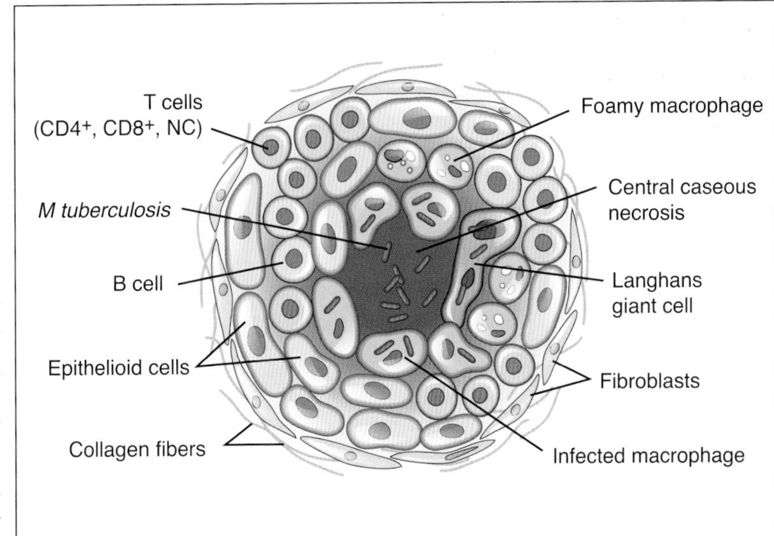

Fig 20-6 The granuloma of primary TB. *(1)* MTB infects the lungs through respiratory droplets generated by infected individuals. *(2)* Alveolar macrophages phagocytose the bacteria but cannot kill them as a result of the inhibition of phagosome-lysosome fusion. Infected macrophages release interleukin-12 and tumor necrosis factor-alpha, which recruit T cells and natural cytotoxic (NC, or natural killer [NK]) cells to the region and induce T-cell differentiation into helper T (T_h1) cells. *(3)* T_h1 cells in turn release interferon gamma, which activates macrophages to kill intracellular bacteria. Infected alveolar epithelial cells release chemokines that attract more macrophages that engulf the bacteria released from the dead macrophages. *(4)* Infected macrophages present antigen to T lymphocytes, which release cytokines that attract more macrophages and initiate inflammation. The tightly packed, infected, epithelioid macrophages form the initial tubercle. $CD4^+$, $CD8^+$, and NC T cells as well as macrophages surround the necrotic mass, forming a granuloma. *(5)* Fibroblasts and collagen are deposited around the epithelioid cells. The macrophages in the center of the tubercle die off, with the cellular proteins and fats producing the caseous (cheese-like) necrosis. *(6)* Rupturing of the tubercle leads to secondary TB, especially in immunocompromised individuals.

dust. Polypeptides in the cell wall act as antigens and are used in skin testing in the form of the purified protein derivative.

MTB produces a protein called exported repetitive protein that prevents the phagosome of the engulfing macrophage from fusing with the lysosome, thereby allowing the organism to escape the degradative enzymes of the lysosome.

MTB is transmitted by close, person-to-person contact, via aerosols and occasionally by ingestion and skin trauma. Large aerosol particles are trapped by the mucosal surfaces and removed by the mucociliary escalator. Smaller particles carrying 1 to 3 mycobacteria can reach the alveoli and initiate the infectious process. It is more common among the urban poor, patients with suppressed immune systems, and immigrants from areas where the incidence is high (Southeast Asia, India, sub-Saharan Africa, Eastern Europe). Health care workers are also at risk for infection.

An estimated 10 to 15 million people in the United States are infected with MTB without displaying symptoms. One in 10 of these individuals is likely to develop active TB at some point in life. Prior to 1984, there was a yearly decline in the number of reported cases of TB in the United States. However, the number of cases started to increase in 1984 and continued until 1993, at which time they started to decline again. The increase in cases is attributed to the human immunodeficiency virus (HIV)/AIDS epidemic; immigration from countries with many TB cases; increased poverty, injection drug use, and homelessness; patients' failure to take antibiotics as prescribed; and the increased number of people in long-term care. Between 1985 and 1992, it is estimated that there were 51,700 cases of TB attributed to the HIV/AIDS epidemic.

Treatment and prevention

The American Thoracic Society recommendations for the treatment of TB are initial treatment with isoniazid (which inhibits mycolic acid biosynthesis), rifampin, pyrazinamide, and ethambutol (which inhibits arabinogalactan synthesis) for 2 months, followed by isoniazid and rifampin for 4 to 6 months. Noncompliance is known to cause the emergence of multidrug-resistant (MDR) strains. In many countries, directly observed therapy is used to ensure that the patients are taking their drugs. In vitro susceptibility testing is important to establish the most effective drug regimen.

MDR strains that are resistant to at least isoniazid and rifampin have become a worldwide problem. The resistance is attributed to one or more chromosomal mutations. One of these mutations is in a gene for mycolic acid synthesis, and another in a gene for catalase-peroxidase, an enzyme required to activate isoniazid within the bacterium. Previous treatment for TB predisposes to the selection of MDR organisms. In addition to MDR TB, extensively drug resistant MTB strains (XDR TB) have emerged throughout the world. These strains are defined as MDR-MTB that are resistant to fluoroqinolones and at least one of the second-line drugs, such as kanamycin, capreomycin, and amikacin.

For persons with significant exposure to MTB or recent conversion of skin test reactivity, isoniazid is used for prophylaxis. In many parts of the world, the bacille Calmette-Guérin (BCG) vaccine, based on attenuated *Mycobacterium bovis*, is used to reduce the severe consequences of TB in infants and children. The vaccine is not considered to be effective in older individuals. It should be considered that all vaccines will develop a positive skin test, which would make the surveillance of health care workers difficult.

Oral aspects

Oral manifestations occur in about 3% of TB cases. The bacteria infect oral tissues and lymph nodes, secondary to active pulmonary TB. Lesions can occur in the soft tissues, including the tongue and palate, and present as painful, ragged ulcers (see Fig 20-5). Infection of the underlying bone may cause TB-related osteomyelitis. Oral TB may resemble oral squamous cell carcinoma, primary syphilis, and oral lesions of pulmonary histoplasmosis, blastomycosis, and coccidioidomycosis. There is a risk of infection via aerosols containing saliva or sputum. MTB survives on surfaces and is resistant to many disinfectants (it is susceptible to Amphyl [Reckitt Benckiser]).

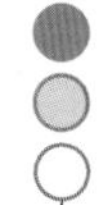

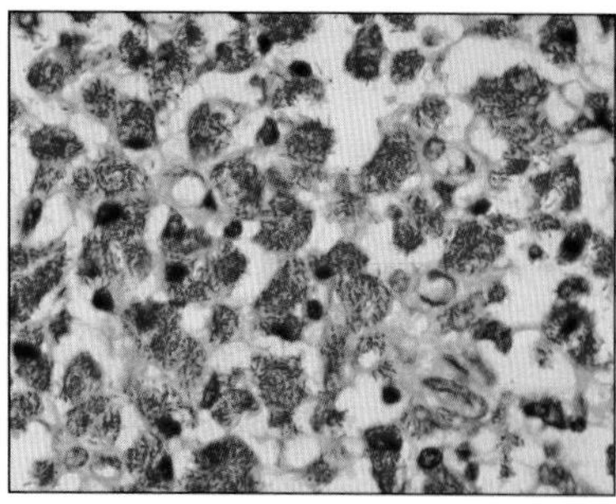
Fig 20-7 Micrograph of a Ziehl-Neelsen–stained lymph node sample from a patient with HIV/AIDS infected with MAC. (Public Health Image Library image 965, courtesy of Dr Edwin P. Ewing, Jr.)

M avium-intracellulare complex

M avium and *M intracellulare* are grouped together as *M avium-intracellulare* complex (MAC) because they are difficult to differentiate physiologically and because they cause identical diseases.

Clinical syndromes and diagnosis

Historically, the disease was restricted to immunocompromised patients and presented similarly to TB, with pulmonary infection being most common. MAC is seen in advanced HIV/AIDS patients and is disseminated. Tissue macrophages of some patients are replete with the mycobacteria, and their blood contains very large numbers of organisms (Fig 20-7). These bacteria must be relatively avirulent to persist in such high concentrations for long periods without clinical evidence of disease. In comparison, one organism per mL of blood in *Escherichia coli* or *Staphylococcus aureus* infection can cause sepsis.

Pathogenesis and epidemiology

Asymptomatic colonization is observed in immunocompetent patients. Localized pulmonary disease is seen in patients with chronic bronchitis or other compromised pulmonary function. In immunocompromised individuals, MAC causes disseminated disease, where the macrophages of the reticuloendothelial system are inundated with the bacteria that survive intracellularly. This as well as the immune response to the infection lead to organ dysfunction.

MAC is acquired primarily through ingestion of contaminated food or water. It is found in soil and water as well as infected poultry and swine. Inhalation of infectious aerosols is believed to play a minor role, except in patients with pulmonary disease. Immunocompromised patients, particularly those with HIV/AIDS, and persons with long-standing pulmonary disease are at greatest risk for the disease. However, the incidence is decreasing because of highly active antiretroviral therapy of HIV/AIDS patients.

Treatment and prevention

MAC is resistant to most antimycobacterial drugs. One recommended combination is clarithromycin (or azithromycin), ethambutol, and clofazimine (or rifampin, ciprofloxacin, or amikacin). Rifabutin as well as clarithromycin (or azithromycin) have been approved for prophylaxis in AIDS patients with low CD4 counts.

M leprae

Clinical syndromes and diagnosis

M leprae causes leprosy, or Hansen disease. The clinical presentation is divided into tuberculoid and lepromatous leprosy. Tuberculoid leprosy is characterized by macules on the skin with hypopigmentation. Lepromatous leprosy is the most infectious form, with large numbers of bacilli in infected tissues, and it causes disfigurations in the skin. Additional symptoms include decreased sensation in the skin lesions, muscle weakness, and numbness in the extremities.

The bacilli can be detected in nasal discharges, scrapings from the nasal mucosa, or incision samples from the skin, using the Ziehl-Neelsen stain. Patients with clinical leprosy but no bacilli in skin samples have paucibacillary Hansen disease (tuberculoid leprosy), and those with positive *M leprae* identification at any site have multibacillary Hansen disease (lepromatous leprosy).

Pathogenesis and epidemiology

Patients with tuberculoid leprosy have a strong cellular immune reaction but a weak humoral response. Infected tissues have many lymphocytes and granulomas but relatively few bacteria. The bacteria induce the production of cytokines such as interferon gamma and interleukin-2 that mediate macrophage activation, phagocytosis, and bacterial clearance. Patients with lepromatous leprosy have a strong antibody response but a specific defect in their cellular response to *M leprae* antigens. Thus, bacilli populate dermal macrophages and Schwann cells of peripheral nerves. This is the most infectious form of leprosy.

More than 12 million cases of leprosy are known worldwide. The largest number of cases in the United States (250 cases annually) are found in California, Texas, Louisiana, and Hawaii, but 90% of infected individuals are immigrants from Mexico, Asia, Africa, and the Pacific Islands. Armadillos can also be infected and represent a potential reservoir of infection. The disease is spread by person-to-person contact, including inhalation of infectious aerosols, and skin contact with respiratory secretions or wound exudates. It is also believed that arthropod vectors are involved.

Treatment and prevention

M leprae infections are treated with dapsone (an antifolate), rifampin, and either clofazimine or ethionamide (an inhibitor of mycolic acid synthesis). Dapsone and rifampin are recommended for paucibacillary disease, and clofazimine is added for multibacillary disease. Therapy is administered for a minimum of 2 years, and it can be lifelong for some patients. If the disease is diagnosed early and treatment is initiated promptly, the clinical response can be satisfactory. Delays in treatment have devastating consequences.

The disease can be controlled by the quick diagnosis and treatment of infected individuals. In regions where the BCG vaccine protects against TB, it appears to protect against *M leprae*, possibly via the induction of immunity against common antigens.

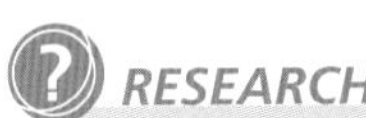

RESEARCH

What is the mechanism of action of clofazimine? What are side effects of this antibiotic?

Other Atypical Mycobacteria

M kansasii is observed in immunocompromised individuals. It is the most common photochromogen responsible for human disease. It presents as chronic pulmonary disease, cervical lymphadenitis, and skin infections. Disseminated disease is observed in immunocompromised patients. Positive PPD tests may be the result of *M kansasii* infection. Combination therapy with rifampin, ethambutol, and isoniazid is effective in most cases.

Mycobacterium marinum and *Mycobacterium ulcerans* grow at cooler temperatures and cause skin diseases. *M marinum* causes "swimming pool granulomas" (nodular lesions along the lymphatics that may progress to ulceration). *M ulcerans* causes extensive ulceration over a period of months.

M bovis infects a variety of animals, most commonly cattle. The disease is controlled in the United States with vaccination, quarantine, and destruction of infected herds. Contaminated milk is the main source of *M bovis* infection.

M fortuitum and *M chelonae* cause disease when introduced subcutaneously by trauma or by catheters, contaminated wound dressing, or a prosthetic device (eg, a heart valve). These infections are considered to be **iatrogenic** (characterized by an abnormal state produced by the physician in a patient by inadvertent or erroneous treatment). These bacteria may also form abscesses at injection sites in injection drug users. *M fortuitum* and *M chelonae* respond to some aminoglycosides, cephalosporins, tetracyclines, and quinolones.

Mycobacterium scrofulaceum is one of the common causes of cervical lymphadenitis, especially in young children, characterized by enlarged lymph nodes that may ulcerate or form a draining sinus to the skin. The condition may be treated by surgical excision of the lesion.

Bibliography

Bauman RW. Microbiology. Boston: Pearson, 2014.

Centers for Disease Control and Prevention. Public Health Image Library. phil.cdc.gov. Accessed 4 August 2015.

Greenwood D, Barer M, Slack R, Irving W. Medical Microbiology, ed 18. Edinburgh: Churchill Livingstone/Elsevier, 2012.

Kwan CK, Ernst JD. HIV and tuberculosis: A deadly human syndemic. Clin Microbiol Rev 2011;24:351–376.

Marx RE, Stern D. Oral and Maxillofacial Pathology: A Rationale for Diagnosis and Treatment, ed 2. Chicago: Quintessence, 2012.

Murray PR, Rosenthal KS, Pfaller MA. Medical Microbiology, ed 6. Philadelphia: Mosby/Elsevier, 2009.

Orme IM, Robinson RT, Cooper AM. The balance between protective and pathogenic immune responses in the TB-infected lung. Nat Immunol 2015;16:57–63.

Ryan KJ, Ray CG. Sherris Medical Microbiology, ed 5. New York: McGraw-Hill, 2010.

Schluger NW, Rom WN. The host immune response to tuberculosis. Am J Respir Crit Care Med 1998;157:679–691.

Take-Home Messages

- Mycobacteria have a thick, lipid-rich cell wall and are stained with the acid-fast staining procedure.
- TB is caused by *M tuberculosis* and is characterized by granuloma formation, most often in the lungs.
- About 90% of infected individuals do not develop disease.
- About one-third of the world's population is infected with MTB, with 100 million people being infected every year.
- Multidrug-resistant and extensively drug-resistant MTB strains have emerged in recent years and require the use of a wide variety of antimycobacterial agents.
- Oral lesions due to MTB can occur in the soft tissues, including the tongue and palate.
- Leprosy is caused by *M leprae*. Tuberculoid leprosy presents with a strong cellular immune response and granulomas, and lepromatous leprosy is characterized by a large bacterial load and minimal immune reactivity.
- MAC is seen in patients with advanced HIV/AIDS and is disseminated.
- Other atypical mycobacteria include *M kansasii, M marinum, M ulcerans, M bovis, M fortuitum, M chelonae*, and *M scrofulaceum*.

Chlamydia, Rickettsia, and Related Bacteria

21

Chlamydia and *Chlamydophila*

The species *Chlamydia trachomatis*, *Chlamydophila psittaci*, and *Chlamydophila pneumoniae*, all of which are responsible for human disease, are classified under the family Chlamydiaceae. They are the agents of trachoma, lymphogranuloma venereum, psittacosis, and pneumonia. They were initially thought to be viruses because they can pass through 0.45-μm filters (ie, similar to "filterable agents"). However, they contain DNA, RNA, and prokaryotic ribosomes; synthesize their own proteins, nucleic acids, and lipids; and are susceptible to antibiotics. They are obligate intracellular bacteria with inner and outer membranes like Gram-negative organisms, but they do not have a peptidoglycan layer or muramic acid in their cell structure. They are not motile and do not have pili.

These species exist in two morphologically distinct forms (Fig 21-1):

1. The extracellular, infectious **elementary body** (about 0.3 μm in diameter) is rigid and resistant to disruption. The outer membrane proteins are cross-linked extensively by disulfide bonds. This membrane enters cells in endocytotic vesicles. Endosomes with elementary bodies are not acidified and fuse with each other but not with lysosomes. If the outer membrane of the elementary body is damaged or the chlamydiae are heat-inactivated or coated with antibodies, endosome-lysosome fusion proceeds.
2. The intracellular, metabolically active, replicating but noninfectious **reticulate body** (0.5 to 1.0 μm in diameter) is osmotically fragile because the cross-linked proteins are absent. The reticulate bodies utilize high-energy phosphate compounds produced by the host cell. Chlamydiae are thus known as **energy parasites**. About 18 to 24 hours after infection, the reticulate bodies reorganize to form elementary bodies, which are released 48 to 72 hours after infection.

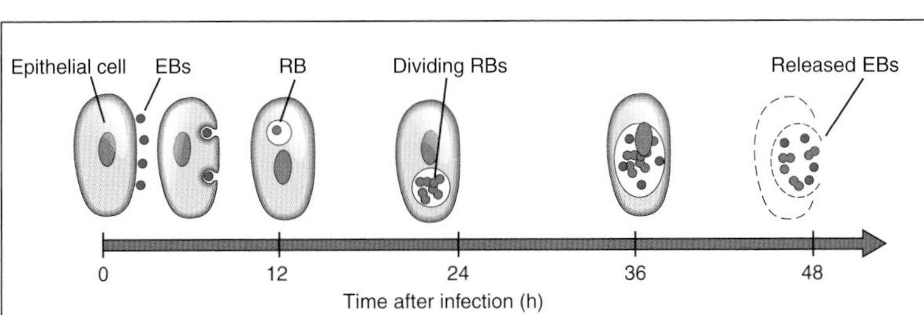

Fig 21-1 The *Chlamydia* life cycle. EB, elementary body; RB, reticulate body. (Adapted from Ryan and Ray.)

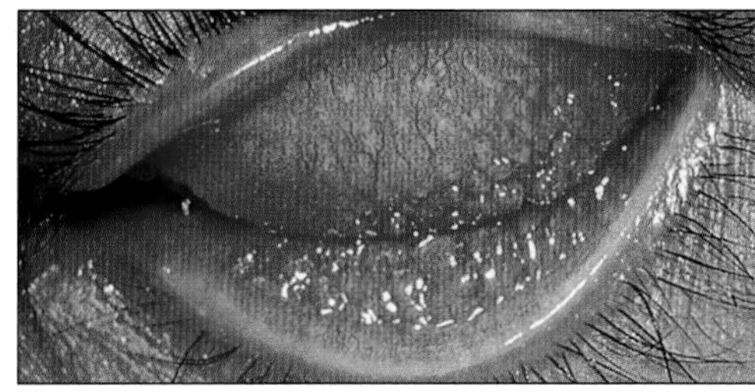

Fig 21-2 *C trachomatis* infection of the lining of the eyelids, causing inclusion conjunctivitis. (Public Health Image Library image 15193, courtesy of Susan Lindsley.)

Chlamydia trachomatis

The major outer membrane protein of *C trachomatis* defines the 18 different serovars of the species.

Clinical syndromes and diagnosis

C trachomatis causes the most common sexually transmitted disease in the United States and possibly worldwide. Most urogenital infections in women are asymptomatic. Clinical syndromes include cervicitis, endometritis, urethritis, salpingitis, bartholinitis, and pelvic inflammatory disease. The symptoms of urethritis are dysuria and urethral discharge. Infection of the cervix may result in a vaginal discharge, but it usually does not produce symptoms. Most genital infections in men are symptomatic. Many cases (35% to 50%) of nongonococcal urethritis are caused by *C trachomatis.* Postgonococcal urethritis results from co-infection with *Neisseria gonorrhoeae* and *C trachomatis.* Tissue scarring may occur as a result of recurrent or chronic infection and may result in sterility and ectopic pregnancy.

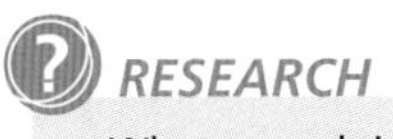

RESEARCH

What are salpingitis and bartholinitis?

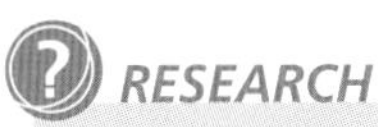

RESEARCH

What is meant by nongonococcal urethritis?

The trachoma biovar of *C trachomatis* is the leading cause of preventable blindness in developing countries (Fig 21-2). Its characteristic is conjunctival scarring, which results in eyelashes turning inward and causing abrasion of the cornea, ulceration, scarring, and loss of vision.

Adult inclusion conjunctivitis is caused by *C trachomatis* strains associated with genital infections. The symptoms include corneal infiltrates, mucopurulent discharge, and keratitis (inflammation of the cornea). Neonatal conjunctivitis occurs as a result of exposure to the bacterium during birth and presents with swollen eyelids and a purulent discharge. If infections are not treated, conjunctival scarring and corneal vascularization can result. Infants are at risk for *C trachomatis* pneumonia if they are not treated or treated only topically. The symptoms of infant pneumonia are rhinitis, followed by a distinctive intermittent cough. The condition lasts for several weeks and is not accompanied by fever.

Lymphogranuloma venereum (LGV) starts with a primary lesion at the site of entry (genital, anorectal, oral) in the form of a vesicle that ruptures, leaving a shallow ulcer that heals. In the second stage of infection, the local lymph nodes, especially the inguinal nodes, become inflamed and enlarged. Systemic symptoms include headache, myalgias, arthralgias, fever, chills, and anorexia. Late complications of the disease include perirectal abscesses and urethral and rectal strictures.

The most specific diagnostic method for *C trachomatis* is cell culture of specimens collected from the site of infection, using susceptible cell lines (such as McCoy cells). Following incubation for 3 to 7 days, the cells are stained with fluorescent monoclonal antibodies against chlamydial antigens. Nucleic acid amplification techniques such as the polymerase chain reaction (PCR) are more sensitive and can be used to detect bacteria in urine samples.

Pathogenesis and epidemiology

Chlamydia infects tissues through abrasions or lacerations on mucosal surfaces. It infects epithelial cells of mucosal surfaces, including the conjunctivae, endocervix, urethra, rectum, endometrium, fallopian tubes, and respiratory tract. The LGV biovar infects lymphoid tissue and replicates in mononuclear phagocytes. Trachoma strains infect epithelial cells. Clinical manifestations arise from cell destruction and the host inflammatory response, with granuloma formation.

Infection leads to the formation of antibodies and cell-mediated immune reactions but not to resistance to reinfection or elimination of the organism. Reinfection induces a strong inflammatory response that can cause tissue damage. The inflammatory response can result in vision loss in patients with eye infections. Sterility and sexual dysfunction in patients with genital infections can also result from the inflammatory response.

C trachomatis serovars (or immunotypes) A, B, and C cause trachoma. Types D to K cause genital tract infections, which are occasionally transmitted to the eyes or the respiratory tract. Serovars L_1, L_2, and L_3 cause LGV. According to the World Health Organization, there are 8 million individuals with irreversible visual impairment due

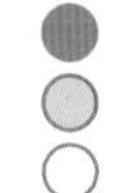

to trachoma, and there are an estimated 84 million cases of active disease requiring treatment. Infections occur predominantly in children. It is transmitted from eye to eye by hands, contaminated clothing, and flies that transmit ocular discharges. It may also be transmitted by respiratory droplets or via feces.

Adult inclusion conjunctivitis occurs mostly in individuals aged 18 to 30 years, with genital infection probably preceding ocular infection. Twenty-five percent of newborns whose mothers have active genital infections develop *C trachomatis* conjunctivitis. Pulmonary infection can also occur in infected infants.

C trachomatis is the most common sexually transmitted bacteria in the United States. In 2012, 1,423,000 cases were reported to the Centers for Disease Control and Prevention. The rate of reported infections increased from 182 to 457 per 100,000 population from 1992 to 2012. The estimated infections per year is 2.9 million. It is estimated that 50 million new cases occur per year worldwide. The incidence of LGV is 200 to 500 cases per year in the United States (mostly observed in gay men), but it is prevalent in Africa, Asia, and South America.

Treatment and prevention

Ocular and genital infections in adults are treated with azithromycin (one dose of 1 g) or doxycycline (100 mg twice a day for 7 days). Alternative treatments are 7-day regimens of erythromycin, levofloxacin, or ofloxacin. Treatment of LGV involves doxycycline for 21 days. Neonatal conjunctivitis and pneumonia can be treated with erythromycin for 10 to 14 days.

Sanitation is important for prevention in areas where trachoma is endemic. Safe sex practices and the immediate treatment of infected individuals and their sexual partners can prevent the transmission of *Chlamydia* genital infections.

C psittaci

C psittaci is transmitted to humans from infected birds via the inhalation of dried bird excrement. The microorganism spreads to the liver, spleen, and lungs and causes lymphocytic inflammation, edema, thickening of the alveolar wall, and infiltration of macrophages. It causes psittacosis (parrot fever), characterized by headache, high fever, and chills. Other symptoms may include malaise, anorexia, myalgia, arthralgia, and a nonproductive cough. Infections are treated with doxycycline and macrolide antibiotics. Untreated psittacosis has a mortality rate of 15% to 20%.

C pneumoniae

This species was first isolated from the conjunctiva of a child in Taiwan and was initially considered to be a psittacosis strain. It was found to be serologically related to strain AR, which led to the designation TWAR strain. DNA homology studies have indicated that it is a species distinct from both *C trachomatis* and *C psittaci.*

C pneumoniae is transmitted by respiratory secretions and causes pneumonia, bronchitis, pharyngitis, sinusitis, and flulike illness. The incubation period for *C pneumoniae* infection is about 21 days. It is spread from person to person, and the disease starts with pharyngitis and laryngitis, progressing to bronchitis and pneumonia 1 to 3 weeks after the onset of initial symptoms. Symptoms such as cough and malaise start gradually but may persist for several weeks or months despite appropriate antibiotic therapy. The clinical course of *C pneumoniae* infections has been likened to that of *Mycoplasma pneumoniae*, and both bacteria are considered the cause of "walking pneumonia." Erythromycin, tetracycline, and doxycycline are used as first-line therapy.

C pneumoniae has been identified in atherosclerotic lesions. However, its relationship to the development of atherosclerosis is not clear.

Rickettsiae and Related Bacteria

Rickettsiae are aerobic, Gram-negative bacilli, but they stain poorly with the Gram stain. Rickettsiae are obligate intracellular parasites that cause typhus, spotted fevers, and Q fever. Four genera are associated with human disease: *Rickettsia, Coxiella, Orientia,* and *Ehrlichia.* There are two diseases of significance in the United States: Rocky Mountain spotted fever caused by *Rickettsia rickettsii* and Q fever caused by *Coxiella burnetii.*

Coxiella and *Ehrlichia* grow in intracellular vacuoles. *Rickettsia* grow in the cytoplasm, and *R rickettsii* can also grow in the nucleus. These bacteria enter the host cells by a process called induced phagocytosis, which requires the expenditure of energy by the microorganisms. The bacterial phospholipase A degrades the phagosome membrane and facilitates the entry of the bacteria into the cytoplasm. The bacteria then utilize the host cell's adenosine triphosphate, coenzyme A, and nicotinamide adenine dinucleotide (NAD). Outside the host cell, the bacteria stop metabolizing and also begin to release small molecules, proteins, and nucleic acids. Thus, most rickettsiae do not survive in the environment. The main exception is *Coxiella,* which can remain in the environment for months to years.

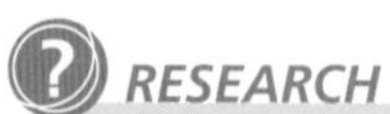

RESEARCH

What are coenzyme A and NAD? What is their relationship to the Krebs cycle?

Pathogenesis and epidemiology

Rickettsiae proliferate at the site of infection and eventually lyse their host cell, and a new round of infection occurs. They spread to the endothelial cells lining small blood vessels, resulting in focal hyperplasia, inflammation, and formation of microthrombi, with localized infarction of organs and tissues.

R rickettsii

R rickettsii is the most common species of *Rickettsia* in the United States and causes Rocky Mountain spotted fever. It damages endothelial cells and causes leakage of blood vessels. It is transmitted by Rocky Mountain wood ticks, dog ticks, and Lone Star ticks (Fig 21-3). It is more common in the Eastern United States. The incidence in 2010 was 6 cases per 1 million people, and it is highest among children and teenagers.

The disease has an abrupt onset following an average of 7 days of incubation. It is characterized by a rash, fever, headache, abdominal pain, vomiting, and myalgia. The rash is macular and first appears on the hands, wrists, feet, and ankles, and then it covers the entire body. However, in some patients the rash does not develop at all. The rash is sometimes found on the oral mucosa, and the local inflammation can cause a swollen throat and tongue. The immune response to infection is by cytotoxic $CD8^+$ T cells that kill infected cells and by antibodies to the outer membrane proteins of the bacterium.

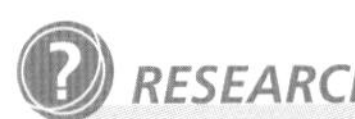

RESEARCH

What are the characteristics of macular, papular, and maculopapular rashes?

The damage to the blood vessels results in vasculitis, as well as bleeding or clotting in the brain or other vital organs. Loss of fluid from the damaged blood vessels may reduce blood circulation to the extremities, which may then damage fingers, toes, or limbs. Patients with severe vasculitis early in the disease process may suffer from permanent health problems, including neurologic deficits and damage to internal organs. Other complications of Rocky Mountain spotted fever in untreated patients are splenomegaly, thrombocytopenia, disseminated intravascular coagulation, and heart failure. The mortality rate is 20% if not treated.

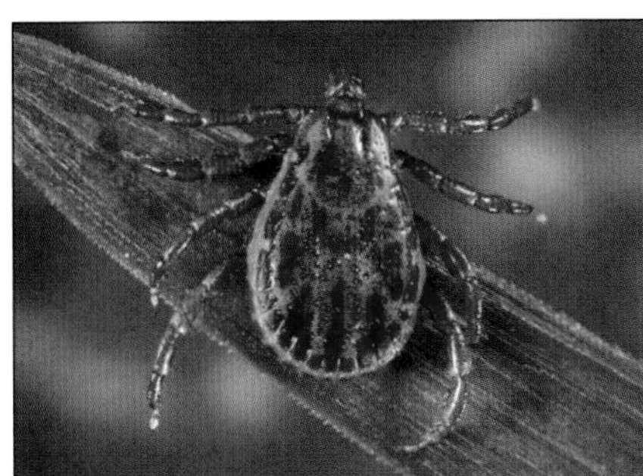

Fig 21-3 The Rocky Mountain wood tick, *Dermacentor andersoni*, the vector for *R rickettsii*. (Public Health Image Library image 10868, courtesy of James Gathany.)

Rickettsia prowazekii

Rickettsia prowazekii causes epidemic typhus, also known as louse-borne typhus. The reservoirs of the bacterium are humans and flying squirrels. It is spread via the human body louse, *Pediculus humanus*. The disease is associated with unsanitary and crowded conditions that favor the spread of body lice. Endemic typhus is present in the Andes regions of South America, in Burundi, and in Ethiopia. The disease can recur years after initial infection, known as Brill-Zinsser disease. Clinical syndromes include high fever, myalgias, and severe headache. A macular rash develops in many patients. The disease may lead to complications, including myocarditis and central nervous system dysfunction. Mortality can be as high as 60% if untreated.

Rickettsia typhi

Rickettsia typhi causes endemic typhus, or murine typhus. It is transmitted primarily via the rat flea (*Xenopsylla cheopsis*) from rodents, but the cat flea (*Ctenocephalides felis*) is thought to be a vector in the United States. The symptoms appear abruptly and include headache, fever, and myalgia. About 50% of infected patients develop a maculopapular rash on the chest and abdomen.

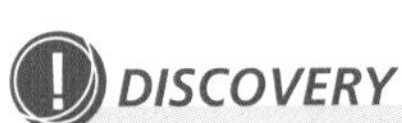

DISCOVERY

Howard Taylor Ricketts received his medical degree in 1897 from Northwestern University and studied in Berlin and the Pasteur Institute in Paris. In 1906, he went to Montana to investigate Rocky Mountain spotted fever, which sometimes had a mortality rate of more than 80%. He was able to detect the etiologic agent of the disease (later called *Rickettsia rickettsii* in his honor) in the blood of infected people and in the tick functioning as vector. Three years later, in 1909, he traveled to Mexico City to study the infectious agent of a major outbreak of typhus (*Typhus exanthematicus*). Ricketts and his assistant, Russell Morse Wilder, thought that the similarities between typhus and spotted fever would provide them with the key to the etiology of the diseases. Unfortunately, the next year Ricketts became infected while isolating the organism causing the disease (*Rickettsia prowazekii*) and died shortly thereafter.

In 1913 and 1914, the Czech microbiologist Stanislaus von Lanov Prowazek, who had received his PhD at the University of Vienna, traveled to Serbia and Constantinople to investigate the typhus epidemics. He studied the etiology, transmission, and life cycle of the microorganism causing the disease. In 1915, he and the Brazilian physician and pathologist Henrique da Rocha-Lima were sent to investigate an epidemic among Russian prisoners in a camp near Cottbus, Germany. Prowazek died of the disease; da Rocha-Lima also contracted the disease but recovered to isolate the causative microorganism, which he called *Rickettsia prowazekii* in honor of both Prowazek and Ricketts.

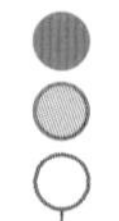

Orientia tsutsugamushi

Formerly in the genus *Rickettsia*, *Orientia tsutsugamushi* causes scrub typhus. "Tsutsugamushi" is Japanese for "dangerous bug fever." It lacks the peptidoglycan layer and lipopolysaccharide in its cell structure. It is transmitted by mites (chiggers) that fall off rodents and live in the scrub brush. The disease is seen primarily in Asia, Australia, Japan, and the Pacific islands. Fever increases gradually within the first week of the onset of symptoms, reaching 40.5°C (or 104.9°F). A macular to papular rash develops on the trunk in less than half of cases. Generalized lymphadenopathy, splenomegaly, central nervous system complications, and heart failure can occur.

In a study conducted in Thailand, it was found that the viral load of HIV patients is lower if they are also infected with *O tsutsugamushi*.

Rickettsia akari

Rickettsia akari is transmitted by mites and causes rickettsialpox. The symptoms include a papular skin lesion at the site of the mite bite (mouse mite), lymphadenopathy, fever, chills, headache, and a generalized papulovesicular rash. In some cases, vesicles develop on the palate, tongue, buccal mucosa, pharynx, and lips.

Laboratory diagnosis

Skin biopsies from rashes are visualized with direct fluorescent antibody or with Gimenez and Giemsa stains. This provides a rapid diagnosis. Serologic testing is used in laboratories with limited resources to diagnose Rocky Mountain spotted fever, epidemic typhus, and scrub typhus using the Weil-Felix agglutination reaction. (Serum from some patients with rickettsial diseases can agglutinate certain strains of *Proteus vulgaris*, an enterobacterium). The indirect fluorescent antibody test is useful for detecting immunoglobulin (Ig) M and IgG antibodies against rickettsia.

Treatment and prevention

Rickettsial infections are treated with doxycycline. Although ciprofloxacin has good in vitro activity, it is not recommended for first-line therapy because of inadequate clinical experience. Prompt diagnosis and initiation of therapy results in a good prognosis. Because serologic diagnosis cannot be made until 2 to 4 weeks into the disease, diagnosis must be based on initial clinical symptoms.

Prevention by vaccines has had limited success. Vaccines are available against epidemic typhus (*R prowazekii*). Hygiene and delousing sprays can control the human body louse. Avoiding tick-infested areas is an important preventive measure. Control of *R typhi* involves controlling the rodent reservoirs. *Orientia* infections can be prevented by avoiding exposure to mites, which involves wearing protective clothing or using insect repellent.

Ehrlichia

Ehrlichiae infect lymphocytes, neutrophils, monocytes, and capillary endothelial cells. Human monocytic ehrlichiosis is caused by *Ehrlichia chaffeensis*, which is transmitted by the Lone Star tick. Infection results in a combination of some of these symptoms that vary from patient to patient: fever, malaise, headache, myalgia, nausea, vomiting, confusion, leukopenia, and thrombocytopenia. A rash is observed in about 60% of children and in less than 30% of adults. Serious cases require prolonged hospitalization and intravenous antibiotics. Infected individuals who are immunocompromised as a result of corticosteroid use, cancer chemotherapy, splenectomy, or human immunodeficiency virus (HIV)/AIDS may develop more severe disease, and the percentage of patients who die from the infection is higher in this group.

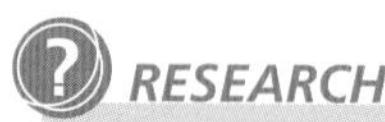

RESEARCH

What are leukopenia and thrombocytopenia?

The treatment of choice is doxycycline and should not be delayed while waiting for definitive laboratory diagnosis. Rifampin can be used in patients who cannot tolerate doxycycline. A microscopic examination of blood smears may show morulae, which are membrane-enclosed microcolonies of ehrlichiae in the cytoplasm of white blood cells (Fig 21-4), in about 20% of patients. The species most often infecting monocytes is *E chaffeensis*, and that entering granulocytes (neutrophils) is *Ehrlichia ewingii*. Nevertheless, these observations cannot produce a definitive identification. DNA amplification tests can detect different species of *Ehrlichia*.

C burnetii

Coxiella is related more to *Legionella* than to *Rickettsia*. The microorganisms are excreted in milk, urine, and feces of infected cattle, sheep, and goats. The bacterium is resistant to heat, desiccation, and many disinfectants. Thus, it can survive for long periods in the environment. Q (query) fever is most commonly caused by inhalation of airborne particles, which are the extracellular infectious form of the microorganism (small cell variant) present in barnyard dust contaminated by dried placental material, birth fluids, and excreta of infected animals. The incubation period is 20 days. It proliferates in the respiratory tract in phagolysosomes of monocytes and macrophages, even at the low pH found in this intracellular compartment; this is the vegetative form (large cell variant).

About 50% of people exposed to *C burnetii* have an asymptomatic infection. As in ehrlichiosis, symptoms vary from person to person and may include high fever, severe headache, muscle aches, chills, nausea, vomiting, nonproductive cough, abdominal pain, and chest pain. In severe cases, Q fever may lead to pneumonia, granulomatous hepatitis, myocarditis, and central nervous system involvement.

Chronic Q fever in the form of endocarditis can develop in patients with underlying heart valve defects or immunosuppression.

The most common method of diagnosis is serology, with indirect immunofluorescence and enzyme-linked immunosorbent assay. PCR-based assays are available in reference laboratories, but the sensitivity of the assay is low for serum samples.

Doxycycline is the antibiotic of choice for acute infections. Failure to respond to this antibiotic is an indication that the patient might be infected with another infectious agent. Chronic infections can be treated for prolonged periods with doxycycline plus hydroxychloroquine that alkalinizes intracellular compartments. An inactivated whole-cell vaccine is efficacious in persons who have not been infected previously.

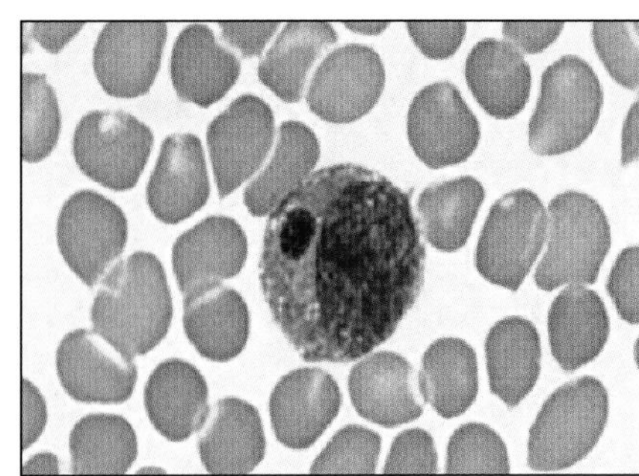

Fig 21-4 Morulae, microcolonies of ehrlichiae, detected in a monocyte on a peripheral blood smear, associated with *E chaffeensis* infection. (Reproduced from the Centers for Disease Control and Prevention. www.cdc.gov/ehrlichiosis/.)

Bibliography

Burillo A, Bouza E. *Chlamydophila pneumoniae.* Infect Dis Clin North Am 2010;24:61–71.

Centers for Disease Control and Prevention. *Chlamydia.* www.cdc.gov/std/stats12/chlamydia.htm. Accessed 16 July 2015.

Centers for Disease Control and Prevention. Ehrlichiosis. www.cdc.gov/ehrlichiosis/. Accessed 16 July 2015.

Centers for Disease Control and Prevention. Public Health Image Library. phil.cdc.gov. Accessed 4 August 2015.

Centers for Disease Control and Prevention. Q Fever. www.cdc.gov/qfever/. Accessed 16 July 2015.

Centers for Disease Control and Prevention. Rocky Mountain Spotted Fever (RMSF). www.cdc.gov/rmsf/. Accessed 16 July 2015.

Eremeeva ME, Dasch GA. Rickettsial (Spotted & Typhus Fevers) & Related Infections (Anaplasmosis & Ehrlichiosis). wwwnc.cdc.gov/travel/yellowbook/2014/chapter-3-infectious-diseases-related-to-travel/rickettsial-spotted-and-typhus-fevers-and-related-infections-anaplasmosis-and-ehrlichiosis. Accessed 16 July 2015.

Groß D, Schäfer G. 100th Anniversary of the death of Ricketts: Howard Taylor Ricketts (1871–1910). The namesake of the Rickettsiaceae family. Microbes Infection 2011;13:10–13.

Murray PR, Rosenthal KS, Pfaller MA. Medical Microbiology, ed 6. Philadelphia: Mosby/Elsevier, 2009.

"Prowazek (Provázek), Stanislaus Von Lanov." Complete Dictionary of Scientific Biography. Encyclopedia.com. 14 March 2014. www.encyclopedia.com/doc/1G2-2830903529.html. Accessed 16 July 2015.

Ryan KJ, Ray CG. Sherris Medical Microbiology, ed 5. New York: McGraw-Hill, 2010.

World Health Organization. Trachoma. www.who.int/blindness/causes/trachoma/en. Accessed 16 July 2015.

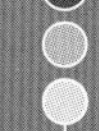

Take-Home Messages

- Chlamydiae are obligate intracellular bacteria with inner and outer membranes, but they do not have a peptidoglycan layer. They have two morphologically distinct forms: the elementary body and the reticulate body.
- *C trachomatis* causes the most common sexually transmitted disease in the United States and possibly worldwide.
- The trachoma biovar of *C trachomatis* is the leading cause of preventable blindness in developing countries.
- *C trachomatis* infects epithelial cells of mucosal surfaces, including the conjunctivae, endocervix, and endometrium.
- *C psittaci* is transmitted to humans from infected birds via the inhalation of dried bird excrement and causes psittacosis.
- *C pneumoniae* is transmitted by respiratory secretions and causes pneumonia, bronchitis, pharyngitis, and sinusitis.
- Rickettsiae are aerobic, Gram-negative, obligate intracellular bacilli.
- *R rickettsii* causes Rocky Mountain spotted fever by damaging endothelial cells and causing leakage of blood vessels. The inflammation can cause a swollen throat and tongue. Infection can result in damage to internal organs and the nervous system.
- *R prowazekii* causes epidemic typhus, with complications including myocarditis and nervous system damage.
- *R akari* can cause lymphadenopathy, generalized papulovesicular rash, and in some cases the appearance of vesicles in the oral cavity.
- Human monocytic ehrlichiosis is caused by *E chaffeensis* and presents with fever, myalgia, confusion, leukopenia, and thrombocytopenia.
- Q fever is most commonly caused by inhalation of airborne particles of *C burnetii.*

Vibrio, *Pseudomonas*, and Related Bacteria

22

Vibrio

The genus contains more than 34 species of comma-shaped bacilli, of which 11 have been associated with human infections. *Vibrio cholerae*, *Vibrio parahaemolyticus*, and *Vibrio vulnificus* are the most prominent among these species. They are Gram-negative, facultatively anaerobic, fermentative bacilli. They are classified as gammaproteobacteria together with enterobacteria. They can be distinguished from Enterobacteriaceae by a positive cytochrome oxidase reaction and the presence of polar flagella (Fig 22-1). *V cholerae* can grow in the absence of salts, while other species require salt. Members of the species are classified on the basis of their somatic O antigens. *V cholerae* O1 and O139 are the causative agents of classic cholera. *V cholerae* O1 can be subdivided into two biotypes: "El Tor" and cholerae.

Clinical syndromes and diagnosis

Cholera presents with an abrupt onset of watery diarrhea and vomiting 2 to 3 days after ingestion. Stool specimens become speckled with mucus flecks, called rice-water stools. Resulting fluid loss can lead to dehydration, metabolic acidosis (bicarbonate loss), and hypovolemic shock (abnormally decreased plasma volume), with cardiac arrhythmia and renal shock. The mortality rate is 60% in untreated patients but less than 1% in patients treated immediately to replace lost fluids and electrolytes.

The clinical syndromes of *V parahaemolyticus* include abdominal cramping, chills, headache, myalgias, and vomiting and may occur within a day of eating contaminated seafood, such as oysters. Exposure of the skin to contaminated water can result in wound infections.

V vulnificus causes wound or soft tissue infections as well as septicemia, especially in patients with liver disease or hematopoietic disease and in those receiving immunosuppressive drugs. The symptoms include fever, chills, low blood pressure, and skin lesions. There are about 95 cases a year in the United States, with a mortality rate of 37%. In normally healthy persons, it causes diarrhea, vomiting, and abdominal pain.

V cholerae and the other *Vibrio* species can be diagnosed definitively by culture from stool or rectal or wound swabs. Thiosulfate citrate bile salts (TCBS) agar is used as a selective medium for the isolation and identification of the microorganism. The serotype is confirmed using specific antisera.

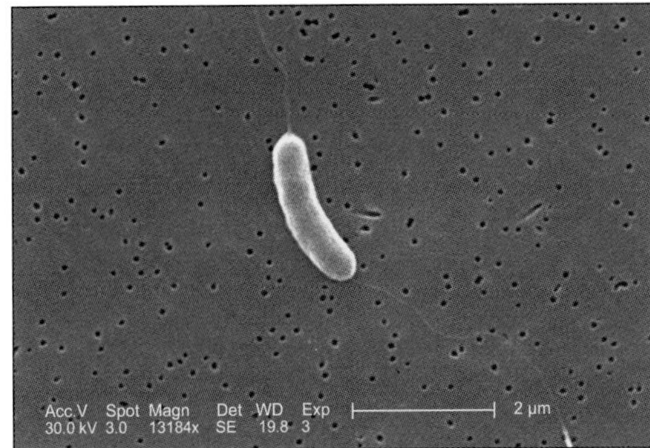

Fig 22-1 Scanning electron micrograph of a flagellated *V vulnificus*. (Public Health Image Library image 6937, courtesy of Janice Haney Carr.)

Pathogenesis and epidemiology

Cholera toxin is an enterotoxin also called choleragen. It is heat labile like the enterotoxin of *Bacillus cereus*. It is encoded by the *ctxA* and *ctxB* genes. It causes hypersecretion of electrolytes and water. This toxin has the A-B structure and binds to gangliosides on mucosal cells via five B subunits. The A subunit adenosine diphosphate (ADP)-ribosylates the stimulatory Gs protein in the plasma membrane of the mucosal cells, locking it in the "on" position. This activates adenyl cyclase, resulting in the accumulation of cyclic adenosine monophosphate, and the active secretion of chloride, bicarbonate, and water out of the cell and into the intestinal lumen. Severely infected patients can lose as much as 1 liter of fluid per hour during the height of the disease.

The bacteria can adhere tightly to the mucosal cell surface by their pili and adhesin molecules. The hemagglutinin-protease (mucinase; *hap* gene) dissolves the protective glycoprotein coating over intestinal cells. The pili that attach the bacteria to the gut mucosa also act as receptors for the bacteriophage CTXø that carries the *ctxA* and *ctxB* genes.

The toxin coregulated pilus (*tcp* gene) mediates the adherence of the bacterium to intestinal mucosal cells. It is also a binding site for bacteriophage CTXø. Colonization factor (*cep* gene) is an adhesin molecule that facilitates adhesion to the mucosal cell surface. Accessory cholera enterotoxin (*ace* gene) mediates increased fluid secretion. The zonula occludens toxin (*zot* gene) loosens the tight junctions of the mucosa of the small intestines.

V parahaemolyticus is invasive and affects the colon. It has a thermostable hemolysin called Kanagawa hemolysin that induces chloride ion secretion and causes β-hemolysis on agar media with human blood.

Vibrio species grow naturally in estuarine and marine environments, particularly those with chitinous shellfish. Cholera is transmitted by contaminated water and food, usually in communities with poor sanitation. Seven major pandemics have occurred since 1817. The seventh pandemic (caused by O1 biotype El Tor) started in Asia in 1961, spread to Africa and Europe in the 1970s and 1980s, and spread to Peru in 1991. This strain has caused disease in most countries in South and Central America. By 1995, more than 1 million cases and 10,000 deaths had been reported. A new epidemic strain emerged in India in 1992, *V cholerae* O139 Bengal. Individuals exposed to O1 are not immune to O139. In 2010, a cholera epidemic started in Haiti and had caused 699,000 cases and more than 8,500 deaths by February 2014. The strain was identified as toxigenic *V cholerae* O1, serotype Ogawa, biotype El Tor.

V parahaemolyticus is transmitted via contaminated seafood. It is the most common cause of bacterial gastroenteritis in Japan and Southeast Asia. It is the most common *Vibrio* species responsible for gastroenteritis in the United States. An outbreak occurred in 2005 in the United States.

Treatment and prevention

Cholera patients must be treated with fluids and electrolytes before the fluid loss leads to hypovolemic shock. Azithromycin can reduce exotoxin production. Control is achieved by improved sanitation, including sewage management and water purification systems. Protection by a killed cholera vaccine is 50% effective and can last up to 2 years. Individuals traveling to endemic areas should not rely on vaccine protection and should avoid consuming contaminated food and water.

V parahaemolyticus infections are usually self-limiting. Fluid and electrolyte therapy should be given. In severe and prolonged cases, tetracycline or ciprofloxacin can be used. Raw oysters should be avoided. *V vulnificus* infections should be treated immediately with doxycycline and a third-generation cephalosporin (eg, ceftazidime). Single-agent treatment with a fluoroquinolone has also been reported to be effective in an animal model of the disease.

Aeromonas

Aeromonas is a facultatively anaerobic, fermentative, Gram-negative bacillus. It can cause diarrheal disease, opportunistic systemic disease, and wound infections. Ingestion of contaminated food or water results in diarrhea accompanied by blood and leukocytes in the stool and se-

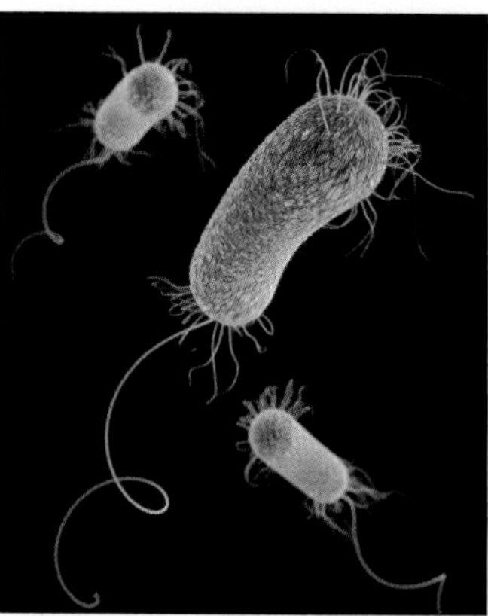

Fig 22-2 Computer-generated image of *P aeruginosa.* (Public Health Image Library image 16876, courtesy of Melissa Brower.)

vere abdominal pain. Wound infections can progress within a day to cause fasciitis, myonecrosis, and bacteremia. The primary species are *Aeromonas hydrophila, Aeromonas caviae,* and *Aeromonas veronii.*

Supportive care is given in the case of acute diarrheal disease. In patients with chronic diarrhea, wound infections, or systemic disease, antibiotics including ciprofloxacin, amikacin, gentamicin, and trimethoprim-sulfamethoxazole can be administered.

Pseudomonas aeruginosa

Pseudomonas aeruginosa are aerobic, Gram-negative bacilli usually arranged in pairs (Fig 22-2). They are classified as gammaproteobacteria and are found in soil, decaying organic matter, vegetation, and water. They also grow in various moist environments in hospitals, including equipment for respiratory therapy and dialysis. They can even survive in disinfectant solutions.

The organisms are nonfermentative (they do not ferment glucose, unlike members of the Enterobacteriaceae) and use relatively few carbohydrates during oxidative metabolism. The presence of cytochrome oxidase also differentiates them from Enterobacteriaceae. Although they utilize oxygen as the terminal electron acceptor, they can also use nitrate as an alternative acceptor and grow anaerobically. Strains with capsules are common in patients with cystic fibrosis. The slime layer facilitates adherence to mucous membranes.

Clinical syndromes and diagnosis

Pseudomonas infections are primarily opportunistic; that is, they are restricted to hosts with compromised immunity, for example with decreased neutrophil counts (< 500/µL). *P aeruginosa* can cause infections anywhere in the body, but urinary tract infections, pneumonia (especially in cystic fibrosis patients), and wound infections (especially burns) are the most common manifestations.

Pulmonary infections can range from benign tracheobronchitis to severe necrotizing bronchopneumonia. Infections in cystic fibrosis patients can exacerbate the underlying disease and lead to involvement of pulmonary parenchyma. Primary skin infections are mostly seen in burn wounds (Fig 22-3). The infection can cause localized vascular damage, tissue necrosis, and bacteremia. Folliculitis and nail infections can also occur in individuals frequently exposed to contaminated water. Urinary tract infections are seen in individuals with urinary catheters.

External ear infections (otitis externa) are most frequently caused by *P aeruginosa.* Swimming is an important risk factor. Malignant external otitis is seen in the elderly and in diabetic patients and leads to damage to the adjacent tissues, including nerves and bone. Surgical and antimicrobial intervention is required treatment. Chronic otitis media may also be caused by *P aeruginosa.*

Eye infections occur after trauma to the cornea followed by exposure to contaminated water and can lead to the development of corneal ulcers. Bacteremia occurs mostly in patients with neutropenia, diabetes, extensive burns, or hematologic malignancies. The mortality rate for *P aeruginosa* sepsis is greater than 50%. Endocarditis is observed mostly in intravenous drug users.

P aeruginosa produces two pigments useful in clinical and laboratory diagnosis: *(1)* Pyocyanin can color blue the pus in a wound. *(2)* Pyoverdin is a yellow-green pigment that fluoresces under ultraviolet light; this property can be used in the early detection of skin infections in burn patients. In the laboratory, these pigments diffuse into the agar and impart a blue-green color that is useful in identification. A positive oxidase reaction, β-hemolytic activity, and pigmentation help with the identification.

Pathogenesis and epidemiology

Attachment of the bacterium to epithelial cells is mediated by pili, flagellae, lipopolysaccharide, and alginate. The capsule formed by the mucoid polysaccharide alginate protects the microorganism against phagocytosis and antibiotics. The lipid A component of lipopolysaccharide has endotoxin activity characteristic of the sepsis syndrome. A bacterial neuraminidase removes sialic acids from the epithelial cell membrane.

Exotoxin A is a secreted protein that inhibits protein synthesis by inactivating eukaryotic elongation factor-2 (EF-2) by ADP-ribosylation, in a manner similar to diphtheria toxin, but it is less potent. It most likely mediates the tissue damage in burn-wound infections and chronic pulmonary infections. Exoenzyme S (ExoS) is an ADP-ribosyltransferase produced by a third of clinical isolates. It interferes with regulatory G proteins that are involved in signaling pathways, the cytoskeleton, and apoptosis. ExoS as well as other proteins are injected into the host cell via the type III secretion system of the bacterium.

A serine protease (LasA) and a zinc metalloprotease (LasB) function as elastases and cause lung parenchymal damage and hemorrhagic lesions (ecthyma gangrenosum). They can also degrade complement components and inhibitors of leukocyte proteases, leading to further tissue

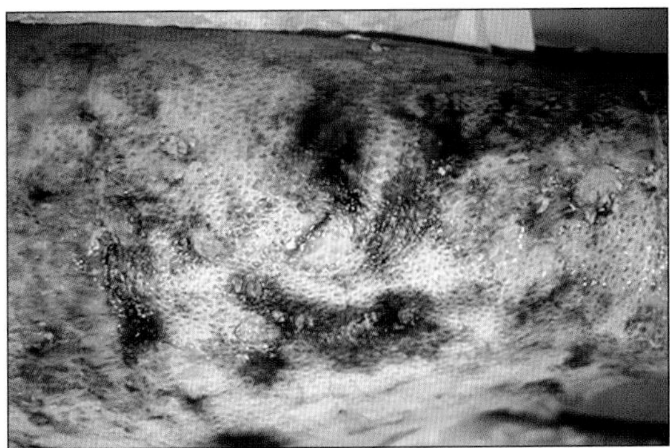

Fig 22-3 Primary skin infection caused by *P aeruginosa*. (Reprinted with permission from Murray et al.)

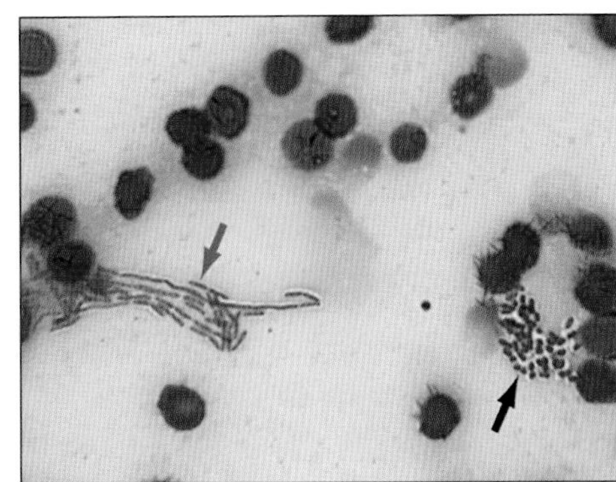

Fig 22-4 Gram stain of *P aeruginosa (red arrow)* and *Acinetobacter baumannii (black arrow)*. (Reprinted with permission from Murray et al.)

damage in acute infections. In chronic *Pseudomonas* infections, antibodies to these proteases are deposited as immune complexes in infected tissues. Phospholipase C degrades lipids, including phosphatidylcholine, producing diacylglycerol, and acts as a hemolysin. Pyocyanin mediates tissue and neutrophil damage by catalyzing the production of superoxide and hydrogen peroxide. It also stimulates the production of interleukin-8 by airway epithelial cells, attracting neutrophils to the infected tissue. In the presence of pyochelin, an iron-binding siderophore, the more toxic hydroxyl radical is formed.

The mutation of porin proteins in *P aeruginosa* is the major mechanism of resistance to antibiotics. The bacterium also produces various β-lactamases that inactivate β-lactam antibiotics. Carbapenems induce the formation of thicker biofilms, and fluoroquinolones and aminoglycosides can induce biofilm formation. Ciprofloxacin treatment enhances the frequency of mutation to carbapenem resistance. Although tetracycline is not very active against *P aeruginosa*, it induces the type III secretion system that facilitates cytotoxicity in vivo. Low concentrations of protein synthesis inhibitors and disinfectants induce multidrug efflux systems through a stress response factor.

P aeruginosa is a ubiquitous opportunistic pathogen. Persistent carriage is uncommon in healthy people but common in hospitalized patients. Risk factors for acquiring infection include prior treatment with broad-spectrum antibiotics, respiratory therapy, prolonged hospitalization, compromised immune function, exposure to contaminated water, diabetes, old age, and intravenous drug use.

RESEARCH

How does the natural peptide cathelicidin help clear pulmonary *P aeruginosa*?

Treatment and prevention

Treatment is challenging because the organism is resistant to most antibiotics, and immunocompromised hosts cannot augment the antibiotic activity. Even susceptible organisms can become resistant during therapy (via β-lactamases or plasmid-mediated resistance transfer). Aminoglycosides have poor activity in the acidic environment of an abscess. Usually a combination of aminoglycosides and β-lactam antibiotics (eg, ticarcillin or piperacillin) with documented activity against the isolate is necessary. Administration of hyperimmune serum or granulocyte transfusions may be beneficial.

Contamination of sterile equipment with *P aeruginosa* and infection of patients by medical personnel must be avoided. Indwelling catheters must be removed promptly. Burned skin must be treated very carefully.

Burkholderia

These organisms were previously classified under the genus *Pseudomonas*. *Burkholderia cepacia* complex are opportunistic microorganisms and can cause bronchopneumonia in patients with granulomatous disease and cystic fibrosis, urinary tract infections in catheterized patients, and septicemia. *Burkholderia pseudomallei* is a highly infectious microorganism that causes pulmonary disease. The clinical syndromes may range from mild bronchitis to necrotizing pneumonia. It can also cause sepsis, which can be deadly and must be treated with antibiotics such as trimethoprim-sulfamethoxazole.

Acinetobacter

Acinetobacter are Gram-negative coccobacilli that sometimes resemble *Neisseria* (Fig 22-4). They do not ferment carbohydrates and do not reduce nitrates, characteristics that distinguish them from Enterobacteriaceae. They are found in moist environments, soaps, and disinfectants. Most human infections are caused by *Acinetobacter baumannii*. They can cause pneumonia, urinary tract infections, as well as soft tissue infections, although their identification does not necessarily indicate infection because they are colonizers of the skin and the respiratory tract. Patients receiving broad-spectrum antibiotics, recovering from surgery, or on respiratory ventilators are at increased risk. *Acinetobacter* infections are rare outside health care settings.

Treatment is complicated, because *Acinetobacter* is resistant to many commonly prescribed antibiotics. Treatment decisions should be made on a case-by-case basis following in vitro antibiotic susceptibility testing. Infection-control procedures, including hand hygiene and environmental cleaning, can prevent transmission.

Moraxella catarrhalis

Moraxella catarrhalis was classified previously with *Neisseria*, based on its coccobacillary morphology, oxidase positivity, and fastidious growth requirements (such as chocolate agar). It can cause bronchopneumonia, sinusitis, and otitis media. The bacterium is resistant to penicillins, but it is susceptible to cephalosporins, tetracycline, erythromycin, and the combination of penicillins with clavulanic acid as a β-lactamase inhibitor.

Bibliography

Centers for Disease Control and Prevention. *Acinetobacter* in Healthcare Settings. www.cdc.gov/HAI/organisms/acinetobacter.html. Accessed 16 July 2015.

Centers for Disease Control and Prevention. Cholera: Diagnosis and Testing in Haiti. www.cdc.gov/haiticholera/diagnosistreatment.htm. Accessed 16 July 2015.

Centers for Disease Control and Prevention. Cholera in Haiti: One Year Later. www.cdc.gov/haiticholera/haiti_cholera.htm. Accessed 16 July 2015.

Centers for Disease Control and Prevention. Cholera Outbreak—Haiti, October 2010. www.cdc.gov/mmwr/preview/mmwrhtml/mm5943a4.htm?s_cid=mm5943a4_w. Accessed 16 July 2015.

Centers for Disease Control and Prevention. Public Health Image Library. phil.cdc.gov. Accessed 4 August 2015.

Centers for Disease Control and Prevention. *Vibrio parahaemolyticus.* www.cdc.gov/vibrio/vibriop.html. Accessed 16 July 2015.

Centers for Disease Control and Prevention. *Vibrio vulnificus.* www.cdc.gov/vibrio/vibriov.html. Accessed 16 July 2015.

Morita Y, Tomida J, Kawamura Y. Responses of *Pseudomonas aeruginosa* to antimicrobials. Front Microbiol 2014;4:422.

Murray PR, Rosenthal KS, Pfaller MA. Medical Microbiology, ed 6. Philadelphia: Mosby/Elsevier, 2009.

Ryan KJ, Ray CG. Sherris Medical Microbiology, ed 5. New York: McGraw-Hill, 2010.

Todar K. Todar's Online Textbook of Bacteriology. http://www.textbookofbacteriology.net. Accessed 16 July 2015.

World Health Organization. Cholera. www.who.int/cholera/en/. Accessed 16 July 2015.

Take-Home Messages

- *Vibrio* are Gram-negative, facultatively anaerobic bacilli with polar flagella.
- *V cholerae* O1 and O139 are the causative agents of classic cholera, which presents with an abrupt onset of watery diarrhea and vomiting a few days after ingestion.
- Cholera toxin causes hypersecretion of electrolytes and water. The hemagglutinin-protease dissolves the protective glycoprotein coating over intestinal cells.
- *V parahaemolyticus* is transmitted via contaminated seafood.
- *V vulnificus* causes wound or soft tissue infections as well as septicemia.
- Cholera patients must be treated with fluids and electrolytes before the fluid loss leads to hypovolemic shock.
- *Aeromonas* is a facultatively anaerobic, Gram-negative bacillus and can cause diarrheal disease, opportunistic systemic disease, and wound infections.
- *P aeruginosa* is an aerobic, Gram-negative bacillus found in soil, decaying organic matter, and equipment for respiratory therapy and dialysis.
- *P aeruginosa* causes urinary tract infections, pneumonia (particularly in cystic fibrosis patients), burn-wound infections, and external ear infections.
- *Pseudomonas* exotoxin A inhibits protein synthesis by inactivating eukaryotic EF-2.
- *B pseudomallei* is a highly infectious bacterium that causes pulmonary disease.
- *A baumannii* can cause pneumonia as well as urinary tract and soft tissue infections, especially in health care settings.
- *M catarrhalis* causes bronchopneumonia, sinusitis, and otitis media.

Oral Microflora and Caries

23

Oral Microflora

Oral microorganisms are referred to as the oral microflora, oral microbiota, and the oral microbiome. The Nobel Laureate Joshua Lederberg originated the term *microbiome* to signify the ecological community of commensal, symbiotic, and pathogenic microorganisms that literally share our body space and have been all but ignored as determinants of health and disease." The oral cavity comprises distinct microbial habitats, including the teeth, gingival sulci, attached gingiva, lips, tongue, cheeks, and hard and soft palate. It is estimated that less than half of the bacterial species in the oral cavity can be cultured using anaerobic microbiologic methods. It is likely that there are 700 to 800 common oral species. About 280 bacterial species have been isolated in culture and named. Molecular methods based on the cloning of the 16S rRNA have confirmed these estimates by identifying about 600 species or "phylotypes." These studies have shown that Firmicutes constitute the largest percentage of oral microflora, with 227 taxa (36.7% of the total). *Taxa* refers to named species and to phylotypes with or without cultivable members. There are 107 Bacteriodetes species, 106 Proteobacteria species, 72 Actinobacteria species, 49 Spirochete species, and 32 Fusobacteria species.

Oral microorganisms have been shown to cause various diseases, including caries, periodontitis, endodontic (root canal) infections, alveolar osteitis, and tonsillitis. Various oral bacteria have been linked to a number of systemic diseases such as cardiovascular disease, diabetes, stroke, preterm birth, and pneumonia. Caries, periodontitis, otitis media, as well as other infections are caused by consortia of organisms in a biofilm rather than by a single microorganism.

Among the normal oral flora, streptococci are the predominant supragingival bacteria. There are four main groups of streptococci: mutans, salivarius, mitis, and anginosus. The predominant cultivable genera in subgingival plaque are *Actinomyces*, *Prevotella*, *Porphyromonas*, *Fusobacterium*, and *Veillonella*.

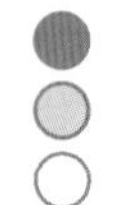

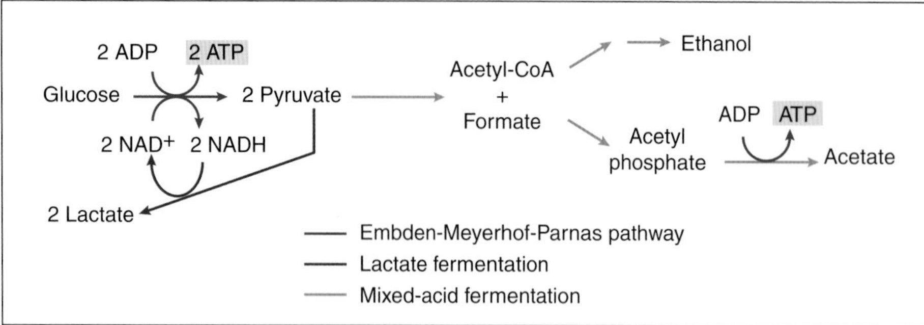

Fig 23-1 Sugar fermentation by *Streptococcus mutans* and the abbreviated pathways of glycolysis *(blue)*, lactate fermentation *(green)*, and mixed-acid fermentation *(orange)*. Bacterial cells may produce lactate only or lactate plus formate, acetate, and ethanol. ADP, adenosine disphosphate; ATP, adenosine triphosphate; NAD/NAPH, nicotinamide adenine dinucleotide; CoA, coenzyme A. (Adapted from Lamont et al.)

Gram-positive cocci

Streptococcus

Oral streptococci have been termed viridans streptococci because many species produce green (viridis, Latin) colonies on blood agar. However, many oral streptococci have strains that cause all three types of hemolysis. The mutans group ("mutans streptococci") colonizes tooth or denture surfaces, rapidly produces acid, and can also grow in an acidic environment (Fig 23-1). *Streptococcus mutans* (serotypes c, e, f, and k) is the primary pathogen in enamel caries in children and young adults and causes root surface caries in the elderly and nursing caries in infants. It derives its species name from the observation that its shape can change into a coccobacillus. *Streptococcus sobrinus* (serotypes d and g) and *Streptococcus criceti* are also in this group. Other mutans streptococci have been identified in rats and monkeys. Mutans streptococci can be identified by growth on a selective medium composed of mitis salivarius agar and bacitracin; however, bacitracin can inhibit the growth of both *S sobrinus* and *S criceti*, rendering it difficult to study the prevalence of these species.

Antigen I/II proteins of *S mutans* are thought to be the surface components of the bacterium that interact with the salivary pellicle. *S mutans* synthesizes both extracellular (glucan, mutan, fructan) and intracellular polysaccharides. The extracellular polymers are involved in biofilm formation, and the intracellular polysaccharides are metabolized to lactic acid when dietary carbohydrates are not available.

RESEARCH

What are the structures of glucan, mutan, fructan, and levan?

The bacteria in the salivarius group are found on mucosal surfaces, including the tongue. *Streptococcus salivarius* produces an extracellular unusual fructan with a levan structure but is not considered to be a significant opportunistic bacterium.

Streptococcus vestibularis does not produce extracellular polysaccharides but generates urease, which generates ammonia, causing an increase in the local pH. It also generates hydrogen peroxide, which contributes to the sialoperoxidase system that produces hypothiocyanite at neutral pH and hypothiacyanous acid at low pH. The products inhibit glycolysis by plaque bacteria.

The mitis group includes *S sanguinis*, *Streptococcus gordonii*, *Streptococcus mitis*, and *Streptococcus oralis*. These bacteria, except *S mitis*, may become opportunistic pathogens and cause infective endocarditis. *S sanguinis* and *S gordonii* are early colonizers of the tooth surface (Fig 23-2). The soluble and insoluble extracellular glucans that they produce facilitate plaque formation. *S sanguinis* produces an immunoglobulin (Ig) A protease, and *S gordonii* can bind α-amylase, the salivary enzyme that breaks down starch, and may appear to the immune system as "self." *S oralis* and *S mitis* are among the most common streptococci in the oral cavity and are also initial colonizers. *S oralis* produces IgA protease and glucans. *Streptococcus pneumoniae*, which can be isolated from the nasopharynx, is also in this group and can transfer antibiotic resistance genes to other mitis group bacteria.

The streptococci in the anginosus group are found in dental plaque and mucosal surfaces, are involved in maxillofacial infections, and are found in abscesses of internal organs, such as the brain and liver. They are also associated with endocarditis, peritonitis, and appendicitis. The species in this group include *Streptococcus anginosus*, *Streptococcus intermedius* (which produces the toxin intermedilysin, which affects neutrophils), and *Streptococcus constellatus*.

Other Gram-positive cocci

Granulicatella adiacens is an early colonizer of teeth and has the property of "satellitism," where growth is seen around colonies of other bacteria that produce growth factors, including cysteine and pyridoxal. Anaerobic cocci such as *Peptostreptococcus stomatis*, *Parvimonas micra*, and *Finegoldia magna* are often found in dental abscesses, carious dentin, infected pulp chambers and root canals, and gingiva with advanced periodontal disease. *Enterococcus faecalis* has been isolated from infected root canals and periodontal pockets that do not respond to therapy. Although staphylococci and micrococci are found abundantly on the skin and in the nose, they are not among the usual microflora in the oral cavity.

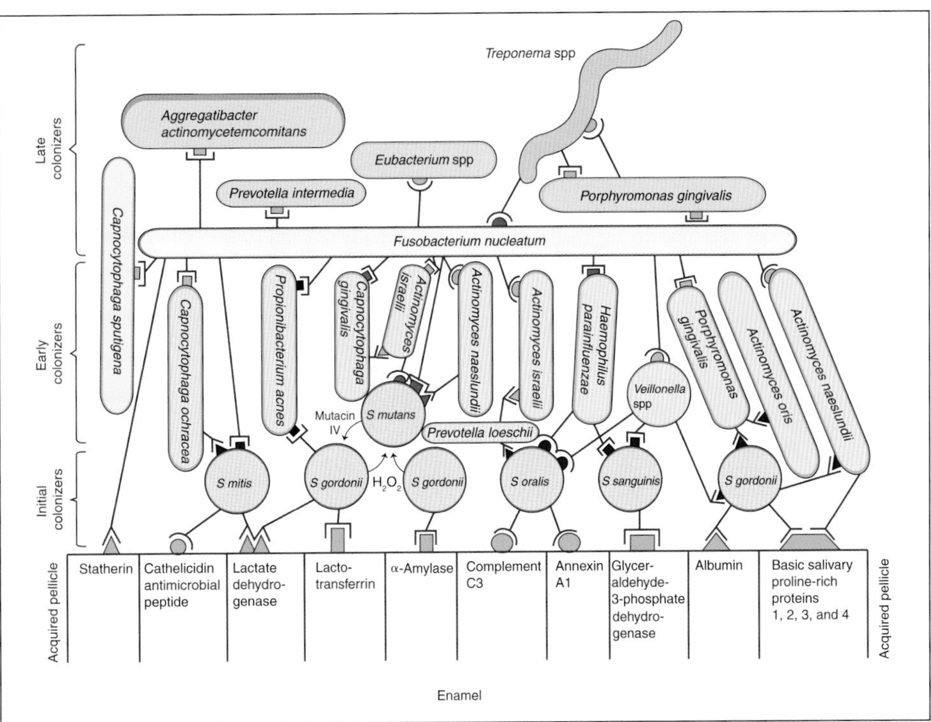

Fig 23-2 Schematic view of the coaggregation (or coadhesion) of bacteria in human dental plaque. Early (or initial) colonizers bind to molecules on the acquired pellicle. Other early colonizers bind to receptors on the surface of the initial colonizers. Adhesins, represented by the symbols with stems, are sensitive to heat and proteases. The receptors, represented by the complementary symbols on the cell surface, are not as sensitive to these treatments. The interaction of the early colonizers with the particular pellicle components is arbitrary in this figure. *S*, *Streptococcus*. (Adapted from Marsh and Martin, with additional data from Kreth et al, Lee et al, and Periasamy and Kolenbrander.)

Gram-positive bacilli and filaments

Lactobacilli constitute about 1% of the total cultivable microflora in the oral cavity. This percentage increases in advanced caries lesions of the enamel and root surface. *Lactobacillus casei*, *Lactobacillus fermentum*, *Lactobacillus rhamnosus*, *Lactobacillus salivarius*, *Lactobacillus acidophilus*, and *Lactobacillus gasseri* are some of the most common species. They are acidogenic and also acid tolerant. Testing for the numbers of lactobacilli in the saliva of patients is one way to monitor patients' dietary intake of carbohydrates.

Eubacteria are pleomorphic, obligate anaerobes found in dental plaque. They constitute more than 50% of the anaerobes of periodontal pockets. Many species previously classified as eubacteria have now been reclassified into genera such as *Mogobacterium*, *Pseudoramibacter*, and *Slackia*, which have all been isolated from infected root canals.

Propionibacterium acnes and *Propionibacterium propionicus* are strict anaerobic bacilli found in dental plaque. *Rothia mucilaginosa* can be isolated from the tongue and produces an extracellular slime layer. *Rothia dentocariosa* and *Bifidobacterium dentium* can be isolated from dental plaque. *R dentocariosa* is occasionally associated with infective endocarditis. *R dentocariosa* and *Scardovia inopinata* are found in about half of caries-active sites and not in caries-free sites. *Scardovia wiggsiae* has been identified as an aciduric and acidogenic species that is associated with early childhood caries.

Actinomyces species, which may appear as short rods or may be pleomorphic with branching, are a major component in dental plaque. *Actinomyces israelii* may be filamentous and can be an opportunistic pathogen and cause actinomycosis, characterized by chronic inflammation in the orofacial region. *Actinomyces naeslundii* has large numbers of fimbriae that mediate attachment and is the most common *Actinomyces* species in dental plaque. It produces an extracellular slime and fructan as well as enzymes that can hydrolyze the polysaccharide. It also synthesizes urease and neuraminidase. It is implicated in root surface caries and gingivitis. *Actinomyces radicidentis* has been found in endodontic infections. *Actinomyces gerensceriae* has been associated with early childhood caries.

Gram-negative cocci

Neisseria species (*Neisseria pharynges*, *Neisseria subflava*, *Neisseria mucosa*, *Neisseria flavescens*) help in plaque formation by consuming oxygen and enabling obligate anaerobes to flourish. Extracellular polysaccharides produced by some *Neisseria* species can be metabolized by some streptococci. The Gram-negative diplococcus *Moraxella catarrhalis* is an opportunistic pathogen found in the nasopharynx of about one-third of the population and can cause otitis media and sinusitis.

Veillonella species, including *Veillonella parvula*, *Veillonella atypica*, and *Veillonella denticariosi*, are anaerobic Gram-negative cocci found mostly in plaque. They lack the initial enzymes in the glycolytic pathway (ie, glucokinase and fructokinase) and thus cannot metabolize carbohydrates. However, they can metabolize lactic acid, the strongest acid produced by oral bacteria. Thus, *Veillonella* can alleviate the enamel-degradative activity of lactic acid (Fig 23-3).

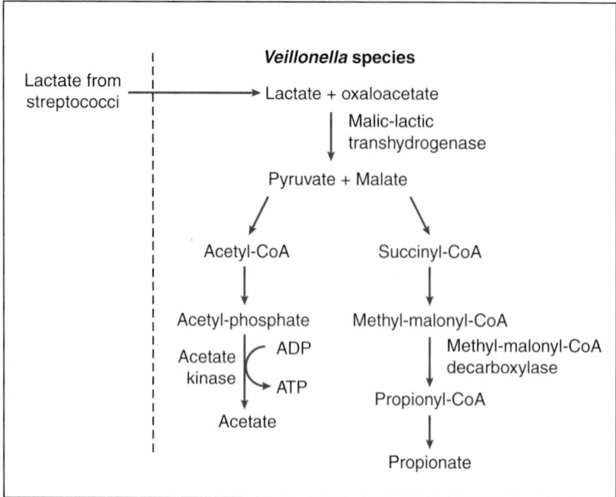

Fig 23-3 Lactate metabolism in *V parvula*, resulting in the production of acetate or propionate. CoA, coenzyme A; ADP, adenosine diphosphate; ATP, adenosine triphosphate. (Adapted from Lamont et al.)

Gram-negative bacilli

Haemophilus parainfluenzae is a facultatively anaerobic Gram-negative bacillus. It requires nicotinamide adenine dinucleotide in laboratory growth media.

Aggregatibacter actinomycetemcomitans is found occasionally in subgingival plaque. It is associated with particularly aggressive forms of juvenile periodontitis and less frequently with adult periodontitis. It grows best in an aerobic atmosphere enriched with 5% to 10% carbon dioxide. Its cell surface molecules stimulate bone resorption. Its virulence factors include leukotoxin, epitheliotoxin, collagenase, and IgG protease. It is also associated with endocarditis, subcutaneous and brain abscesses, and osteomyelitis.

Capnocytophaga are carbon dioxide–dependent ("capnophilic"), fusiform rods with "gliding" motility, and they are found in subgingival plaque. They are associated with destructive periodontal disease. Some strains produce IgA1 protease. The species include *Capnocytophaga gingivalis, Capnocytophaga sputigena, Capnocytophaga ochracae, Capnocytophaga granulosa*, and *Capnocytophaga haemolytica*.

Eikenella corrodens is found in dental plaque and is associated with dentoalveolar abscesses, infective endocarditis, and some forms of chronic periodontitis.

Fusobacterium species are strict anaerobes with a slender "cigar" shape. *Fusobacterium nucleatum* subspecies *polymorphum* is found in the normal gingival crevice. *F nucleatum* subspecies *nucleatum* is isolated mainly from periodontal pockets. Fusobacteria catabolize amino acids, including histidine, lysine, and aspartate. They coaggregate with most other oral bacteria and are thought to be an important bridging organism between early and late colonizers during plaque formation (see Fig 23-2). These bacteria remove sulfur from cysteine and methionine to produce hydrogen sulfide and methyl mercaptan, which are highly odorous and cause halitosis. Together with spirochetes, they are involved in inflammatory periodontal disease. The "fusospirochetal complex" is thought to cause necrotizing ulcerative gingivitis and necrotic oral ulcers, particularly in human immunodeficiency virus (HIV)/AIDS patients. The spirochete *Treponema denticola* decreases the *F nucleatum*–induced expression of human β-defensins and interleukin-8 in gingival epithelial cells by interfering with endosome-lysosomal maturation and with reactive oxygen species–dependent activation of Toll-like receptors.

Porphyromonas species are pleomorphic, asaccharolytic bacilli that utilize proteins and peptides for their metabolism. They are strict anaerobes that require vitamin K and hemin. They produce black-pigmented colonies on blood agar; the pigment may be involved in protection from the effects of oxygen. *Porphyromonas gingivalis* is found almost exclusively at subgingival sites, especially in advanced periodontal lesions. In experimental animals, *P gingivalis* is highly virulent. It produces proteases specific for peptide bonds adjoining arginine (arg-gingipains) or lysine (lys-gingipains) that degrade complement proteins, immunoglobulins, and proteins that sequester iron and heme. It also has a hemolysin and collagen-degrading enzymes. Its fimbriae mediate attachment to oral epithelial cells and to tooth surfaces coated with saliva. *Porphyromonas endodontalis* has been identified primarily in infected root canals.

Prevotella are also pleomorphic, strict anaerobes. The species *Prevotella intermedia, Prevotella melaninogenica, Prevotella nigrescens*, and *Prevotella loescheii* form black-pigmented colonies. They require vitamin K and hemin for growth and can convert glucose into acetic acid and succinic acid, among others. *P intermedia* is associated with chronic periodontitis and endodontic infections.

Campylobacter rectus (formerly classified as *Wolinella recta*) is a curved bacillus with polar flagellae. It is a strict anaerobe and is often found in sites of periodontal disease, particularly in immunocompromised patients. Some strains produce a toxin with some homology to the leukotoxin of *A actinomycetemcomitans*.

Treponema are motile, helical cells that have endoflagellae in the periplasmic space. They are strict anaerobes that require culturing in certain epithelial cells. They can be observed by dark-field microscopy. *T denticola* has arginine-specific protease activity and can degrade collagen and gelatin. Some oral spirochetes can attach to the oral epithelium by one of their poles, facilitate the destruction of the cells, and penetrate into deeper tissues. Their number increases in advanced periodontal disease. Whether spirochetes cause the disease or increase in number as a result of the disease is still under investigation.

Mycoplasma

Mycoplasmas are the smallest free-growing cells and do not have a peptidoglycan layer. *Mycoplasma salivarium, Mycoplasma pneumoniae*, and *Mycoplasma hominis* have been isolated from saliva, and *Mycoplasma buccale, Mycoplasma oralis*, and *M pneumoniae* have been found in the oral mucosa and dental plaque. Mycoplasmas may play a role in salivary gland hypofunction and in periodontal disease.

Fungi

Candida species constitute the largest fraction of fungi in the mouth. The prevalence of *Candida* in asymptomatic adults is in the wide range of 2% to 71%; this value approaches 100% in immunocompromised individuals and those on broad-spectrum antibiotics. The most common site of isolation of *Candida* is the dorsum of the tongue. The use of dentures and orthodontic appliances, particularly in the maxilla and on fitting surfaces, increases the incidence of *Candida*, which binds avidly to denture acrylic. *Candida albicans* is the most common species, but many other species are also isolated. These include *Candida glabrata*, *Candida tropicalis*, *Candida krusei*, and *Candida parapsilosis*.

Viruses

Herpes simplex virus type 1 is the most frequently found virus in saliva and the orofacial region. The virus is the cause of cold sores, which occur when the latent virus in the trigeminal nerve is activated by stress or ultraviolet light. Occasional isolation from saliva indicates periodic shedding of the virus. Various strains of Coxsackievirus have been detected in saliva and the oral epithelium. Human papillomavirus types 2, 4, 6, 11, and 16 are detected in oral lesions of patients with HIV/AIDS. Cytomegalovirus has also been detected in the saliva of adults without disease symptoms. The presence of hepatitis B and HIV in saliva may pose a cross-infection threat, emphasizing the need for universal precautions.

Protozoa

Two protozoans have been found frequently in the oral cavity: *Trichomonax tenax* and *Entamoeba gingivalis*. Their prevalence has been estimated by conventional detection techniques to be in the range of 4% to 52% in the healthy population. Studies using detection of 16S rRNA sequences by polymerase chain reaction have indicated that only 2% of the healthy population carries *T tenax*, but this increases to 21% in patients with periodontal disease.

The Oral Ecosystem and Dental Plaque

Many diseases of the oral cavity have a polymicrobial etiology. There are several factors that contribute to the ability of an assembly of microorganisms (such as those in dental plaque) to cause disease. These include the salivary flow rate and medications that can affect this rate, diet, tobacco use, and the integrity of the immune system. Understanding oral ecology is essential for understanding the pathogenesis of caries and periodontal disease caused by oral bacteria. The habitat of a microorganism is the location where it grows. A microbial community is the set of microorganisms, or microflora, living in a particular habitat. The ecosystem comprises the microbial community and the surrounding microenvironment. The niche is the location, or role, of a microorganism living in a particular habitat in which it thrives best.

Oral habitats

The main oral habitats are the mucosal surfaces, teeth, saliva, and gingival crevicular fluid. The dorsum of the tongue has papillary structures that provide a niche for bacteria that would otherwise be removed by salivary flow. This habitat also has a low redox potential that is suitable for Gram-negative, obligately anaerobic bacteria that are involved in periodontal disease and malodor (halitosis).

Teeth constitute a nonshedding surface for bacterial colonization. Bacteria and their polysaccharide products accumulate on tooth surfaces to produce dental plaque, which is generated both in health and in disease. Smooth surfaces are colonized by a limited number of species compared with those present in pits and fissures. Subgingival surfaces are in a more anaerobic environment than supragingival surfaces. The topography of the teeth, for example occlusal fissures, and inadequate restorations present areas that are difficult to clean by the natural flushing action of saliva.

Saliva can clear the potentially damaging acids produced by plaque bacteria after metabolizing carbohydrates. Saliva buffers the pH between 6.75 and 7.25 by means of bicarbonate, phosphate, and peptides. The proteins and glycoproteins in saliva generate the acquired pellicle on tooth surfaces, provide nutrients for normal oral microflora, aggregate microorganisms to facilitate their removal by swallowing, and inhibit the growth of exogenous microorganisms, for example by the action of lysozyme, lactoferrin, and histatins.

Gingival crevicular fluid can remove non-adherent bacteria, introduce IgG and neutrophils, and provide peptides and carbohydrates that bacteria can use for their metabolism. The pH of gingival crevicular fluid increases in the presence of gingivitis and periodontitis, providing a favorable environment for periodontopathogens such as *P gingivalis* and *P intermedia*.

Prosthodontic and orthodontic appliances may act as reservoirs for bacteria and yeasts. One of the causes of *Candida*-associated denture stomatitis is poor denture hygiene.

Microorganisms in the oral cavity can promote or suppress neighboring bacteria by prior occupation of colonizing sites, thus preventing the attachment of "latecomers." Bacteriocins are toxins produced by some bacteria that kill bacteria of the same or other species. For example, colicin E1 produced by certain strains of *Escherichia coli* can kill other strains of *E coli*. *S salivarius* produces the molecule enocin, which inhibits *Streptococcus pyogenes*. The production of metabolic end products, such as short-chain carboxylic acids, lowers the local pH, rendering the environment unsuitable for certain bacteria. Metabolic end products of certain bacteria can be used by others for nutritional purposes, as in the case of *Veillonella* species utilizing metabolic acids produced by *S mutans*. The coaggregation of bacteria within the same species or with bacteria of different species can

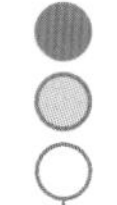

affect the microenvironment. An interesting manifestation of this phenomenon is the "corncob" arrangement of cocci bound to filamentous microorganisms.

Oral microbial colonization is also affected by the local pH, which can vary between a mean of 7.3 on the palate and 6.3 on the buccal mucosa. The local pH can vary because of the production of H^+ by fermenting bacteria, food intake, and the buffering capacity of saliva. The oxidation-reduction potential, or redox potential (Eh), of the environment determines which microorganisms can survive in the niche. Oxygen is a strong electron acceptor, and its environment becomes oxidized. Anaerobic microorganisms need reduced conditions for their metabolism. If the Eh is too high, some microorganisms will not grow even if oxygen is removed completely from the microenvironment. Oxygen tension, or the percentage of oxygen in the mouth, is generally low, about 12% on the posterior surface of the tongue and 0.3% to 0.4% on the buccal folds of the maxilla and mandible. Tolerance to oxygen by microorganisms requires the ability to reduce oxygen radicals, achieved by the expression of superoxide dismutase and catalase. The use of antibiotics or antiseptics, as well as diet, will also influence the colonization and growth of microorganisms.

Dental plaque

Dental plaque is a complex microbial community that forms on tooth surfaces and contains living, dead, and dying bacteria and their products, as well as salivary compounds. Calcified plaque is termed *calculus* (or *tartar*). Microorganisms in dental plaque are surrounded by an organic matrix, sometimes referred to as the *glycocalyx*, which is derived from both the host and microorganisms. The matrix acts as a food reserve and as a glue that binds organisms to each other and to surfaces. The composition of plaque is variable, depending on the sites on the same tooth, the same site on different teeth, and different times on the same tooth site. Communities of microorganisms attached to a surface form a biofilm. Biofilms may protect microorganisms from host defenses and antimicrobial agents and can render them more pathogenic.

Dental plaque may be categorized as supragingival plaque, fissure plaque (mainly on molar fissures), approximal plaque (at contact points of teeth), smooth-surface plaque (on buccal and palatal surfaces and mucosal surfaces), subgingival plaque, and prosthodontic (denture plaque) or orthodontic appliance–associated plaque.

Within minutes of exposure to the oral microenvironment, a layer of glycoproteins, lipids, and glycolipids (called the pellicle) derived from saliva, gingival crevicular fluid, and bacteria is deposited on the tooth surface. Single bacteria, called pioneer organisms, are deposited initially on the pellicle. The total interactive energy of particles approaching each other is the sum of the attractive van der Waals energy due to fluctuating dipoles within the molecules of the particles and the repulsive electrostatic energy. The particles can achieve equilibrium at a net attractive energy either in the "primary minimum" (at very short distances) or in the "secondary minimum" (at distances of 10 to 20 nm apart). Because the initial interactions between bacteria and the tooth surface, or between bacteria, are reversible, the two surfaces are most likely in the secondary minimum. These initial interactions can transform into more stable associations within the primary minimum via the specific interaction between adhesins on the microbial cell surface and receptors in the acquired pellicle. At this stage, hydrophobic interactions also contribute to the total energy of interaction. Adhesin-receptor recognition also contributes to the tropism of an organism for a particular surface or habitat. Different categories of bacteria sequentially colonize the plaque. An extracellular matrix composed of microbial polysaccharides and layers of salivary glycoproteins is produced. The predominant organisms at this initial stage are streptococci, particularly *S salivarius*, *S mitis*, and *S oralis*.

New colonizers start inhabiting the plaque as the microenvironment is changed as a result of the metabolic products of the pioneer organisms. This may include the creation of a low redox potential suitable for anaerobes, change of local pH, expression of new receptors for attachment, and generation of end products of metabolism (eg, lactate) or breakdown products (eg, peptides, hemin), which can be used as primary nutrients by other organisms. This results in the growth of microbial complexity, size, and thickness. The plaque mass reaches a critical size with a balance between the deposition and loss of bacteria, forming a climax community. The degenerating bacteria in a climax community may act as seeding agents for mineralization; this results in the formation of a calcified mass called calculus. The bacteria near the enamel surface have a reduced cytoplasm–cell wall ratio, most likely because they are metabolically inactive. Cocci can attach to filamentous microorganisms, especially on the outer layer of plaque, giving rise to a "corncob" structure.

The specific interaction of adhesins on the microbial cell surface with receptors in the acquired pellicle contributes to the tropism of an organism for a particular surface or habitat. *S mutans* and *P gingivalis* adhere preferentially to hydroxyapatite treated with proline-rich proteins. Colonization of *S sobrinus* may involve the interaction of glucans with receptors (glucan-binding proteins). The *P gingivalis* 150-kD adhesin binds to fibrinogen. The *F nucleatum* 42-kD protein mediates co-aggregation with *P gingivalis*, contributing to the extended structure of dental plaque. Type 1 fimbriae on *A naeslundii* mediate adherence to surface-bound proline-rich proteins, while type 2 fimbriae interact with surface sugars on already attached bacteria (ie, lectin-like activity). *A naeslundii* binds to acidic proline-rich proteins when the latter are bound to a surface but not when they are in solution. It is thought that a conformational change occurs when these proteins bind to hydroxyapatite. Such hidden receptors for bacterial adhesins are called cryptitopes. Members of the *S mitis* group bind to fibronectin when complexed to collagen, but not in solution. This may be a mechanism by which certain oral streptococci colonize damaged heart valves in endocarditis.

Caries

Caries is the localized destruction of the tissues of the tooth by bacterial fermentation of dietary carbohydrates. The key factors in the development of caries include a susceptible tooth surface, the nature of saliva flow, plaque bacteria, and the consumption of fermentable carbohydrates. Several hypotheses have been put forth to explain the initiation of caries. The specific plaque hypothesis emphasizes the importance of mutans streptococci in caries initiation. The nonspecific plaque hypothesis states that heterogeneous groups of bacteria that can produce acids as end products of fermentation are involved in the initiation of caries.

There is a significant correlation between *S mutans* counts in saliva and plaque and the prevalence and incidence of caries. (*Prevalence* is the number of cases of a disease present in a specified population at a given time. *Incidence* is the frequency of occurrence of any disease over a period of time in relation to the population in which it occurs). *S mutans* can be isolated from precise sites on the tooth surface before the development of caries. There is a correlation between the progression of caries lesions and *S mutans* counts. *S mutans* produces cell surface protein antigen I/II and extracellular polysaccharides from sucrose that facilitate microbial adhesion to tooth surfaces and to other bacteria. In experimental rodents and nonhuman primates on a sucrose-rich diet, *S mutans* is the most effective *Streptococcus* species that causes caries. It has the ability to initiate and maintain growth and continue acid production (primarily lactic acid via the action of lactate dehydrogenase on pyruvate) in sites with a low pH.

Lactobacillus species are present in increased numbers in most caries lesions on enamel and root surfaces. Their numbers in saliva correlate to the presence of caries. Some strains produce caries in gnotobiotic rats. They initiate and maintain growth at low pH (they are aciduric). *Lactobacillus* species produce lactic acid in conditions below pH 5 (they are acidogenic). Although these properties suggest that lactobacilli are involved in the initiation of caries, their affinity for the tooth surface is low, their numbers in dental plaque in early caries lesions are usually low, and their population size is a poor predictor of the number of future plaques. It is thought that their numbers in saliva increase only after the development of caries. Thus, lactobacilli may not be involved in the initiation of dental caries, but they are involved in the progression of caries deep into enamel and dentin. They are pioneer organisms in the advancing carious process.

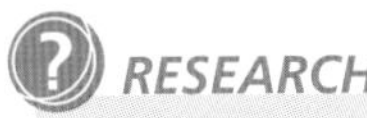

RESEARCH

How are gnotobiotic animals used in medical and dental research?

Lactobacilli inhibit the growth of mutans streptococci in culture. The main *Lactobacillus* species are *L fermentum*, *Lactobacillus plantarum*, *L salivarius*, and *Lactobacillus paracasei*. Other species include *L acidophilus* and *L gasseri*.

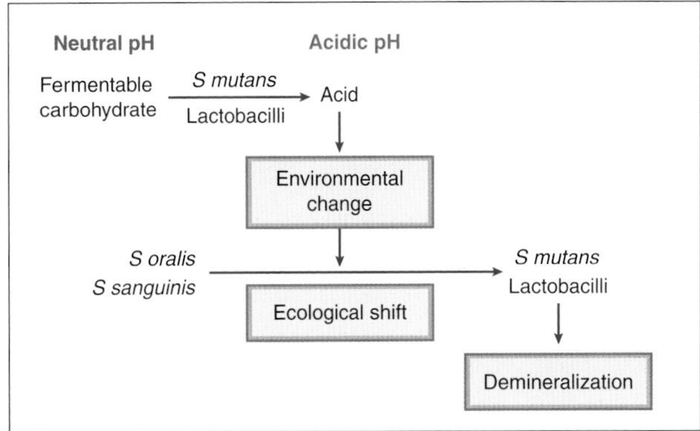

Fig 23-4 Schematic flow of events leading to demineralization, as proposed by the ecological plaque hypothesis.

L salivarius and *L gasseri* inhibit the growth of *Staphylococcus aureus*, *E faecalis*, *S pneumoniae*, and *Salmonella* Enteritidis.

Low pH causes demineralization by reducing the concentration of the tribasic phosphate (PO_4^{3-}), which is needed to form hydroxyapatite:

$$10Ca^{2+} + 6PO_4^{3-} + 2H_2O \rightarrow 2H^+ + \underset{\text{[hydroxyapatite]}}{Ca_{10}(PO_4)_6(OH)_2}$$

Low pH tends to reduce the concentration of tribasic phosphate by adding H^+ to phosphate:

$$6PO_4^{3-} + H^+ \underset{pK = 7.0}{\rightarrow} 6HPO_4^{2-} + H^+ \underset{pK = 4.0}{\rightarrow} 6H_2PO_4^{1-}$$

Recent research has indicated that the microbial composition at the initial stage of caries that affects enamel is different from the composition at subsequent stages of caries as well as different from that in dental plaque on the intact tooth surface. The relative proportion of *S mutans* increases from 0.12% in dental plaque to 0.72% in enamel caries; however, *S mitis* and *S sanguinis* appear to be the dominant streptococci in these lesions. The bacterial genes involved in tolerance to acid stress fermentation of dietary sugar are overexpressed only at the enamel caries stage. By contrast, genes encoding collagenases and other proteases are overexpressed in dentin cavities and are likely involved in the degradation of dentin. Thus, low pH and diet influence the onset of caries via the degradation of enamel; however, both acidogenic and proteolytic bacteria appear to be involved in dentin caries where the cavity expands.

The ecological plaque hypothesis tries to account for some of the shortcomings of the specific and nonspecific plaque hypotheses (Fig 23-4). Cariogenic flora found in natural plaque are weakly competitive and comprise only a minority of the total community. The increase in fermentable carbohydrates results in prolonged low pH, promoting the growth of acid-tolerant bacteria and initiating demineralization. The balance in the plaque community turns in favor of mutans streptococci and lactobacilli. There is a dynamic

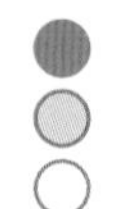

relationship between the bacteria and the host, and changes in major host factors, including salivary flow, can affect plaque development.

The extended caries ecological hypothesis proposes that the caries process consists of three reversible stages:

1. Intact enamel surfaces harbor mainly nonmutans streptococci and *Actinomyces*, causing only mild and infrequent acidification. This is the stage of dynamic stability where demineralization and remineralization rates are in equilibrium, or there is a net mineral gain.
2. There is more extensive and frequent acidification with a frequent supply of sugar. Nonmutans streptococci may adapt to these conditions by increasing their acidogenicity and acidurance. This, in turn, shifts the balance between demineralization and remineralization toward net mineral loss and initiation of caries.
3. When acidic conditions are prolonged, more aciduric bacteria are selected, and the more dominant microorganisms are mutans streptococci, lactobacilli, aciduric nonmutans streptococci, bifidobacteria, *Actinomyces*, and yeasts.

In the extended ecological plaque hypothesis, not only mutans streptococci but also the entire population of acidogenic and aciduric bacteria participate in the development of the caries process. Thus, the removal of specific aciduric bacteria, such as mutans streptococci, by means of antibiotics, vaccination, or gene therapy may not be sufficient for the control of caries in the long term. Control of the microflora may be achieved by preventing the acidification of the plaque biofilm via mechanical removal, reduction of sugary foods in the diet, and the stimulation of saliva to help neutralize the pH.

Genomics approaches to oral biofilms

Oral microbial communities have often been studied by microbiologic culture methods. In recent years, sequencing of the DNA encoding 16S rRNA has been used to determine the microbial content of oral biofilms. Metagenomics and metatranscriptomics methods employing high-throughput sequencing can more readily provide information on the composition and function of biofilms. The metabolic activity of the biofilm is important in the onset of caries, and metabolome analysis can evaluate this activity. Biofilm samples should be taken from precise sites on teeth, without pooling samples.

Prevention of caries

Strategies to control or prevent caries include the use of sugar substitutes, fluoridation, and fissure sealants, as well as the control of cariogenic flora by antimicrobials and other currently experimental techniques.

Fluoride ions substitute for the hydroxyl groups in hydroxyapatite. The resulting fluoroapatite is less soluble in acid and promotes the remineralization of early caries lesions. Fluoride ions reduce glycolysis by inhibiting enolase that catalyzes the conversion of phosphoglycerate to phosphoenolpyruvate. Fluoride ions also inhibit respiration (the electron transport chain). Xylitol inhibits the sugar metabolism of mutans streptococci. Use of xylitol gum (but not sorbitol gum) decreases the mutans streptococcus counts and percentage in plaque. However, salivary levels of mutans and total streptococci and lactobacilli are not affected.

Chlorhexidine is an antimicrobial that inhibits sugar transport in streptococci, amino acid uptake and catabolism in *S sanguinis*, and the protease activity of *P gingivalis*. Chlorhexidine affects membrane functions, such as adenosine triphosphate synthase and maintenance of ion gradients in streptococci, and inhibits the binding of plaque-forming bacteria to tooth surfaces. Mutans streptococci are especially susceptible to chlorhexidine. Triclosan inhibits acid production by streptococci and a protease of *P gingivalis*. Its activity is enhanced by copolymer or zinc citrate. Like chlorhexidine, triclosan is substantive (ie, it binds effectively to oral surfaces). However, an important environmental concern with triclosan is that it can be converted to polychlorinated dibenzodioxin under ultraviolet light. Thus, extensive use of antimicrobial soaps and toothpaste can result in the accumulation of triclosan and its byproducts in groundwater.

Antibodies against antigen I/II of mutans streptococci by passive immunization can inhibit recolonization after chlorhexidine treatment. In experimental replacement therapy, low-virulence mutants of mutans streptococci deficient in glucosyltransferase or lactate dehydrogenase activity are introduced into the oral cavity. Introduction of excess *S salivarius* in the mouth can displace *S mutans*, thereby reducing the probability of the initiation of caries.

Bibliography

Aas JA, Paster BJ, Stokes LN, Olsen I, Dewhirst FE. Defining the normal bacterial flora of the oral cavity. J Clin Microbiol 2005;43:5721–5732.

Atanasova KR, Yilmaz Ö. Prelude to oral microbes and chronic diseases: Past, present and future. Microbes Infection 2015;17:473–483.

Dewhirst FE, Chen T, Izard J, et al. The human oral microbiome. J Bacteriol 2010;192:5002–5017.

Genco R, Hamada S, Lehner T, McGhee J, Mergenhagen S (eds). Molecular Pathogenesis of Periodontal Disease. Washington, DC: ASM, 1994.

Kayalar C, Düzgüneş N. Membrane action of colicin E1: Detection by the release of carboxyfluorescein and calcein from liposomes. Biochim Biophys Acta 1986;860:51–56.

Kreth J, Zhang Y, Herzberg MC. Streptococcal antagonism in oral biofilms: *Streptococcus sanguinis* and *Streptococcus gordonii* interference with *Streptococcus mutans*. J Bacteriol 2008;190:4632–4640.

Kolenbrander PE (ed). Oral Microbial Communities: Genomic Inquiry and Interspecies Communication. Washington, DC: ASM, 2011.

Lamont RJ, Hajishengallis GN, Jenkinson HF. Oral Microbiology and Immunology, ed 2. Washington, DC: ASM, 2014.

Lee YH, Zimmerman JN, Custodio W, et al. Proteomic evaluation of acquired enamel pellicle during in vivo formation. PLoS One 2013;8:e67919.

Marsh PD, Martin MV. Oral Microbiology, ed 5. Edinburgh: Churchill Livingstone Elsevier, 2009.

Nir S, Bentz J, Düzgüneş N. Two modes of reversible vesicle aggregation: Particle size and the DLVO theory. J Colloid Interface Sci 1981;84:266–269.

Nyvad B, Crielaard W, Mira A, Takahashi N, Beighton D. Dental caries from a molecular microbiological perspective. Caries Res 2013;47:89–102.

Periasamy A, Kolenbrander PE. Mutualistic biofilm communities develop with Porphyromonas gingivalis and initial, early, and late colonizers of enamel. J Bacteriol 2009;191:6804–6811.

Rogers AH (ed). Molecular Oral Microbiology. Norfolk, UK: Caister Academic, 2008.

Samaranayake L. Essential Microbiology for Dentistry, ed 4. Edinburgh: Churchill Livingstone Elsevier, 2012.

Shin JE, Baek KJ, Choi YS, Choi Y. A periodontal pathogen *Treponema denticola* hijacks the *Fusobacterium nucleatum*-driven host response. Immunol Cell Biol 2013;91:503–510.

Simón-Soro A, Belda-Ferre P, Cabrera-Rubio R, Alcaraz LD, Mira A. A tissue-dependent hypothesis of dental caries. Caries Res 2013;47:591–600.

Söderling E, Hirvonen A, Karjalainen S, Fontana M, Catt D, Seppä L. The effect of xylitol on the composition of the oral flora: A pilot study. Eur J Dent 2011;5:24–31.

Takahashi N, Nyvad B. The role of bacteria in the caries process: Ecological perspectives. J Dent Res 2011;90:294–303.

Tanner AC, Mathney JM, Kent RL, et al. Cultivable anaerobic microbiota of severe early childhood caries. J Clin Microbiol 2011;49:1464–1474.

Take-Home Messages

- Oral microorganisms cause various diseases, including caries, periodontitis, endodontic infections, alveolar osteitis, and tonsillitis.
- Estimates of the number of common oral species are between 700 and 800, only about 280 of which have been isolated in culture.
- Streptococci are the predominant supragingival bacteria. The four main groups of streptococci are mutans, salivarius, mitis, and anginosus.
- Other Gram-positive cocci include *Peptostreptococcus*, *Parvimonas*, and *Enterococcus*.
- Gram-positive bacilli in the oral cavity include *Lactobacillus*, *Eubacterium*, *Propionibacterium*, *Rothia*, and *Actinomyces*.
- *Neisseria*, *Veillonella*, and *Moraxella* are the main Gram-negative cocci.
- Gram-negative bacilli including *A actinomycetemcomitans*, *Capnocytophaga*, *Porphyromonas*, and *Prevotella* are associated with various forms of periodontal disease.
- The main oral habitats are the mucosal surfaces, teeth, saliva, and gingival crevicular fluid.
- Oral microbial colonization is affected by the local pH and the oxidation-reduction potential.
- Initial interactions between bacteria and the tooth surface can transform into more stable associations via the specific interaction between adhesins on the microbial cell surface and receptors in the acquired pellicle.
- The bacterial species in plaque become increasingly anaerobic and Gram-negative with time as the plaque matures.
- The key factors in the development of caries include a susceptible tooth surface, the nature of saliva flow, plaque bacteria, and the consumption of fermentable carbohydrates.
- There is a significant correlation between *S mutans* counts in saliva and plaque and the prevalence and incidence of caries.
- *Lactobacillus* species are present in increased numbers in most caries lesions on enamel and root surfaces.
- Low pH generated by acid production by bacteria causes demineralization by reducing the concentration of the tribasic phosphate (PO_4^{3-}), which is needed to form hydroxyapatite.
- In the extended ecological plaque hypothesis, not only mutans streptococci but also the entire population of acidogenic and aciduric bacteria participate in the development of the caries process.

Periodontal and Endodontic Infections

24

Periodontal Disease

Periodontitis is a chronic inflammatory disease of the tissues surrounding and supporting teeth (the periodontium) (Fig 24-1). The destruction of the periodontium is the most common cause of tooth loss. In healthy tissue, the host immune response is active. Disruption or imbalance of the production of inflammatory mediators facilitates the destruction of the periodontal tissue and alveolar bone. Both commensal and pathogenic bacteria can activate the innate immune responses via pattern-recognition receptors.

Periodontal disease can be broadly categorized into gingivitis and periodontitis. The clinical features of plaque-related gingivitis include redness, edema, and bleeding. Periodontitis usually develops from preexisting gingivitis; however, not all cases of gingivitis lead to periodontitis. Periodontitis can be classified into two main groups: *(1)* chronic periodontitis, which is the most prevalent form, and *(2)* aggressive periodontitis, which can be localized or generalized.

Microorganisms in the **healthy gingival sulcus** are generally Gram-positive and facultatively anaerobic organisms. In **chronic periodontitis**, the microorganisms are approximately 75% Gram-negative, 90% of which are strict anaerobes, as well as motile bacilli and spirochetes (Fig 24-2). The pathogenic potential of periodontal microorganisms is determined by their ability to colonize the host, evade host defenses, and damage host tissues. The currently recognized key periodontopathogens include *Porphyromonas gingivalis*, *Prevotella intermedia*, *Tannerella forsythia* (formerly *Bacteroides forsythus*), *Aggregatibacter actinomycetemcomitans* (formerly *Actinobacillus actinomycetemcomitans*), *Fusobacterium nucleatum*, *Capnocytophaga* species, and *Treponema denticola*. The colored fonts refer to the designation introduced by Soc-

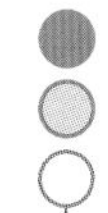

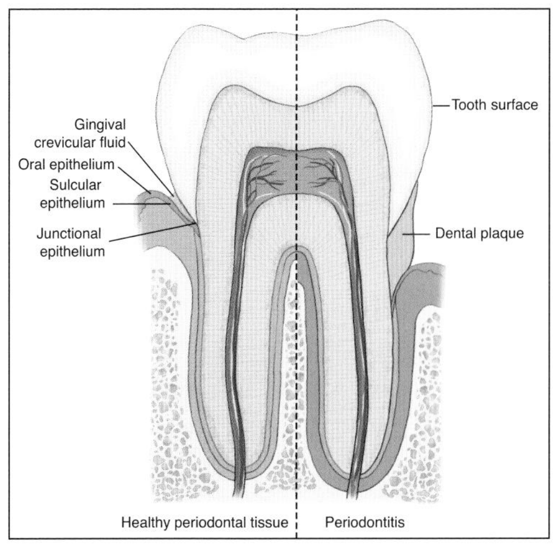

Fig 24-1 The normal periodontium and the effects of periodontal disease. Healthy periodontal tissue *(left)* has connective tissue and alveolar bone, both of which support the tooth root. The oral epithelium covers this tissue, and the junctional epithelium connects it to the tooth. The region between the epithelium and the tooth surface is the sulcus, which is filled with gingival crevicular fluid. In periodontitis *(right)*, the tooth and root surfaces are covered with dental plaque, which, together with the inflammatory response, causes the destruction of the periodontal tissue and bone. (Adapted from Darveau.)

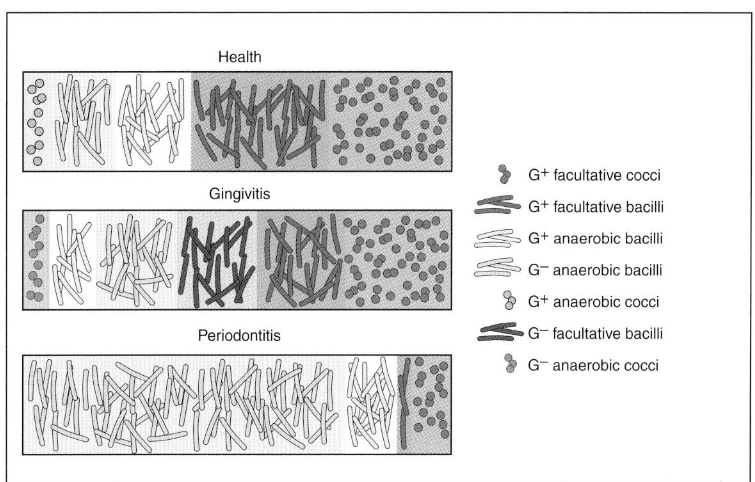

Fig 24-2 Predominant plaque bacterial morphotypes in health, gingivitis, and periodontitis. (Data from Samaranayake.)

ransky et al (Fig 24-3). The red complex, according to the Socransky grouping, includes *P gingivalis*, *T forsythia*, and *T denticola*, which are found most frequently in deep periodontal pockets. Sites containing none of these bacteria have the shallowest mean pocket depth. Increased colonization with the orange complex, which includes *P intermedia*, *F nucleatum*, and *Peptostreptococcus micros*, leads to more sites being colonized by the red complex.

The symptoms of chronic periodontitis include gingival inflammation; loss of attachment between the root surface, the gingivae, and alveolar bone; and increased depth and bleeding on probing. These symptoms may be accompanied by bone loss. Large numbers of obligately anaerobic Gram-negative rods and filament-shaped bacteria are observed in the periodontal pockets. Many are proteolytic and asaccharolytic; ie, they are unable to produce energy from carbohydrates.

Some of the predominant Gram-positive bacteria are *Eubacterium brachy*, *Eubacterium nodatum*, *Parvimonas micra*, and *Peptostreptococcus stomatis*. The predominant Gram-negative bacteria are *T forsythia*, *F nucleatum*, *P gingivalis*, *P intermedia*, *Prevotella loescheii*, *Campylobacter rectus*, and *Treponema* species.

New species emerge in chronic periodontitis as a result of the ecological change arising from the host inflammatory response, increased flow of gingival crevicular fluid, presence of new nutrients, increase in proteolytic metabolism, and rise in pH. *Treponema socranskii*, *P gingivalis*, and *Porphyromonas endodontalis* are recovered almost exclusively from diseased sites.

Aggressive periodontitis can be localized or generalized and was previously designated as *localized* or *generalized juvenile periodontitis*. It is strongly associated with the presence of *A actinomycetemcomitans*. This Gram-negative coccobacillus is found in 97% of affected sites and constitutes 70% of the cultivable microflora. Aggressive periodontitis patients have elevated serum antibodies to *A actinomycetemcomitans*. Reduction in the number of this bacterium in the periodontium results in the resolution of the disease. The recurrence of aggressive periodontitis is related to the re-emergence of *A actinomycetemcomitans*. However, it can also be isolated from healthy sites. *A actinomycetemcomitans* is not found in some sites with the disease. Infection with this bacterium causes neutrophil abnormalities, including signal transduction, reduced chemotaxis, and phagocytosis, and increased superoxide production.

A actinomycetemcomitans is facultatively anaerobic and can colonize the buccal mucosa and dental plaque. Its virulence factors include leukotoxin, which kills human macrophages and neutrophils by inducing the release of lysosomal enzymes; immunosuppressive factor, which inhibits B-cell growth; collagenase; and lipopolysaccharide, which activates the alternative complement pathway and stimulates bone resorption.

The main microorganisms associated with generalized aggressive periodontitis are *Treponema* species, *F nucleatum*, *Lactobacillus* species, *Eubacterium* species, *Parvimonas* species, *P intermedia*, and *Selenomonas* species.

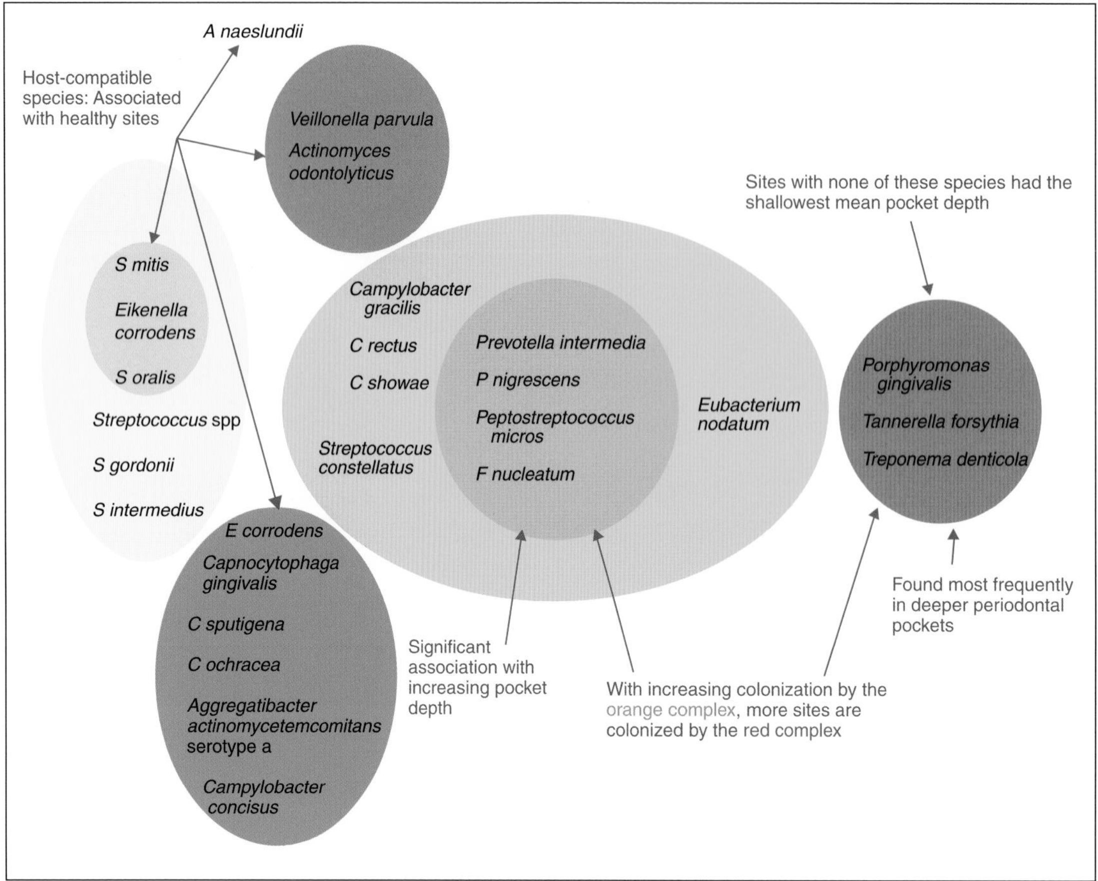

Fig 24-3 The Socransky grouping of bacteria into complexes to reflect their interaction with the host in health and periodontal disease. The red complex is found most frequently in deep periodontal pockets and is usually preceded by bacteria in the orange complex. Members of the yellow, green, and purple complexes are usually found in healthy sites. (Adapted from Marsh and Martin and from Haffajee et al.)

Necrotizing ulcerative gingivitis is a specific, anaerobic, polymicrobial infection of gingival tissue by oral spirochetes (*Treponema* species) and a range of "fusiform" bacteria (*Fusobacterium* species), which together form a "fusospirochetal complex" (Fig 24-4). The other bacteria associated with this condition include *Leptotrichia*, *Capnocytophaga*, *Tannerella*, *P intermedia*, *P gingivalis*, and *Selenomonas sputigena*.

P gingivalis is one of the red complex bacteria. It is a Gram-negative, nonmotile, obligately anaerobic bacillus. It requires hemin (which carries iron and protoporphyrin) and vitamin K for growth. Its virulence factors include the capsular polysaccharide, collagenase, trypsin-like proteases (gingipain), keratinase, hemolysins, fibrinolysins, hyaluronidase, and phospholipase. *P gingivalis* can interact with *Actinomyces naeslundii*, *F nucleatum*, *T denticola*, and *T forsythia*. It can bind to epithelial cells, fibroblasts, erythrocytes, and the extracellular matrix. These interactions are mediated by fimbriae and may be facilitated by proteolytic enzymes.

P intermedia is one of the orange complex bacteria. It is a Gram-negative, pleomorphic bacillus. It is a strict anaerobe and requires vitamin K and hemin for growth. It is associated with chronic periodontitis and dentoalveolar abscesses. Its virulence factors include phospholipase A, immunoglobulin (Ig) A/IgG proteases, mercaptans, and hydrogen sulfide.

Oral spirochetes are long, thin, corkscrew-like, Gram-negative, anaerobic, highly mobile bacteria. They are killed by oxygen and are difficult to grow in media. Their virulence factors include endotoxin, the ability to penetrate tissue, a factor that inhibits lymphocyte activation, and their propensity to block the fusion of phagosomes with lysosomes. The spirochete *T denticola* is part of the red complex.

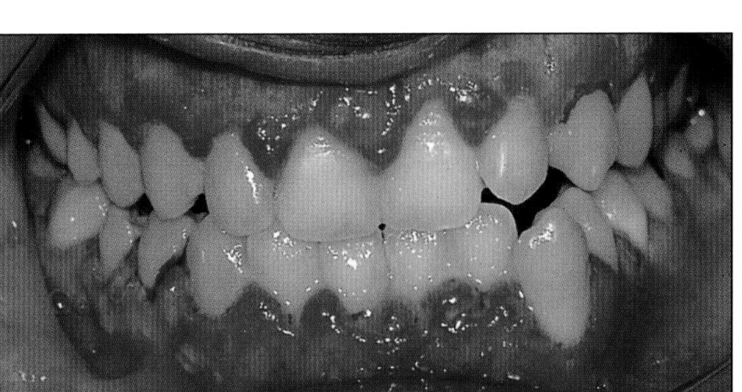

Fig 24-4 Necrotizing ulcerative gingivitis is a severe inflammation limited to the gingiva, with ulcerations and necrosis of the interdental papillae. (Reprinted with permission from Marx and Stern.)

Role of Bacterial Products in Periodontal Disease

Periodontal bacteria produce different products that damage the periodontium (Table 24-1). Endotoxin, or lipopolysaccharide, is present on the surface of all Gram-negative organisms and causes cytotoxicity, bone resorption, complement activation, and local inflammation. Activated complement induces macrophage activation and secretion of prostaglandins. Prostaglandin E stimulates lymphocytes to produce osteoclast-activating factor, which results in bone resorption.

Collagenase, produced by *P gingivalis* and *A actinomycetemcomitans*, degrades connective tissue. Hyaluronidase, secreted by *Streptococcus mitis* and some Gram-positive rods, destroys sulcus attachment and increases tissue permeability to invasive bacteria.

Proteases are produced by *P gingivalis* and some fusobacteria, and they damage cell membranes. Phospholipase A, produced by *P gingivalis* and *P intermedia*, damages cell membranes and induces prostaglandin-mediated bone resorption. Nucleases produced by *F nucleatum* and some streptococci degrade nucleic acids.

IgA/IgG proteases are produced by *P gingivalis*, *P intermedia*, and *Capnocytophaga* species, and they degrade immunoglobulins. Catalase generated by *Actinomyces viscosus* and *A actinomycetemcomitans* decreases neutrophil peroxide-mediated killing activity. Mercaptans produced by *P gingivalis* and *P intermedia* cause cytotoxicity to host cells. Hydrogen sulfide generated by *F nucleatum*, *P gingivalis*, *P intermedia*, and *C rectus* causes cytotoxicity to epithelial cells.

Fibrinolysin, secreted by *P gingivalis* and some spirochetes, destroys the fibrin barrier to local infection. Leukotoxin produced by *A actinomycetemcomitans* and *C rectus* results in leukocyte cytotoxicity. Chemotaxis inhibitors produced by *P gingivalis* decrease neutrophil defenses. The capsule in a number of organisms decreases phagocytosis. Immunosuppressive factors are produced by *A actinomycetemcomitans*, *T denticola*, *F nucleatum*, and *T socranskii* and inhibit lymphocyte proliferation.

Table 24-1 Bacterial factors implicated in the etiology of periodontal disease

Stage of disease	Bacterial factor(s)
Attachment to host tissues	Surface components, including adhesins
	Fimbriae
Replication at susceptible site	Proteases to obtain nutrients
	Development of food chains
	Bacteriocins to compete with other bacteria
Evasion of host defenses	Capsule
	Neutrophil receptor blockers
	Leukotoxin
	Immunoglobulin-specific proteases
	Complement-degrading proteases
	Induction of suppressor T cells
Direct tissue damage	Arginine-specific proteases (gingipain)
	Collagenase
	Hyaluronidase
	Chondroitin sulfatase
	Lipoteichoic acid
	Lipopolysaccharide
	Butyric and propionic acids
	Indole
	Ammonia
	Volatile sulfur compounds
Indirect tissue damage	Inflammatory response to plaque antigens
	Prostaglandins
	Elastase
	Cathepsin B

(Adapted from Marsh and Martin.)

The Host Immune System in Periodontitis

Periodontal bacteria also induce host inflammatory responses that cause damage to host tissues (see Table 24-1 and Fig 24-5). The glycoprotein Del-1 was observed in animal studies to turn down the inflammatory immune response. Del-1 is an endogenous inhibitor of neutrophil adhesion dependent on the integrin leukocyte function antigen-1 (LFA-1) and on reciprocal higher expression of interleukin-17 (IL-17). A breakdown in the normal control of the cytokine IL-17 by Del-1 can facilitate the onset of periodontitis, partic-

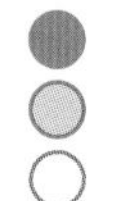

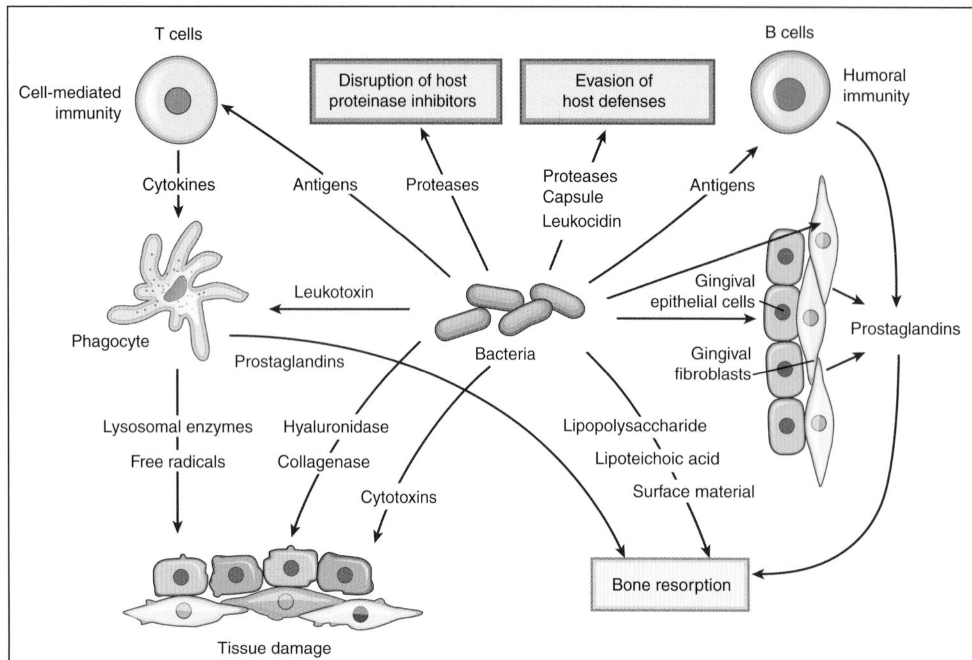

Fig 24-5 Mechanisms by which bacteria in dental plaque can cause damage to host tissues by direct and indirect routes. (Adapted from Marsh and Martin.)

ularly in older individuals. Thus, periodontitis may be characterized as a disruption of homeostasis, which then allows infectious and inflammatory conditions to proceed on their destructive paths.

In periodontitis, microbial communities that are out of balance (dysbiotic) have synergistic interactions with each other to protect themselves from host defenses, to acquire nutrients, and to thrive in an inflammatory environment. Periodontitis-associated bacteria are thought to be "inflammophilic"; ie, they have evolved to both endure inflammation and take advantage of it. Thus, inflammation can stimulate the selection of these pathogenic communities by providing tissue breakdown products as nutrients, such as collagen peptides and heme compounds. The species that do not benefit from the altered ecological conditions or those that are negatively impacted by inflammation are competed out. Periodontitis-associated biofilms increase in biomass as periodontal inflammation increases, consistent with the hypothesis that inflammation facilitates the growth of dysbiotic microbial communities. By contrast, anti-inflammatory treatments in animal models of periodontitis reduce the periodontal bacterial load as well as inhibit bone loss. The selection of inflammophilic bacteria will stimulate inflammatory tissue destruction and disease progression. Thus, controlling inflammation is crucial to the treatment of periodontitis, because it will most likely control both dysbiosis and disease progression.

Ecological Plaque Hypothesis

In vitro experiments indicate that serum promotes the growth of plaque bacteria species associated with periodontal disease. Slightly alkaline pH increases the proportion of *P gingivalis* from less than 1% to greater than 99% of a community of black-pigmented anaerobes. Bacteria most adapted to the changing ecology will be selected, upregulating virulence factors. There is a spiraling escalation of the inflammatory challenge followed by an increasingly destructive host response. Gingival crevicular fluid flow increases, bringing host molecules like transferrin and hemoglobin that can be catabolized, leading to an increase in pH and more anaerobic conditions. These changes will upregulate the production of virulence factors, such as proteases by *P gingivalis* (Fig 24-6). According to the ecological plaque hypothesis, disease can be prevented by targeting the putative pathogens, interfering with inflammation, and altering the redox potential of the periodontal pocket to prevent the growth of obligate anaerobes.

Endodontic and Dentoalveolar Infections

Dentoalveolar infections are pus-producing (pyogenic) infections associated with the teeth and surrounding supporting structures, such as the periodontium or alveolar bone. A dentoalveolar abscess usually develops by the extension of the initial caries lesion into dentin and spread of the bacteria to the pulp via the dentinal tubules. The pulp responds either by rapid acute inflammation involving the whole pulp, which quickly becomes necrosed, or by the development of a chronic localized abscess, with most of the pulp remaining viable. Microorganisms can also reach the pulp by traumatic tooth fracture, by traumatic exposure during dental treatment (iatrogenic infection), through the periodontal mem-

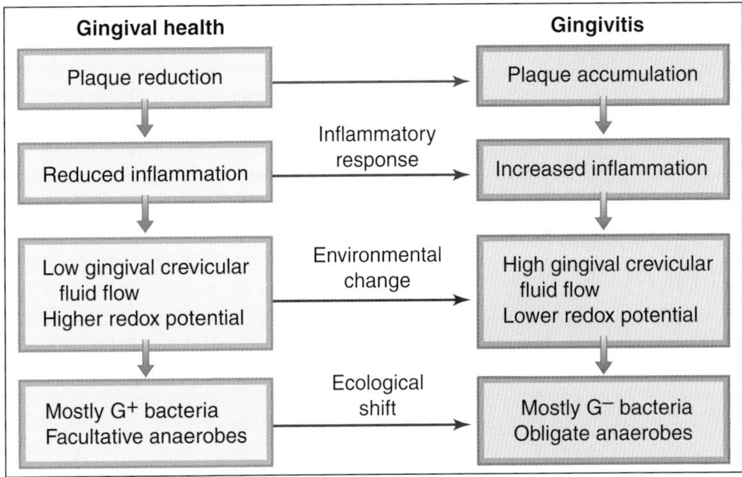

Fig 24-6 The ecological plaque hypothesis regarding the onset of periodontal disease. Plaque accumulation may stimulate an inflammatory response, changing environmental conditions within the periodontal pocket and allowing the overgrowth of proteolytic and anaerobic Gram-negative bacteria. (Adapted from Marsh and Martin.)

brane and accessory root canals, and rarely by anachoresis (ie, infection via the pulpal blood supply during bacteremia, caused for example by tooth extraction at a different site). Dentoalveolar infections are usually polymicrobial in nature.

Bacteria involved in endodontic disease are opportunistic pathogens that are part of the normal oral flora that gain access to the otherwise sterile pulp tissue and cause inflammatory reactions. Dentinal tubules may be exposed to bacterial invasion after a breach in the integrity of enamel or cementum. Bacterial molecules that diffuse into the pulp through dentinal tubules induce an inflammatory reaction, which may be able to eliminate the bacteria. Inability to block the bacterial invasion results in infection of the root canal system, pulpitis, pulp necrosis, and periapical disease. Although the number of bacterial species in the oral cavity is very large, only a small number of species invade dentinal tubules and the root canals. The majority of tubule microflora are anaerobic Gram-positive bacteria including *Eubacterium*, *Propionibacterium*, *Veillonella* and *Bifidobacterium* species, and *P micra*, indicating that the microenvironment is favorable for these bacteria. Gram-negative, obligately anaerobic bacilli, including *Porphyromonas* species, are seen less frequently. Streptococci may recognize molecules in dentinal tubules, including collagen type I, that mediate bacterial adhesion and growth. Interactions of other oral microflora with these streptococci may facilitate dentinal invasion by particular bacteria. Dental pulp infections usually involve complexes of anaerobic bacteria such as *Prevotella*, *Parvimonas*, and the recently discovered genera *Olsenella* and *Dialister*. The various phyla and species identified in infected pulp are given in Box 24-1. *P endodontalis* is detected more frequently than *P gingivalis*. These microorganisms are found in both symptomatic and asymptomatic infections. There appears to be less microbial diversity in symptomatic infections, with higher levels of *Fusobacterium*, *Dialister*, *Prevotella*, and *Eubacterium*. Fungi including *Candida albicans* and *Aspergillus* have also been detected in root canals.

The bacteria may exist as aggregates or biofilms on the dentin surface; this renders them resistant to antimicrobial agents. The virulence factors of the bacteria enable them to break down both the pulp and periradicular tissues (ie, the tissue around the roots). Pulp cells produce chemokines, including IL-8 (also known as CXCL8), that attract neutrophils and mononuclear cells. The inflammation may spread to the apical regions if not treated. This, in turn, may result in the destruction of periapical alveolar bone. An *abscess* is a collection of pus into a cavity formed by the liquefaction of tissue. *Dental abscess*, *dentoalveolar abscess*, and *odontogenic abscess* are synonymous and describe the abscesses formed in the tissues around the tooth. These abscesses may be caused by an endodontic infection (acute apical abscess) or a periodontal infection (periodontal abscess and pericoronitis). Acute abscess in the apical area stimulates nerve endings, thereby causing severe pain that can only be relieved by draining the pus via the pulp chamber or by an incision to the apical region.

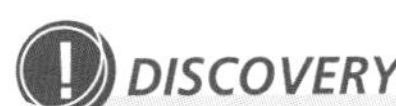

The ancient Chinese believed that tooth abscesses were caused by a white worm with a black head that lived in the tooth. In the 17th century, Antonie van Leeuwenhoek described the microorganisms in the root canal of an extensively carious tooth. In 1894, W. D. Miller published his findings on the bacterial infection of root canals. Further studies in the 1930s led to the perception that Gram-positive facultative bacteria were the endodontic pathogens. The development of anaerobic culturing methods in the 1960s revealed that the endodontic microbiota were mostly anaerobes. Later studies focused on the pathogenicity of black-pigmented Gram-negative bacteria. The use of an anaerobic medium of transport such as VMGA III (Viability medium, Göteborg, anaerobically prepared and sterilized) and molecular assays have led to the identification of new species that are difficult to culture.

The Gram-positive coccus *Enterococcus faecalis* has been identified as the major microorganism in failed end-

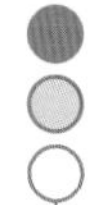

Box 24-1 The prevalent phyla, genera, and species found in root canal infections

Actinobacteria
Actinomyces species
Propionibacterium acnes
Propionibacterium propionicum

Bacteroidetes
Tannerella forsythia
Porphyromonas endodontalis
Porphyromonas gingivalis
Prevotella species

Firmicutes
Enterococcus faecalis
Eubacterium species
Lactobacillus species
Parvimonas micra
Peptostreptococcus species
Selenomonas species
Streptococcus species
Veillonella parvula

Fusobacteria
Fusobacterium nucleatum

Proteobacteria
Eikenella corrodens
Campylobacter gracilis
Campylobacter rectus

Spirochetes
Treponema denticola
Treponema maltophylum
Treponema parvum
Treponema socranskii

Red, most abundant; *blue*, abundant; *purple*, less abundant. (Data from Lamont et al.)

odontic treatments. It is resistant to high temperature and high pH and appears to gain access to the pulp chamber during treatment or infiltration into a temporary or permanent restoration. Other species that are not as easy to culture as *E faecalis* have also been identified in dentinal canals. Human immunodeficiency virus (HIV) has also been detected in vital pulp as well as herpesviruses in endodontic infections and abscesses.

Treatment of endodontic infections involves extirpating the pulp, enlarging the root canal, irrigating the canal system with antimicrobial agents, and obturating (sealing) the canals. Sodium hypochlorite is a highly effective antimicrobial agent that also dissolves necrotic tissue. Chlorhexidine is often used to clean the canal system; its substantivity (ie, its ability to bind dentin for prolonged antimicrobial activity) is an advantage.

Ludwig's angina is a bilateral infection of the sublingual and submandibular spaces that causes swelling of the tissues at the front of the neck. *Prevotella* and *Porphyromonas* species, fusobacteria, and anaerobic streptococci are common sources of this infection, which is life-threatening due to airway obstruction. Prompt intervention and maintenance of the airway is of critical importance. High-dose, empirical, systemic antibiotic therapy (usually intravenous penicillin, with or without metronidazole) is also essential.

Periodontal abscess is an endogenous, polymicrobial infection with predominantly anaerobic, periodontopathic flora such as *Porphyromonas* and *Prevotella* species, fusobacteria, hemolytic and anaerobic streptococci, spirochetes, and *Capnocytophaga* and *Actinomyces* species. It is an acute or chronic destructive process in the periodontium, resulting in a localized collection of pus that connects with the oral cavity through the gingival sulcus and/or other periodontal sites.

Osteomyelitis is the inflammation of the medullary bone in the maxilla and mandible. It is uncommon and is seen mostly in immmunocompromised patients. Anaerobes such as *Porphyromonas* and *Prevotella* species, fusobacteria, and streptococci are the most common isolates. Exogenous bacteria such as *Treponema pallidum* and *Mycobacterium tuberculosis* are rarely associated with osteomyelitis of the jaws. It requires both medical and surgical intervention.

Cervicofacial actinomycosis is an endogenous granulomatous disease, usually presenting at the angle of the mandible and related to trauma or a history of tooth extraction (see Fig 13-4). It is mainly caused by *Actinomyces israelii*. The pus associated with actinomycosis contains yellow visible granules called "sulfur granules." The infection can be treated with penicillin after drainage of the facial abscess. Erythromycin, tetracycline, or clindamycin can be used as an alternative if the patient is allergic to penicillin.

Bibliography

Darveau RP. Periodontitis: A polymicrobial disruption of host homeostasis. Nature Rev Microbiol 2010;8:481–490.

Eisen D, Lynch DP. The Mouth: Diagnosis and Treatment. St Louis: Mosby, 1998.

Eskan MA, Jotwani R, Abe T, et al. The leukocyte integrin antagonist Del-1 inhibits IL-17-mediated inflammatory bone loss. Nat Immunol 2012;13:465–473.

Genco R, Hamada S, Lehner T, McGhee J, Mergenhagen S (eds). Molecular Pathogenesis of Periodontal Disease. Washington, DC: ASM, 1994.

George M, Ivančaková R. Root canal microflora. Acta Medica (Hradec Kralove) 2007;50:7–15.

Haffajee AD, Socransky SS, Patel MR, Song X. Microbial complexes in supragingival plaque. Oral Microbiol Immunol 2008;23:196–205.

Hajishengallis G. The inflammophilic character of the periodontitis-associated microbiota. Mol Oral Microbiol 2014;29:248–257.

Kolenbrander PE (ed). Oral Microbial Communities: Genomic Inquiry and Interspecies Communication. Washington, DC: ASM, 2011.

Lamont RJ, Hajishengallis GN, Jenkinson HF. Oral Microbiology and Immunology, ed 2. Washington, DC: ASM, 2014.

Love RM, Jenkinson HF. Invasion of dentinal tubules by oral bacteria. Crit Rev Oral Biol Med 2002;13:171–183.

Marsh PD, Martin MV. Oral Microbiology, ed 5. Edinburgh: Churchill Livingstone Elsevier, 2009.

Marx RE, Stern D. Oral and Maxillofacial Pathology: A Rationale for Diagnosis and Treatment, ed 2. Chicago: Quintessence, 2012.

National Institute of Dental and Craniofacial Research. Gum (Periodontal) Diseases. nidcr.nih.gov/OralHealth/Topics/GumDiseases/. Accessed 20 July 2015.

Rogers AH (ed). Molecular Oral Microbiology. Norfolk, UK: Caister Academic, 2008.

Samaranayake L. Essential Microbiology for Dentistry, ed 4. Edinburgh: Churchill Livingstone Elsevier, 2012.

Siqueira JF, Roças IN. Microbiology and treatment of acute apical abscesses. Clin Microbiol Rev 2013;26:255–273.

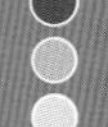

Take-Home Messages

- Periodontitis is a chronic inflammatory disease of the tissues surrounding and supporting teeth.
- Periodontitis usually develops from preexisting gingivitis; however, not all cases of gingivitis lead to periodontitis.
- In chronic periodontitis, the microorganisms are approximately 75% Gram-negative, 90% of which are strict anaerobes.
- The "red complex" bacteria, according to the Socransky grouping, includes *P gingivalis*, *T forsythia*, and *T denticola*, which are found most frequently in deep periodontal pockets. Sites containing none of these bacteria have the shallowest mean pocket depth.
- Increased colonization by the orange complex, which includes *P intermedia*, *F nucleatum*, and *P micros*, leads to more sites being colonized by the red complex.
- Aggressive periodontitis is strongly associated with the presence of *A actinomycetemcomitans*.
- Periodontal bacteria produce molecules that damage the periodontium, including endotoxin, collagenase, hyaluronidase, proteases, phospholipase A, mercaptans, and leukotoxin.
- Periodontitis-associated bacteria are thought to be inflammophilic (ie, they have evolved to both endure inflammation and take advantage of it).
- Controlling inflammation is crucial to the treatment of periodontitis.
- According to the ecological plaque hypothesis, periodontal disease can be prevented by targeting the putative pathogens, interfering with inflammation, and altering the redox potential of the periodontal pocket.
- The majority of dentinal tubule microflora are anaerobic Gram-positive bacteria including *Eubacterium*, *Propionibacterium*, *Veillonella* and *Bifidobacterium* species, and *P micra*.
- Dental pulp infections usually involve complexes of anaerobic bacteria such as *Prevotella*, *Parvimonas*, and the recently discovered genera *Olsenella* and *Dialister*.
- Dentoalveolar abscesses can be generated in the tissues around the tooth following an endodontic or periodontal infection.
- The Gram-positive coccus *E faecalis* has been identified as the major microorganism in failed endodontic treatments.

Fungal Structure, Replication, and Pathogenesis

25

Fungi are a diverse group of free-living eukaryotic microorganisms that may be unicellular or may differentiate into multicellular, branching filamentous structures. Although there are more than 200,000 species of fungi, less than 200 of them are associated with human disease.

Fungi normally survive by degrading organic matter and may be classified as saprobes, symbionts, commensals, or parasites. Saprobes (or saprophytes) live on dead or decaying organic matter. Symbionts live together with their host, and this relationship generates a mutual advantage for each organism. Commensals live in a close relationship with their host, whereby the fungi benefits and the host neither benefits nor is harmed. Parasites live on or within a host and benefit from this association, whereas the host is usually harmed.

Diseases

Pathogenic fungi can cause a large range of diseases, including mycotoxicoses, hypersensitivity diseases, and mycoses resulting from colonization of the host. The latter include superficial, cutaneous, and subcutaneous mycoses. Superficial mycoses are limited to the outer layers of the skin and are not considered to be destructive. For example, pityriasis versicolor is a skin discoloration and scaling caused by *Malassezia furfur*. Infections of the keratinized skin, hair, and nails by fungi are classified as cutaneous mycoses and are caused by dermatophytes, which include the genera *Epidermophyton*, *Trichophyton*, and *Microsporum*. The symptoms include itching, scaling, ringlike patches on the skin (called "ringworm," although they have nothing to do with worms), and discolored nails. Subcutaneous mycoses are caused by trauma to the skin, involve the deeper skin layers, and include lymphocutaneous sporotrichosis (caused by *Sporothrix schenckii*).

Some fungi, including *Histoplasma capsulatum* and *Coccidioides immitis*, cause systemic mycoses that start with infection of the lungs and then spread to other parts of the body. Opportunistic mycoses are seen in immunosuppressed or debilitated individuals, or those with catheters, and are caused by normally commensal fungi, includ-

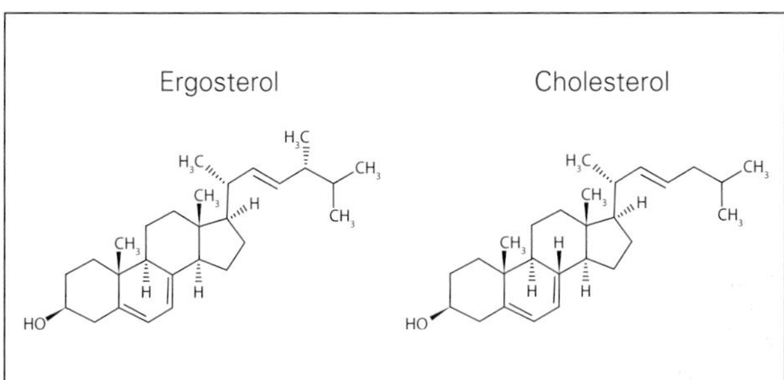

Fig 25-1 Structures of ergosterol and cholesterol. (Adapted from Vanegas et al.)

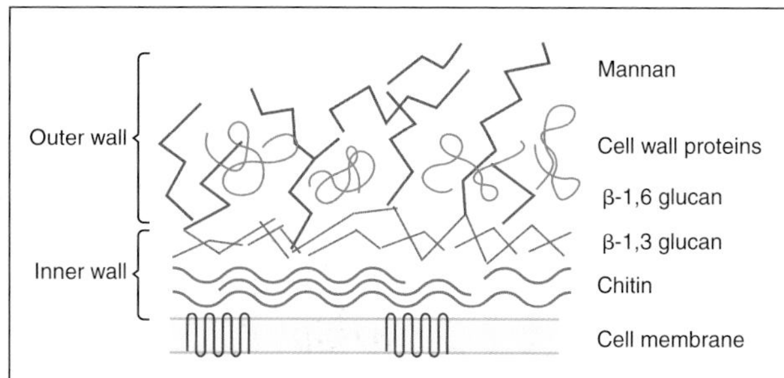

Fig 25-2 Schematic structure of the *Candida albicans* cell wall, showing the carbohydrate-rich layers comprising mannan (mannosylated proteins), β-glucan, and chitin. (Adapted from Gow et al.)

ing *Candida* and *Aspergillus*. *Cryptococcus neoformans* can cause systemic mycoses in healthy individuals, but disease is seen more often in immunocompromised patients.

Structure and Replication

The fungal cell structure is similar to that of other eukaryotic cells, except that the cell membrane contains **ergosterol** instead of cholesterol (Fig 25-1) and the cell is surrounded by a rigid **cell wall** whose composition differs from that of bacterial and plant cell walls (Fig 25-2). The components of the cell wall include galactomannan, **mannan** (α-1,6-linked polymer of D-mannose, with α-1,2 and α-1,3-linked branches of 1 to 5 residues), **α-glucan** (α-1,3- and α-1,4-linked polymer of D-glucose), **β-glucan** (β-1,3-linked polymer of D-glucose, with β-1,6-linkages at branch points), **cellulose** (β-1,4-linked polymer of D-glucose), **chitosan** (β-1,4-linked polymer of D-glucosamine), and **chitin** (β-1,4-linked unbranched polymer of N-acetylglucosamine). The cell wall is a dynamic structure that changes during the morphologic transitions of many fungi. Some of the internal components of the cell wall, such as β-glucans, can be exposed on the cell surface in some locations (eg, the bud scar in *Candida albicans*). The composition of the cell wall also varies between different fungal species. For example, the predominant cell wall polysaccharides in Zygomycetes (*Rhizopus* and *Mucor*) are chitin and chitosan, whereas those in Ascomycetes (*Aspergillus*, *Candida*, *Histoplasma*, and *Coccidioides*) are β-glucans and mannans, and those in Basidiomycetes (*Cryptococcus*) are chitin and mannans.

Fungi can exist as **yeasts** (also known as *blastospores*) or as **molds**. Yeasts reproduce by budding, via the formation of blastoconidia, which is part of the parent cell. They may also reproduce by fission, which is essentially like classical eukaryotic cell division. **Pseudohyphae** may form when daughter cells elongate. Molds are multicellular structures with tubular, elongated structures called **hyphae**. Hyphae elongate by growth at their tips (known as *apical extension*) and may be hollow and multinucleated (coenocytic) or divided (septate) (Fig 25-3). Septate hyphae have cross-walls that differ among species and may enable communication between the elements of the hypha through pores or incomplete walls. The conglomeration of hyphae results in the formation of a **mycelium**.

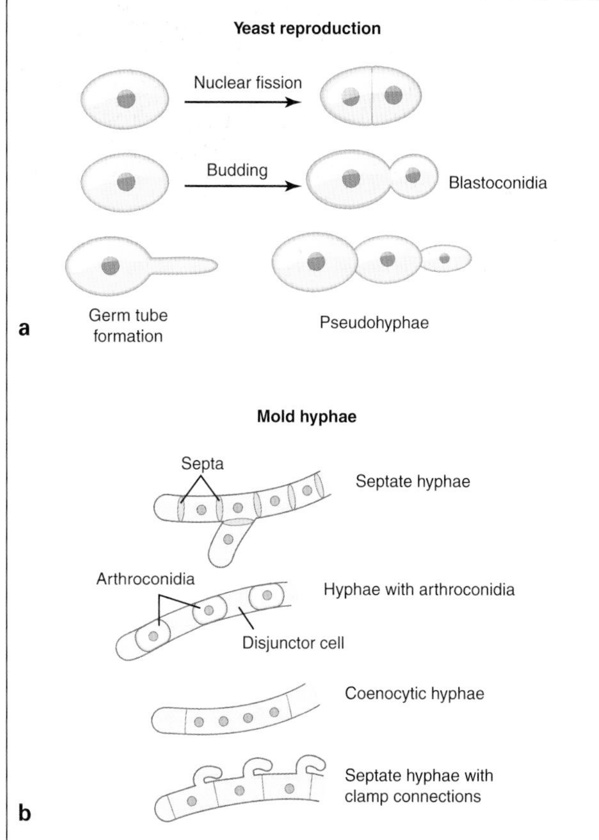

Fig 25-3 Morphology of fungal cells. *(a)* Yeasts reproducing by nuclear fission and by the formation of blastoconidia and the generation of pseudohyphae. *(b)* Different types of hyphae. (Adapted from Murray et al.)

Vegetative hyphae grow on or below the surface of a "solid" growth medium like agar, whereas **aerial hyphae** extend above the surface of the medium and can produce asexual reproductive structures called **conidia** (in *Aspergillus* species) or **sporangiophores** (in *Rhizopus* species) (Fig 25-4). These structures can become readily airborne and

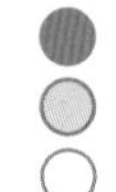

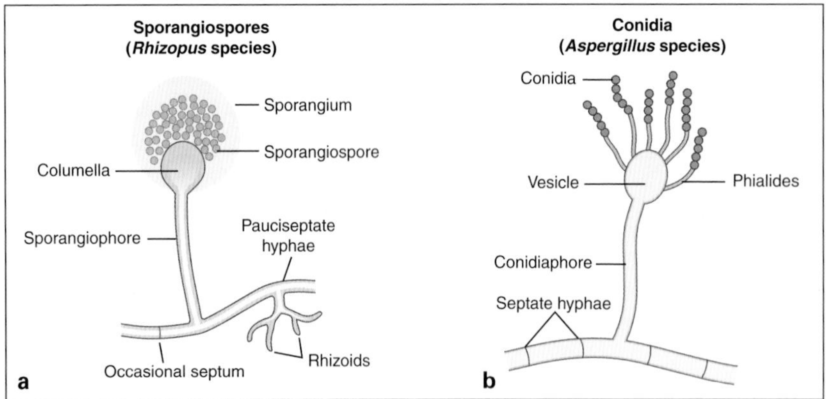

Fig 25-4 Structures associated with the formation of sporangiospores *(a)* and conidia *(b)*. (Adapted from Murray et al.)

can spread the fungus. Many classes of fungi produce both asexual and sexual spores. The fungal form producing asexual spores is known as an anamorph, and that producing sexual spores is known as a teleomorph. The morphology of the conidia, the conidiophore that holds the conidia, or the chlamydoconidia that form bulging structures within hyphae is used in the identification of fungi.

Some fungi can switch between the mold and yeast phases and are known as dimorphic fungi. Some pathogenic fungi convert to the yeast phase when they infect a tissue, whereas they grow as molds in the environment. When *H capsulatum* is converting to the yeast phase at 37°C, the heat shock response is induced, oxidative phosphorylation is uncoupled, and RNA and protein synthesis is stopped. When the yeast phase is achieved, a new set of enzymes, proteins, and cell wall glucans are produced.

Pathogenesis

Fungi cause disease by adhering to mucosal surfaces, invading tissues, producing extracellular products, and evading destruction by phagocytes. The primary fungal pathogens that can infect apparently healthy, immunocompetent hosts and avoid the immune system include *Blastomyces dermatitidis*, *H capsulatum*, *C immitis*, and *Paracoccidioides brasiliensis*. These pathogens have both a saprobic phase, in which they produce hyphae that generate the infectious cells, and a parasitic phase, in which they reproduce in the hospitable environment of the respiratory epithelium. This dimorphism is considered to be one of the virulence factors of these microorganisms.

Adhesion

Adhesion is an important first step in the initiation of fungal infections. *Candida* species (Fig 25-5) and other pathogenic fungi have an unusual ability to adhere to human skin and to endothelial and epithelial tissues (Fig 25-6). *Candida* can form biofilms alone or in conjunction with other microorganisms on these surfaces, creating a medically challenging condition, because the biofilms have reduced susceptibility to antifungal agents. Mannoproteins on the surface of *C albicans* act as adhesins that interact with fibronectin and other components of the extracellular matrix of host cells. Agglutinin-like sequence (Als) proteins (Als1–Als7, Als9) on *C albicans* mediate attachment to a variety of surfaces, including endothelial and epithelial cells as well as abiotic surfaces such as plastic, and contribute to biofilm formation. The hypha-associated, glycophosphatidylinositol-anchored protein Hwp1 is a substrate for the transglutaminase on mammalian cell surfaces, and this reaction may mediate the attachment of the fungus to host cells.

Invasion

The yeast-to-hyphal transformation (phenotypic switching) of *C albicans* is instrumental in its penetration through epithelial cell surfaces and adaptation to changes in the microenvironment. Secreted aspartyl proteases degrade host tissue proteins, enabling several *Candida* species to penetrate connective tissue barriers. Certain fungal cell surface proteins (invasins), such as Als3 (which is also an adhesin), can interact with E-cadherin on epithelial cells and N-cadherin on endothelial cells and induce endocytosis.

The conidial cells of *C immitis* produce an extracellular protease that can break down immunoglobulin (Ig) G, IgA, hemoglobin, collagen, and elastin. The degradation of secretory antibodies helps the microorganism in establishing an infection in the host mucosa. An alkaline protease produced by *C immitis* can degrade lung structural proteins and may be an important virulence factor in tissue invasion.

Intracellular survival

Although *C immitis* endospores are phagocytosed readily by alveolar macrophages, they can survive in phagosomes, producing an alkaline layer resulting from the production of ammonia or ammonium ions. It is thought that a fungal intracellular urease is involved in the production of ammonia. The arthroconidia of *C immitis* have an outer wall containing small, cysteine-rich peptides called hydrophobins that have antiphagocytosis properties. *H capsulatum* prevents the acidification of phagolysosomes in alveolar macrophages, thereby interfering with enzymatic digestion and antigen processing and helping the survival of the fungus. Maintenance of the phagolysosomal pH in

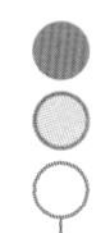

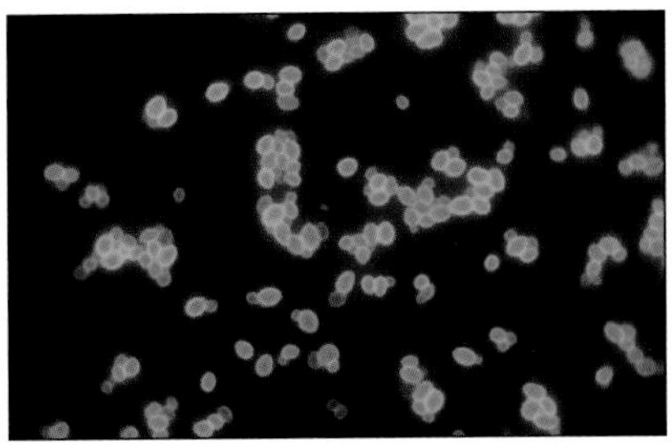

Fig 25-5 *Candida albicans.* (Public Health Image Library image 291, courtesy of Maxine Jalbert and Dr Leo Kaufman.)

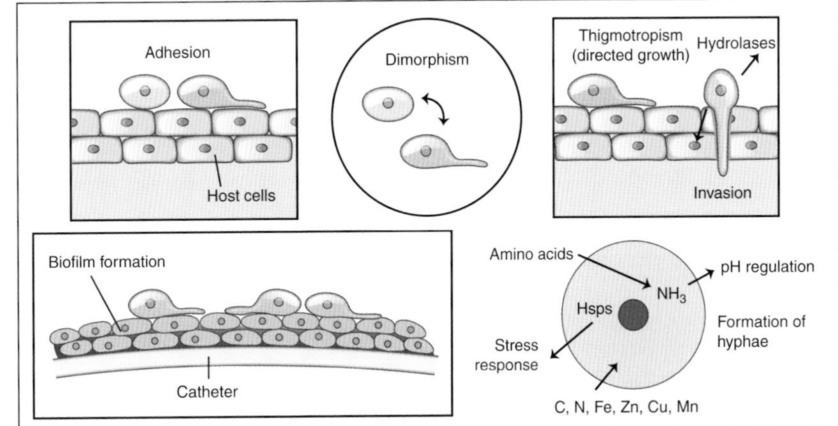

Fig 25-6 Selected *C albicans* pathogenicity mechanisms. Yeasts adhere to host cells via adhesins. This triggers the yeast-to-hyphal transformation and thigmotropism (directed growth). Invasins induce the endocytotic uptake of the fungus by the host cell. The penetration into host cells and tissues is facilitated by adhesion, exertion of physical forces, and secretion of fungal hydrolases. Biofilms are formed by the attachment of fungal cells to artificial surfaces (such as catheters) or host cell surfaces; yeasts are adjacent to the surface, and hyphal cells are found in the outer part of the biofilm. Phenotypic switching of the fungus may affect antigenicity and biofilm formation. A number of "fitness traits" affect the pathogenicity of the fungi, including a stress response (via heat shock proteins, Hsps), hyphae formation by amino acid uptake, extracellular alkalinization via the export of ammonia (NH_3), the uptake of compounds such as carbon and nitrogen sources, and the uptake of essential trace metals. (Adapted from Mayer et al.)

the range 6 to 6.5 also enables the uptake of iron by the microorganism. *H capsulatum* releases a calcium-binding protein, CBP-1, that enables the acquisition of calcium while the yeast cell is inside a macrophage vacuole.

Wild-type *H capsulatum* with cell walls that contain α-(1,3)-glucan not only survive within macrophages but also undergo cell division, eventually killing the host cell. Mutants without the α-(1,3)-glucan are still able to survive within macrophages. Neutrophils can more readily digest *P brasiliensis* strains that lack the α-(1,3)-glucan. A high content of this glucan is associated with increased virulence.

Hormonal factors

The observation that the rate of symptomatic disease caused by *P brasiliensis* is 78 times greater in males than in females has led to the hypothesis that hormones are important in the pathogenesis of this fungus. Mammalian estrogen binds specifically to proteins of *P brasiliensis* and blocks specifically the transition from the saprophytic form to the invasive form of the microorganism in vitro. This block also occurs in vivo. These observations point to the involvement of estrogen-fungus receptor binding in the pathogenesis of *P brasiliensis*.

Heat shock proteins

Heat shock proteins (Hsps) are expressed in fungi in response to exposure to high temperature and other adverse conditions such as starvation. They act as chaperonins by preventing the unfolding and aggregation of other proteins. In *C albicans*, the protein Hsp90 regulates morphogenesis, drug resistance, and biofilm formation; Hsp78 is produced in response to phagocytosis by macrophages; and Ssa1 acts as an invasin.

Evasion of the immune system

After inhalation, *B dermatitidis* undergoes thermal dimorphism from the small conidia into the larger yeast form (8 to 30 μm) that is difficult for neutrophils to phagocytose. The yeast cells also shed their immunodominant antigen, thereby modifying their cell wall composition and evading recognition by macrophages. Virulent strains of *B dermatitidis* shed a component of the cell wall glycoprotein WI-1, which binds to macrophage receptors and to opsonizing antibodies and complement. Thus, opsonizing antibodies and complement cannot facilitate the phagocytosis of the fungus itself, and the fungus thus avoids phagocytosis. Cell-bound WI-1, however, induces a strong cellular and humoral immune response. *C albicans* binding to complement can inhibit phagocytosis.

Immune response to fungal pathogens

Fungal infections tend to be progressive and debilitating in individuals with depressed immune systems, such as those with impaired neutrophil function and depressed helper T cell (T_h1) immune responses resulting from leukemia, Hodgkin disease, steroid treatment, or AIDS. Fungi bind to the Toll-like receptors (TLR2 and TLR4) and lectin-like receptors (eg, dectin-1) on phagocytes. Antigenic stimulation of the immune system in the form of antigen presentation to T_h cells can result in the generation of T_h1 cells that secrete interleukin-2 (IL-2) and interferon gamma (IFN-γ) or T_h2 cells that generate IL-4, IL-5, and IL-10. In experimental animals, generation of a T_h2 response is not protective against *B dermatitidis* infection, whereas a T_h1 response limits the spread of the infection and enables antifungal therapy to clear the infection. Similarly, *C immitis* antigens may elicit a strong T_h2 response, thereby directing the immune response away from the T_h1 response that would have been able to resolve the infection, as deduced from animal experiments. In *P brasiliensis*, the β-(1,3)-glucan induces an intense inflammatory response, and the gp43 protein elicits a strong humoral as well as a delayed-type hypersensitivity response.

Humoral immune responses to *C neoformans* can help resolve the infection, although T_h1 responses appear to be more important in this process. Antibodies against *C albicans* enhance the uptake of the yeast into phagocytes. In *C immitis* infections, however, a strong antibody response is associated with the dissemination of the fungus.

Activation of naïve T cells along the T_h1 pathway results in the production of IFN-γ, IL-2, IL-12, and IL-18 that stimulate phagocytosis and the production of cytotoxic $CD8^+$ T cells and opsonizing antibodies, resulting in a protective effect against fungal infections.

Bibliography

Centers for Disease Control and Prevention. Candidiasis. www.cdc.gov/fungal/diseases/candidiasis/index.html. Accessed 21 July 2015.

Centers for Disease Control and Prevention. Public Health Image Library. phil.cdc.gov. Accessed 4 August 2015.

Engleberg NC, DiRita V, Dermody TS. Schaechter's Mechanisms of Microbial Disease. Baltimore and Philadelphia: Lippincott Williams & Wilkins, 2007.

Deus Filho A. Chapter 2: Coccidioidomycosis. J Bras Pneumol 2009;35:920–930.

Gow NA, van de Veerdonk FL, Brown AJ, Netea MG. *Candida albicans* morphogenesis and host defence: Discriminating invasion from colonization. Nat Rev Microbiol 2011;10:112–122.

Hardison SE, Brown GD. C-type lectin receptors orchestrate antifungal immunity. Nature Immunol 2012;13:817–822.

Huang SH, Wu CH, Chang YC, Kwon-Chung KJ, Brown RJ, Jong A. *Cryptococcus neoformans*-derived microvesicles enhance the pathogenesis of fungal brain infection. PLoS One 2012;7:e48570.

Joklik WK, Willett HP, Amos DB, Wilfert CM. Zinsser Microbiology, ed 20. Norwalk, CT: Appleton & Lange, 1992.

Levinson W. Review of Medical Microbiology and Immunology, ed 11. New York: McGraw-Hill, 2010.

Marsh PD, Martin MV. Oral Microbiology, ed 5. Edinburgh: Churchill Livingstone Elsevier, 2009.

Mayer FL, Wilson D, Hube B. *Candida albicans* pathogenicity mechanisms. Virulence 2013;4:119–128.

Mosby's Dictionary of Medicine, Nursing and Health Professions, ed 9. Philadelphia: Mosby/Elsevier, 2012.

Murray PR, Rosenthal KS, Pfaller MA. Medical Microbiology, ed 6. Philadelphia: Mosby/Elsevier, 2009.

Ryan KJ, Ray CG. Sherris Medical Microbiology, ed 5. New York: McGraw-Hill, 2010.

Vanegas JM, Contreras MF, Faller R, Longo ML. Role of unsaturated lipid and ergosterol in ethanol tolerance of model yeast biomembranes. Biophys J 2012;102:507–516.

Take-Home Messages

- The fungal cell membrane differs from that of other eukaryotic cells in that it contains ergosterol and is surrounded by the cell wall.
- Fungi can exist as yeasts (blastospores) or as molds. Molds are multicellular structures with tubular, elongated structures called *hyphae*. The conglomeration of hyphae results in the formation of a mycelium.
- Some pathogenic fungi grow as molds in the environment and convert to the yeast phase when they infect tissues.
- The main fungal pathogens that can infect apparently healthy hosts and avoid the immune system include *B dermatitidis, H capsulatum, C immitis*, and *P brasiliensis*.
- *Candida* species and other pathogenic fungi have an unusual ability to adhere to human skin and to endothelial and epithelial tissues.
- Mannoproteins on the surface of *C albicans* act as adhesins that interact with fibronectin and other components of the extracellular matrix of host cells.
- The yeast-to-hyphal transformation of *C albicans* is central to its penetration through epithelial cell surfaces.
- *C immitis* conidial cells produce an extracellular protease that can break down immunoglobulins, hemoglobin, collagen, and elastin.
- *C immitis* endospores can survive in phagosomes by producing an alkaline layer.
- *H capsulatum* prevents the acidification of phagolysosomes in alveolar macrophages, thereby inhibiting degradative enzymes.
- Mammalian estrogen binds to proteins of *P brasiliensis* and blocks the transition from the saprophytic form of the fungus to the invasive form.
- Virulent strains of *B dermatitidis* shed a component of their cell wall glycoprotein that binds to macrophage receptors, opsonizing antibodies and complement and thereby inhibiting phagocytosis.
- Activation of the T_h1 pathway stimulates phagocytosis and the production of cytotoxic $CD8^+$ T cells and opsonizing antibodies, resulting in a protective effect against fungal infections.

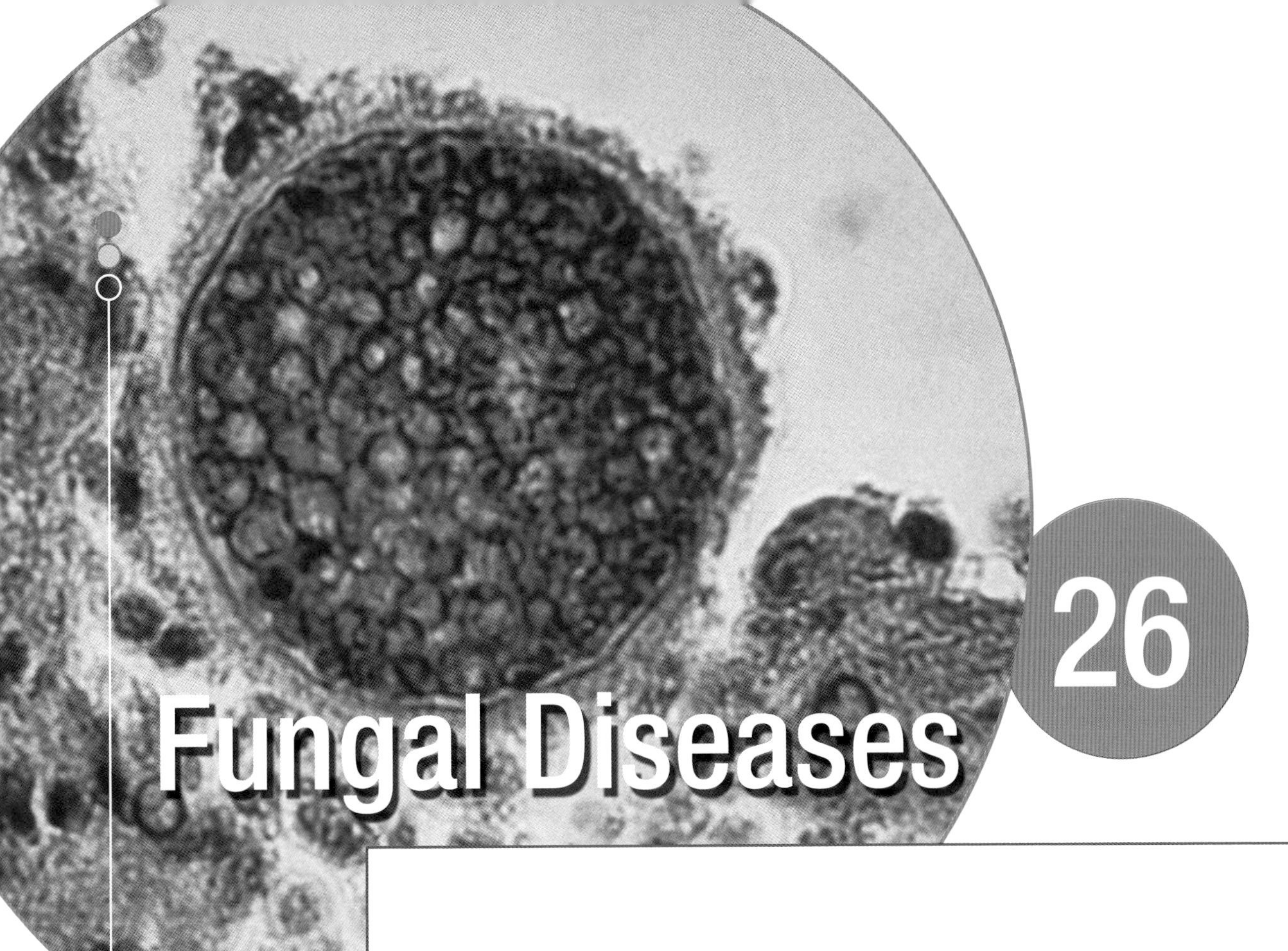

26 Fungal Diseases

Pathogenic fungi can cause mycotoxicoses, hypersensitivity diseases, and mycoses by colonizing the host. Mycoses can be superficial, cutaneous, and subcutaneous. Superficial mycoses occur in the outer layers of the skin and are not destructive. For example, *Malassezia furfur causes* pityriasis versicolor, which is a skin discoloration and scaling. Dermatophytes, which include the genera *Epidermophyton*, *Trichophyton*, and *Microsporum,* cause cutaneous mycoses involving keratinized skin, hair, and nails. The symptoms include itching, scaling, ringlike patches on the skin (called "ringworm," although they are not caused by worms), and discolored nails. Trauma to the skin can cause subcutaneous mycoses, including lymphocutaneous sporotrichosis, which is caused by *Sporothrix schenckii.*

Systemic mycoses are caused by fungi, including *Histoplasma capsulatum* and *Coccidioides immitis*, starting with infection of the lungs and spreading to other parts of the body. Opportunistic mycoses are seen in immunosuppressed or debilitated individuals, or those with catheters, and are caused by normally commensal fungi, including *Candida* and *Aspergillus*. Although *Cryptococcus neoformans* can cause systemic mycoses in healthy individuals, the disease is seen more often in immunocompromised patients.

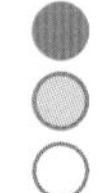

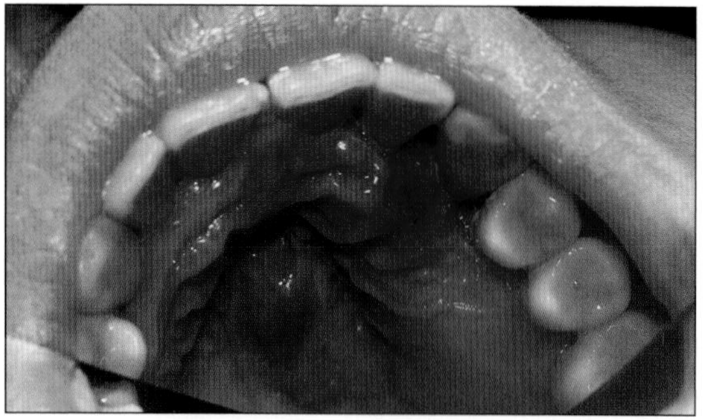

Fig 26-1 Chronic progressive histoplasmosis. An oral lesion of histoplasmosis presents as a fleshy red mass in the palatal mucosa and ulcerations around several teeth. (Reprinted with permission from Marx and Stern.)

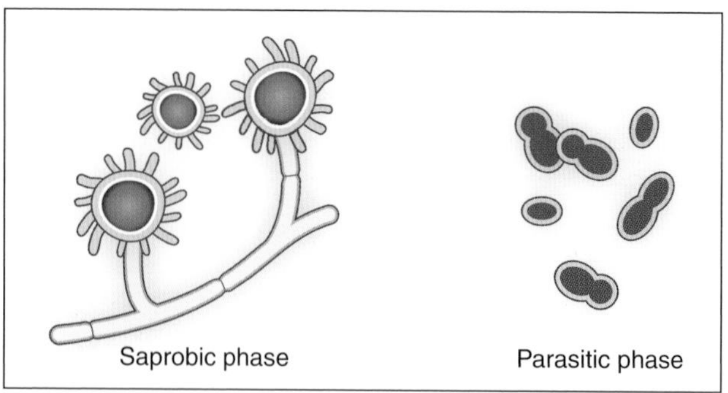

Fig 26-2 Saprobic (at 25°C) and parasitic (at 37°C) phases of *H capsulatum*. (Adapted from Murray et al.)

Systemic Mycoses

Primary fungal pathogens can colonize immunocompetent hosts, avoid the immune system, and find an environment with a source of nutrition. The major primary pathogens, all in the phylum Ascomycota, are *H capsulatum*, *Blastomyces dermatitidis*, *C immitis*, and *Paracoccidioides brasiliensis*. They all have a saprobic phase when they are in the form of filamentous, septate hyphae. In the parasitic phase, they reproduce asexually at body temperature.

H capsulatum

Clinical syndromes and diagnosis

There are two varieties of *H capsulatum* that cause histoplasmosis. *H capsulatum* variant *capsulatum* causes disseminated and pulmonary disease, whereas *H capsulatum* variant *duboisii* infections cause bone and skin lesions.

Exposure to low levels of *H capsulatum* var *capsulatum* results in asymptomatic infection in 90% of individuals. Exposure to high levels of the microorganism can cause a flulike illness, with fever, chills, myalgia, headache, cough, and chest pain. Hilar and mediastinal lymphadenopathy are seen in chest radiographs. Some patients develop severe pneumonia. Disseminated disease is rare (1 in 2,000 adults with acute infection) but can result in fatigue, fever, and weight loss, with hepatosplenomegaly and oropharyngeal ulcers (Fig 26-1). Oral ulcers are mildly painful and are fleshy, slightly elevated tissues. This chronic progressive histoplasmosis arises from chronic lung infection that can spread hematogenously or by coughed-up sputum. Mucosal lesions may be the primary clinical finding in a seemingly healthy individual. Ulcerated lesions on the tongue are typical for disseminated disease in AIDS patients. Individuals with chronic obstructive pulmonary disease may develop chronic cavitary pulmonary histoplasmosis, which can be fatal.

Localized *H capsulatum* var *duboisii* infections cause regional lymphadenopathy, papular or nodular skin lesions that lead to ulceration, and bone lesions with the involvement of draining sinuses and overlying abscesses. A disseminated form of the disease is seen in severely immunodeficient patients, leading to anemia, fever, organomegaly, weight loss, and death if untreated.

Infection can be diagnosed by histology of samples from lymph nodes, bone marrow, liver, or lung, following special staining (eg, with Gomori methenamine silver [GMS] or periodic acid Schiff [PAS] stain). *H capsulatum* var *duboisii* cells are larger (8 to 15 µm) than var *capsulatum* cells (2 to 4 µm). The cell wall polysaccharide antigen in serum or urine samples is detected by enzyme-linked immunosorbent assay (ELISA). The mold phase of *H capsulatum* is characterized by thin, branching, septate hyphae that produce microconidia and typical tuberculate macroconidia (Fig 26-2). Detection of anti–*H capsulatum* antibodies is also helpful in diagnosis in immunocompetent individuals.

Pathogenesis and epidemiology

H capsulatum transforms into the yeast phase when it enters the lungs, where it is phagocytosed by macrophages and neutrophils. Infection activates cell-mediated immunity, leading to the release of cytokines like interferon gamma that activate macrophages to kill the intracellular fungi. While the immune system is being activated, the yeasts in macrophages spread to the local lymph nodes and then to the reticuloendothelial system via the bloodstream. Cell-mediated immunity results in the formation of granulomas, which can calcify subsequently. The microorganism can survive in the granulomas and spread again if cell-mediated immunity declines.

The microorganism grows in soil with a high nitrogen content in areas frequented by birds and bats. Natural infection occurs in bats, whereas birds are not infected. The fungus is found commonly in the Midwestern United States.

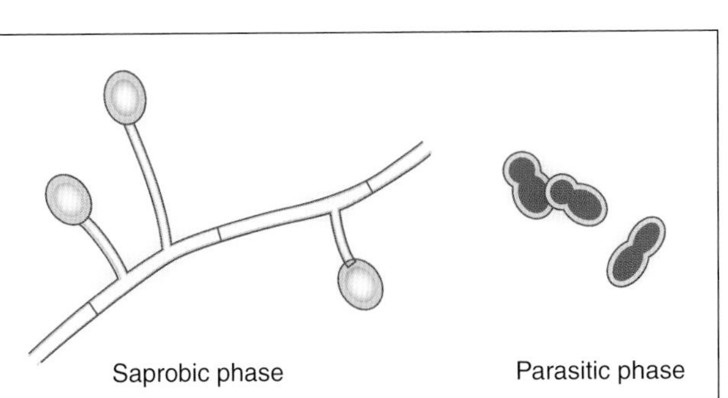

Fig 26-3 Saprobic (at 25°C) and parasitic (at 37°C) phases of *B dermatitidis*. (Adapted from Murray et al.)

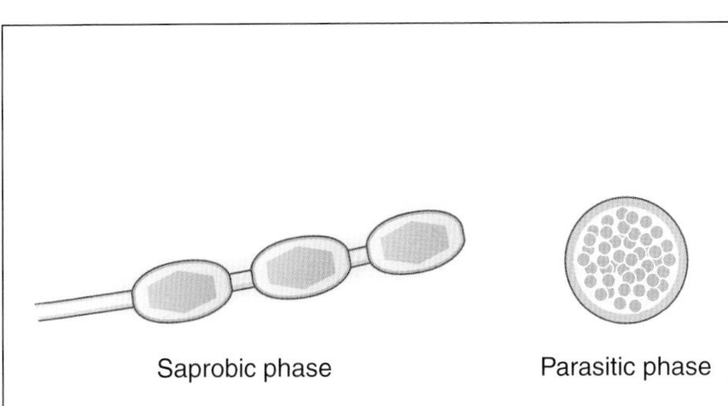

Fig 26-4 Saprobic (at 25°C) and parasitic (at 37°C) phases of *C immitis*. (Adapted from Murray et al.)

Treatment and prevention

Most patients recover without therapy. In more severe cases, itraconazole can be administered. In patients with acute respiratory distress syndrome, therapy should start with amphotericin B, followed by itraconazole for 12 weeks. Infection can be prevented by taking respiratory precautions (eg, using respirators) when working in potentially infected surroundings (eg, barns, chicken coops, etc).

B dermatitidis

Clinical syndromes and diagnosis

B dermatitidis infection causes symptomatic pulmonary disease in less than half of the individuals exposed to the fungus. Pulmonary disease may be resolved without the involvement of other organs or may lead to systemic disease; alternatively, it may develop into pneumonia with high fever, cough, anorexia, fatigue, and diffuse infiltrates. Acute respiratory distress syndrome can develop with extensive exposure. The microorganism can also cause skin lesions after spreading from the lungs via the bloodstream (hematogenous dissemination) and may present as papular, pustular, ulcerative-nodular lesions or wartlike growths with crusted surfaces. They may be seen on the face, neck, scalp, and hands.

B dermatitidis can be diagnosed by culturing samples from sputum, bronchoalveolar lavage, or tissue biopsy. At 25°C, round, oval, or pear-shaped conidia 2 to 10 µm in diameter are observed; at 37°C, broad-based, budding yeasts 8 to 15 µm in diameter are seen (Fig 26-3). The conidia are infectious and should be handled in a biosafety cabinet.

Pathogenesis and epidemiology

Inhaled *B dermatitidis* conidia convert to yeasts and are phagocytosed by macrophages that may be instrumental in carrying the fungus to other organs. The fungus is spread by exposure to conidia from soil and leaf litter. It is endemic in southeastern, south central, and Midwestern states, the Great Lakes region, and Africa.

Treatment and prevention

Mild and moderate blastomycosis is treated with itraconazole for 6 to 12 months. Fluconazole is an alternative for patients who cannot tolerate itraconazole. Amphotericin B is used initially in severe cases; this is followed by itraconazole treatment. The newer antifungals voriconazole and posaconazole are being evaluated for the treatment of blastomycosis.

C immitis

C immitis and *Coccidioides posadasii* cause coccidioidomycosis, the former in California and the latter elsewhere. Besides their geographic location, these two fungi are very similar. They are dimorphic; in nature and at room temperature in the laboratory, they form barrel-shaped "arthoconidia" molds separated by disjunctor cells. When they enter the lungs, they form round spherules 20 to 60 µm in diameter that contain endospores, which are released upon rupture and form new spherules (Fig 26-4).

Clinical syndromes and diagnosis

Infections caused by *C immitis* include coccidioidomycosis, coccidioidal granuloma, and San Joaquin Valley fever and result in a variety of lesions, thereby earning *C immitis* the label "the great imitator." In about 60% of patients, infection causes asymptomatic pulmonary disease. It may also cause a flulike illness with symptoms including chest pain, fever, cough, and weight loss. The fungus can cause disseminated disease in patients who are symptomatic for 6 weeks or longer, with manifestations in the skin, bones, joints, and meninges (Fig 26-5). If untreated, disseminated disease is fatal in 90% of cases. The most serious complication of *C immitis* infection is chronic meningitis, which requires continuous therapy.

The best method for diagnosis is the visualization of endosporulating spherules in sputum, tissues, or exudates, using calcofluor white for exudates and hematoxylin and eosin, GMS, or PAS stain for biopsies. If samples are cultured, care must be taken to keep the cultures properly contained to avoid infection of laboratory personnel.

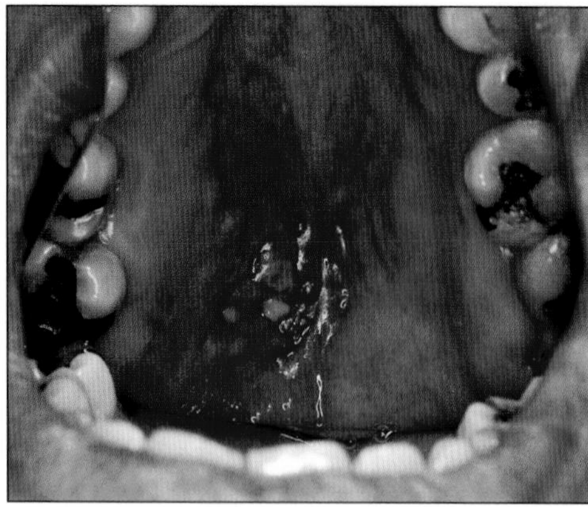

Fig 26-5 Coccidioidomycosis of the palate secondary to hematogenous spread from pulmonary coccidioidomycosis. (Reprinted with permission from Marx and Stern.)

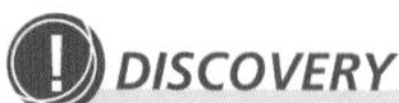

Coccidioidomycosis was first identified in Argentina in 1891 by Alejandro Posadas, who was a medical student at the time. A patient presented with recurring skin tumors. Together with the pathologist Robert Wernicke, Posadas described the organism found in the lesions as a parasite that was similar to coccidian protozoa. The first two cases in the United States were found in 1894 by Emmet Rixford among immigrants who were working in the fields in the San Joaquin Valley. Rixford and T. C. Gilchrist identified a parasite similar to that reported by Posadas, describing it as a protozoan of the order Coccidia, class Sporozoa, and calling it *C immitis*. In 1900, William Ophüls and Herbert Moffitt described a third case in North America and observed that when a sample from the lesion was cultured, it produced a mold, thus identifying the microorganism as a fungus.

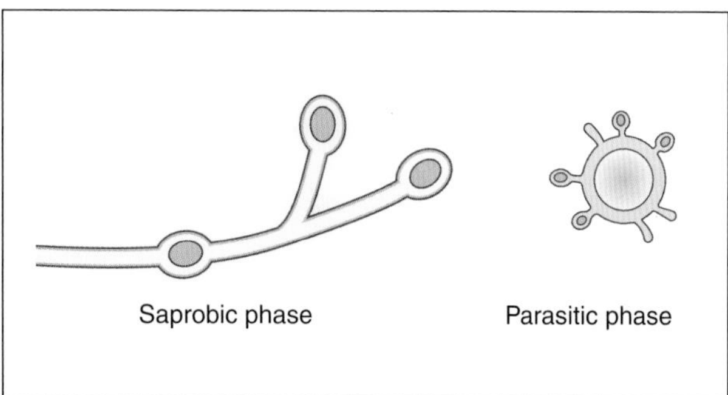

Fig 26-6 Saprobic (at 25°C) and parasitic (at 37°C) phases of *P brasiliensis*. (Adapted from Murray et al.)

Pathogenesis and epidemiology

C immitis is thought to be the most virulent of fungal infections, with only a few arthroconidia causing primary coccidioidomycosis. Immune complex formation with the microorganism can cause allergic reactions such as an erythematous macular rash.

It is found in soil, especially in environments rich in rodent and bat droppings, and is endemic to the southwestern United States, northern Mexico, and Central and South America. Rain facilitates the growth of the fungus, and subsequent drought and wind increases the probability of aerosolization of the arthroconidia. It is transmitted via inhalation.

Treatment and prevention

Itraconazole and fluconazole are used for the treatment of mild to moderate coccidioidomycosis but for periods of 12 to 24 months. Amphotericin B is necessary for the treatment of severe disease. Because the organism is readily airborne in endemic areas, it is difficult to control transmission, but avoiding dust storms in these areas is a preventive measure.

P brasiliensis

P brasiliensis causes paracoccidioidomycosis, which is also known as South American blastomycosis. The yeast form of this fungus is in the range of 3 to 30 µm in diameter and has a characteristic shape, with multiple blastoconidia budding from the surface (Fig 26-6).

Clinical syndromes and diagnosis

Pulmonary infections are often asymptomatic. However, in some infected individuals, chronic pulmonary symptoms, including purulent sputum, chest pain, and cough, are seen. Disseminated disease can result in cutaneous and mucocutaneous ulcers, the latter mostly in the mouth, lips, gingiva, buccal mucosa, and palate. The infection can be diagnosed by serology (ie, detection of specific antibodies), microscopic examination of specimens from infected tissues, and culture of the microorganism.

Pathogenesis and epidemiology

The route of infection is believed to be respiratory. Infection results in the depression of T cell–mediated immunity. *P brasiliensis* primarily infects males, which may be the result of the inhibition of mold-to-yeast conversion by estrogens but not by androgens. The gp43 protein of the yeast phase of the fungus mediates adhesion to laminin-1 and thus may be involved in attachment to the basement membrane. It also elicits a strong humoral and delayed-type hypersensitivity response in the host. The α-(1,3)-glucan in the cell wall is also a virulence factor.

Treatment and prevention

The treatment of choice is itraconazole for at least 6 months. Severe infections need to be treated with amphotericin B followed by itraconazole or sulfonamides.

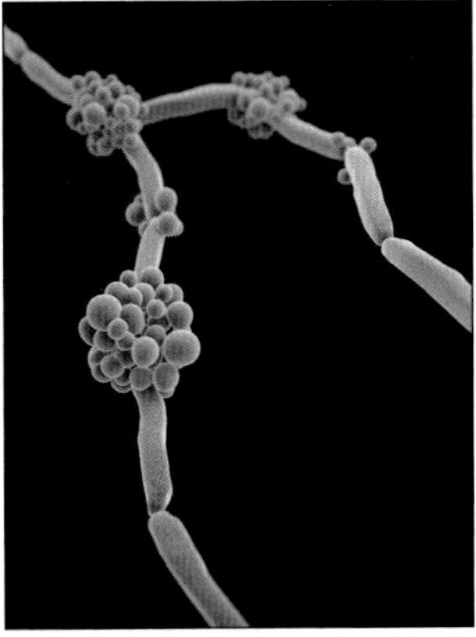

Fig 26-7 Computer-generated image of *Candida* based on a scanning electron micrograph. There are clusters of blastoconidia as well as single blastoconidia produced by budding that are attached to the septate hyphal filaments. (Public Health Image Library image 16871, courtesy of Melissa Brower.)

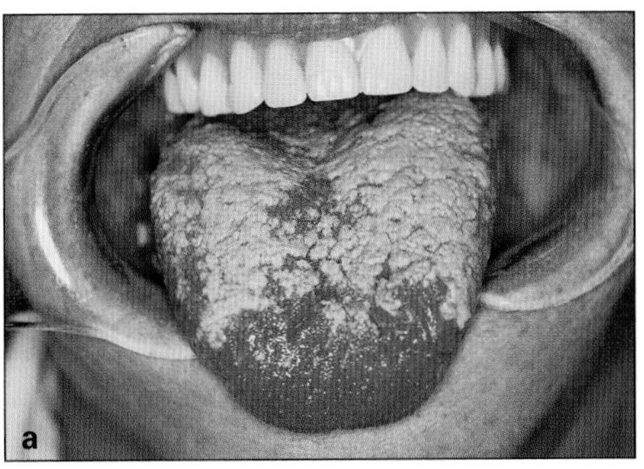

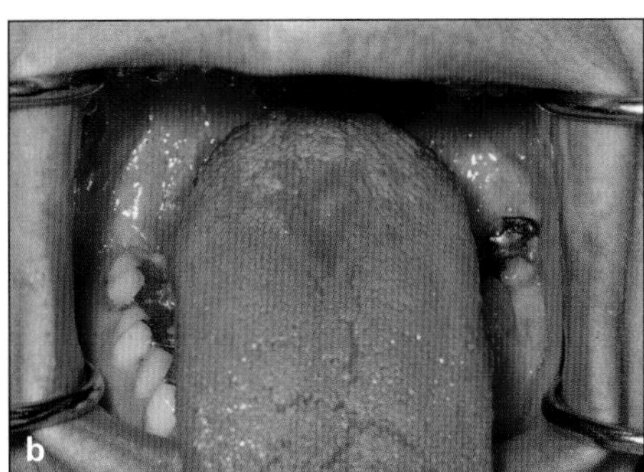

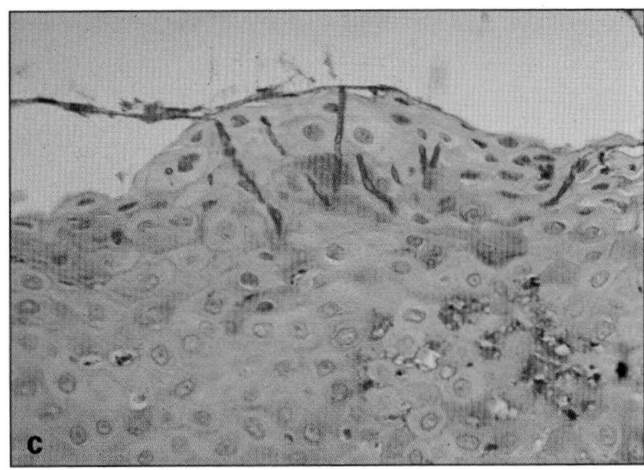

Fig 26-8 Presentation of oral candidiasis. *(a)* Pseudomembranous candidiasis (thrush). The *Candida* colonies may be scraped with a tongue scraper. The remainder of the dorsal tongue appears inflamed. *(b)* Median rhomboid glossitis, caused by a superficial *Candida* infection that produces a focal inflammation and atrophy of the papillae. *(c)* PAS-stained median rhomboid glossitis biopsy, revealing burrowing, nonseptate, nonbranching *Candida* organisms. (Reprinted with permission from Marx and Stern.)

Opportunistic Mycoses

Opportunistic fungal infections occur in individuals whose immune systems are compromised, including patients with diabetes, malignancy, or AIDS; those undergoing marrow and organ transplantation; the elderly; patients who have had immunosuppressive therapy; and premature infants. *Candida albicans*, *Aspergillus fumigatus*, and *C neoformans* are the most common opportunistic fungi.

Candida

The *Candida* species most frequently isolated from mucosal and bloodstream infections is *C albicans*. The other major species associated with bloodstream infections are *Candida glabrata*, *Candida parapsilosis*, and *Candida tropicalis*. *Candida* species are part of the normal human flora and are found on mucosal surfaces of the oral cavity, vagina, and the gastrointestinal tract. They are oval yeasts in the range of 3 to 5 μm in diameter that reproduce by budding (Fig 26-7). They can also form hyphae called germ tubes attached to the yeast cell or other elongated structures called pseudohyphae that do not have the walls and septae of true hyphae. Under some culture conditions, thick-walled chlamydoconidia are formed by *C albicans* but not by the other species. *Candida* microorganisms can undergo phenotypic switching to different morphotypes, which may be one reason why they can survive in many different environments in the host.

Clinical syndromes and diagnosis

Candida species can cause superficial cutaneous and mucosal disease, as well as disseminated infections of the liver, spleen, heart, kidneys, and brain. They are also present as commensal microorganisms on the skin and in the vagina and urethra. Mucosal infections, generally referred to as thrush, may present in different forms:

- White patches on the mucosa
- Erythematous infection with red and sore areas
- Pseudomembranous type that displays a bleeding surface after scraping
- Leukoplakia, a white, thick epithelium
- Perlèche, or angular cheilitis, characterized by fissures and cracks at the corners of the mouth

Disseminated infection usually presents as fever, candidemia, or organ dysfunction. It can cause meningitis, esophagitis, chorioretinitis (inflammation of the choroid and retina), vertebral osteomyelitis, hepatosplenic and renal abscesses, vulvovaginal infections, pneumonia, bone and joint infections, or pericarditis and endocarditis. Skin lesions appearing during dissemination of *Candida* are useful in diagnosis.

Oral candidiasis (sometimes called *candidosis*) presents in various forms (Fig 26-8). Pseudomembranous candidiasis involves the presence of white plaque-like lesions in the mouth (oral thrush) (see Fig 26-8a). When the lesions are removed by gentle scraping, an erythematous mucosal surface is exposed. The removed "pseudomembranes" consist of epithelial cells and fungi. In immunocompromised patients, esophageal tissues are also infected, leading to difficulty in swallowing.

Acute erythematous candidiasis is usually seen on the dorsum of the tongue following therapy with a broad-spectrum antibiotic that causes a decrease in the bacterial community and allows the overgrowth of *Candida*. "Antibiotic sore mouth" is sometimes used to describe this condition. Patients complain of a burning mouth, and a reddened mucosa is observed without white flecks.

Chronic hyperplastic candidiasis is seen most often in the buccal commissure region as white patches, primarily in middle-aged men who smoke. If untreated, 5% to 10% of cases progress to dysplasia and oral cancer. The white patches cannot be removed without bleeding. The lesions can be homogenous or heterogenous, the latter having regions of erythema, giving a nodular appearance to the lesion.

Chronic erythematous candidiasis, also known as ***Candida*-associated denture stomatitis**, presents as redness on the mucosa apposed to dentures, especially on the palate. This condition is attributed to the formation of *Candida* biofilms on both the dentures and the mucosal surfaces, poor oral hygiene, and poorly fitting dentures.

Angular cheilitis is seen as erythematous lesions or cracking at the corners of the mouth and is usually associated with other forms of oral candidiasis. *Candida* may not be the only cause of these lesions, because *Staphylococcus aureus* or streptococci are also found at these sites. **Median rhomboid glossitis** results from atrophied papillae at the middle and dorsum of the tongue (see Figs 26-8b and 26-8c) and may be associated with the use of inhaled steroids and smoking.

Chronic mucocutaneous candidiasis is associated with impaired T cell (possibly helper T [T_h17] cell)–mediated immunity against *Candida* and presents as white patches on mucosal surfaces and crusted lesions on the skin.

Candida species have been isolated from 93% of patients with denture stomatitis. The microorganisms adhere directly to denture acrylic (polymethyl methacrylate) or through a layer of bacterial plaque. Denture stomatitis is reestablished soon after treatment is stopped; thus, denture plaque may be a protected reservoir for *Candida*.

For diagnosis, samples from mucosal or skin lesions can be examined by microscopy for budding yeasts and pseudohyphae. PAS or GMS stains are used to visualize the fungi. Samples can also be plated on selective medium containing chromogenic substrates (CHROMagar *Candida*). *C albicans* shows up as green colonies and *C tropicalis* as blue colonies. *C albicans* and *Candida dubliniensis* can be distinguished by the production of germ tubes and chlamydospores. Identification of the different species of *Candida* is useful in the choice of antifungal agents, considering their different susceptibilities to them.

Pathogenesis and epidemiology

The virulence factors of *Candida* species include **adherence** to oral tissues and biomaterials via both specific (via adhesins) and nonspecific processes, morphology, phenotypic switching, **secreted aspartyl proteases**, and **phospholipases**. The switching of *C albicans* from its yeast morphology to a filamentous form may enable it to penetrate the tissue epithelial cell layer and confer resistance to phagocytosis. Phenotypic switching may alter the antigenicity and adhesiveness of the cell surface and resistance to phagocytosis and antifungals. Secreted aspartyl proteases may degrade the extracellular matrix proteins of the host and induce apoptosis in epithelial cells.

The main source of infection by *Candida* is the body itself. When the defensive barrier to *Candida* is breached, the microorganism causes an **opportunistic infection**. *Candida* may also be transmitted exogenously from contaminated parenteral fluids, corneas, or cardiac valves as well as from other patients or health care workers. Most bloodstream infections in the United States are caused by *C albicans*, followed by *C glabrata*. The age of the patient, his or her exposure to certain antifungals, and the nature of infection control may affect the prevalence of a particular species in a particular patient. When fluconazole is used as a prophylactic antifungal, species that are relatively resistant to this agent, such as *C glabrata* and *Candida krusei*, tend to predominate.

Invasive candidiasis is the fourth most common cause of **hospital-acquired bloodstream infections** in the United States, behind coagulase-negative staphylococci, *S aureus*, and enterococci. This high prevalence may have been caused by the suppression of indigenous bacterial flora by antibiotics and the use of immunosuppressive drugs, catheters, and implanted devices.

Treatment and prevention

Candidal skin infections may be treated with topically applied antifungals, including nystatin and clotrimazole. Ketoconazole (Nizoral, Janssen) may be used for the treatment of mucocutaneous *Candida* infections. Oropharyngeal and esophageal thrush is treated with the triazole fluconazole (Diflucan, Pfizer). **Oral lesions** respond well to the topical antifungal agents nystatin (Mycostatin pastilles, Bristol-Myers Squibb) and clotrimazole (Mycelex troches [lozenges], Ortho-McNeil-Janssen). Disseminated *Candida* is generally treated with amphotericin B or fluconazole.

Prevention measures include the use of fluconazole in high-risk individuals, including bone-marrow transplant patients; avoiding the use of broad-spectrum antibiotics; and adherence to infection-control procedures. Long-term use of fluconazole, however, can lead to the emergence of *C glabrata* and *C krusei* that are resistant to this antifungal. In this case, an echinocandin or amphotericin B can be used. It is important to drain abscesses and remove vascular catheters that are likely to be the source of infection.

C neoformans

C neoformans is a spherical/oval microorganism that multiplies by budding and is usually covered with a polysaccharide capsule, which is visualized clearly in preparations with India ink. The budding occurs via a narrow base, in contrast to the broad-based budding observed in *B dermatitidis*.

Clinical syndromes and diagnosis

Cryptococcal pneumonia varies from an asymptomatic infection to bilateral pneumonia, with nodular infiltrates. Clinical symptoms of cryptococcal meningitis include headache, fever, impaired vision, mental disorders, and seizures. The symptoms are more severe in AIDS patients and other immunocompromised individuals. Disseminated cryptococcosis may also present with skin lesions, chorioretinitis, and invasion of the ocular nerve.

Diagnosis involves the culture of samples from blood or the cerebrospinal fluid. Microscopic examination after staining with India ink reveals encapsulated budding yeast cells. Other stains that can be used include mucicarmine and GMS. The capsular polysaccharide antigen can be detected in serum samples by ELISA or latex agglutination.

Pathogenesis and epidemiology

Cryptococcus is found in soil with bird droppings and infects humans via the lungs. It is not transmitted between humans. Infection is often asymptomatic but can cause disseminated disease in immunocompromised patients. Cryptococcus is the most common cause of fungal meningitis. About half the cases of cryptococcal meningitis, however, occur in immunocompetent individuals. AIDS patients with a CD4⁺ cell count less than 200/µl are at high risk for cryptococcal meningitis and disseminated disease.

The capsule may downregulate the T_h1 arm of the immune response and thus inhibit T-cell immunity, which is normally essential in controlling the infection. Microvesicles derived from the fungus appear to enhance the penetration of *C neoformans* through the blood-brain barrier.

Treatment and prevention

Treatment of *C neoformans* infections involves the combined use of amphotericin B and flucytosine for an initial 2-week period (induction therapy), followed by 8 weeks of treatment with fluconazole or itraconazole (consolidation therapy). The cerebrospinal fluid should be monitored to assess the success of therapy. Long-term suppression of meningitis in AIDS patients is achieved by the administration of fluconazole.

Aspergillus

Aspergillus organisms are very common in the environment. *A fumigatus* and *Aspergillus flavus* can cause aspergillosis. They have septate hyphae, and they reproduce by conidia that form on conidiophores.

Clinical syndromes and diagnosis

The clinical symptoms of invasive pulmonary aspergillosis are pleuritic chest pain, dyspnea, cough, hemoptysis (coughing up blood), and fever. Chest radiographs show multiple nodules, hemorrhage around the nodules, and necrotic tissue. Sinus invasion may cause acute facial pain. Disseminated *Aspergillus* infections manifest as necrotic skin lesions (Fig 26-9) and brain abscesses leading to stroke or seizures. Diagnosis involves culture and the observation of septate hyphae in tissue specimens.

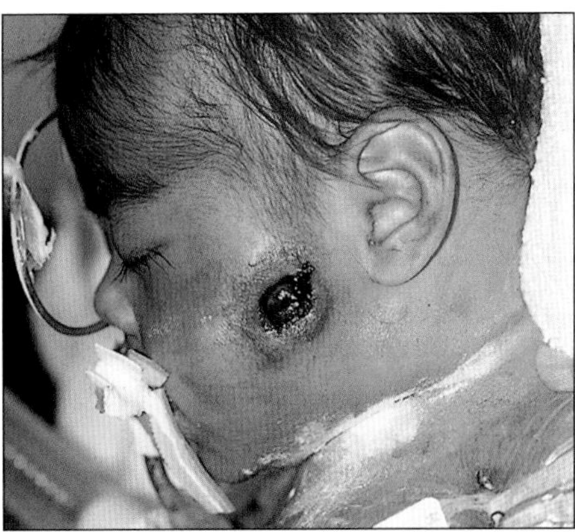

Fig 26-9 Ulceration seen in aspergillosis as a complication in an immunocompromised organ transplant patient. (Reprinted with permission from Marx and Stern.)

Pathogenesis and epidemiology

Healthy individuals are not susceptible to aspergillosis, which is an opportunistic infection. The type of disease depends on the local or general physiologic and immunologic state of the host. Transplant recipients, neutropenic patients, and those on corticosteroids are the common hosts. In contrast to candidiasis, the fungal organisms in aspergillosis are not part of the normal flora of humans but are found in the environment. The microorganism is found in soil, decomposing vegetation, and manure. Conidia enter the body by inhalation and then germinate into hyphae. The conidia are phagocytosed by macrophages, which kill them; but the macrophages cannot kill hyphae. Neutrophils line up along hyphae and secrete reactive oxygen species that can kill the hyphae. *Aspergillus* is angioinvasive, with the hyphae invading tissues through the endothelial barrier and causing necrosis and hemorrhage.

Treatment and prevention

Treatment has to be started early, before extensive invasion of tissues, and involves the administration of voriconazole, amphotericin B, or caspofungin. Prevention can be achieved by filtering the air in hospital rooms of at-risk individuals and by reducing exposure to construction dust and other potential environmental sources.

Zygomycetes

Zygomycetes include the genera Rhizopus and Mucor; they behave similarly to *Aspergillus* in that they are angioinvasive,

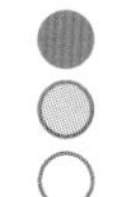

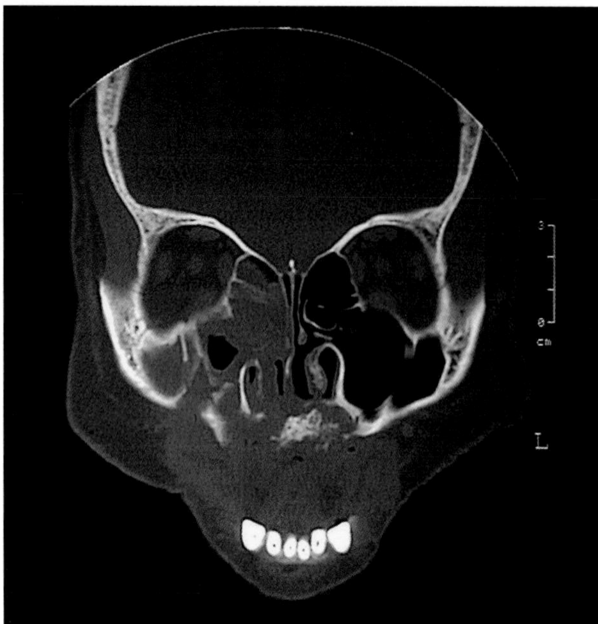

Fig 26-10 Mucormycosis of the nasal cavity and perinasal sinuses. (Reprinted with permission from Marx and Stern.)

but they are broader and do not have septae. Predisposing conditions for zygomycosis (or mucormycosis) include hematologic malignancies, diabetes mellitus with ketoacidosis, neutropenia, human immunodeficiency virus (HIV)/AIDS, and use of corticosteroids. Rhinocerebral mucormycosis is the most common presentation in diabetic patients and involves the spread of the fungi from the nares and paranasal sinuses (Fig 26-10) into the palate, ocular orbit, facial soft tissues, and eventually the brain. Mucormycosis is also seen in the lungs, the gastrointestinal tract, and subcutaneous tissues of immunosuppressed patients. Zygomycetes can also colonize the damaged tissues in severely burned patients and become invasive. They can invade major blood vessels, causing emboli that result in ischemia (hemorrhagic infarction) and necrosis of adjacent tissues.

Amphotericin B and aggressive surgical debridement are used to treat zygomycosis.

Pneumocystis jirovecii

Formerly named *Pneumocystis carinii* and thought to be a protozoan, this microorganism is now classified as a fungus, based on ribosomal RNA analysis. Its ecological niche is not known, but it is likely that individuals are exposed early in life. It causes pneumonia in immunocompromised individuals with T-cell deficiency and was the most common opportunistic infection during the early years of HIV/AIDS. The clinical symptoms include dyspnea, fatigue, and dry cough. Foamy proteinaceous material, sloughed-off alveolar cells, and the fungus fill the alveolar space. The organism can be diagnosed by silver stain of lung biopsies, direct fluorescence antibody testing, and polymerase chain reaction. The infection can be treated with trimethoprim-sulfamethoxazole, which can also be used for prophylaxis.

Superficial, Cutaneous, and Subcutaneous Mycoses

These mycoses are the most common fungal infections in humans. They do not often lead to serious disease. Intact skin and mucosal surfaces serve as barriers to infection by these fungi, with the fatty acid content, pH, epithelial turnover of the skin, and normal bacterial flora contributing to host resistance.

Superficial mycoses

Superficial mycoses are limited to the keratinized layers of the skin, nails, and hair. They usually do not elicit a cellular response from the host because they colonize tissues that are not living. They are easy to diagnose and treat.

M furfur

The organism appears in skin samples as clusters of yeasts 3 to 8 µm in diameter, with occasional short hyphae, and causes pityriasis versicolor, which manifests as macules with hypo- or hyperpigmentation. The lesions occur primarily on the upper torso, arms, shoulders, neck, and face and interfere with melanin production. Transmission is thought to be via the transfer of infected keratinous layers of skin from person to person. The disease is treated by the topical application of azoles or selenium sulfide. If the infection is widespread, it may be treated with oral ketoconazole or itraconazole.

Hortaea werneckii

The fungus causes tinea nigra, which is most prevalent in tropical and subtropical areas. The lesions are brown to black and are most often seen on the palms of the hands and the soles of the feet. Examination of skin scrapings show septate hyphae that are branched frequently. The condition can be treated with topical azoles or terbinafine.

Trichosporon

Several species of *Trichosporon* cause white piedra, an infection of hairs in the groin and the axillae in which the hair shafts bear a white to brown, soft, nodular mass of fungi. Topical azoles and hygiene are useful in treating the condition.

Piedraia hortae

The fungus forms brown to reddish-black mold that surrounds the hair shaft and is held together by a hard substance, causing the black piedra. This condition is not common and can be treated by a haircut and regular hygiene.

Cutaneous mycoses

Cutaneous mycoses are caused by a group of closely related fungi including *Microsporum*, *Trichophyton*, and *Epidermophyton*, also known as the dermatophytes ("skin plants"). They colonize only the outer dead layers of the skin, hair, and nails, and their optimal temperature for growth is 25°C. They are keratinophilic and keratinolytic; they can break down keratin, which is a principal constituent of the epidermis, hair, and nails and a highly insoluble protein with a large percentage of cysteine. *Microsporum* can be identified by its macroconidia and *Trichophyton* by its microconidia. *Epidermophyton* produces smooth-walled macroconidia of several units.

The diseases caused by these microorganisms manifest as a "ringworm" or "tinea" (Latin for "worm") in the superficial layers of the skin following penetration through the stratum corneum. The spread of the infection and the associated inflammation cause the appearance of what looks like a circular worm. Infection of feet is termed *tinea pedis* (athlete's foot); that of the scalp, *tinea capitis*; the beard and hair, *tinea barbae*; the body, *tinea corporis*; the nail beds, *tinea unguium*, causing onychomycosis; and the hands, *tinea manus*. A rapidly progressive form of onychomycosis involving the upper and underside of nails is seen in AIDS patients.

Laboratory diagnosis involves culture and microscopic examination. Some dermatophyte species, such as *Microsporum audouinii*, fluoresce under ultraviolet illumination (Wood lamp).

Many skin infections are self-limiting. Persistent infections can be treated with topical tolnaftate, allylamines, or azoles. Nail-bed and extensive infections require systemic therapy with griseofulvin, itraconazole, fluconazole, or terbinafine. The azoles and terbinafine are particularly effective in the treatment of onychomycosis.

Subcutaneous mycoses

Although certain systemic fungi can produce subcutaneous manifestations, the subcutaneous mycoses described here are caused by fungi that grow in soil and on vegetation and are introduced into subcutaneous tissue through trauma. Patients can usually associate a splinter, thorn, or bite with the site of the infection. Subcutaneous mycoses occur in parts of the body that are prone to trauma, such as feet, legs, hands, and arms. The main subcutaneous mycoses are sporotrichosis, chromoblastomycosis, and mycetoma. Bacterial infections can mimic such fungal infections, and it is important to establish the etiologic agent, because most bacterial infections can be treated with antibiotics.

Most infections are chronic and are resistant to many antifungal agents. In the United States, most subcutaneous fungal infections are rare, except for lymphocutaneous sporotrichosis.

S schenckii

This dimorphic fungus is found in soil, hay, moss, and decaying vegetation. The disease is seen frequently in farmers, gardeners ("rose garden disease"), and laborers. The conidia and yeasts can bind to proteins of the extracellular matrix, including laminin, fibronectin, and collagen. Lymphocutaneous sporotrichosis is characterized by nodular and ulcerative lesions that develop along lymphatics draining the primary site of infection. The disease is treated with itraconazole. Pulmonary and systemic infections require the use of amphotericin B.

Bibliography

Centers for Disease Control and Prevention. Candidiasis. www.cdc.gov/fungal/diseases/candidiasis/index.html. Accessed 21 July 2015.

Centers for Disease Control and Prevention. Public Health Image Library. phil.cdc.gov. Accessed 4 August 2015.

Deus Filho A. Chapter 2: Coccidioidomycosis. J Bras Pneumol 2009;35:920–930.

Dorocka-Bobkowska B, Konopka K. Susceptibility of *Candida* isolates from denture-related stomatitis to antifungal agents in vitro. Int J Prosthodont 2007;20:504–506.

Engleberg NC, DiRita V, Dermody TS. Schaechter's Mechanisms of Microbial Disease. Baltimore and Philadelphia: Lippincott Williams & Wilkins, 2007.

Gow NA, van de Veerdonk FL, Brown AJ, Netea MG. *Candida albicans* morphogenesis and host defence: Discriminating invasion from colonization. Nat Rev Microbiol 2011;10:112–122.

Hardison SE, Brown GD. C-type lectin receptors orchestrate antifungal immunity. Nature Immunol 2012;13:817–822.

Huang SH, Wu CH, Chang YC, Kwon-Chung KJ, Brown RJ, Jong A. *Cryptococcus neoformans*-derived microvesicles enhance the pathogenesis of fungal brain infection. PLoS One 2012;7:e48570.

Joklik WK, Willett HP, Amos DB, Wilfert CM. Zinsser Microbiology, ed 20. Norwalk, CT: Appleton & Lange, 1992.

Levinson W. Review of Medical Microbiology and Immunology, ed 11. New York: McGraw-Hill, 2010.

Marsh PD, Martin MV. Oral Microbiology, ed 5. Edinburgh: Churchill Livingstone Elsevier, 2009.

Marx RE, Stern D. Oral and Maxillofacial Pathology: A Rationale for Diagnosis and Treatment, ed 2. Chicago: Quintessence, 2012.

Mosby's Dictionary of Medicine, Nursing and Health Professions, ed 9. Philadelphia: Mosby/Elsevier, 2012.

Murray PR, Rosenthal KS, Pfaller MA. Medical Microbiology, ed 6. Philadelphia: Mosby/Elsevier, 2009.

Ryan KJ, Ray CG. Sherris Medical Microbiology, ed 5. New York: McGraw-Hill, 2010.

Vanegas JM, Contreras MF, Faller R, Longo ML. Role of unsaturated lipid and ergosterol in ethanol tolerance of model yeast biomembranes. Biophys J 2012;102:507–516.

Take-Home Messages

- *H capsulatum, B dermatitidis, C immitis*, and *P brasiliensis* cause systemic mycoses.
- Exposure to high levels of *H capsulatum* var *capsulatum* can cause a flulike illness and severe pneumonia. Disseminated disease is rare but can cause fever, weight loss, hepatosplenomegaly, and oropharyngeal ulcers.
- *B dermatitidis* infection causes symptomatic pulmonary disease in less than half of the individuals exposed to the fungus. If it spreads, it can cause pustular, ulcerative-nodular lesions.
- *C immitis* is likely to cause the most virulent of fungal infections, with only a few arthroconidia causing primary coccidioidomycosis or San Joaquin Valley fever. It can cause disseminated disease, with manifestations in the skin, bones, joints, and meninges.
- Disseminated disease due to *P brasiliensis* can result in cutaneous and mucocutaneous ulcers, the latter mostly in the oral cavity.
- *C albicans, A fumigatus*, and *C neoformans* are the most common opportunistic fungi.
- *Candida* species can cause superficial cutaneous and mucosal disease, as well as disseminated infections of the liver, spleen, heart, kidneys, and brain.
- Pseudomembranous candidiasis involves the presence of white plaque-like lesions in the mouth.
- Acute erythematous candidiasis, also known as "antibiotic sore mouth," is seen on the dorsum of the tongue following antibiotic therapy that causes a decrease in the bacterial community and allows the overgrowth of *Candida*.
- *Candida*-associated denture stomatitis presents as redness on the mucosa apposed to dentures, especially on the palate, and is attributed to *Candida* biofilms on both the dentures and the mucosal surfaces.
- The virulence factors of *Candida* species include adherence to oral tissues and biomaterials, morphology, phenotypic switching, secreted aspartyl proteases, and phospholipases.
- Invasive pulmonary aspergillosis presents with pleuritic chest pain, dyspnea, cough, bloody cough, and fever. Disseminated *Aspergillus* infections manifest as necrotic skin lesions and brain abscesses leading to stroke or seizures.
- *C neoformans* can cause cryptococcal pneumonia and cryptococcal meningitis.
- *Pneumocystis jirovecii* was the most common opportunistic infection during the early years of HIV/AIDS. It causes pneumonia in immunocompromised individuals with T-cell deficiency.
- *M furfur, H werneckii*, and *Trichosporon* cause superficial mycoses.
- Cutaneous mycoses are caused by the dermatophytes *Microsporum, Trichophyton*, and *Epidermophyton*.
- The main subcutaneous mycoses are sporotrichosis, chromoblastomycosis, and mycetoma.

27 Antifungal Chemotherapy

Similar to antibacterial agents, antifungal agents are characterized by their antifungal spectrum, fungistatic and fungicidal activities, antifungal synergism and antagonism, and mechanisms of resistance by fungi.

The antifungal spectrum of an antifungal indicates the range of fungi that are inhibited by the agent. If an antifungal agent inhibits a large variety of fungi, including yeasts and molds, it is considered a broad-spectrum antifungal. If it inhibits a limited range of fungi, it is considered a narrow-spectrum antifungal. Antifungal drugs can be fungistatic (inhibiting the growth of fungi) or fungicidal (causing cytotoxicity in fungi). The minimum inhibitory concentration is the lowest concentration of the drug that will inhibit the growth of the microorganism in a standardized assay. The minimum fungicidal concentration is the lowest concentration of the drug that will reduce the number of organisms by 99.9% (1,000-fold) in a standardized assay. In this chapter, various antifungal agents are reviewed with respect to their cellular targets.

Cytoplasmic Membrane

The polyenes amphotericin B and nystatin form complexes with ergosterol in the fungal cell membrane and alter the permeability of the membrane (Fig 27-1). Amphotericin B can also become oxidized and initiate a cascade of oxidation reactions that damage the membrane. Amphotericin B (Fungizone, Bristol-Myers Squibb) is administered intravenously because it is not absorbed via the gastrointestinal tract. Because it can also interact with cholesterol in human cell membranes, it is relatively toxic and causes fever, chills, myalgias, hypotension, dyspnea (a sensation of uncomfortable breathing), and headache. It can cause renal dysfunction, and thus its dosage has to be titrated in each patient. AmBisome (Gilead) is a liposomal preparation of amphotericin B, and Abelcet (Sigma-Tau) is an amphotericin B–lipid complex, both of which have lower toxicity than the free drug. Treatment with amphotericin B is limited to dangerous fungal infections because of its toxicity. It has a broad spectrum of activity and is effective against *Aspergillus* species, most *Candida* species, *Cryptococcus neoformans*, *Blastomyces dermatitidis*, *Histoplasma capsulatum*, and *Coccidioides immitis*, among others.

Nystatin is structurally similar to amphotericin B, and its mechanism of action is the same. However, it is quite toxic and is used topically for the treatment of mucocutaneous, oropharyngeal, and vaginal candidiasis.

The azoles are synthetic compounds used systemically, and they are classified into imidazoles and triazoles (see Fig 27-1). They inhibit the cytochrome P450 enzyme 14α-lanosterol demethylase involved in the biosynthesis of ergosterol, a major component of the fungal membrane. This inhibition causes the accumulation of lanosterol and the disruption of the structure of the cell membrane. Ketoconazole (an imidazole), itraconazole, and fluconazole are first-generation systemic azoles. Because of its side effects and drug interactions, ketoconazole (Nizoral, Janssen) has limited clinical use and has been replaced by itraconazole. Itraconazole (Sporanox, Janssen) is lipophilic, can be given orally or intravenously, and has a broad spectrum of activity, including *Candida* species, *C neoformans*, and endemic dimorphic pathogens. Fluconazole (Diflucan, Pfizer) is used in treating *Candida*, *Cryptococcus*, and *Coccidioides* infections as well as maintenance therapy for cryptococcal meningitis in AIDS patients. Clotrimazole (Mycelex, Ortho-McNeil-Janssen) and miconazole are used topically. Miconazole is used in the treatment of oropharyngeal candidiasis and denture stomatitis.

Voriconazole (Vfend, Pfizer) is a second-generation antifungal triazole with fungistatic activity against yeasts, including *Candida*, and fungicidal activity against *Aspergillus*. It can penetrate into the central nervous system and other tissues; thus, it can be used in the treatment of *Aspergillus*-induced brain abscesses.

Allylamines inhibit squalene epoxidase, which is required for ergosterol synthesis, resulting in an increase in the mol fraction of squalene in the cytoplasmic membrane. Terbinafine (Lamisil, Novartis) is a broad-spectrum antifungal that is effective against dermatophytes, *Candida* species, *Cryptococcus*, and *Aspergillus*. Naftifine (Naftin, Merz) and butenafine (Lotrimin Ultra, Bayer) can be used in the treatment of dermatophyte infections.

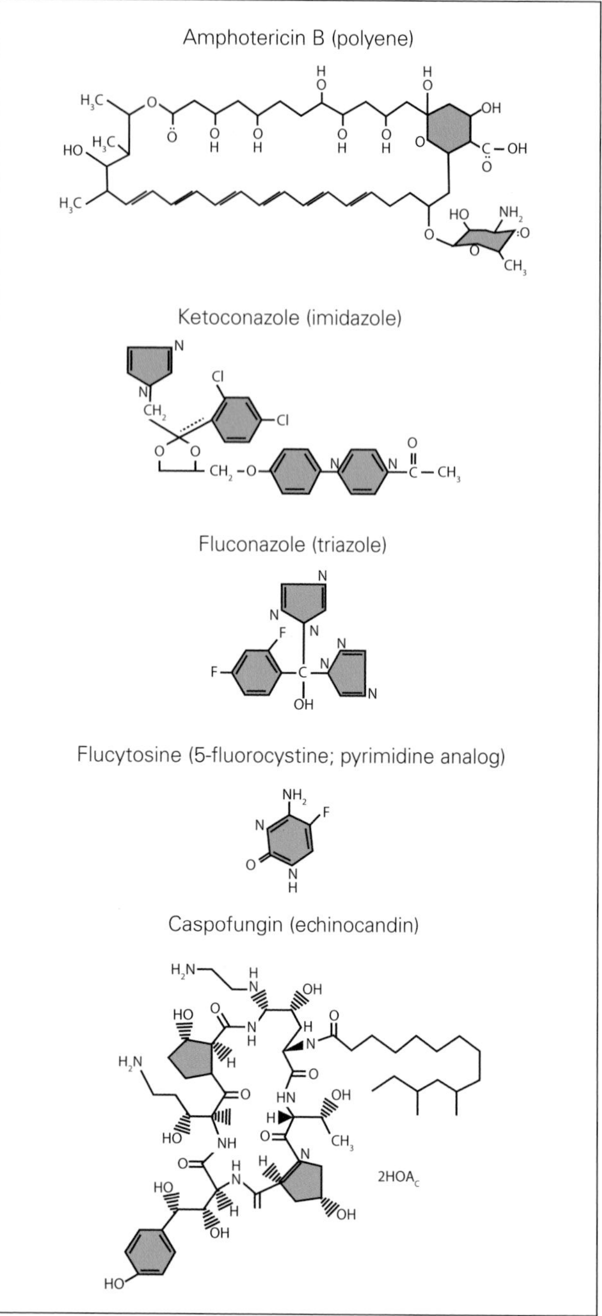

Fig 27-1 Chemical structures of representative antifungals. (Adapted from Murray et al.)

RNA and DNA Synthesis

The pyrimidine analog 5-fluorocytosine (flucytosine; Ancobon, Valeant) is used orally for the treatment of systemic infections caused by *Candida*, *Cryptococcus*, and *Aspergillus* (see Fig 27-1). It is taken up by yeast cells by the action of cytosine permease and is converted into 5-fluorouracil by cytosine deaminase. 5-fluorouracil is converted to 5-fluorouridine triphosphate, which is incorporated into fungal RNA, thereby altering the aminoacylation of tRNA and disrupting the amino acid pool and protein synthesis. It may also be converted to 5-fluorodeoxyuridine monophosphate, which inhibits thymidylate synthetase and thus DNA synthesis. It is generally used in combination with an azole. Fungi lacking cytosine deaminase or having a mutation in the enzyme are resistant to the drug. 5-fluorouracil can cause dose-related bone marrow suppression and hepatotoxicity.

Cell Wall

Echinocandins are a new class of lipopeptide antifungals that inhibit the synthesis of 1,3-β-D-glucan, resulting in the disruption of the cell wall (see Fig 27-1). Because mammalian cells do not have this molecule, these agents are highly selective in their toxicities for particular fungi that have relatively high amounts of this glucan in their cell walls, such as *Candida* and *Aspergillus*. Glucans are involved in maintaining the osmotic integrity of the fungal cell as well as in cell division and growth. Echinocandins have fungicidal activity against *Candida* species and fungistatic activity against *Aspergillus* species. They have to be administered intravenously, and they localize in the major organs. Caspofungin can be used for the treatment of invasive candidiasis and for aspergillosis that is resistant to other antifungals. Micafungin (Mycamine, Astellas) and anidulafungin (Eraxis, Pfizer) are used in the treatment of candidemia and esophageal candidiasis.

Mitosis

Griseofulvin, produced by *Penicillium griseofulvum*, is thought to interact with microtubules and inhibit mitosis. It is administered orally and used in the treatment of dermatophyte infections. It is selectively incorporated into keratin-containing tissues such as the skin, hair, and nails, interfering with dermatophyte cell division.

Combination Antifungals

A combination of antifungal agents may be useful in the treatment of fungal diseases. These drugs may be chosen based on the following considerations:

- Drugs that inhibit different stages of a metabolic pathway may ensure the inhibition of the end product, such as the cell membrane.
- One drug may cause the permeabilization of the cell membrane, enabling the cellular entry of another drug.
- A drug that inhibits the efflux pumps of the microorganism may increase the retention of an antifungal agent.
- Two drugs that affect different targets in the fungal cells are likely to be more effective, and the development of drug resistance is less likely.

Bibliography

Antachopoulos C, Katragkou A, Roilides E. Immunotherapy against invasive mold infections. Immunotherapy 2012;4:107–120.

de Groot PW, Bader O, de Boer AD, Weig M, Chauhan N. Adhesins in human fungal pathogens: Glue with plenty of stick. Eukaryot Cell 2013;12:470–481.

Dorocka-Bobkowska B, Düzgüneş N, Konopka K. AmBisome and Amphotericin B inhibit the initial adherence of Candida albicans to human epithelial cell lines, but do not cause yeast detachment. Med Sci Monit 2009;15:BR262–BR269.

Engleberg NC, DiRita V, Dermody TS. Schaechter's Mechanisms of Microbial Disease. Baltimore and Philadelphia: Lippincott Williams & Wilkins, 2007.

Mayer FL, Wilson D, Hube B. *Candida albicans* pathogenicity mechanisms. Virulence 2013;4:119–128.

Mosby's Dictionary of Medicine, Nursing and Health Professions, ed 9. Philadelphia: Mosby/Elsevier, 2012.

Murray PR, Rosenthal KS, Pfaller MA. Medical Microbiology, ed 6. Philadelphia: Mosby/Elsevier, 2009.

Ryan KJ, Ray CG. Sherris Medical Microbiology, ed 5. New York: McGraw-Hill, 2010.

Shankar J, Restrepo A, Clemons KV, Stevens DA. Hormones and the resistance of women to paracoccidioidomycosis. Clin Microbiol Rev 2011;24:296–313.

Vermes A, Guchelaar HJ, Dankert J. Flucytosine: A review of its pharmacology, clinical indications, pharmacokinetics, toxicity and drug interactions. J Antimicrob Chemother 2000;46:171–179.

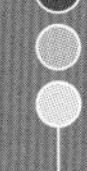

Take-Home Messages

- Amphotericin B and nystatin form complexes with ergosterol in the fungal cell membrane and alter the permeability of the membrane.
- Azoles inhibit the enzyme 14α-lanosterol demethylase involved in the biosynthesis of ergosterol.
- Allylamines inhibit squalene epoxidase, which is required for ergosterol synthesis.
- Fungal cytosine deaminase converts 5-fluorocytosine into 5-fluorouracil, which gets incorporated into RNA and disrupts protein synthesis.
- Echinocandins inhibit the synthesis of 1,3-β-D-glucan, resulting in the disruption of the cell wall.
- Griseofulvin is thought to interact with microtubules and to inhibit mitosis.

Virus Structure, Replication, and Pathogenesis

28

Viruses are obligate intracellular "parasites" in that they need the machinery of their host cell to replicate. They were originally identified as microorganisms that can pass through filters that normally retain bacteria and that can cause cytopathology in cell cultures. They were thus termed "filterable agents." Viruses are generated by the assembly of individual components encoded by viral genetic material that are synthesized in the host cell. They are either RNA or DNA viruses and normally do not contain both types of nucleic acid. Some viruses, such as the ubiquitous rhinoviruses that cause the common cold, have a protein coat, or capsid, around the nucleic acid and are described as **naked capsid viruses**. The capsid or nucleic acid–protein complexes called *nucleoproteins* may be encapsulated in a lipid bilayer membrane derived from the plasma membrane of the host cell, forming **enveloped viruses**. Herpesviruses and influenza virus are examples of enveloped viruses.

Virus Structure

Viruses range in size from 18 nm in the case of parvoviruses to about 300 nm as with poxviruses. Adenovirus is about 90 nm, and human immunodeficiency virus (HIV) is about 100 nm in diameter. Naked capsid viruses contain a DNA or RNA genome and nucleic acid binding proteins packaged in an assembly of structural proteins. Protein subunits of the capsid assemble into protomers that then form pentameric **capsomeres**. The latter then form the procapsid and eventually the complete capsid (Fig 28-1). Many naked capsid viruses are icosahedral, with 20 equilateral triangular faces and 12 vertices. In the hierarchical viral classification system of A. Lwoff, R. W. Horne, and P. Tournier proposed in 1962, RNA viruses are further classified into icosahedral and helical viruses. For example, picornaviruses are icosahedral naked capsid viruses. Tobacco mosaic virus is an example of a helical virus.

Naked capsid viruses are relatively stable at elevated temperatures, in acidic or dry conditions, and in the presence of detergents and proteases. They are released from their host cell by the lysis of the cell. They are spread readily on fomites, from hand to hand, and by small droplets. They can dry out and still retain infectivity, and they can survive in the gastrointestinal system because of their resistance to low pH and bile detergents. Antibodies are generally sufficient for protection against naked capsid virus infections.

An icosahedral or helical nucleocapsid can be surrounded by a lipid bilayer membrane containing structural (matrix) proteins and spike glycoproteins, thus forming an enveloped virus (see Fig 28-1). An example of an enveloped virus containing an icosahedral capsid is herpesvirus, whereas that containing a helical nucleocapsid is paramyxovirus (eg, mumps virus). Their shape is usually round or pleomorphic, the exceptions being rhabdoviruses and poxviruses. They are released from the cell by budding and in some cases by exocytosis or cell lysis. Enveloped viruses are relatively sensitive to environmental conditions, such as heat, drying, and the presence of solvents and detergents. Thus, they are not expected to cause infections via the gastrointestinal tract. They are spread in large droplets and secretions or by organ transplantation and blood transfusion. In general, they must stay hydrated, but some viruses such as coronaviruses can survive on dry surfaces for 1 to 3 hours; therefore, such surfaces in a hospital setting must be disinfected.

The genome size of enveloped viruses is related to the size of the envelope. The inside surface of the membrane is usually lined with the matrix proteins that confer structural strength, facilitate the assembly of the viral components at the host cell surface, and also determine the shape of the virus. Glycoproteins embedded in the viral membrane form spikes on the virus that are visible in electron micrographs; these spikes can mediate the attachment of the virus to host cell receptors for the virus or cause the agglutination of red blood cells (in which case they are termed hemagglutinins) (see Fig 28-1). Some envelope glycoproteins have neuraminidase activity, as in the case of influenza virus, and are the target of antiviral drugs such as oseltamivir (Tamiflu, Gilead). The spike proteins also act as antigens for immunity. Both antibody- and cell-mediated immunity are generally needed for protection against enveloped viruses. Enveloped viruses can cause hypersensitivity reactions and inflammation, which can be pathogenic to the host.

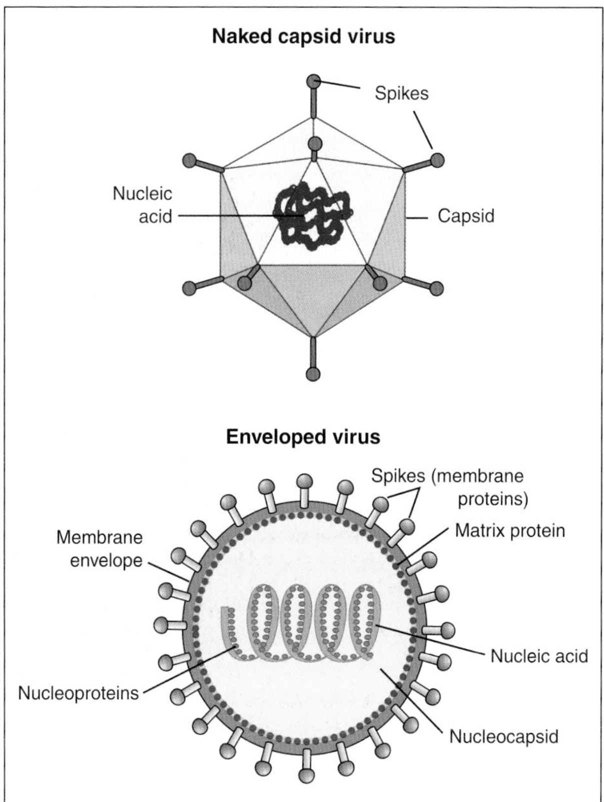

Fig 28-1 Schematic structure of naked capsid and enveloped viruses.

Virus Classification

Viruses have been named according to a variety of criteria. For example, based on the size, morphology, and nucleic acid of the virus, picornaviruses are small RNA viruses, and togaviruses have a "cloak." Some viruses are named based on the disease they cause (eg, encephalitis viruses and hepatitis viruses). Arboviruses (arthropod-borne) and respiratory viruses are named for the means of transmission. The names *adenovirus* and *enterovirus* describe the tissue tropism of these microorganisms.

There are three major classification systems for viruses. In the hierarchical system, viruses are grouped by their shared properties instead of their tissue tropism or the diseases they cause. They are classified into RNA or DNA viruses and are further divided according to capsid symmetry into icosahedral and helical viruses. The next steps of the classification are according to the presence or absence of an envelope and the structure of the genome (eg, double or single stranded). The International Committee on Taxonomy of Viruses extended the hierarchical classification system to include several orders, which contain families that in turn have subfamilies, followed by genera. A more simplified version of this system described originally in Baron's *Medical Microbiology* is shown in Table 28-1.

The Baltimore classification is based on the pathways by which families of viruses produce mRNA, which is essential for the production of viral proteins and viral replication (Fig 28-2):

- Group I: Double-stranded DNA: adenoviruses, herpesviruses, poxviruses, papillomaviruses, polyomaviruses
- Group II: Single-stranded positive-strand (sense) DNA: parvoviruses
- Group III: Double-stranded RNA: reoviruses

Table 28-1 **Classification of major groups of viruses of medical significance**

Family	Genus or subfamily	Typical member
DNA viruses		
Parvoviridae	Erythrovirus	B19 parvovirus
	Dependovirus	Adeno-associated virus 2
Papovaviridae	Papillomavirus	Human papillomavirus (HPV)
	Polyomavirus	JC and BK viruses
Adenoviridae	Mastadenovirus	Adenovirus (serotypes 1–47)
Herpesviridae	Alphaherpesvirinae	Herpes simplex virus (HSV) 1 and 2
	Varicellovirus	Varicella zoster virus (VZV)
	Gammaherpesvirinae	Epstein-Barr virus (EBV)
	Betaherpesvirinae	Cytomegalovirus (CMV)
	Roseolovirus	Human herpesvirus 6 (HHV-6)
	Betaherpesvirinae	Human herpesvirus 7 (HHV-7)
Poxviridae	Orthopoxvirus	Vaccinia virus; Variola virus (eradicated)
	Molluscipoxvirus	Molluscum contagiosum virus
Hepadnaviridae	Orthohepadnaviruses	Hepatitis B virus (HBV)
RNA viruses		
Picornaviridae	Enterovirus	Poliovirus (67 serotypes)
	Rhinovirus	Human rhinovirus (> 100 serotypes)
	Hepatovirus	Hepatitis A virus (HAV)
	Aphthovirus	Foot and mouth disease virus
Caliciviridae	Calicivirus	Norwalk virus; Hepatitis E virus (HEV)
Astroviridae	Astrovirus	Human astrovirus (7 serotypes)
Togaviridae	Alphavirus	Eastern equine encephalitis virus
	Rubivirus	Rubella virus
Flaviviridae	Flavivirus	Yellow fever virus; Dengue virus
	Hepatitis C viruses	Hepatitis C virus (HCV)
Reoviridae	Reovirus	Reovirus
	Orbivirus	Colorado tick fever virus
	Rotavirus	Human rotavirus (groups A, B, C)
Orthomyxoviridae	Influenza virus A, B	Influenza A and B viruses
	Influenza virus C	Influenza C virus
Paramyxoviridae	Paramyxovirus	Newcastle disease virus; Parainfluenza virus
	Morbilivirus	Measles virus
	Rubulavirus	Mumps virus
	Pneumovirus	Respiratory syncytial virus (RSV)
Rhabdoviridae	Vesiculovirus	Vesicular stomatitis virus; Chandipura virus
	Lyssavirus	Rabies virus
Bunyaviridae	Bunyavirus	La Crosse virus
	Hantavirus	Hantaan virus; Puumula virus
	Nairovirus	Crimean-Congo hemorrhagic fever virus
	Phlebovirus	Rift Valley fever virus; Uukuniemi virus
Coronaviridae	Coronavirus	SARS coronavirus
Arenaviridae	Arenavirus	Lassa virus

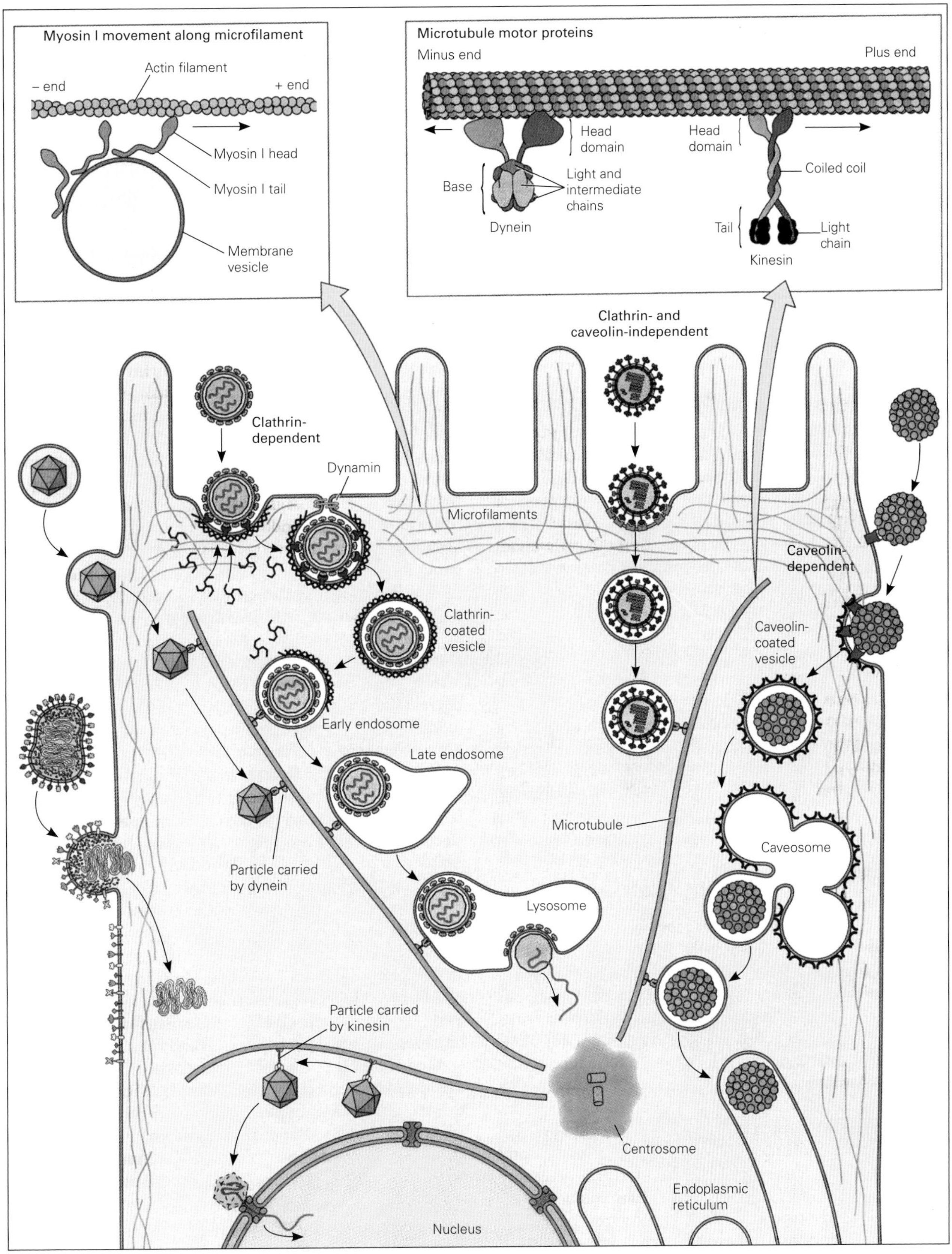

Myosin I movement along microfilament
Actin filament
– end
+ end
Myosin I head
Myosin I tail
Membrane vesicle

Microtubule motor proteins
Minus end
Plus end
Head domain
Base
Light and intermediate chains
Dynein
Head domain
Coiled coil
Tail
Light chain
Kinesin

Clathrin- and caveolin-independent
Clathrin-dependent
Dynamin
Microfilaments
Caveolin-dependent
Clathrin-coated vesicle
Caveolin-coated vesicle
Early endosome
Late endosome
Particle carried by dynein
Microtubule
Caveosome
Lysosome
Particle carried by kinesin
Centrosome
Endoplasmic reticulum
Nucleus

Fig 28-4 Mechanisms of cellular entry of viruses and their intracellular movement. (Reprinted with permission from Flint et al.)

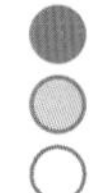

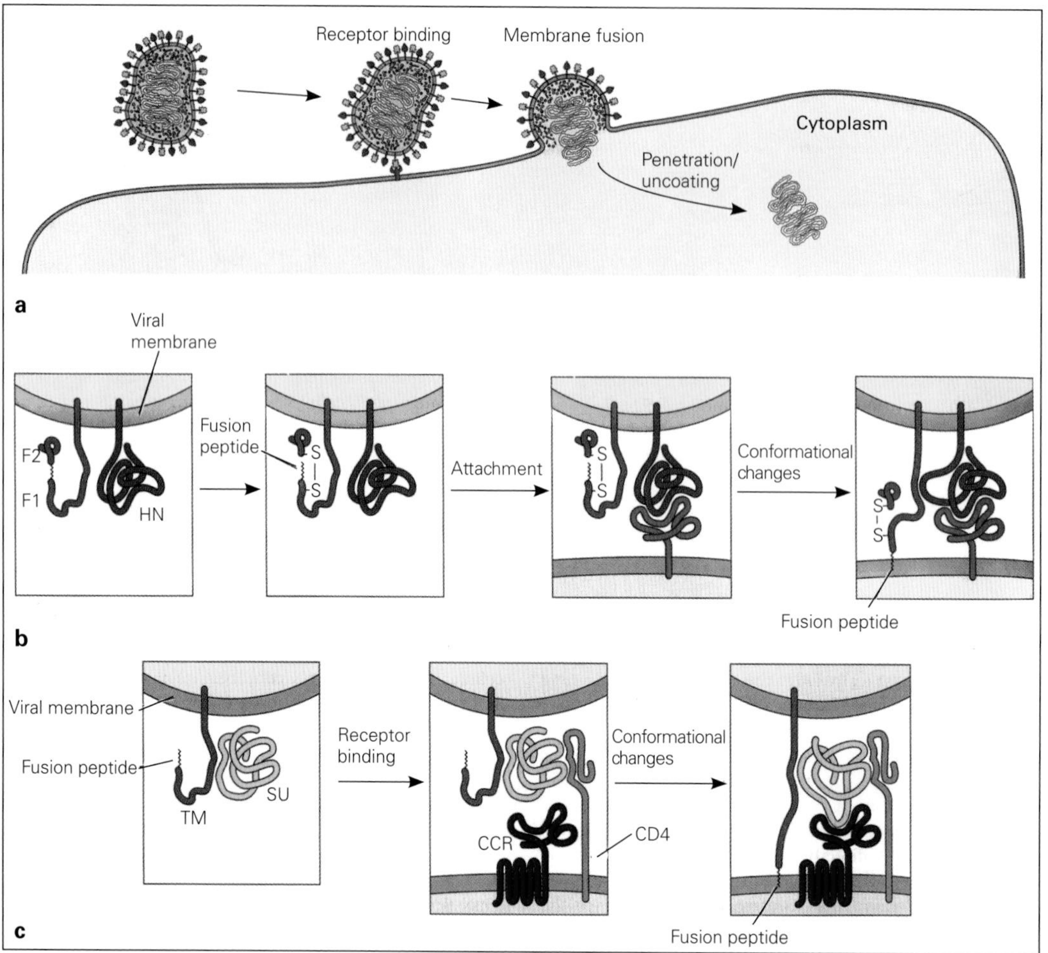

Fig 28-5 Mechanisms of entry of paramyxoviruses and HIV by fusion at the plasma membrane. *(a)* Paramyxoviruses bind to cell surface receptors via their HN (parainfluenza virus), H (measles virus), or G (respiratory syncytial virus) glycoproteins. The fusion protein, F, mediates the fusion reaction at neutral pH, and the viral ribonucleoprotein is released into the cytoplasm. *(b)* Molecular mechanism of membrane fusion induced by the F protein. The F protein is composed of two subunits that are produced by the cleavage of the precursor F0 protein by a cellular protease, exposing the N-terminal hydrophobic fusion peptide of the F1 subunit. The fusion peptide is hidden between the proteins of the trimeric structure of the F proteins. Binding of the HN to the cellular receptor (shown in *red*), induces a conformational change of the F protein, resulting in the insertion of the fusion peptide into the host membrane and eventual merging of the viral and cellular membranes. *(c)* Molecular mechanism of the involvement of chemokine receptors (CCR) in HIV fusion with the host cell membrane. TM (gp41) and SU (gp120) are the transmembrane and surface protein components of HIV Env, respectively. Binding of SU to the primary cellular receptor, CD4, leads to the exposure of an SU site with high affinity for the CCR co-receptor. This in turn results in a conformational change in TM that causes the insertion of the hydrophobic N-terminal peptide of TM into the host membrane, facilitating membrane fusion. (Reprinted with permission from Flint et al.)

Viral assembly is carried out by specific interactions between proteins, between proteins and nucleic acids, and between proteins and the cell membrane. With the exception of poxviruses, DNA viruses assemble in the nucleus. The protein components of DNA viruses must have basic amino acid sequences to facilitate nuclear localization. RNA viruses and poxviruses are assembled in the cytoplasm. The assembly process is not perfect, and errors can lead to the formation of virions that do not have all the components necessary for infection and replication. These virions are known as *defective interfering particles* because they can compete with infectious virions for binding sites on potential host cells.

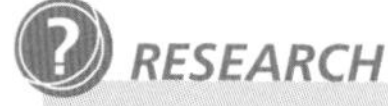

How can you assess how many defective interfering particles there are in a suspension of virions?

Viral Pathogenesis

Following transmission of the virus to the new host, the virus infects the cells that have receptors for the virus. The infection can take various forms. In lytic infections, virus multiplication in the host cell results in the lysis of the cell and the release of the newly synthesized virions. In persistent infections, the virus survives in the host cell by synthesizing a small number of virions that do not kill the cell. Viral entry can be followed by a latent infection where the viral genome is maintained in the cell, for example, as an unintegrated episome in the host nucleus (as in herpesvirus infections), and no virions are produced. The viral genome may be activated at a later time point to produce new virions that may result in cytopathology. Infections are said to be abortive when they do not result in the production of virions and there is no harmful effect on the cell. Some viruses can transform the host cell into a cancer cell that can divide without the regular control mechanisms in a normal cell.

Viral infections can cause acute infections or different types of persistent infections. The common cold, caused by rhinoviruses, coronaviruses, some adenoviruses, and influenza C virus, is an acute infection, where viral infection is followed by the disease episode and then the virus is eliminated. Measles virus infection is an example of an acute infection that can sometimes result years later in a complication called *subacute sclerosing panencephalitis*. After causing chickenpox, varicella zoster virus becomes latent in nerve cells and can be activated a long time later by stress, manifesting itself as zoster. Hepatitis B virus causes chronic infection, with constant shedding of the virus from infected cells following an initial disease episode.

Viruses can cause cytopathology by various mechanisms. Poliovirus and herpes simplex virus inhibit the synthesis of cellular proteins. Enveloped viruses alter the structure of the cell membrane as they are budding from it and by inserting their glycoproteins into the membrane. Enveloped viruses like paramyxoviruses, herpesviruses, and HIV can cause polykaryon (syncytium) formation. Syncytium formation may enable viral spread from cell to cell and may enable the virus to escape detection by antibodies. Herpesviruses inhibit the synthesis of cellular DNA. Herpes simplex virus and naked capsid viruses can disrupt cytoskeletal structure. Cell membrane permeability is altered by togaviruses and herpesviruses.

Viruses can generate intracellular inclusion bodies that may arise from altered membrane or chromosomal structures or may be a conglomeration of viral capsids synthesized in the cell. Rabies virus–infected cells develop Negri bodies in the cytoplasm, and cytomegalovirus infection results in owl's eye inclusion bodies in the nucleus. Basophilic (having an affinity for basic dyes) nuclear inclusion bodies are formed by adenoviruses, and acidophilic (having an affinity for acidic dyes) cytoplasmic inclusion bodies are formed by poxviruses.

Oncogenic viruses include some DNA viruses and retroviruses that transform or immortalize the infected cells, increasing the cell growth rate and causing the loss of contact-inhibition of growth, removing growth suppressor molecules in the cell, and altering cellular morphology. For example, adenovirus proteins E1A and E1B bind to and inhibit the function of the retinoblastoma gene product (RB) and the "tumor suppressor" protein p53, respectively. This results in the enhancement of cell proliferation by cytokines, hormones, transcriptional activators, and proto-oncogenes (a set of cellular genes that cause normal cells to become cancerous when they undergo mutations). A similar effect is observed in human papillomavirus–infected cells, where viral E6 and E7 proteins inactivate p53 and RB, respectively. Inactivation of p53 prevents the growth arrest and apoptosis (programmed cell death) of the infected cells when DNA is damaged, because p53 is involved in DNA repair. Epstein-Barr virus acts as a B-cell mitogen, stimulating cell division, and induces the *bcl-2* oncogene of the cells that acts as an inhibitor of apoptosis, thus facilitating uncontrolled growth. Human T-cell lymphotropic virus type 1 (HTLV-1) is a retrovirus that transactivates via its Tax protein the expression of genes, such as that for the cytokine interleukin-2 (IL-2), which stimulates the growth of lymphocytes. Hepatitis B virus, hepatitis C virus, and human herpesvirus 8 (HHV8) are also oncogenic viruses.

Antiviral immunity can cause some of the pathologic symptoms of viral infection (viral immunopathogenesis). Induction of interferon-α and cytokines can cause flulike symptoms including fever, headache, and malaise that are common in respiratory viral infections. Cell-mediated immunity is induced as a result of viral infection and can cause serious immunopathology, especially in the case of enveloped viruses such as measles and mumps viruses. T cell–mediated hypersensitivity reactions and inflammation result in the classical symptoms of infection by these viruses. Infection by hepatitis B virus can result in the presence of large amounts of viral antigen in the blood that can then form complexes with antivirus antibodies, with the ensuing activation of the complement system and tissue damage (Type III hypersensitivity). Hemorrhagic diseases caused by yellow fever and dengue viruses are caused by the immune system primed from a previous infection and highly activated by a subsequent exposure.

Bibliography

Baron S. Medical Microbiology, ed 4. Galveston, TX: University of Texas Medical Branch at Galveston, 1996.

Düzgüneş N (ed). Mechanisms and Specificity of HIV Entry into Host Cells. New York: Plenum, 1991.

Düzgüneş N. Molecular mechanisms of membrane fusion. In: Pedroso de Lima MC, Düzgüneş N, Hoekstra D (eds). Trafficking of Intracellular Membranes: From Molecular Sorting to Membrane Fusion. Berlin: Springer Verlag, 1995:97–129.

Düzgüneş N, Shavnin SA. Membrane destabilization by N-terminal peptides of viral envelope proteins. J Membrane Biol 1992;128:71–80.

Flint SJ, Enquist LW, Racaniello VR, Skalka AM. Principles of Virology, ed 3. Washington, DC: ASM, 2009.

Hogle JM. Poliovirus cell entry: Common structural themes in viral cells entry pathways. Annu Rev Microbiol 2002;56:677–702.

Murray PR, Rosenthal KS, Pfaller MA. Medical Microbiology, ed 6. Philadelphia: Mosby/Elsevier, 2009.

Rockefeller University. Destroying Dogma: The Discovery of Reverse Transcriptase. Centennial.rucares.org/index.php?page=Destroying_Dogma. Accessed 23 July 2015.

Ryan KJ, Ray CG Sherris Medical Microbiology, ed 5. New York: McGraw-Hill, 2010.

Strauss JH, Strauss EG. Viruses and Human Disease, ed 2. Burlington, MA: Academic, 2008.

Swiss Institute of Bioinformatics. ViralZone. viralzone.expasy.org/all_by_species/254.html. Accessed 23 July 2015.

Take-Home Messages

- Naked capsid viruses are relatively stable at elevated temperatures, in acidic or dry conditions, and in the presence of detergents and proteases.
- Naked capsid viruses are released from their host cell by the lysis of the cell.
- Enveloped viruses are relatively sensitive to environmental conditions, such as heat, drying, and the presence of solvents and detergents.
- Enveloped viruses are released from the cell by budding and in some cases by exocytosis or cell lysis.
- The spike proteins of enveloped viruses act as antigens for immunity.
- The Baltimore classification of viruses is based on the pathways by which families of viruses produce mRNA.
- The early phase of virus replication comprises attachment, penetration, and uncoating. The late phase consists of macromolecular synthesis, viral assembly, and release.
- The early gene products during the macromolecular synthesis stage of DNA viruses are DNA-binding proteins and enzymes that facilitate the production of viral macromolecules.
- The late gene products are the structural proteins of the viruses.
- In positive-strand RNA viruses, the genetic material acts as mRNA, which binds ribosomes and is translated into viral proteins.
- In negative-strand RNA viruses, the RNA is first transcribed into mRNA via the RNA-dependent RNA polymerase.
- Viruses can cause lytic, persistent, or latent infections.
- Viruses can cause cytopathology by various mechanisms, including syncytium formation and the inhibition of cellular protein synthesis.
- Oncogenic viruses transform or immortalize the infected cells.
- In human papillomavirus–infected cells, viral E6 inactivates the cellular tumor suppressor protein p53, and E7 inactivates the retinoblastoma protein RB.
- Viral induction of interferon-α and cytokines in the host can cause flulike symptoms. Induction of cell-mediated immunity can cause serious immunopathology, especially in the case of enveloped viruses.

29 Antiviral Chemotherapy

Because viruses utilize the host cell machinery to replicate, the discovery of antiviral agents has been much slower than that of antibacterial drugs. Two of the earliest antiviral agents that came into use in the 1960s were idoxuridine for the treatment of herpetic keratitis and methisazone for the prophylaxis of smallpox in persons in contact with smallpox-infected patients and the treatment of the infective complications of smallpox vaccination. Idoxuridine has now been replaced by acyclovir.

Targets for Antiviral Drugs

Attachment

Viral attachment to cell surface receptors can be blocked by neutralizing antibodies and receptor antagonists. Passive immunization is the oldest form of antiviral therapy. Recombinant soluble CD4 (rsCD4) was shown to inhibit infection by laboratory isolates of human immunodeficiency virus type 1 (HIV-1). Later studies, however, showed that primary isolates of HIV-1 obtained from patients were not inhibited by rsCD4 or required very high concentrations of the molecule to prevent viral entry into host cells. Other receptor antagonists include dextran sulfate in the case of HIV-1 and herpes simplex virus (HSV) and peptide analogs of HIV-1 co-receptors such as CXCR5-derived peptides (maraviroc; Selzentry, Pfizer).

Penetration and uncoating

Amantadine and rimantadine inhibit the uncoating of influenza A and also inhibit the assembly of functional virions by facilitating the irreversible conformational change of the hemagglutinin. Tromantadine inhibits HSV penetration. Peptide T20 (enfuvirtide; Fuzeon, Trimeris/Roche) inhibits HIV fusion with the cell membrane. Pleconaril fits into the receptor-binding canyon of the picornavirus capsid and prevents capsid disassembly.

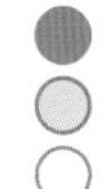

RNA synthesis

Ribavirin inhibits nucleoside biosynthesis and mRNA capping. It also promotes hypermutation. Ribavirin is used against respiratory syncytial virus and hepatitis C virus (HCV) infections. Interferon-α and interferon inducers inhibit mRNA synthesis. Interferon-α coupled to poly(ethylene glycol) to increase its circulation time in blood is used in the treatment of hepatitis B virus (HBV) and HCV infections. Antisense oligonucleotides are used in the inhibition of cytomegalovirus (CMV) retinitis.

Viral DNA polymerases

Viral DNA polymerases are a prime target for many antiviral drugs because they are essential for viral replication and are different from host enzymes. Nucleoside analogs that cause DNA chain termination because of their modified sugar residue include acyclovir and ganciclovir. Zidovudine, dideoxycytidine, and dideoxyinosine also have modified sugar groups and are inhibitors of RNA-dependent DNA polymerase (reverse transcriptase). Nucleoside analogs that alter recognition and base pairing because of a modified nucleoside base include 5'-iododeoxyuridine and trifluridine. Phosphonoformate (foscarnet) binds to the pyrophosphate binding site of DNA polymerase and is effective against herpesviruses (CMV, HSV-1, and HSV-2).

Post-translational modification of proteins

Viral proteases are essential to the assembly of certain viruses, such as HIV-1. They cleave polyproteins translated from large mRNAs into individual functional proteins. The first HIV-1 protease inhibitors were saquinavir, ritonavir, and indinavir.

Neuraminidase

The neuraminidase (sialidase) enzyme of influenza virus is essential for viral release from host cells. Zanamivir (Relenza, GlaxoSmithKline) and oseltamivir (Tamiflu, Gilead) are inhibitors of neuraminidase.

Viral envelope

Detergent-like compounds, such as nonoxynol-9, can disrupt the envelope of HIV and HSV. Antibodies directed against the viral envelope proteins can neutralize the virus and facilitate its clearance by macrophages via their Fc receptors. Such passive immunization is used for post-exposure prophylaxis of rabies, hepatitis A, and hepatitis B viruses.

Antiviral Agents

Nucleoside analogs

One of the important aspects of acyclovir (acylguanosine; Zovirax, GlaxoSmithKline) has been the demonstration that a compound could prevent the DNA replication of a DNA virus at concentrations much lower than those that affect cellular DNA synthesis. This observation paved the way for the synthesis of many antiviral drugs that were available when HIV emerged in the 1980s, as well as other drugs afterward.

Acyclovir is a prodrug that is activated by monophosphorylation through the action of virally encoded thymidine kinase (TK) (Fig 29-1). There is no initial phosphorylation in uninfected cells; thus, no active drug is produced to inhibit cellular DNA synthesis or cause cytotoxicity. The activity of acyclovir correlates with the capacity of the particular herpesvirus to produce TK and decreases in the sequence HSV-1 & HSV-2 > Epstein-Barr virus (EBV) = varicella zoster virus (VZV) >> CMV. The monophosphorylated acyclovir is then triphosphorylated by cellular TKs. This compound is then incorporated into viral (or cellular) DNA and causes chain termination. Further antiviral specificity of acyclovir is caused by the viral DNA polymerase being more sensitive than cellular polymerases to acyclovir triphosphate. In addition, viral DNA polymerase, but not the cellular polymerase, is inactivated by acyclovir triphosphate.

Resistance to acyclovir develops upon mutation of TK, such that activation of acyclovir cannot occur, and mutation of DNA polymerase, thus preventing drug binding.

Valacyclovir (Valtrex, GlaxoSmithKline) is a derivative of acyclovir that is absorbed more efficiently after oral administration. It is converted into acyclovir, thus increasing the bioavailability of the drug for the treatment of HSV and serious VZV infections, whose treatment requires higher concentrations of the drug. Penciclovir persists inside cells to a greater extent than acyclovir and inhibits VZV and HSV in a manner similar to acyclovir. Famciclovir (Famvir, Novartis) is a prodrug of penciclovir that is better absorbed orally; it is then converted to the active drug in the liver or intestinal lining.

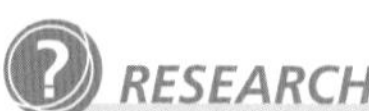

What are the molecular structures of valacyclovir, penciclovir, and famciclovir?

Ganciclovir (9-[1,3-dihydroxy-2-propoxymethyl]guanine; Cytovene, Genentech) differs from acyclovir by the presence of a hydroxymethyl group. It is phosphorylated to a greater degree than acyclovir in CMV-infected cells. The viral DNA polymerase has a 30-fold greater affinity to ganciclovir than cellular DNA polymerase. It is effective in treatment of CMV retinitis, but it has the potential to cause bone marrow toxicity.

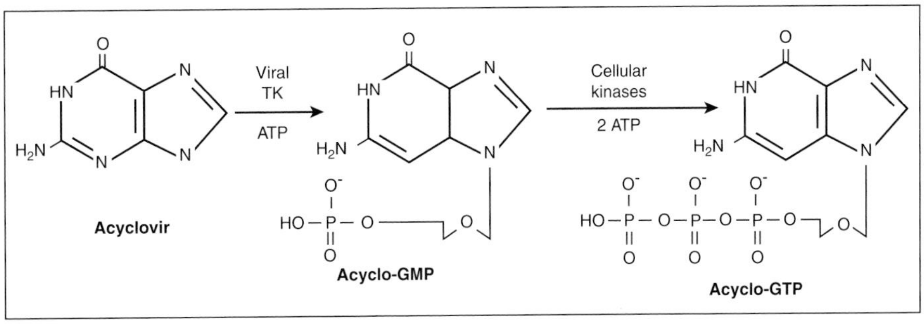

Fig 29-1 The phosphorylation of acyclovir. The drug is monophosphorylated by viral TK and di- and triphosphorylated by cellular kinases, resulting in the formation of acycloguanosine triphosphate (acyclo-GTP). (Adapted from Murray et al.)

Acyclovir
Viral TK
ATP
Acyclo-GMP
Cellular kinases
2 ATP
Acyclo-GTP

Ganciclovir is being used in suicide gene therapy applications. A replication-deficient adenovirus encoding HSV TK (HSV-*tk*) ("Cerepro" or "sitimagene ceradenovec") is delivered to the wound bed of a resected brain tumor (glioblastoma). Tumor cells encoding TK are susceptible to ganciclovir. Early studies have indicated an increase in the mean survival time of 18 to 30 weeks. Unfortunately, larger clinical trials have not shown significant efficacy in this experimental approach.

Entecavir (Baraclude, Bristol-Myers Squibb) is a novel deoxyguanosine derivative cleared for the treatment of HBV infection. It inhibits reverse transcription, DNA replication, and transcription.

Azidothymidine (AZT, zidovudine; Retrovir, GlaxoSmithKline) was the first antiviral used against HIV-1 (Fig 29-2). It needs to be phosphorylated after entering cells. It inhibits reverse transcriptase by inhibiting chain elongation, because the 3′-OH on deoxyribose is replaced with an azido group. Host cell DNA polymerase is about 100 times less sensitive to AZT-triphosphate than reverse transcriptase. AZT treatment of pregnant HIV-infected women can prevent the transmission of the virus to the baby. However, the babies must not be breastfed, because the virus can still be transmitted by this route.

Dideoxyinosine (didanosine; Videx, Bristol-Myers Squibb), dideoxycytidine (zalcitabine; Hivid, Roche), d4T (stavudine), and lamivudine (3TC; Epivir, GlaxoSmithKline) are used in treating HIV-1 infections. Lamivudine (Epivir-HBV) in conjunction with interferon-α is also used for the treatment of HBV infections. Epivir as well as the other nucleoside analog drugs can cause severe liver toxicity.

Ribavirin (Virazole, Valeant) inhibits the synthesis of guanine nucleotides and 5′-capping of viral mRNA. Ribavirin triphosphate inhibits RNA polymerases. It is administered in aerosol form for the treatment of children with severe respiratory syncytial virus bronchopneumonia. In oral or intravenous form, it may be useful for the treatment of other viral diseases, including influenza, measles, Lassa fever, Rift Valley fever, and various hemorrhagic fevers. It is cleared for the therapy of HCV in combination with interferon-α.

The thymidine analogs idoxuridine, trifluorothymidine, and fluorouracil inhibit thymidine biosynthesis or get incorporated into the viral DNA in place of thymidine, causing misreading of the viral genome, mutations, and viral inactivation. HSV-infected cells that are undergoing DNA replication are affected preferentially by these drugs. Trifluridine is currently preferred over idoxuridine, which was the first cleared antiherpes drug. Fluorouracil is cytotoxic to rapidly dividing cancer cells and also effective against human papillomaviruses.

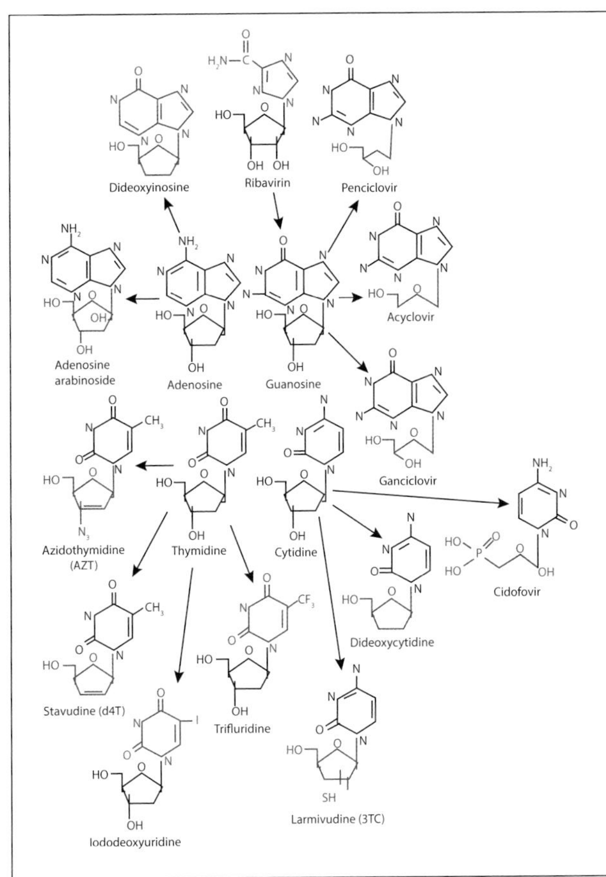

Fig 29-2 Nucleoside analog antiviral drugs. (Reprinted from Murray et al.)

Cidofovir (Vistide, Gilead) is one of the phosphonyl methylester acyclic nucleoside analogs that inhibit viral DNA polymerase (see Fig 29-2). Because it is already phosphorylated, it does not have to be monophosphorylated after entry into a cell. It is cleared for treatment of CMV retinitis in AIDS patients. It is currently being studied for potential emergency treatment of smallpox. It is also effective against herpesviruses, polyomavirus, papillomavirus, and adenoviruses. Because cidofovir is nephrotoxic, patients must be monitored for renal failure.

Adefovir dipivoxil is a prodrug of adefovir, which is a nucleotide analog of adenosine, and mediates chain termination of HBV DNA.

Non-nucleoside analog DNA polymerase inhibitors

Phosphonoformic acid (foscarnet) and phosphonoacetic acid inhibit viral replication by binding to the site on DNA polymerase that binds the pyrophosphate moiety of nucleotides, thereby blocking nucleotide binding. Phosphonoformic acid also inhibits HIV reverse transcriptase but is only used in the treatment of CMV retinitis in AIDS patients.

The non-nucleoside reverse transcriptase inhibitors nevirapine, delavirdine, and efavirenz do not bind to the active site of the enzyme but rather to a different site. The mechanism of resistance of these inhibitors is different from that of nucleoside inhibitors that bind to the active site. Therefore, they are used in combination with nucleoside analogs to prevent the emergence of drug resistance.

Protease inhibitors

Retroviral protease is used by lentiviruses to process, or cleave, the polyprotein precursor into the individual viral proteins (Fig 29-3).

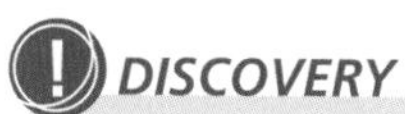

DISCOVERY

To guide the rational design of drugs against the protease, it was necessary to determine the three-dimensional structure of the enzyme. Initial attempts to clone the protein in bacteria were not successful, and the virions contained too little protease to be useful. Instead, in the late 1980s and early 1990s, scientists at NCI-Frederick, including Alexander Wlodawer, Maria Miller, and colleagues, pursued the alternative of total protein chemical synthesis. The first accurate structure of the protease and the first co-crystal structure of its complex with an inhibitor, an isostere hexapeptide called MVT-101, were determined using the synthesized protein. The molecular coordinates of the crystal structure were made available to other scientists who used them to solve the x-ray structures of the enzyme complexes with a large number of potential inhibitors that mimicked the tripeptide in the protease active site.

The first inhibitor of the HIV protease, saquinavir (Invirase, Roche), was cleared in 1995. This was followed by indinavir (Crixivan, Merck) and ritonavir (Norvir, Abbott) in 1996. Subsequently developed protease inhibitors include nelfinavir (Viracept, Agouron), amprenavir (Agenerase, Vertex; Prozei, Kissei), lopinavir + ritonavir (Kaletra, Abbott; Aluvia, Abbott), fosamprenavir (Lexiva/Telzir, GlaxoSmith-

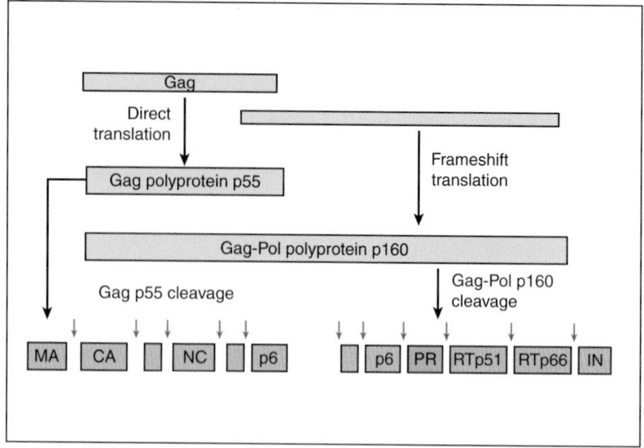

Fig 29-3 The Gag and Gag-Pol polyproteins of HIV-1 and the protease cleavage sites *(red arrows)* producing the individual proteins. MA, p17 matrix protein; CA, p24 capsid protein; NC, p9 nucleocapsid; PR, p11 protease; RT, p51 and p66 reverse transcriptase; IN, p31 integrase. (Adapted from Bioafrica HIV bioinformatics in Africa; www.bioafrica.net/proteomics/proteasesites.gif.)

Kline), atazanavir (Reyataz, Bristol-Myers Squibb/Novartis; Zrivada, Bristol-Myers Squibb/Novartis), tipranavir (Aptivus, Boehringer Ingelheim), and darunavir (Prezista, Tibotec). Protease inhibitors may cause hepatotoxicity and inhibit the P450 enzyme, causing drug-drug interactions. Ritonavir and saquinavir inhibit the chymotrypsin-like activity of the proteasome and block the formation and presentation of peptides by major histocompatibility complex class I proteins to cytotoxic T cells.

Highly active antiretroviral therapy (HAART) uses a combination of nucleoside reverse transcriptase inhibitors, non-nucleoside reverse transcriptase inhibitors, and protease inhibitors. The particular combination and dose depend on the pattern of drug resistance in the strain(s) of HIV-1 in the patient. Some of the potential problems with HAART include intolerable side effects and the inability to metabolize drugs in patients co-infected with hepatitis C.

Inhibitors of the hepatitis C virus proteases have been developed recently. Simepravir (Olysio, Janssen) inhibits the NS3/4A protease, and ABT-450 (Paritaprevir, Enanta) inhibits the NS3 protease.

Influenza virus inhibitors

Amantadine (Symmetrel, Endo) and rimantadine (Flumadine, Forest) inhibit influenza A virus infection by two distinct mechanisms: *(1)* They buffer the pH of endosomes, thereby inhibiting virus-endosome membrane fusion and uncoating. *(2)* At lower concentrations, they block the channel formed by the matrix M2 protein. If influenza hemagglutinin encounters a low pH environment during viral biosynthesis, it is expected to undergo an irreversible conformational change and denaturation. Normally, the M2 channel prevents the acidification of Golgi bodies and other cytoplasmic vesicles, allowing the transport of newly synthesized intact hemagglutinins to the cell surface. Blocking the M2 channel results in the denaturation of the hemagglutinin and inactivation of the virus.

Amantadine and rimantadine have to be taken within 48 hours of exposure to influenza A virus. Since 2001, however, the number of drug-resistant strains has increased sharply, thus obviating the use of these antivirals. Nevertheless, the improvement of the symptoms of a Parkinson's disease patient receiving amantadine for influenza virus has led to further studies and to the use of this drug as an alternative therapy for this condition.

Zanamivir (Relenza) and oseltamivir (Tamiflu) inhibit the neuraminidase of influenza A and B viruses. Zanamivir is an inhalation drug, while oseltamivir is administered orally. Neuraminidase normally cleaves sialic acid (neuraminic acid) residues on the surface of the infected cells, thereby allowing the virus to be released. When this enzyme is inhibited, the hemagglutinin of the virus binds to the cell surface sialic acid and cannot be released, thereby preventing the infection of new cells.

Antisense oligonucleotides

Fomivirsen (Vitravene, Isis) is the first antisense-based therapeutic product for use in human medicine. It is complementary to a segment of the CMV mRNA and is employed in the treatment of CMV retinitis in patients who have failed other therapies. To enable its proper localization to infected cells, it is delivered via intravitreal injection. Antisense oligonucleotides against HIV can be effective if delivered efficiently into infected macrophages.

Interferon

Interferon-α induces cellular enzymes that interfere with viral protein synthesis. It is active against hepatitis C when given in the PEGylated form together with ribavirin. It has also been cleared for the treatment of genital warts associated with human papillomavirus, via direct injection. It prevents Ebola virus infection in experimental animals if administered early. However, the virus can interfere with the signal transduction involved in the expression of interferon-responsive proteins.

A summary of antiviral agents is given in Table 29-1.

Table 29-1 Antiviral agents, their mechanisms of action, and their applications

Mechanism of action	Antiviral agent	Viral spectrum
Inhibition of viral uncoating	Amantadine	Influenza A
	Rimantadine	Influenza A
Neuraminidase inhibition	Oseltamivir	Influenza A, B
	Zanamivir	Influenza A, B
Inhibition of viral DNA polymerase	Acyclovir	HSV, VZV
	Famciclovir	HSV, VZV
	Penciclovir	HSV
	Valacyclovir	HSV, VZV
	Ganciclovir	CMV, HSV, VZV
	Foscarnet	CMV, resistant HSV
	Cidofovir	CMV, adenovirus?
	Trifluridine	HSV, VZV
Inhibition of viral entry/fusion	Maraviroc	HIV-1
	Enfuvirtide	HIV-1
Inhibition of reverse transcriptase	Zidovudine	HIV-1
	Dideoxyinosine	HIV-1
	Dideoxycytidine	HIV-1
	Stavudine	HIV-1
	Lamivudine	HIV-1, HBV*
	Nevirapine	HIV-1
	Delavirdine	HIV-1
	Efavirenz	HIV-1
Inhibition of viral DNA integration	Raltegravir	HIV-1
Inhibition of viral protease	Saquinavir	HIV-1
	Indinavir	HIV-1
	Ritonavir	HIV-1
	Nelfinavir	HIV-1
	Lopinavir	HIV-1
	Darunavir	HIV-1
Inhibition of viral RNA polymerase	Ribavirin	RSV, HCV,* Lassa fever
Antisense inhibition of viral mRNA	Fomivirsen	CMV
Inhibition of viral protein synthesis	Interferon-α	HBV, HCV, HPV

HPV, human papillomavirus; RSV, respiratory syncytial virus.
*Used in combination with interferon-α.
(Adapted from Ryan and Ray.)

Resistance to Antiviral Agents

Viral replication, especially that of RNA viruses, is replete with errors, and there is no RNA repair mechanism available to correct errors in replication. Higher rates of replication, as in HIV-1, HBV, and HCV, result in higher rates of mutations. CMV and VZV do not replicate as fast. Selective pressure of the antiviral agent may increase the probability of mutations arising to such an extent that viral replication is diminished. The rate of mutation is generally higher in single-stranded RNA viruses, such as HIV-1 and influenza, than in double-stranded DNA viruses, including HSV. The rates of mutation may differ in different viral genes. The rate of mutation in genes involved in phosphorylating nucleosides (such as the UL97 gene in CMV) tends to be higher than that in the genes for viral DNA polymerase.

Bibliography

Bauer DJ. A history of the discovery and clinical application of antiviral drugs. Br Med Bull 1985;41:309–314.

Cheng YC, Huang ES, Lin JC, et al. Unique spectrum of activity of 9-[(1,3-dihydroxy-2-propoxy)methyl]-guanine against herpesviruses in vitro and its mode of action against herpes simplex virus type 1. Proc Natl Acad Sci USA 1983;80:2767–2770.

De Clercq E. The design of drugs for HIV and HCV. Nat Rev Drug Discov 2007;6:1001–1018.

De Clercq E. The nucleoside reverse transcriptase inhibitors, nonnucleoside reverse transcriptase inhibitors, and protease inhibitors in the treatment of HIV infections (AIDS). Adv Pharmacol 2013;67: 317–358.

Düzgüneş N. Sitimagene ceradenovec, a gene therapeutic for the treatment of glioma. Curr Opin Mol Ther 2008;10:187–195.

Düzgüneş N, Simões S, Slepushkin V, et al. Enhanced inhibition of HIV-1 replication in macrophages by antisense oligonucleotides, ribozymes and acyclic nucleoside phosphonate analogs delivered in pH-sensitive liposomes. Nucleosides Nucleotides Nucleic Acids 2001;20:515–523.

Elion GB. Acyclovir: Discovery, mechanism of action, and selectivity. J Med Virol Suppl 1993;1:2–6.

Ghosh AK, Pretzer E, Cho H, Hussain KA, Düzgüneş N. Antiviral activity of UIC-PI, a novel inhibitor of the human immunodeficiency virus type 1 protease. Antiviral Res 2002;54:29–36.

Greenwood D, Barer M, Slack R, Irving W. Medical Microbiology, ed 18. Edinburgh: Churchill Livingstone/Elsevier, 2012.

Miller M. The early years of retroviral protease crystal structures. Biopolymers 2010;94:521–529.

Murray PR, Rosenthal KS, Pfaller MA. Medical Microbiology, ed 7. Philadelphia: Mosby/Elsevier, 2013.

Ryan KJ, Ray CG. Sherris Medical Microbiology, ed 5. New York: McGraw-Hill, 2010.

Yee M, Konopka K, Balzarini J, Düzgüneş N. Inhibition of HIV-1 Env-mediated cell-cell fusion by lectins, peptide T-20, and neutralizing antibodies. Open Virol J 2011;5:44–51.

Take-Home Messages

- The targets for antiviral agents include the viral envelope, virus attachment, penetration, RNA synthesis, viral DNA polymerases, and post-translational modification.
- Acyclovir is a prodrug that is activated by monophosphorylation through the action of virally encoded thymidine kinase, particularly in herpesviruses.
- Valacyclovir, penciclovir, and famciclovir are newer-generation derivatives of acyclovir.
- Azidothymidine was the first antiviral used against HIV-1.
- Ribavirin is administered as an aerosol for the treatment of children with severe respiratory syncytial virus bronchopneumonia. It is also used in the treatment of hepatitis C together with interferon-a.
- Interferon-a induces cellular enzymes that interfere with viral protein synthesis.
- Dideoxyinosine, dideoxycytidine, d4T, and lamivudine are used in treating HIV-1 infections.
- Inhibitors of the HIV protease include saquinavir, indinavir, ritonavir, nelfinavir, amprenavir, atazanavir, and darunavir.
- Zanamivir and oseltamivir inhibit the neuraminidase of influenza A and B viruses.
- High rates of replication of viruses such as HIV-1, HBV, and HCV result in higher rates of mutations and the onset of drug resistance.

30 Naked Capsid DNA Viruses

Adenoviruses, papillomaviruses, polyomaviruses, and parvoviruses are all naked capsid DNA viruses.

Adenoviruses

Adenoviruses most commonly cause respiratory illness but can also cause fever, diarrhea, conjunctivitis ("pink eye"), rash, gastroenteritis, and cystitis (bladder infection). They are frequently recovered from tonsils or adenoids resected from healthy children, indicating that they do not always cause disease. They are shed for long periods after initial infection from the pharynx and intestines.

Adenoviruses are non-enveloped, icosahedral viruses (diameter: 70–90 nm), with 20 triangular faces and 12 vertices (Fig 30-1). The 5-mer penton proteins are located at the vertices, where the viral attachment proteins are connected via a fiber (Fig 30-2). There are approximately 100 immunologically distinct types, 52 of which can infect humans.

Adenoviral genes (36,000 bp) are transcribed from both the Watson and Crick strands of DNA and in both directions. The early proteins include a DNA polymerase that replicates the genome. The virus encodes proteins that suppress host immune responses and apoptosis.

The viral attachment proteins usually bind to a cell surface protein in the immunoglobulin superfamily called the coxsackie adenovirus receptor because it also binds coxsackie B virus. Some adenoviruses bind to the major histocompatibility complex class I. The penton proteins interact with an α_v integrin in the cell membrane, promoting the internalization of the virus in clathrin-coated vesicles. The virus lyses the endosomal vesicles, and the capsid delivers the DNA genome to the nucleus. The penton and fiber proteins of the capsid are toxic to the cell and can inhibit cellular macromolecular synthesis.

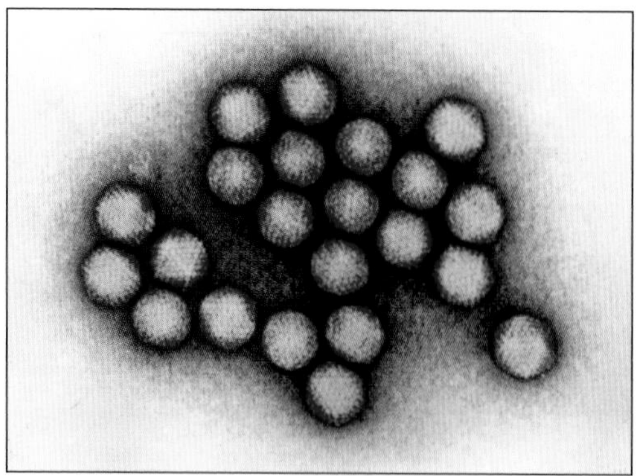

Fig 30-1 Colorized transmission electron micrograph of adenovirus. (Public Health Image Library image 10010, courtesy of Sherif Zaki, MD, PhD; and Wun-Jun Shieh, MD, PhD, MPH.)

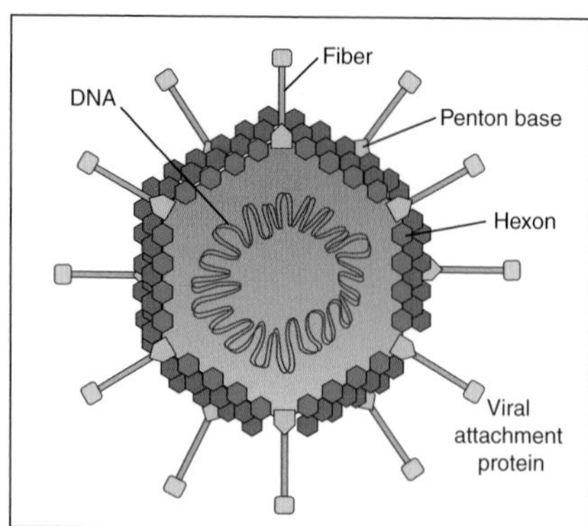

Fig 30-2 Schematic structure of adenovirus, showing the arrangement of the penton and hexon proteins.

The immediate early E1A transactivator protein is necessary for the transcription of the early proteins of the virus, including the DNA polymerase. E1A stimulates cell growth by binding to the retinoblastoma gene product (p105RB). E1B binds to the cellular growth suppressor protein (or tumor suppressor protein), p53.

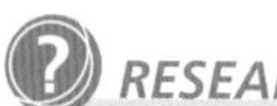

RESEARCH

How do adenoviruses lyse the endosomes in which they are internalized? What is the molecular basis of the cytotoxicity of the penton and fiber proteins?

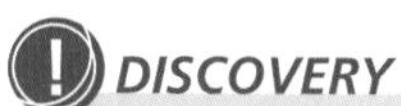

DISCOVERY

Wallace Rowe, a postdoctoral fellow, and Robert Huebner at the National Institutes of Health were working in 1953 on isolating the virus that caused the common cold. They used "explants" of adenoids and tonsils grown in cell culture. Rowe noted that some cultures of adenoid cells became rounded and clumped within a week, so he decided to determine whether this cytopathic effect was the result of a viral infection. He showed that the causative agent could be passaged in cell culture and that it was a virus that was present in the original tissue.

Clinical syndromes and diagnosis

Different adenovirus serovars or types are associated with different clinical syndromes. Acute febrile pharyngitis and pharyngoconjunctival fever are caused by adenoviruses 2, 3, 4, 5, 6, and 7. In children younger than 3 years of age, pharyngitis alone is seen and may present symptoms similar to streptococcal infection. Older school-age children are at risk for pharyngoconjunctival fever, which is caused by serotypes 3 and 7. Acute respiratory disease is caused by types 4, 7, 14, 14a, and 21. Infants are at risk for pneumonia, attributed to serotypes 1, 2, 3, and 7. Some adenovirus infections can present as whooping cough, croup, and bronchitis.

Adenovirus serotypes 40 and 41 cause endemic childhood diarrhea. By contrast, outbreaks of diarrhea are usually caused by noroviruses. Cytotoxicity to cells lining the gut caused by these serotypes may lead to malabsorption. Acute hemorrhagic cystitis is caused by serotypes 11 and 21. Adenoviruses may cause a "septic shock"–like syndrome in newborns and systemic infection in bone marrow transplant patients.

Diagnosis involves the use of fluorescent antibody or enzyme immunoassay, DNA probe analysis, polymerase chain reaction, electron microscopy, or light microscopy of intranuclear inclusions. Adenovirus can be cultured in human embryonic kidney cells, HeLa cells, and human epidermal carcinoma cells.

Pathogenesis and epidemiology

Adenovirus infects epithelial cells lining respiratory and enteric organs. Replication results in dense intranuclear inclusions. After localizing in lymph nodes, it can spread to multiple organs by viremia. It becomes latent in lymphoid tissues, including tonsils, adenoids, and Peyer's patches.

Adenovirus is spread by aerosols, close contact, or the fecal-oral route. It infects mucoepithelial cells in the respiratory or gastrointestinal tract, the conjunctiva, and the cornea. Antibodies are important for prophylaxis and for resolution of the infection. It is stable to drying, detergents, and mild chlorine treatment. Infected fingers can readily spread the virus to the eyes. Adenoviruses (types 1, 2, and 5) account for 5% to 10% of pediatric respiratory infections. Persons in day-care centers and military training camps and those who frequent public swimming pools are susceptible to infection.

Treatment and prevention

Treatment of adenoviral infections is symptomatic. Antiviral agents such as ganciclovir, ribavirin, and cidofovir have shown efficacy in vitro and, in some cases, in patients. Cidofovir has been used to treat severe infections in immunocompromised patients. A live oral vaccine has been developed to counter serotypes 4 and 7 that cause disease in military recruits.

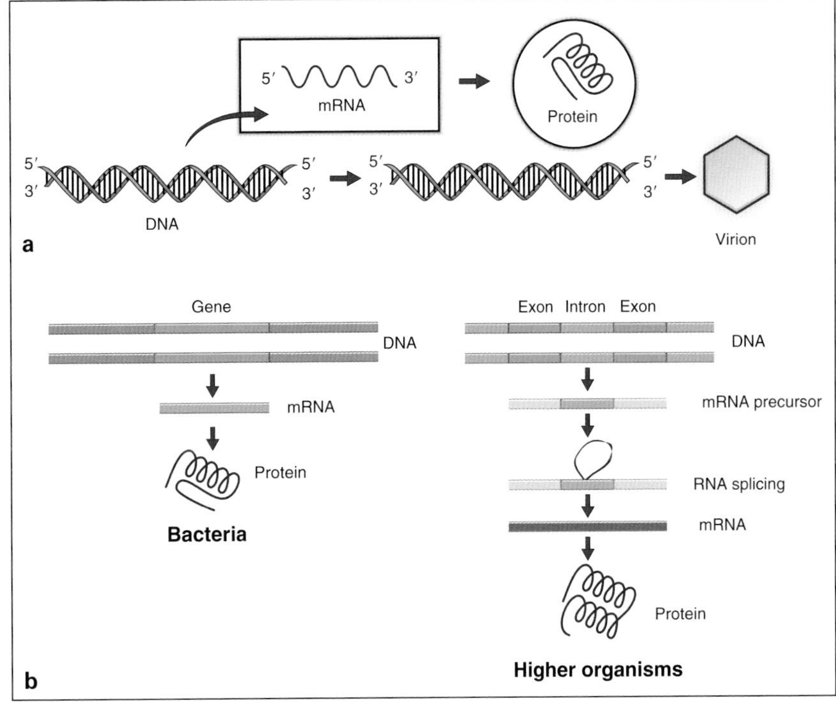

Fig 30-3 *(a)* Adenovirus encodes proteins to promote mRNA and DNA synthesis, including its own DNA polymerase. *(b)* The gene structure and flow of genetic information in bacteria *(left)* and higher organisms *(right)*. In bacteria, the genetic information is encoded as a continuous segment of DNA, and the transcribed mRNA is translated into protein. In eukaryotes, the gene is usually split into exons and intervening introns, and the mRNA has to be "spliced" before it can be translated into a protein. (Adapted from http://www.nobelprize.org/nobel_prizes/medicine/laureates/1993/press.html.)

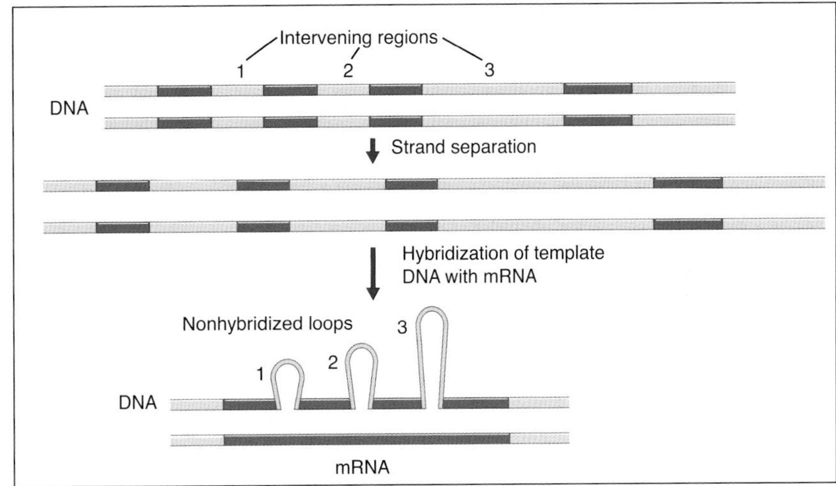

Fig 30-4 The experiment that demonstrated that adenovirus DNA contains split genes. The genetic information in the mRNA is derived from the DNA as four segments that are separated by three intervening regions (1, 2, and 3). When mRNA is hybridized with the template DNA strand, the intervening sequences in the DNA strand appear as loops because they do not have counterparts in the RNA. The hybrid was visualized by electron microscopy. (Adapted from http://www.nobelprize.org/nobel_prizes/medicine/laureates/1993/press.html.)

DISCOVERY

In the mid-1970s, the prevailing general concept of hereditary material was that a gene is a continuous segment within a DNA molecule. When the gene is turned on, its information is copied into an mRNA molecule and is subsequently translated into a protein (Fig 30-3a). In 1977, however, Richard J. Roberts at the Cold Spring Harbor Laboratory and Phillip A. Sharp at the Massachusetts Institute of Technology discovered independently that genes could be discontinuous, with several well-separated segments. As their experimental model system, both scientists used adenovirus, whose genome is a single DNA molecule. They wanted to find out where the different genes were located in the genome. They showed biochemically that one end of an adenovirus mRNA did not behave as expected. One possibility was that the DNA segment corresponding to this segment of RNA was not located next to the rest of the gene. Using electron microscopy to determine where this segment was located on DNA, they discovered that a single RNA molecule corresponded to four well-separated segments in the DNA molecule (Fig 30-3b). Thus, an individual gene may contain several DNA segments separated by "irrelevant" DNA (Fig 30-4). Soon after this discovery, it was shown that this discontinuous (or split) structure was the most common gene structure in eukaryotes. Roberts and Sharp were awarded the Nobel Prize in Physiology or Medicine in 1993.

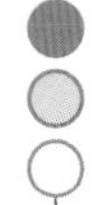

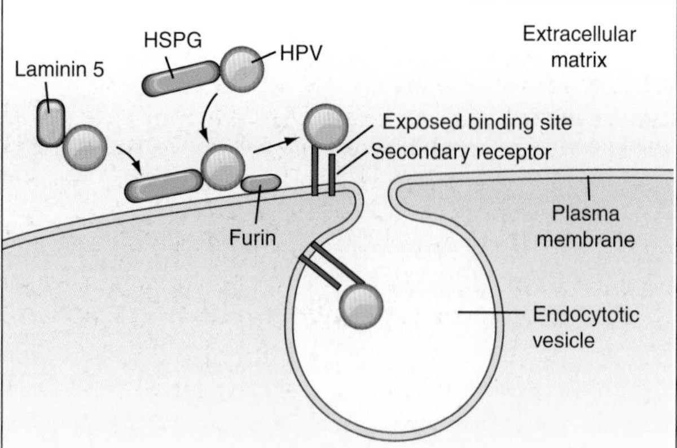

Fig 30-5 Interaction of human papillomavirus (HPV) with the extracellular matrix (ECM) and cell surface. Heparan sulfate proteoglycan (HSPG) is thought to be the initial attachment receptor for HPV. It is found in the ECM and on the surface of many types of cells. HPV binds to laminin 5 in the ECM, although this interaction may not be that important for productive infection. A secondary receptor is likely to be involved in the infectious entry of HPV after the interaction with HSPG. The virions are transferred to the putative secondary receptor on the cell surface. Capsid interaction with HSPG results in a conformational change that in turn exposes a furin (a serine endoprotease) cleavage site. Following this proteolytic cleavage, an additional conformational change exposes the binding site for the secondary cell surface receptor or lowers the affinity for the primary receptor. This results in the transfer of the capsid to the secondary receptor, which then triggers endocytosis. (Adapted from Horvath et al.)

Human Papillomaviruses

Papillomaviruses were the first DNA viruses associated with malignant transformation. They are icosahedral viruses 52 to 55 nm in diameter, with double-stranded DNA containing 8,000 bp. They replicate in cutaneous and mucosal epithelial cells and induce cell proliferation, forming benign tumors. Some lesions develop carcinomas. In vivo, the L1 major capsid protein in the capsid binds heparan sulfate proteoglycans in the extracellular matrix, a process that exposes the L2 minor capsid protein that binds to a receptor on epithelial cells (Fig 30-5). The entry of human papillomavirus (HPV) in vitro is initiated by binding directly to a cell surface receptor. Most HPV strains that have been studied seem to enter the cell via clathrin-dependent endocytosis, but the conclusions are not unequivocal. The productive entry of HPV is a slow process with an unusually extended residence time on the cell surface. The genome enters the nucleus after the nuclear membrane breaks down during mitosis.

The virus replicates by using the cell's DNA polymerase in the more differentiated epithelial cells. In the fully differentiated keratinocytes, the capsid proteins are synthesized, the DNA is replicated, and the assembled virus particles are released by cell lysis.

Clinical syndromes and diagnosis

HPV infection causes skin or genital warts that can resolve spontaneously, possibly because of the immune response. Laryngeal papillomas, also termed *recurrent respiratory papillamatosis*, are usually associated with HPV-6 and HPV-11 and are found mostly in young children and middle-aged adults. In children, these papillomas present a danger of airway obstruction. Laryngeal and pharyngeal cancers are associated with HPV-16 and HPV-18 infection. HPV types 13 and 32 can also cause multifocal papillomavirus epithelial hyperplasia, especially in children and young adults (Fig 30-6). These soft, fleshy papules range in color from pink to white and can occur on the lips, buccal mucosa, and lateral borders of the tongue.

HPV-16 and HPV-18 also cause cervical papillomas and dysplasia. Cervical dysplasia may become cancerous through the action of co-factors. At least 85% of cervical carcinomas contain integrated HPV DNA (rather than plasmid-like, or episomal, DNA). More than 99% of invasive cervical cancers contain HPV DNA. HPV-16 is the most common high-risk HPV, and it is the cause of more than 50% of invasive cervical cancers worldwide. The mean incidence of cervical cancer is 35 per 100,000, and it is the second most common cancer in women. A subset of oropharyngeal squamous cell cancers (OSCC), especially in the lingual and palatine tonsils, are caused by high-risk HPV. However, HPV-associated OSCC has a better prognosis than HPV-negative OSCC.

Common cutaneous warts are caused by HPV types 2, 4, and 7 and usually disappear spontaneously. Regrowth of warts after treatment is most likely the result of infection of the adjoining skin. Anogenital warts, known as condylomata acuminate, are seen in sexually active adults. Vulvar and vaginal warts, as well as those on the penis and perianal skin, are readily visible, whereas cervical warts require the aid of a colposcope that magnifies the epithelium. Application of 5% acetic acid to the epithelium induces whitening of the flat, or noncondylomatous, warts in which there is a high concentration of nuclear material.

Histologic examination reveals hyperplasia of prickle cells, which are cells with rod-shaped processes, and the production of excess keratin. Papanicolaou-stained cervical smears (Pap smears) show koilocytotic cells with perinuclear vacuolization (Fig 30-7). Intraepithelial cervical neoplasia and cancer can ensue following infection of the female genital tract by HPV-16 and HPV-18. The initial neoplastic changes observed by light microscopy are called dysplasias. Fortunately, 40% to 70% of the mild dysplasias regress spontaneously. The most reliable methods for establishing HPV infection is DNA probe analysis and the polymerase chain reaction. HPV antigens in infected cells can be detected and localized by immunofluorescence, and the viral particles can be visualized by electron microscopy.

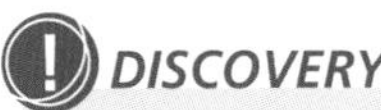

DISCOVERY

In the 1970s, Harald zur Hausen postulated a role for HPV in cervical cancer, against the prevailing view. He reasoned that if the tumor cells contained an oncogenic virus, they should contain viral DNA integrated into their genomes, and the HPV genes associated with cell proliferation should be detectable by examining tumor cells for this DNA. He looked for different HPV types that could be associated with cervical cancer. Interestingly, only parts of the viral DNA were integrated into the host cell genome. In 1983, zur Hausen discovered novel HPV DNA in cervical cancer biopsies belonging to HPV type 16. HPV-16 and HPV-18 were found in about 70% of cervical cancer biopsies. Vaccines were ultimately developed that provide greater than 95% protection from infection by the high-risk HPV-16 and HPV-18.

Harald zur Hausen was awarded half of the Nobel Prize in Physiology or Medicine in 2008 for his discovery that HPV causes cervical cancer, the other half being shared by Luc Montagnier and Françoise Barré-Sinoussi for their discovery of human immunodeficiency virus (HIV).

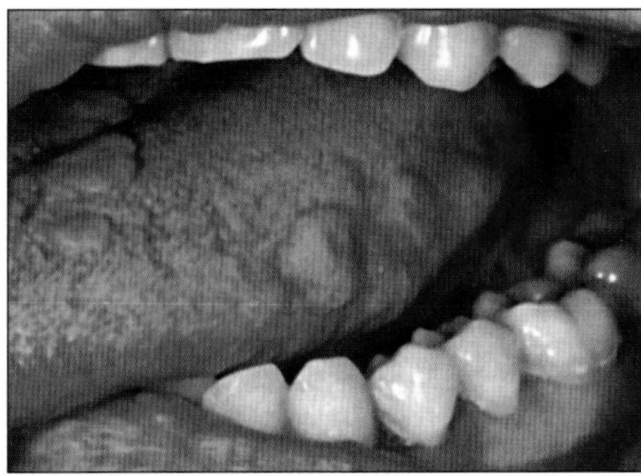

Fig 30-6 Multifocal papillomavirus epithelial hyperplasia, presenting as numerous papules and plaques caused by HPV infection. (Reprinted with permission from Eisen and Lynch.)

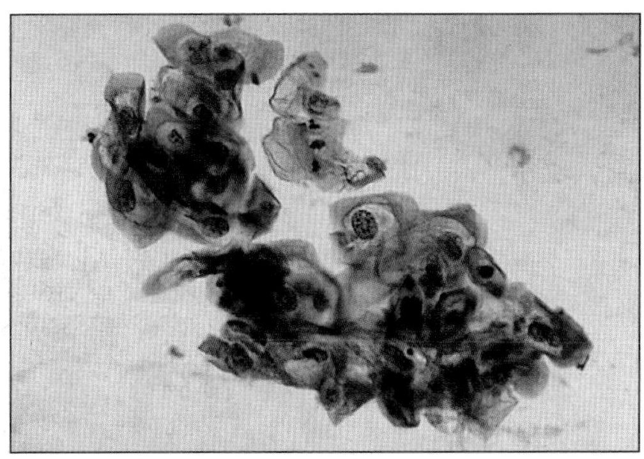

Fig 30-7 Papanicolaou stain of exfoliated cervicovaginal squamous epithelial cells, showing the perinuclear cytoplasmic vacuolization (koilocytosis) that is characteristic of HPV infection. (Reprinted with permission from Murray et al.)

Pathogenesis and epidemiology

E6 and E7 proteins of these viruses have been identified as oncogenes. They bind and inactivate cellular growth suppressor (transformation suppressor) proteins p53 and p105 (the retinoblastoma gene product, p105RB). E6 binds the p53 protein and targets it for degradation. E7 binds and inactivates p105RB. Cervical dysplasia may become cancerous through the action of co-factors. Transformation of the infected cells depends on the type of HPV, the location and duration of infection, the strength of the immune response, and environmental and other risk factors. Regression of HPV infections depends on the action of helper T cell (T_h1)–driven cytotoxic T cells and subsequent protection from infection by antibodies generated by T_h2-stimulated B cells. HPV resists inactivation and can be transmitted on fomites or by direct contact with infected individuals through breaks in the skin or mucosa. It infects epithelial cells in the skin or mucosa.

Treatment and prevention

Warts may be destroyed by surgical cryotherapy with liquid nitrogen or dry ice, although topical treatment with salicylic acid is also successful. Genital warts are more difficult to treat. Antiproliferative agents such as 5-fluorouracil and podophyllin, chemical treatment with trichloroacetic acid, and cryotherapy can be used. Topical application of immunomodulators, such as imiquimod (Aldara, 3M) and interferon, stimulate innate and inflammatory responses. Intralesional delivery of cidofovir is also an alternative. Laryngeal papillomas can be removed by surgery.

The HPV vaccine Gardasil (Merck) is a mixture of four HPV type-specific, virus-like particles composed of the capsid L1 proteins from types 6, 11, 16, and 18. It is recommended for females 9 to 26 years of age. It is given in three doses: an initial dose followed by boosters at 2 months and 6 months. It is not known if the vaccine can prevent cancers of the oropharynx, but most HPV-associated cancers of the oropharynx are caused by the HPV types that are prevented by the vaccine. The Cervarix (GlaxoSmithKline) vaccine is used to prevent infection by types 16 and 18.

Polyomaviruses

Polyomaviruses ("many tumor viruses") are about 45 nm in diameter, and their DNA contains 5,100 bp. Initial infection is via the respiratory tract. They are then spread by viremia and establish persistent and latent infection in the kidneys and lungs. They can be reactivated in immunocompromised patients.

The most common human polyomaviruses are JC virus and BK virus, which were discovered in 1971 and named after the initials of the patients from whom they were isolated. Merkel cell polyomavirus was discovered in 2009 and is associated with Merkel cell carcinoma, which is a rare human neuroendocrine malignant tumor of the skin in immunocompromised individuals or those overexposed to sunlight. SV40 is a simian virus that has contaminated early

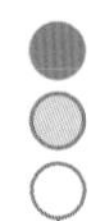

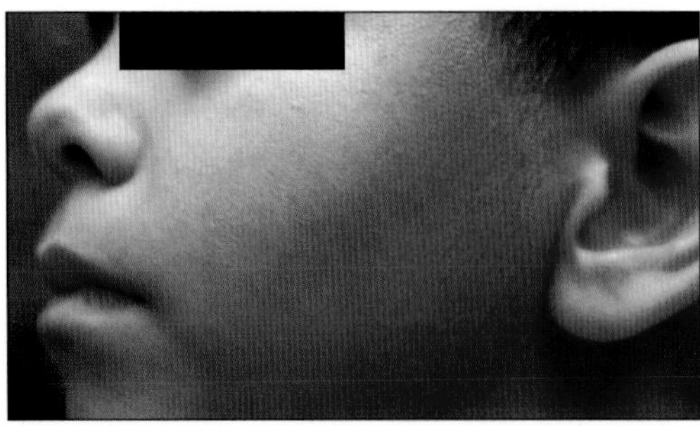

Fig 30-8 Left side of a boy's face showing signs of erythema infectiosum, or fifth disease, caused by parvovirus B19. (Public Health Image Library image 4508, courtesy of Dr Philip S. Brachman.)

poliovirus vaccines; however, no adverse effects such as induction of tumors have been reported. SV40 is used in the laboratory to transform cultured cells.

The early region of the genomes of JC, BK, and SV40 viruses code for nonstructural T (transformation) proteins, and the late region codes for the viral capsid proteins. Similar to adenovirus, both strands of DNA code for proteins.

JC virus infects glial cells by binding to sialic acid–containing carbohydrates and serotonin receptors and enters the cells via endocytosis. The T antigen of SV40 controls gene transcription and DNA replication and inactivates the cellular growth suppressor proteins p53 and p105RB.

JC virus establishes infection in the kidneys, monocyte-lineage cells, and B cells, but replication is blocked by the action of the immune system. In immunocompromised patients, most commonly in those with advanced HIV infection, it causes progressive multifocal leukoencephalopathy (PML), where astrocytes are transformed partially and oligodendrocytes are killed, resulting in demyelination. PML presents with multiple neurologic symptoms, including impairment of speech, vision, and coordination, and paralysis of arms and legs. PML also afflicts patients receiving the monoclonal antibodies rituximab (to treat rheumatoid arthritis and B-cell non-Hodgkin lymphoma) and natalizumab (used to treat relapsing multiple sclerosis) as therapy.

BK virus multiplies in the urinary tract. It is associated with ureteral stenosis (narrowing of the ureter) in renal transplant patents and hemorrhagic cystitis in bone marrow transplant patients.

JC virus can be diagnosed by polymerase chain reaction amplification of viral DNA in cerebrospinal fluid. The pathology caused by PML can be detected by magnetic resonance imaging or computed tomography. BK and JC viruses can be detected by cytology of urine that shows enlarged cells with basophilic nuclear inclusions. In situ immunofluorescence and DNA probe analysis are also useful in detecting viral components.

Polyomavirus infections can be treated with cidofovir, which acts on cellular DNA polymerase. However, it is nephrotoxic. Reversing the immunosuppression that causes the activation of the virus can also be useful.

Parvoviruses

Parvoviruses are naked capsid, single-stranded DNA viruses 18 to 26 nm in diameter, and thus they are among the smallest viruses. Only one member of the parvoviruses—human parvovirus B19—causes disease in humans.

Clinical syndromes and diagnosis

Human parvovirus B19 causes erythema infectiosum, or fifth disease, with a characteristic rash on the cheek ("slapped cheek disease") (Fig 30-8). It is the fifth of the childhood exanthems, the first four being varicella, rubella, roseola, and measles. It is observed more often in children than in adults. Illness usually starts within 4 to 14 days, but sometimes up to 20 days, after getting infected with parvovirus B19. About 20% of people who get infected do not develop symptoms.

B19 infection in adults causes polyarthritis, with painful or swollen joints of the hands, wrists, knees, and ankles. It can also inhibit the synthesis of red blood cells, leading to transient aplastic crisis, hydrops fetalis (edema in the fetus), congenital anemia, pure red cell aplasia, or persistent anemia. Infection of seronegative pregnant women increases the risk for fetal death by causing anemia and congestive heart failure.

Diagnosis may involve immune electron microscopy, enzyme immunoassay, and nucleic acid hybridization. A low reticulocyte count is consistent with B19 infection.

Pathogenesis and epidemiology

Parvovirus B19 attaches to the glycolipid globoside (blood group P antigen) on various cells. This lipid is found on erythroid progenitors, erythrocytes, megakaryocytes, vascular endothelial cells, placental cells, and fetal myocardial and liver cells. The virus causes upper respiratory tract infections and viremia and infects erythroid precursor cells. Reticulocytopenia in chronic hemolytic anemia patients (aplastic crisis) is the most serious complication. Infection causes a rash (erythema infectiosum) (see Fig 30-8).

Parvovirus B19 is transmitted by respiratory secretions, such as saliva, sputum, or nasal mucus, as well as by blood transfusion or blood products. Infected persons are most contagious when it seems like they have a cold, before the development of the rash or joint pain and swelling.

Treatment and prevention

B19 infection is usually mild and self-limiting, requiring only symptomatic relief for joint pain. Blood transfusion is called for in transient aplastic crisis, until the virus is cleared by the immune response. Blood transfusion and immunoglobulin treatment over a 5- to 10-day period is necessary in immunocompromised individuals. In congenital anemia or hydrops, intrauterine transfusion decreases the mortality rate of the fetus.

Take-Home Messages

- Adenoviruses cause respiratory illness, diarrhea, conjunctivitis, rash, gastroenteritis, and cystitis.
- Acute febrile pharyngitis and pharyngoconjunctival fever are caused by adenoviruses 2, 3, 4, 5, 6, and 7.
- Acute respiratory disease is caused by adenoviruses 4, 7, 14, 14a, and 21.
- Adenovirus serotypes 40 and 41 cause endemic childhood diarrhea.
- Papillomaviruses were the first DNA viruses associated with malignant transformation.
- Laryngeal papillomas are usually associated with HPV-6 and HPV-11 and present a danger of airway obstruction in children.
- Laryngeal and pharyngeal cancers are associated with HPV-16 and HPV-18 infection.
- HPV-16 and HPV-18 also cause cervical papillomas and dysplasia.
- In HPV infection, Papanicolaou-stained cervical smears show koilocytotic cells with perinuclear vacuolization.
- The most common human polyomaviruses are JC virus and BK virus. In immunocompromised patients, JC virus causes progressive multifocal leukoencephalopathy.
- Human parvovirus B19 causes erythema infectiosum, or fifth disease. In chronic hemolytic anemia patients, it can cause aplastic crisis, which is the most serious complication.

Bibliography

Centers for Disease Control and Prevention. Adenovirus. www.cdc.gov/adenovirus/index.html. Accessed 24 July 2015.

Centers for Disease Control and Prevention. Parvovirus B19 and Fifth Disease. www.cdc.gov/parvovirusB19/fifth-disease.html. Accessed 24 July 2015.

Centers for Disease Control and Prevention. Public Health Image Library. phil.cdc.gov. Accessed 4 August 2015.

Eisen D, Lynch DP. The Mouth: Diagnosis and Treatment. St Louis: Mosby, 1998.

Ginsberg HS. Discovery and classification of adenoviruses. In: Seth P (ed). Adenoviruses: Basic Biology to Gene Therapy. Austin, TX: Landes Bioscience, 1999.

Greenwood D, Barer M, Slack R, Irving W. Medical Microbiology, ed 18. Edinburgh: Churchill Livingstone/Elsevier, 2012.

Horvath CA, Boulet GA, Renoux VM, Delvenne PO, Bogers JP. Mechanisms of cell entry by human papillomaviruses: An overview. Virol J 2010;7:11.

Murray PR, Rosenthal KS, Pfaller MA. Medical Microbiology, ed 7. Philadelphia: Mosby/Elsevier, 2013.

Nobelprize.org. The Nobel Prize in Physiology or Medicine 1993 Press Release. http://www.nobelprize.org/nobel_prizes/medicine/laureates/1993/press.html. Accessed 24 July 2015.

Nobelprize.org. The Nobel Prize in Physiology or Medicine 2008 Press Release. http://www.nobelprize.org/nobel_prizes/medicine/laureates/2008/press.html. Accessed 24 July 2015.

Ryan KJ, Ray CG. Sherris Medical Microbiology, ed 5. New York: McGraw-Hill, 2010.

San Martin C. Latest insights on adenovirus structure and assembly. Viruses 2012;4:845–877.

Human Immunodeficiency Virus and Other Retroviruses

31

Retroviruses are enveloped viruses with a positive-strand RNA genome. They replicate through a DNA intermediate, which requires an enzyme that can transcribe RNA into DNA. This enzyme, an RNA-dependent DNA polymerase, was first described by David Baltimore, Howard Temin, and Satoshi Mizutani in 1970 and termed reverse transcriptase (RT). This mechanism was a new addition to what had been known as the "central dogma of molecular biology," originally described by Francis Crick in 1958, which stated that genetic information flows in one direction, from DNA to RNA to protein.

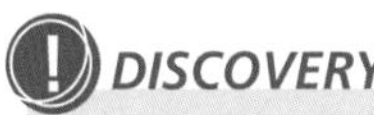

DISCOVERY

A previously unknown disease emerged in the early 1980s, afflicting groups of individuals in certain risk groups in the United States who were dying of opportunistic infections. It is now known that this disease—acquired immunodeficiency syndrome (AIDS)—can develop in any individual exposed to the etiologic agent. The agent was isolated from patients with lymphadenopathy (abnormal enlargement of the lymph nodes) and AIDS by Françoise Barré-Sinoussi and Luc Montagnier at the Pasteur Institute in 1983. It was a virus, initially called *lymphadenopathy-associated virus (LAV)*. Robert Gallo and collaborators in 1984 showed the presence of antibodies to a virus they called HTLV-III in the blood of patients with AIDS. Jay Levy also isolated a virus from AIDS patients in 1984 and called it *AIDS-associated retrovirus (ARV)*. The virus was later designated as *human immunodeficiency virus type 1 (HIV-1)*. A related virus that is prevalent in West Africa, related to simian immunodeficiency virus, was isolated subsequently and designated as HIV-2.

Françoise Barré-Sinoussi and Luc Montagnier were awarded half of the Nobel Prize in Physiology or Medicine in 2008.

Human Immunodeficiency Virus

Structure and replication

The HIV envelope has two glycoproteins that are produced by cleavage of the precursor gp160 by cellular proteases. The highly glycosylated surface protein (SU) gp120 binds to the host cell surface receptor CD4, which is found on helper T lymphocytes, monocytes, and macrophages. Mutations in gp120 occur over time in an infected individual, preventing the immune system from completely clearing the virus and also rendering difficult the generation of an effective vaccine. Gp120 is attached noncovalently to the transmembrane glycoprotein (TM) gp41, which mediates virus-cell and cell-cell fusion.

The envelope surrounds the capsid, a truncated cone-shaped structure composed primarily of the viral p24 protein (Fig 31-1). Inside the capsid are two copies of viral RNA and two tRNA molecules that hybridize to the RNA and act as primers to facilitate reverse transcription of the genome once the contents of the capsid are in the host cell cytoplasm. The capsid also contains RT, integrase, and protease. The genome is flanked by RNA sequences called long terminal repeat (LTR) that comprise promoter and enhancer gene sequences that bind transcription factors.

The replication cycle of HIV-1 begins with binding of gp120 to CD4 (via a constant region on gp120) and to a secondary receptor (via the variable V3 loop region on gp120). Tissue tropism and the host range of the virus depend primarily on binding to the receptor. Membrane fusion and viral entry is dependent on the secondary receptor, which is a G-protein–coupled chemokine receptor. Early in the infection of a person, this co-receptor is the chemokine receptor CCR5, expressed primarily on macrophages and dendritic cells (Fig 31-2). Thus, the virus is initially "M-tropic" or an "R5 virus." Later, during chronic infection of a person, the gp120 gene undergoes mutations and the new gp120 binds to the chemokine receptor CXCR4, expressed primarily on T cells; the virus is then said to be "T-tropic" or an "X4 virus." The interaction of gp120 with the co-receptor displaces gp120 to a sufficient extent that the trimeric transmembrane gp41 can insert its hydrophobic N-terminus into the host cell membrane, thereby mediating membrane fusion.

HIV-1 can also infect cells that are CD4-negative, such as fibroblasts and certain brain cells, most likely via its interaction with a co-receptor and the fusion activity of gp41. HIV-1 binds to the cellular adhesion molecule $\alpha4\beta7$ integrin, which is found on gut-associated lymphoid tissue, and to the DC-SIGN receptor (dendritic cell–specific intercellular adhesion molecule-3–grabbing nonintegrin) expressed on dendritic cells. HIV-1 can fuse with certain negatively charged liposomes with no receptors, and the fusion product has a greatly impaired ability to infect cells.

Once it enters the cytoplasm, the viral RNA genome is reverse transcribed by RT; a complementary, negative-strand DNA (cDNA) is produced; and the RNA template is degraded by the ribonuclease H activity of the RT. A positive-strand DNA is generated by the DNA-dependent DNA polymerase activity of the RT. The U3 and U5 sequences from each end of the genome are duplicated and become part of the LTRs on both ends of the genome (see Fig 31-2). Therefore, the DNA genome is longer than the RNA genome of the virus. Reverse transcription does not faithfully transcribe the viral genome, introducing mutations at a rate of about 1 in 2,000 bases copied, thereby leading to the emergence of new strains and allowing the virus to escape immune recognition.

The double-stranded cDNA is circularized and then complexes with cellular and viral proteins to form a preintegration complex, which is transported through the nuclear pore complex into the nucleus (see Fig 31-2). If the cell is in a growth phase, the complex is integrated into the host chromosome via the action of the viral integrase, forming the provirus. The provirus may stay dormant or enter a productive cycle. In the latter case, the viral genome is transcribed into a full-length RNA by the RNA polymerase II of the host cell.

The HIV genome has three main gene clusters: *gag*, *pol*, and *env*. The group-specific antigen gene, gag, encodes the capsid (p24), nucleocapsid (p7), and matrix (p17) genes. The polymerase, pol, gene encodes RT, integrase, and protease. The envelope, env, gene codes for the transmembrane gp41 protein and the surface protein gp120, which form trimers and are trafficked to the plasma membrane.

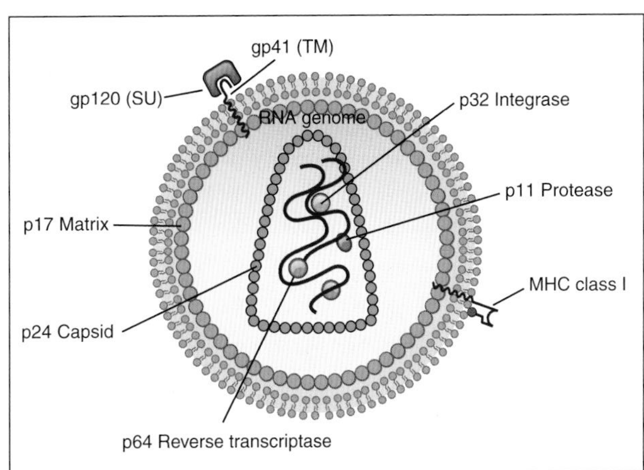

Fig 31-1 Schematic diagram of an HIV virion. The envelope, which is derived from the host cell plasma membrane, incorporates the spike glycoproteins gp120 and the transmembrane gp41, which are associated noncovalently. The envelope may also incorporate host membrane proteins such as major histocompatibility complex (MHC) class I and class II molecules. The matrix protein generates the shape of the virion. The capsid protein p24 forms the nucleocapsid structure that encloses two copies of genomic RNA. Two molecules of reverse transcriptase are bound to the RNA. The nucleocapsid includes the protease and the integrase. The protease cleaves the HIV polyproteins into individual proteins, causing virion maturation following virus budding from the host cell. The integrase is necessary for the incorporation of the reverse-transcribed HIV DNA genome into the host cell chromosome following infection.

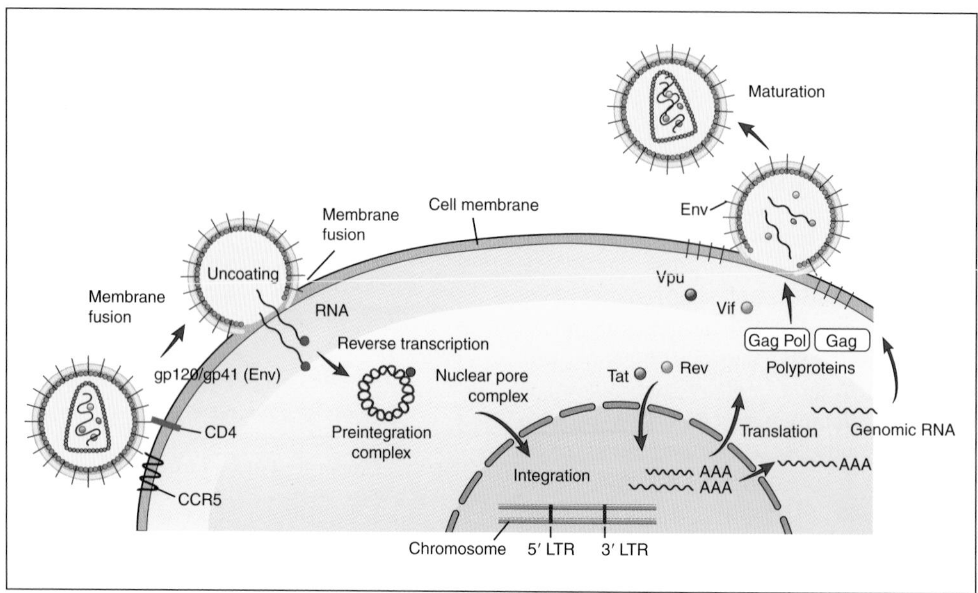

Fig 31-2 The replication cycle of HIV. The infection begins when the envelope glycoproteins gp120/gp41 (Env) bind to the CD4 receptor and the chemokine receptor (CCR5), leading to a conformational change and exposing the gp41 N-terminus. This hydrophobic peptide segment is inserted into the host cell membrane and facilitates the fusion of the viral membrane with that of the cell. The nucleocapsid is uncoated, the viral RNA genome enters the cytoplasm, and reverse transcription results in a double-stranded DNA copy of the viral genome. A preintegration complex is formed with the participation of viral and cellular proteins, including the integrase and capsid, and mediates the entry of the viral genome into the nucleus. Integrase facilitates the integration of the viral DNA into the chromosome, with the participation of a host protein. The integrated, proviral DNA is transcribed by the host RNA polymerase II. The mRNA transcripts are translated into polyproteins, and the genome-length RNA and the proteins are incorporated into the HIV virions. After virus budding from the cell membrane, the protease produces the individual proteins in a process known as *maturation*.

These genes are initially in the form of polyproteins, which are cleaved by proteases to form the final protein products. In the case of Gag and Pol, the HIV protease carries out this function within the newly synthesized virion. All of the viral components are assembled at the plasma membrane, and the virus buds, taking with it some cellular membrane proteins, including the major histocompatibility complex (MHC). The HIV genome can be transferred from cell to cell via cell-cell fusion, leading to multinucleated syncytia.

HIV gene expression is regulated by six gene products called *auxiliary proteins* or *accessory gene products*:

1. Tat is a transcriptional activator that acts at a site (TAR) near the onset of mRNA transcription by recruiting cellular proteins to the RNA polymerase and enabling the complete transcription of the HIV genome.
2. Rev promotes the transport of unspliced mRNA into the cytoplasm. Only Rev, Tat, and Nef are synthesized from fully spliced mRNA. The RNAs encoding the other genes are not spliced and hence would not normally be transported into the cytoplasm. Thus, Rev plays a crucial role in the production of viral proteins by binding to the Rev-responsive element in the *env* region of the viral RNA and transporting the latter into the cytoplasm.
3. Nef downregulates cellular CD4 and MHC class I proteins.
4. Vif (virion infectivity factor) increases the ability of HIV to infect primary T cells and some nonpermissive cells in culture. Vif inhibits APOBEC-3G, a cellular RNA-editing enzyme that hypermutates the HIV genome.
5. Vpu complexes with CD4 in the endoplasmic reticulum to enable the newly synthesized gp120 to reach the plasma membrane and mediates the release of the virus at the plasma membrane.
6. Vpr is essential for virus replication in nondividing cells like macrophages and enables the viral DNA to reach the nucleus.

Clinical syndromes and diagnosis

The initial HIV infection may be asymptomatic or may be followed within 2 to 4 weeks by the "acute phase," characterized by flulike or mononucleosis-like symptoms and continuing for up to 6 weeks. The symptoms of this phase include malaise, fever, hepatosplenomegaly, lymphadenopathy, rash, and arthralgias. Mild, aseptic meningitis is sometimes observed. After this phase, the infection may become asymptomatic or turn into ongoing generalized lymphadenopathy as a result of virus multiplication in lymph nodes. The pathogenesis of the virus involves the gradual depletion of $CD4^+$ T cells. Thus, immune responses controlled by T cells decline. The clinical syndromes associated with this decline include opportunistic infections by fungi, herpes simplex virus, and intracellular bacteria (Box 31-1). At this stage, the $CD4^+$ T-cell count in blood is below 350/µL,

Box 31-1 Common opportunistic infections and malignancies in patients with untreated AIDS

Fungal
- *Pneumocystis jirovecii* pneumonia
- Cryptococcosis
- Candidiasis
- Disseminated histoplasmosis
- Disseminated coccidioidomycosis

Mycobacterial
- Disseminated *Mycobacterium tuberculosis*
- *Mycobacterium avium-intracellulare* complex infections

Protozoan
- Toxoplasmosis
- Cryptosporidiosis
- *Isospora belli* infection
- *Entamoeba histolytica* infection

Viral
- Persistent mucocutaneous herpes simplex virus infection
- Cytomegalovirus retinitis or disseminated virus infection
- Persistent or disseminated varicella zoster virus infection
- Progressive multifocal leukoencephalopathy (reactivated JC virus)
- Molluscum contagiosum poxvirus
- Epstein-Barr virus hairy leukoplakia

Malignancies
- Kaposi sarcoma (human herpesvirus 8)
- Lymphoma

(Adapted from Ryan and Ray.)

and the number of virions is increased compared with the asymptomatic phase. When the CD4$^+$ T-cell concentration falls below 200/µL and the virus load is above 75,000 RNA copies/mL, "full-blown AIDS" is manifested, with HIV wasting syndrome, neurologic symptoms, and malignancies. About 50% of infections result in significant disease within 10 years. In 1993, the Centers for Disease Control and Prevention (CDC) established AIDS-defining conditions as HIV seropositivity and CD4$^+$ lymphocyte counts less than 200/mm^3 (normal levels are 800 to 1,200/mm^3).

One of the first opportunistic infections recognized early in the HIV epidemic was *Pneumocystis carinii* pneumonia (see Box 31-1). The organism has been recently renamed *Pneumocystis jirovecii*. The main oral manifestations of HIV/AIDS are oral candidiasis (thrush; see Fig 26-8) and hairy leukoplakia caused by Epstein-Barr virus (see Fig 33-6). Other opportunistic infections include cerebral toxoplasmosis, cryptococcal meningitis, cryptosporidium, progressive multifocal leukoencephalopathy caused by reactivation of JC virus, herpes simplex virus and varicella zoster virus recurrence, cytomegalovirus retinitis, and gastrointestinal disease. The main bacterial opportunistic infections are caused by *Mycobacterium tuberculosis*, *Mycobacterium avium-intracellulare* complex, and the gastrointestinal pathogens *Salmonella*, *Shigella*, and *Campylobacter*.

Certain malignancies are also observed in HIV/AIDS. Human herpesvirus 8–associated Kaposi sarcoma was one of the unusual manifestations of HIV infection in the early 1980s, afflicting about 25% of patients. The incidence of Kaposi sarcoma in the United States declined from 1,838.9 cases per 100,000 person-years in 1990–1995 to 334.6 in 1996–2002. The incidence of non-Hodgkin lymphoma also declined from 1,066.2 cases per 100,000 person-years in 1990–1995 to 390.1 cases in 1996–2002. These declines may be the result of the restoration of CD4$^+$ lymphocyte levels in HIV-seropositive individuals following highly active antiretroviral therapy (HAART).

HIV infection of macrophages and microglial cells of the brain may result in inflammation that can damage the brain and spinal cord. Some of the symptoms are headaches, progressive weakness, confusion, memory loss, behavioral changes, and loss of sensation in the extremities.

Both the disease and the use of antiretroviral drugs can result in seizures, spinal cord dysfunction, lack of coordination, difficult or painful swallowing, anxiety disorder, depression, fever, pain, loss of vision, and coma. Neurologic complications are seen in more than 50% of adults with AIDS in the United States.

HIV infection can be diagnosed by the presence of antibodies against viral components, using enzyme-linked immunosorbent assay (ELISA) and whole viral lysates. The results have to be confirmed using Western blot analysis of the presence of antibodies to particular HIV proteins. For this analysis, HIV proteins are electrophoresed and then transferred to nitrocellulose paper. Sera from patients are added to the paper, and to visualize the antibodies bound to the HIV proteins, enzyme-labeled antihuman immunoglobulin (Ig) G antibodies are added, followed by the chromogenic substrate. HIV-specific antibodies can be detected rapidly in blood or in oral fluid obtained via swabbing the gums.

Plasma levels of HIV are recorded to study the course of the disease and to measure the effectiveness of antiviral treatments. The viral RNA is reverse transcribed into cDNA, which is then amplified with the polymerase chain reaction. The number of viral RNA copies per milliliter of plasma is termed the viral load.

Pathogenesis and epidemiology

The pathogenesis of AIDS is directly related to the tropism of the virus for CD4$^+$ cells and myeloid cells, which results in the gradual decline in the number of CD4$^+$ T cells and the subsequent impairment of the immune system. Nevertheless, apparently CD4-negative cells such as renal and gastrointestinal cells and astrocytes in the brain may also be infected, possibly via alternative receptors or via cell-cell fusion. The type of HIV that initially infects a person, for example via sexual contact, is the R5 virus, which binds to both the CD4 receptor and the CCR5 chemokine receptor that are found on monocytes, macrophages, and dendritic cells. The virus enters through a break in the mucosal surface and infects the mucosa-associated lymphoid tissue. Monocytes, macrophages, and dendritic cells, as well as memory T cells that get infected later, act as reservoirs of the virus. HIV bound on the surface of dendritic cells via the DC-SIGN molecule may infect CD4+ T cells that interact with the dendritic cell during antigen presentation. Mutations in the structure of CCR5 may prevent virus entry, as in individuals with the Δ32 deletion mutation. As the viral gp120 mutates late in the course of the disease, the virus becomes T-tropic and binds to both CD4 and the CXCR4 chemokine receptor. This shift correlates with the progression of the disease, most likely because of the more rapid destruction of helper T lymphocytes.

The destruction of CD4+ T cells is caused by a number of factors:

- The budding of a large number of virions from the cell surface may compromise the integrity of the plasma membrane. The large amounts of viral proteins and nucleic acids produced in the cell may affect the proper functioning of cellular processes.
- When HIV proteins distort cellular regulation, or when nonintegrated circular viral DNA accumulates in nonpermissive (nonactivated) CD4 T cells, the cells may undergo programmed cell death (apoptosis). The HIV envelope alone, or that bound to antibodies, may impart an inappropriate signal to CD4+ cells, forcing them to initiate apoptosis.
- Uninfected cells ("innocent bystanders") may be killed by cytotoxic T cells that recognize HIV bound to the surface of the cell in a process known as *antibody-dependent cellular cytotoxicity.* Cytotoxic T cells may also destroy uninfected cells that have taken up HIV particles and present viral fragments on their surface.
- CD4+ T cells may be unable to respond to immune stimulation when they are "deactivated" by signals from HIV, resulting in a state known as anergy.
- HIV can kill hematopoietic precursor cells and damage the microenvironment needed for the differentiation of these cells in the bone marrow and thymus. These tissues may not be able to regenerate, thus adversely affecting the immune system.
- Chronic activation of helper T cells in response to the large amounts of HIV antigen produced may lead to the terminal differentiation and death of the cells.

HIV establishes latency in memory T cells, which do not express the virus. There is an extended period of clinical latency, without apparent evidence of disease. However, HIV still replicates in lymph nodes and is trapped by follicular dendritic cells that are located in germinal centers. These cells trap microorganisms, including HIV, as B cells initiate their response after recognizing antigens of the trapped pathogen. During periods of undetectable virus in the blood (usually less than 50 RNA copies/mL), large numbers of HIV accumulate in the lymph nodes. CD4+ T cells in the germinal centers and their vicinity become activated by cytokines secreted by other immune cells in the lymphoid tissue; this enables productive infection of the CD4+ cells by HIV and increases virus production by infected cells.

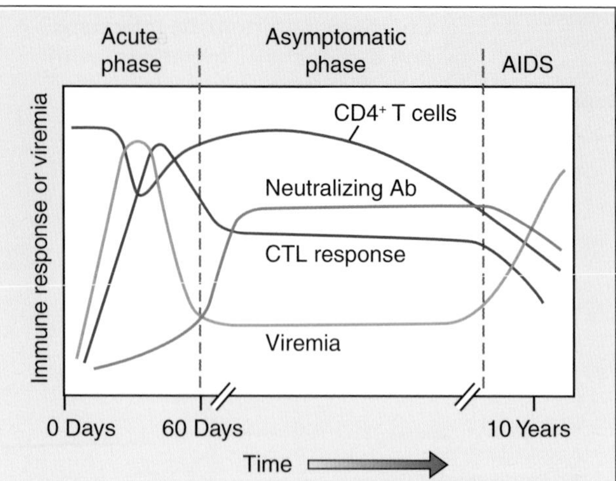

Fig 31-3 The approximate time course of viremia, the production of neutralizing antibodies (Ab), the number of CD4+ T cells in blood, and the CTL response to HIV infection. (Adapted from Ryan and Ray.)

As a result of the chronic secretion of cytokines and activation of immune cells, the complex fine structure of the lymph node deteriorates and scar tissue is formed. This in turn causes breakdown in the proper communication between the cells, impairing the immune response. Cells in the lymph node cannot communicate, so the immune system cannot function properly. Although antiretroviral therapy can reduce virus production and infection of new cells, the immune system may not be able to recover completely as a result of the damaged lymph node architecture.

CD8+ cytotoxic T lymphocytes (CTLs) recognize and kill actively infected cells that are producing virions and are a very important component of the immune response to infection. A successful HIV vaccine will have to elicit both CTLs and neutralizing antibodies. CTLs secrete chemokines such as RANTES, MIP-1α, and MIP-1β that bind the chemokine co-receptors for HIV, thereby restricting HIV entry and replication. The CD8 antiviral factor and the defensins released by these cells also inhibit viral replication to some extent. CTLs have to be activated by helper T cells; thus, when the number of CD4+ T cells declines, CTL numbers also decline, contributing to disease progression. Figure 31-3 shows the approximate time course of viremia, the production of neutralizing antibodies, the number of CD4+ T cells in blood, and the cytotoxic T-cell response to HIV infection.

It has been estimated that the plasma half-life of HIV is 5 to 6 hours, 10 billion virions are produced every day, and up to 1 billion CD4+ cells are generated each day in response to the infection. The HIV RT enzyme is error prone while making DNA copies from viral RNA, and thus new strains of HIV emerge that may avoid detection by antibodies or CTLs. Strains of HIV from patients with advanced disease are more virulent and infect more cell types than strains obtained earlier from the same individual. One explanation may be that HIV develops the ability to use co-receptors in addition to CCR5 (eg, CXCR4).

There are three major routes of HIV transmission:

1. Sexual transmission: Among adults, HIV is transmitted most commonly via sexual intercourse with an infected partner. The virus can penetrate the epithelial layers of the vagina, vulva, penis, or rectum. The risk of transmission is increased by factors that may damage the epithelia, especially other sexually transmitted infections that cause ulcers or inflammation. The virus can traverse the vaginal mucosa and interact with dendritic projections of Langerhans cells and infect macrophages, dendritic cells, and helper T lymphocytes in the submucosal layers. Dendritic cells in the mucosa may bind to and carry the virus from the site of infection to the local lymph nodes, where other cells may become infected. The DC-SIGN molecule on the surface of dendritic cells may be involved in this transmission process.
2. Transmission via blood: Sharing of needles contaminated with HIV-infected blood is a major route of transmission among injection drug users. Because all blood products in the United States are tested for HIV and other viruses, the risk of transmission via blood transfusions is very low. However, at the beginning of the AIDS epidemic, many individuals receiving clotting factors were exposed to HIV. Clotting factors are now genetically engineered. Health care workers are at risk for transmission from accidental needlestick injuries or from exposure of broken skin and mucosal membranes to infected blood. However, the rate of seroconversion from such incidents is fortunately less than 1% of those exposed to HIV-positive blood. This may be because the amount of infectious virus in the needle is very small, and larger volumes and repeated exposure are necessary for a significant probability of infection. Nevertheless, extreme care is necessary in handling needles and sharp instruments. Although the virus has been detected in tears, saliva, and urine, these sources have not been demonstrated to be infectious. Breast milk, however, is a source of infection of neonates.
3. Vertical transmission: HIV transmission to children in the United States is mostly before or during birth. The use of a specific regimen of azidothymidine (zidovudine) reduces the chance of transmission by about two-thirds, and combinations of antiretroviral drugs further reduce the rate of mother-to-child transmission. The azidothymidine regimen has greatly reduced vertical transmission in resource-poor developing countries. However, the virus may also be transmitted via breastfeeding, and thus affordable alternatives to breastfeeding are needed.

HIV is not transmitted by touching, kissing, coughing, sneezing, insect bites, water, food, or via swimming pools.

At the end of 2012, approximately 1.2 million individuals, including an estimated 156,000 persons whose infections had not been diagnosed, were living with AIDS in the United States. It is estimated that 13,700 people diagnosed with AIDS died in 2012. Since the beginning of the AIDS epidemic in the early 1980s, an estimated 658,507 people have died of the disease. Worldwide, there are approximately 35 million people living with AIDS. In the United States, there were about 47,000 new infections in 2013. There were an estimated 2.1 million new cases around the world in 2013.

Treatment and prevention

Many of the antiretroviral drugs tested initially against HIV infection had been developed previously for the potential treatment of cancer. Azidothymidine (AZT) was the first successful anti-HIV therapy. The initial clinical trial was halted early because the treatment group had a significantly lower death rate than the placebo group. AZT is still given to infants born to HIV-positive mothers for 6 weeks after birth. However, the single use of nucleoside analog antivirals is declining. Antiretroviral drugs are currently given as a combination, called highly active antiretroviral therapy (HAART), because the likelihood of the development of drug resistance is lower and the blood levels of HIV can be reduced to undetectable levels (Box 31-2). HAART can be customized for individual patients depending on the susceptibility of the viral strains and the tolerability of the drugs. It is recommended that therapy be initiated if the patient has AIDS-defining illnesses or if the level of helper T cells drops to less than 200/μL. If the viral load is high (greater than 100,000 RNA copies/mL), therapy can be considered even if the helper T cell numbers are greater than 350/μL. Postexposure prophylaxis, for example following a needlestick injury, is essential to prevent infection.

Anti-HIV drugs have a number of different viral targets (see Box 31-2). Binding of gp120 to the CCR5 co-receptor is inhibited with a receptor agonist (maraviroc). Gp41-mediated virus-cell fusion is inhibited by a peptide drug (T-20, enfuvirtide). RT is inhibited by nucleoside analog drugs, including AZT, dideoxyinosine, and dideoxycytidine, that are phosphorylated by cellular enzymes and incorporated into the cDNA, thereby causing DNA chain termination. RT is also inhibited by other mechanisms by non-nucleoside inhibitors (efavirenz). Raltegravir inhibits viral integrase, preventing the incorporation of the viral genome into the cell chromosome. Protease inhibitors such as ritonavir and indinavir block the cleavage of the Gag and Gag-Pol polyproteins, thereby preventing the maturation of the virus structure (Fig 31-4). The protease inhibitor shown in Fig 31-5 is darunavir, a prototype of which was first shown to inhibit HIV-1 replication in the author's laboratory.

Although antiviral drugs inhibit HIV replication or infection, they cannot cure HIV/AIDS. Early investigations of HIV led to the belief that HIV infection was not curable because of the presence of the proviral genome in the chromosomes of infected cells. However, this defeatist belief has been questioned during the last decade, and scientists have begun to investigate methods by which latently infected cells can be activated to express HIV so that these cells can be recognized by the immune system.

Box 31-2 Antiviral drugs for HIV infection

Nucleoside analog reverse transcriptase inhibitors (NRTIs)
- Azidothymidine (AZT, zidovudine; Retrovir, GlaxoSmithKline)
- Dideoxycytidine (ddC, zalcitabine; Hivid, Roche)
- Dideoxyinosine (ddI, didanosine; Videx, Bristol-Myers Squibb)
- Stavudine (d4T; Zerit, Bristol-Myers Squibb)
- Tenofovir disoproxil fumarate (Viread, Gilead)
- Lamivudine (3TC; Epivir, GlaxoSmithKline)
- Abacavir sulfate (ABC; Ziagen, GlaxoSmithKline)
- Emtricitabine (Emtriva, Gilead)

Non-nucleoside reverse transcriptase inhibitors (NNRTIs)
- Nevirapine (Viramune, Boehringer Ingelheim)
- Efavirenz (Sustiva, Bristol-Myers Squibb)
- Etravirene (Intelence, Janssen)
- Rilpivirine (Edurant, Janssen)
- Delavirdine (Rescriptor, Pfizer)

Protease inhibitors (PIs)
- Saquinavir mesylate (Invirase, Roche)
- Tipranavir (Aptivus, Boehringer Ingelheim)
- Darunavir (Prezista, Tibotec)
- Ritonavir (Norvir, Abbott)
- Indinavir (Crixivan, Merck)
- Lopinavir + ritonavir (Kaletra, Abbott)
- Nelfinavir (Viracept, Agouron)
- Fosamprenavir (Lexiva, GlaxoSmithKline)
- Atazanavir (Reyataz, Bristol-Myers Squibb/Novartis)
- Nelfinavir mesylate (Viracept, Agouron)

Binding and fusion inhibitors
- Maraviroc (CCR5 inhibitor; Selzentry, Pfizer)
- Enfuvirtide (T-20; Fuzeon, Trimeris/Roche)

Integrase inhibitors
- Raltegravir (Isentress, Merck)
- Dolutegravir (Tivicay, GlaxoSmithKline)

Combinations used in highly active antiretroviral therapy (HAART)
- Efavirenz + tenofovir + emtricitabine (Atripla, Bristol-Myers Squibb)
- Ritonavir-boosted atazanavir + tenofovir/emtricitabine
- Ritonavir-boosted darunavir + tenofovir/emtricitabine
- Raltegravir + tenofovir/emtricitabine
- Abacavir + zidovudine + lamivudine (Trizivir, GlaxoSmithKline)
- Emtricitabine + rilpivirine + tenofovir (Complera, Gilead)
- Elvitegravir + cobicistat + emtricitabine + tenofovir (Stribild, Gilead)
- Lamivudine + zidovudine (Combivir, GlaxoSmithKline)
- Abacavir + lamivudine (Epzicom, GlaxoSmithKline)
- Tenofovir + emtricitabine (Truvada, Gilead)

(Adapted from Murray et al.)

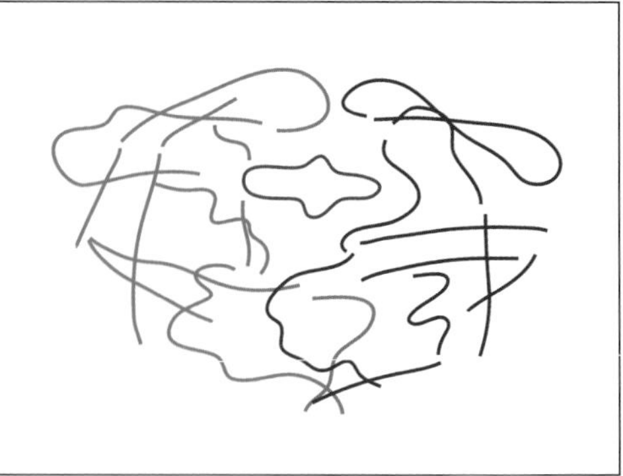

Fig 31-4 The schematic homodimeric structure of the HIV-1 protease and the location of darunavir in between the dimers. Darunavir has a high affinity for the protease and prevents its dimerization. Binding of the inhibitor is favored by the interactions between the apolar residues of the inhibitor and the hydrophobic amino acid side chains.

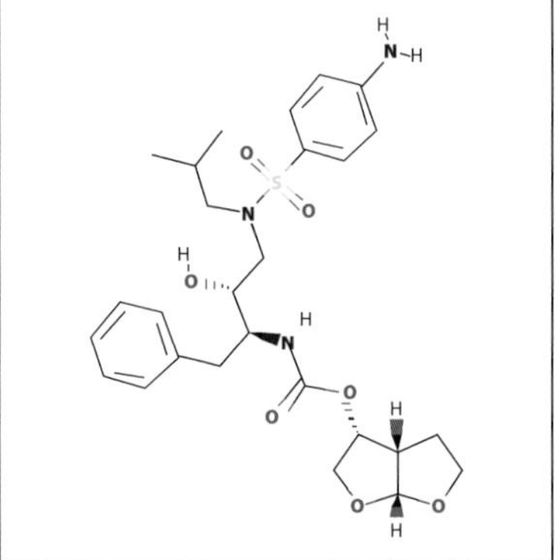

Fig 31-5 The structure of darunavir. (Adapted from the NIH PubChem Open Chemistry Database.)

One enzyme involved in enabling histone proteins to compact DNA is **histone deacetylase** (HDAC), which removes acetyl groups bound to lysines. The exposed lysines as well as arginines can interact with negatively charged DNA and condense it, thereby preventing transcription. Inhibitors of HDAC can induce the acetylation of histones, enabling transcriptional activation, including that of the HIV proviral genome. Inhibitors such as **vorinostat**, panobinostat, and romidepsin are being tested in clinical trials. Initial results indicate that mere activation of HIV in latently infected cells is not sufficient for the immune system to recognize and kill the cells and hence eliminate the reservoir. Additional strategies may include:

- Administration of cytokines, antibodies, and components of a therapeutic vaccine to stimulate the immune system.
- Ex vivo (outside the body) activation of immune cells, such as cytotoxic T lymphocytes, γδ T cells, or natural cytotoxic cells (also known as *natural killer [NK] cells*), by cytokines or HIV peptides.
- Genetic modification of patient peripheral blood cells to express T-cell receptors that can efficiently recognize viral antigens.
- Use of antibody-toxin conjugates that can recognize and kill virus-infected cells.
- Lentivirus-mediated delivery to infected cells of suicide gene constructs that are activated only in HIV-expressing cells.

Prevention of HIV infection requires a number of approaches:

• Educating the population as to how HIV is transmitted and explaining prevention measures, such as the practicing of safe sex, the proper use of condoms, monogamous relationships, and not sharing or reusing needles.
• Screening blood, blood products, and organs for HIV.
• Infection-control measures, including universal precautions based on the assumption that all patients are infectious for HIV. These include wearing protective gloves, mask and gown, and other barriers to prevent exposure to blood products. Contaminated surfaces should be disinfected with 10% household bleach, 70% ethanol or isopropanol, 2% glutaraldehyde, and 4% formaldehyde (or 6% hydrogen peroxide).
• Use of contraceptive creams with anti-HIV drugs and male circumcision. These procedures only reduce the risk of infection.

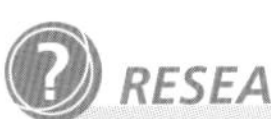

What are the different approaches that have been tried in developing an HIV vaccine? What are the difficulties in producing a highly efficacious vaccine?

Other Retroviruses

The three human retrovirus subfamilies are the Oncovirinae, which includes human T-cell lymphotropic virus type 1 (HTLV-1) and HTLV-2; the Lentivirinae, which includes HIV-1 and HIV-2; and the Spumavirinae. The first human retrovirus to be isolated was a spumavirus, but it does not cause human disease. Endogenous retroviruses have been found throughout the human chromosomes, but they do not produce virions. The first oncoretrovirus, HTLV-1 was discovered in the 1970s and was shown to cause a rare cancer restricted to Japan, Africa, and the Caribbean.

Human T-cell lymphotropic virus

The HTLV Tax protein is a transcriptional activator of the viral LTR, and Rex facilitates the transport of mRNA encoding structural proteins into the cytoplasm. Gp46 and gp21 are the envelope proteins of the virus, and p24 is the capsid protein. Although HTLV-1 can penetrate and infect different cell types, productive infection is restricted to a few cell types, including T lymphocytes.

Clinical syndromes and diagnosis

HTLV-1 causes adult T-cell leukemia/lymphoma in 1% to 2.5% of infected individuals, following a decades-long latency. The syndromes include hepatosplenomegaly, lymphadenopathy, and lesions in the skin and bones. Fungal and viral opportunistic infections are seen in these patients, especially following treatment with chemotherapy. HTLV-1 also causes HTLV-associated myelopathy/tropical spastic paraparesis, whose symptoms include weakness in the lower limbs, low back pain, and spasticity during walking. HTLV-2 causes hairy cell leukemia of T-cell origin.

Pathogenesis and epidemiology

HTLV-1 infection of CD4 T cells can lead to malignant transformation after many years. The Tax protein of the virus binds to the LTR of HTLV-1 and enhances the transcription of proto-oncogenes, which leads to transformation. Tax also causes an increase in the production of interleukin-2 (IL-2) and IL-2 receptor, causing uncontrolled growth. Syncytia formation of infected T lymphocytes has been observed. HTLV-associated myelopathy/tropical spastic paraparesis is a demyelinating disease, especially in motor neurons, most likely via an autoimmune reaction and CTL-mediated killing of neurons.

HTLV-1 is transmitted via blood, including sexual intercourse, blood transfusion, and intravenous drug use. HTLV-1 is prevalent in Japan, the Caribbean, and Hawaii. In parts of Japan, the prevalence of seropositivity has been as high as 27%. In Western Europe and the United States, the incidence is increasing among intravenous drug users. Breastfeeding appears to be the main source of mother-to-child transmission.

Treatment and prevention

Adult T-cell leukemia/lymphoma is usually treated with anticancer medicines. Patients with HTLV-associated myelopathy/tropical spastic paraparesis may benefit from a combination of interferon and antiretroviral agents such as AZT and lamivudine.

Bibliography

Archin NM, Sung JM, Garrido C, Soriano-Sarabia N, Margolis DM. Eradicating HIV-1 infection: Seeking to clear a persistent pathogen. Nat Rev Microbiol 2014;12:750–764.

Barré-Sinoussi F, Chermann JC, Rey F, et al. Isolation of a T-lymphotropic retrovirus from a patient at risk for acquired immune deficiency syndrome (AIDS). Science 1983;220:868–871.

Biggar RJ, Chaturvedi AK, Goedert JJ, Engels EA; HIV/AIDS Cancer Match Study. AIDS-related cancer and severity of immunosuppression in persons with AIDS. J Natl Cancer Inst 2007;99:962–972.

Centers for Disease Control and Prevention. (2014) HIV/AIDS: Basic Statistics. www.cdc.gov/hiv/basics/statistics.html. Accessed 28 July 2015.

Engelman A, Cherepanov P. The structural biology of HIV-1: Mechanistic and therapeutic insights. Nat Rev Microbiol 2012;10:279–290.

Gallo RC, Salahuddin SZ, Popovic M, et al. Frequent detection and isolation of cytopathic retroviruses (HTLV-III) from patients with AIDS and at risk for AIDS. Science 1984;224:500–503.

Gebremedhin S, Au A, Konopka K, Milnes M, Düzgüneş N. A gene therapy approach to eliminate HIV-infected cells. J Calif Dent Assoc 2012;40:403–406.

Ghosh AK, Pretzer E, Cho H, Hussain KA, Düzgüneş N. Antiviral activity of UIC-PI, a novel inhibitor of the human immunodeficiency virus type 1 protease. Antiviral Res 2002;54:29–36.

Hamer DH. Can HIV be cured? Mechanisms of HIV persistence and strategies to combat it. Curr HIV Res 2004;2:99–111.

Huang D, Caflisch A. How does darunavir prevent HIV-1 protease dimerization? Chem Theory Comput 2012;8:1786–1794.

Konopka K, Davis BR, Larsen CE, Düzgüneş N. Anionic liposomes inhibit human immunodeficiency virus type 1 (HIV-1) infectivity in CD4⁺ A3.01 and H9 cells. Antiviral Chem Chemother 1993;4:179–187.

Konopka K, Düzgüneş N. Expression of CD4 controls the susceptibility of THP-1 cells to infection by CCR5- and CXCR4-dependent HIV type 1 isolates. AIDS Res Hum Retroviruses 2002;18:123–131.

Larsen CE, Nir S, Alford DR, Jennings M, Lee KD, Düzgüneş N. Human immunodeficiency virus type 1 (HIV-1) fusion with model membranes: Kinetic analysis and the effects of pH and divalent cations. Biochim Biophys Acta 1993;1147:223–236.

Levy JA, Hoffman AD, Kramer SM, Landis JA, Shimabukuro JM, Oshiro LS. Isolation of lymphocytopathic retroviruses from San Francisco patients with AIDS. Science 1984;225:840–842.

Mosby's Dictionary of Medicine, Nursing and Health Professions, ed 9. Philadelphia: Mosby/Elsevier, 2012.

Murray PR, Rosenthal KS, Pfaller MA. Medical Microbiology, ed 7. Philadelphia: Mosby/Elsevier, 2013.

National Institute of Allergy and Infectious Diseases. More on How HIV Causes AIDS. www.niaid.nih.gov/topics/HIVAIDS/Understanding/howHIVCausesAIDS/pages/howhiv.aspx. Accessed 28 July 2015.

National Institute of Neurological Disorders and Stroke. Neurological Complications of AIDS Fact Sheet. http://www.ninds.nih.gov/disorders/aids/detail_aids.htm. Accessed 28 July 2015.

Ryan KJ, Ray CG. Sherris Medical Microbiology, ed 5. New York: McGraw-Hill, 2010.

Sarngadharan MG, DeVico AL, Bruch L, Schüpbach J, Gallo RC. HTLV-III: The etiologic agent of AIDS. Princess Takamatsu Symp 1984;15:301–308.

US Food and Drug Administration. Antiretroviral drugs used in the treatment of HIV infection. http://www.fda.gov/ForPatients/Illness/HIVAIDS/Treatment/ucm118915.htm. Accessed 28 July 2015.

Take-Home Messages

- Retroviruses are enveloped viruses with a positive-strand RNA genome that is transcribed into DNA by reverse transcriptase. The DNA is then integrated into the host cell genome.
- Human immunodeficiency virus type 1 (HIV-1) is the etiologic agent of acquired immunodeficiency syndrome (AIDS), currently designated as HIV/AIDS.
- The replication cycle of HIV-1 begins with binding of the viral envelope surface glycoprotein (SU) gp120 to CD4 and to a secondary receptor, which is normally a chemokine receptor.
- The transmembrane glycoprotein (TM) gp41 undergoes a conformational change and inserts its hydrophobic N-terminus into the host cell membrane and facilitates membrane fusion.
- The HIV genome has three main gene clusters: *gag*, *pol*, and *env*.
- The initial HIV infection may be asymptomatic or may be followed within 2 to 4 weeks by the acute phase.
- After this phase, the infection may become asymptomatic or turn into ongoing generalized lymphadenopathy.
- The pathogenesis of the virus involves the gradual depletion of $CD4^+$ T cells.
- The clinical syndromes associated with this depletion include opportunistic infections with fungi, herpes simplex virus, and intracellular bacteria.
- The AIDS-defining conditions set by the CDC are HIV seropositivity and $CD4^+$ lymphocyte counts less than 200/mm^3.
- HIV-1 enters the host through a break in mucosal surfaces and infects the mucosa-associated lymphoid tissue. Monocytes, macrophages, and dendritic cells, as well as memory T cells that get infected later, act as reservoirs of the virus.
- The destruction of $CD4^+$ T cells is caused by a number of factors, including virus budding, apoptosis, cytotoxic T-cell action on uninfected cells, and chronic activation.
- During clinical latency, HIV-1 still replicates in lymph nodes and is trapped by follicular dendritic cells located in germinal centers. The complex, fine structure of the lymph node deteriorates, and scar tissue is formed.
- HIV is transmitted primarily by sexual contact, blood transfusion, and mother-to-child transmission.
- HAART reduces the likelihood of the development of drug resistance and can reduce the blood levels of HIV to undetectable levels.
- Anti–HIV-1 drugs include RT inhibitors dideoxycytidine and dideoxyinosine, the co-receptor antagonist maraviroc, the fusion inhibitor enfuvirtide, the integrase inhibitor raltegravir, and the protease inhibitors saquinavir and darunavir.
- The retrovirus HTLV-1 causes adult T-cell leukemia/lymphoma in a low percentage of infected individuals after a decades-long latency.

32 Hepatitis Viruses

Inflammation of the liver, or hepatitis, can be caused by viruses, bacteria, protozoa, toxins, and drugs. There are six viruses that cause hepatitis (Table 32-1). The structures and nucleic acids of these viruses are different from one another. Hepatitis A virus (HAV) is a picornavirus that causes infectious hepatitis. Hepatitis B virus (HBV) causes "serum hepatitis"; it is an enveloped DNA virus. Hepatitis C virus (HCV) was known as *non-A, non-B hepatitis* before the agent was identified in 1989; it is an enveloped flavivirus. Hepatitis D virus (HDV) is also known as the *delta agent* and requires co-infection with HBV as a helper virus. Hepatitis E virus (HEV) is an enteric non-A, non-B hepatitis virus. Hepatitis G virus (HGV) is a new, parenterally transmitted virus.

Hepatitis A Virus

HAV (genus: *Hepatovirus*) is a naked capsid picornavirus with a positive-sense, single-strand RNA that was identified in 1973 by immunoelectron microscopy. The genomic viral protein VPg is attached to the RNA at the 5′ end. The capsid contains the VP1 to VP4 proteins (Fig 32-1). Upon binding to its receptor (HAV cell receptor 1 glycoprotein, or T-cell immunoglobulin and mucin domain protein), the VP4 protein is released, causing the virion structure to weaken. The VP1 protein at one of the vertices of the capsid forms a channel across the plasma membrane, and the viral RNA enters the cytoplasm through this channel. The RNA is translated into a polyprotein, which is then cleaved into individual proteins by virus-encoded proteases. The assembled virus is released by exocytosis, unlike other picornaviruses.

Clinical syndromes and diagnosis

The incubation period for HAV is 15 to 45 days. Initial symptoms are malaise, headache, myalgia, abdominal pain, poor appetite, and low-grade fever. Jaundice develops in 70% to 80% of adults and 10% of children, with concomitant improvement of symptoms. Many infected individuals have a subclinical illness, as indicated by the low number of reported cases and the relatively high seropositivity (about 40%). The incidence of fulminant hepatitis is only 1 to 3 per 1,000 individuals. Infection does not lead to chronic liver disease.

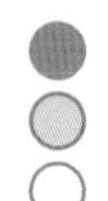

Table 32-1 Hepatitis viruses

Abbreviation	Common name	Virus structure	Transmission
HAV	Infectious hepatitis	Picornavirus; RNA	Fecal-oral
HBV	Serum hepatitis	Hepadnavirus; DNA	Parenteral; sexual
HCV	Non-A, non-B posttransfusion hepatitis	Flavivirus; RNA	Parenteral; sexual
HDV	Delta agent	Viroid-like; circular RNA	Parenteral; sexual
HEV	Enteric non-A, non-B hepatitis	Calicivirus-like, RNA	Fecal-oral
HGV	Hepatitis G virus	Flavivirus; RNA	Parenteral

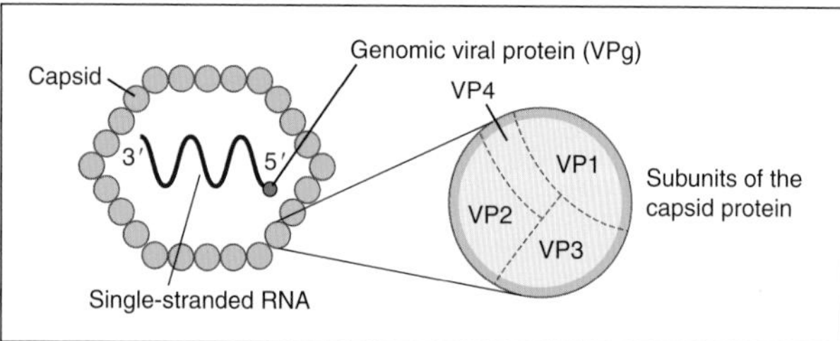

Fig 32-1 Schematic diagram of HAV, which is 27 nm in diameter, and the possible arrangement of the VP1–VP4 subunits of the capsid. The virus contains a single-stranded RNA molecule with a genomic viral protein attached at the 5′ end of the RNA.

Diagnosis is usually based on the clinical course of infection. Acute HAV infection can be demonstrated by the detection of anti-HAV immunoglobulin (Ig) M antibodies.

Pathogenesis and epidemiology

Following ingestion, HAV is most likely taken up through the epithelial cells of the oropharynx and the intestines and enters the bloodstream to reach the liver. HAV multiplies in hepatocytes and Kupffer cells. It is shed into the bile and the stool and can be found in large quantities by electron microscopy 10 to 14 days before the symptoms appear. Infection induces lymphocyte infiltration, followed by the elimination of infected cells by natural cytotoxic (or *natural killer*) cells, cytotoxic T cells, and antibody-dependent cellular cytotoxicity. This immune response causes immunopathology.

The virus is prevalent in communities with poor sanitation, as expected because of its fecal-oral route of transmission. Contaminated food, particularly shellfish from coastal areas close to sewage outlets, causes outbreaks. Shellfish can act as a filter for the virus and concentrate it, and in 1988 it caused an outbreak in China that infected 300,000 people. Because most infected people are contagious during the asymptomatic incubation period, HAV can spread rapidly. Day-care centers may be a source of virus spread. The number of acute hepatitis A cases in the United States reported to the Centers for Disease Control and Prevention (CDC) has declined from 13,397 in 2000 to 1,398 in 2011.

Treatment and prevention

Treatment is supportive, such as rest and adequate nutrition. Prevention measures include avoiding contaminated water and food, hand washing, and chlorine treatment of drinking water. Administration of immune serum globulin before or soon after exposure is highly effective in reducing the symptoms of the disease. A killed-virus vaccine (Havrix, GlaxoSmithKline; Vaqta, Merck) is recommended for children and adults who are at high risk for infection (eg, in the same household or having intimate contact with an infected person). It may even be given shortly after exposure to the virus.

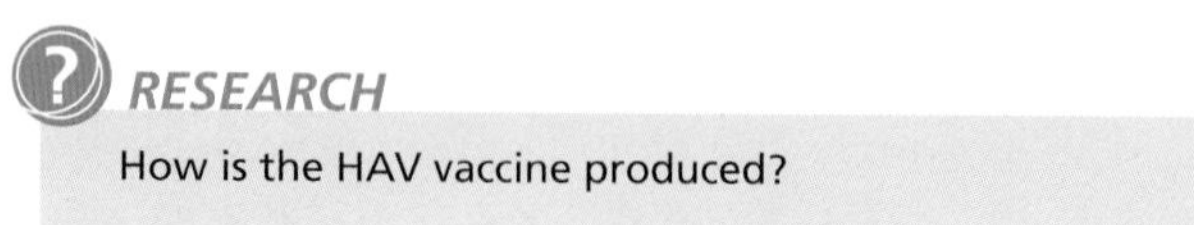

How is the HAV vaccine produced?

Hepatitis B Virus

The genus *Orthohepadnavirus* of the Hepadnaviridae family includes HBV ("serum hepatitis"), which is a major cause of chronic liver disease. It is an enveloped DNA virus that was first identified in 1965. HBV is a double-layered virus, with a 27-nm inner core, made up of the core antigen HBcAg enclosing the viral DNA and the polymerase, and an outer envelope 42 nm in diameter, containing the surface antigen HBsAg (Fig 32-2). The virion is termed the *Dane particle* in honor of David S. Dane. The sodium taurocholate co-transporting polypeptide (found exclusively in hepatocytes) acts as the cell uptake receptor for HBV. The virus is internalized in clathrin-coated endocytotic vesicles. Fusion of the viral and endosomal membranes appears to be pH-independent, unlike influenza virus. In chronically infected individuals, spherical and filamentous "subviral" particles are formed from HBsAg, lipid, and carbohydrate, without the viral DNA (Fig 32-3). As many as 10^{13} particles/mL and 10^{10} infectious virions/mL can be detected in blood. The virus also produces the HBeAg protein that is secreted from infected cells into the bloodstream. Its presence is an indicator of active viral infection. Hepadnaviruses are the only viruses that produce a DNA genome by reverse transcription of an intermediate RNA as a template (Fig 32-4).

Clinical syndromes and diagnosis

In the prodrome phase of acute infection, the symptoms include weakness, lack of appetite, nausea, and vomiting. The symptoms of hepatitis are jaundice, pain in the upper right quadrant of the abdomen, pale stools, and dark urine. Liver damage can be assessed by elevated levels of alanine transaminase (ALT) in the blood.

Immune complexes of antibody and HBsAg can lead to arthritis, maculopapular rash, glomerulonephritis, and acute necrotizing vasculitis. About 1% of acute infections can become fulminant and result in liver failure.

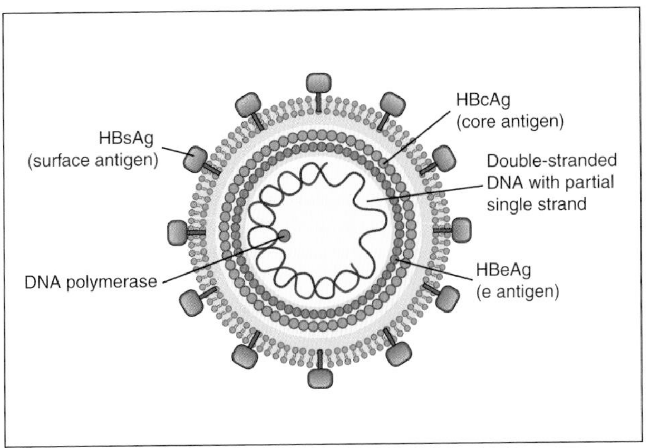

Fig 32-2 Schematic diagram of HBV (the Dane particle), with a diameter of 42 nm.

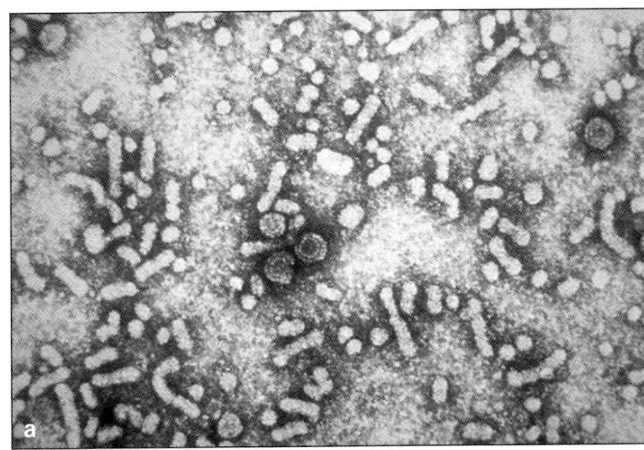

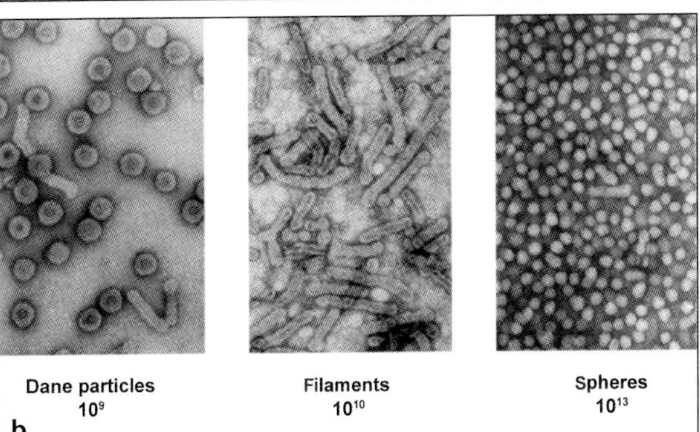

Fig 32-3 *(a and b)* Negative-stain electron microscopy images and approximate numbers of HBV-associated particles in 1 mL of serum from a highly viremic, chronically infected HBV carrier. In this image, the Dane particles appear to be 52 nm in diameter, the spheres are 17 to 25 nm in diameter, and the filaments have the same diameter as the spheres but different lengths. *(a)* (Public Health Image Library image 5631, courtesy of the CDC.) *(b)* (Reprinted from Gerlich.)

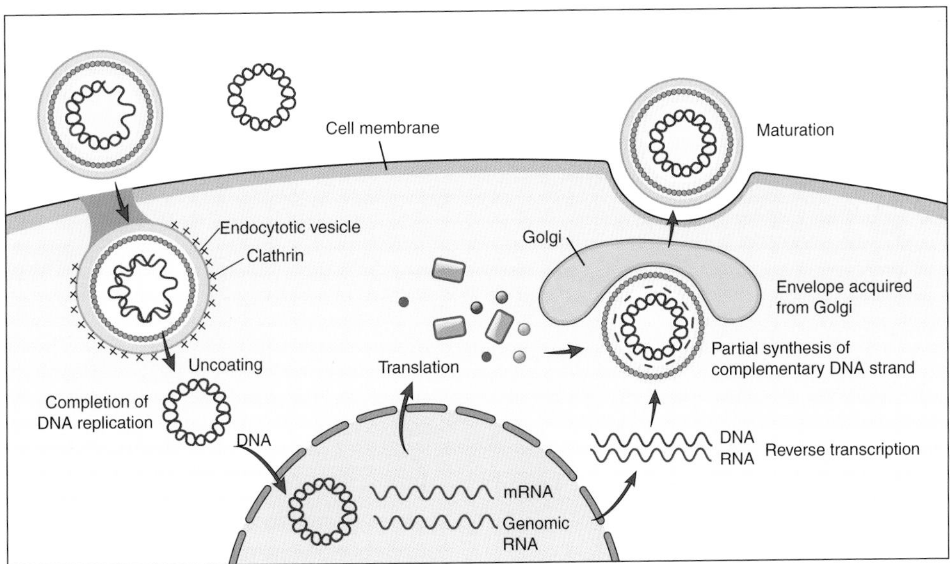

Fig 32-4 The replication cycle of HBV.

Although 90% to 95% of adults with acute infection recover completely, the remaining 5% to 10% of adults, 20% to 50% of children younger than 6 years of age, and 90% of newborns with acute infection develop a chronic HBV infection. These individuals have an insufficient cell-mediated immunity, which would normally clear the acute infection completely. The initial phase of chronic infection is referred to as the immune tolerance phase, where the virus replicates to very high levels. Patients in this phase are highly infectious. HBeAg is present in serum, and ALT levels are normal, indicating normal liver function, as corroborated by the lack of inflammation and fibrosis in liver biopsies (Fig 32-5). The tolerance phase is followed by the immune clearance phase; for young patients, this generally occurs at adulthood. In this phase, the ALT levels are elevated, and there are still high levels of HBV DNA in serum and moderate to severe liver inflammation and fibrosis.

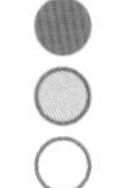

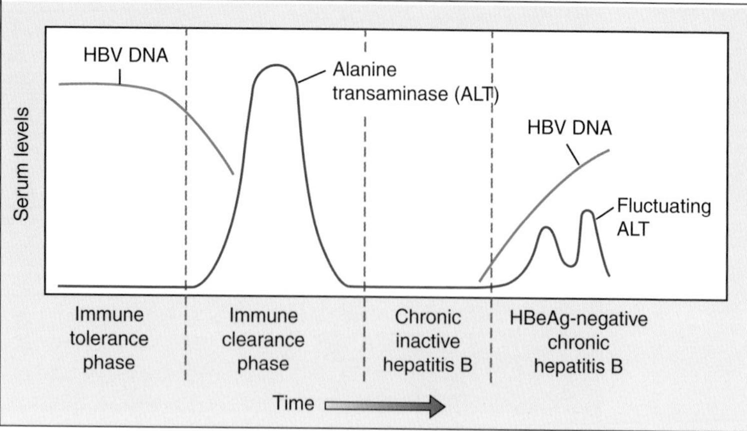

Fig 32-5 Serum markers seen in the different phases of chronic HBV infection. (Adapted from Greenwood et al.)

The next phase is inactive chronic hepatitis B in patients who eliminate active HBV infection. These patients, called "healthy hepatitis B carriers," have a relatively favorable long-term prognosis and have normal ALT levels but still have HBsAg in blood.

Persistent carriage of HBV is associated with primary hepatocellular carcinoma. Viral nucleic acid sequences are integrated into the tumor cell genome, and the cells express HBV antigens. Primary liver cancer constitutes 20% to 30% of all malignancies in parts of Africa and Asia but only 1% to 2% in the Americas and Europe. Primary hepatocellular carcinoma is a vaccine-preventable cancer, as is cervical cancer.

Detection of various antigens and antibodies in blood provides detailed information on the stage of infection. HBsAg is detected during acute or chronic HBV infection. Its presence means that a person has an acute or chronic infection and can pass the virus to others. Its absence indicates that the person does not have HBV. HBsAg is the most important laboratory test for the detection of early HBV infection. Donated blood is screened for HBsAg. If a person is HBsAg-positive on two occasions at least 6 months apart, he or she is considered a chronic carrier. Anti-HBs is an antibody produced by the body in response to HBsAg, and it means that a person is protected or immune from getting HBV because he or she was successfully vaccinated against HBV or recovered from an acute infection and will not get hepatitis B again. Total anti-HBc is produced by the body in response to core antigen, and its presence means that a person is either infected currently with HBV or was infected in the past.

IgM antibody to the core antigen (IgM anti-HBc) is used to detect an acute infection, and a positive test indicates that a person was infected within the last 6 months. HBeAg is found in the blood when the virus is present during an active HBV infection. A positive test for HBeAg means that a person has high levels of virus in the blood and can readily infect others. This test can also be used to determine the effectiveness of treatment for chronic hepatitis B.

The presence of HBeAg is the best indicator for the presence of infectious virus; ie, it is a marker of active infection. Anti-HBe antibody indicates that a person has chronic HBV infection but is at lower risk for liver problems because there are lower levels of HBV in the blood. A positive test for HBV DNA indicates that the virus is multiplying and that the person is highly contagious. The presence of viral DNA in a person with chronic HBV infection means that a person is possibly at increased risk for liver damage. The efficacy of drug therapy for chronic HBV infection can be monitored by this test.

Pathogenesis and epidemiology

In acute infection, the portal tracts are inflamed, and there is lymphocyte infiltration. Infected hepatocytes have a ballooning appearance and contain acidophilic bodies. There are high levels of virus in the blood. Viral antigens on the hepatocyte surface induce both B-cell and T-cell responses. Antibody-dependent natural cytotoxic cells and cytotoxic T cells can cause damage to hepatocytes. Induction of interferons can increase the expression of major histocompatibility class I molecules on hepatocytes, leading to enhanced antigen recognition by the immune system and cytotoxicity to the target cells.

In chronic hepatitis, necrosis, inflammation, and fibrosis are observed, leading to the development of cirrhosis. Liver damage results from immune system attack on hepatocytes expressing viral antigens, as well as autoimmune reactions to liver antigens. Progression to chronic hepatitis is associated with the inefficiency of the immune response, as indicated by the increased probability of chronic hepatitis in the very young and in immunocompromised persons. Increased risk of cirrhosis is associated with older age, higher levels of HBV DNA, longer duration of infection, infection with HBV genotype C, alcohol consumption, and co-infection with HCV, HDV, and human immunodeficiency virus (HIV).

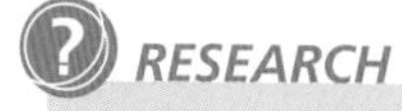

What are the characteristics of cirrhosis?

It is estimated that 80% of primary hepatocellular carcinoma can be attributed to chronic HBV infection. The introduction of universal vaccination against HBV in Taiwan has reduced the incidence of hepatocellular carcinoma in young adults in that country. Hepatocellular carcinoma is one of the most common causes of cancer mortality.

The virus is transmitted through transfusion of blood and blood products, accidental injection of contaminated blood, contaminated needles and syringes, exchange of fluids (such as blood, semen, and vaginal secretions), and organ and tissue transplantation. Vertical transmission from mother to child occurs when the mucous membranes of the baby are contaminated by maternal blood during birth. Close contact between family members involving saliva and blood, such as biting or scratching or sharing of household items, can also lead to infection.

It is estimated by the World Health Organization that 350 million persons worldwide are infected chronically. High prevalence areas are sub-Saharan Africa, most of Asia, and the Pacific islands. Intermediate prevalence areas are Southern Europe, the Middle East, and the Indian subcontinent.

Health care providers and laboratory workers are at risk for exposure. Surgery, dental surgery, and obstetrics and gynecology are high-risk occupations involving working in restricted areas with sharp instruments. Infected health care workers can also accidentally infect patients.

Treatment and prevention

For acute hepatitis B, the treatment is supportive. For chronic hepatitis B, the aim of treatment is to inhibit viral replication, liver disease, and cirrhosis. Pegylated interferon-α is used over a period of 24 to 48 weeks to inhibit viral replication but has adverse side effects including neutropenia, thrombocytopenia, and flulike symptoms.

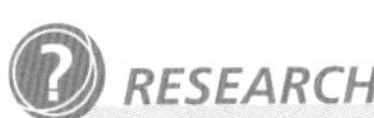

RESEARCH

What is pegylation, and what is its function?

Lamivudine (3TC; 2′,3′-dideoxy-3′-thiacytidine) is a potent reverse transcriptase inhibitor originally developed for the treatment of HIV. It reduces HBV DNA, sometimes to undetectable levels, in 40% of HBeAg-positive patients and in 60% to 70% of HBeAg-negative patients. However, drug-resistant virus emerges with prolonged use. Thus, lamivudine is now used more often as a prophylactic drug to prevent reactivation of HBV in immunocompromised individuals. Adefovir is a nucleotide analog that can decrease HBV DNA levels and normalize liver function. Entecavir is a guanosine analog with potent activity against HBV (Fig 32-6). It is phosphorylated intracellularly and acts by competing with guanosine for interaction with the HBV DNA polymerase. It is incorporated into the growing HBV DNA molecule, and this results in the inhibition of polymerase activity and in chain termination. Treatment with entecavir results in the loss of HBV DNA in serum in 70% to 90% of patients, and ALT levels are normalized in 70% to 80% of the patients. Tenofovir is similar in structure to adefovir but has less kidney toxicity; thus, a higher dose can be used and better antiviral activity can be achieved. The loss of HBV DNA is achieved in 80% to 90% of patients after about a year of therapy, and ALT levels return to normal in 70% to 80% of the patients.

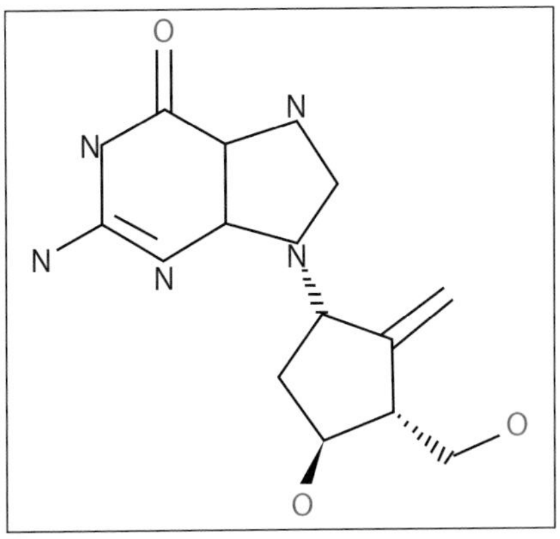

Fig 32-6 The structure of entecavir. (Reproduced from the National Library of Medicine.)

The HBV vaccine is based on recombinant HBsAg produced in yeast; the product is similar to the small particles seen in patients. It is administered in three injections into the deltoid muscle of the upper arm at 0, 1, and 6 months. Greater than 95% of young females develop protective antibodies; the efficacy rate is only 80% in older males. A postvaccination level of greater than 10 mIU Anti-HBs/mL is considered to be protective. In some cases, individuals may not develop immunity even after two courses of the vaccine. For these vaccine nonresponders, hepatitis B immune globulin (Anti-HBsAg) should be administered following accidental exposure. Passive immunization should also be employed even in vaccine responders after exposure and in infants born of HBsAg-positive mothers.

Hepatitis C Virus

It is estimated that there are 170 million carriers of HCV worldwide and 4 million in the United States. HCV is transmitted in a manner similar to HBV but can more readily establish chronic infection.

The virus is classified in the Flavivirus family, which also includes dengue virus serotypes 1 to 4 and yellow fever virus. Flaviviruses are enveloped, positive-strand RNA viruses with an icosahedral capsid or core consisting of the C protein. HCV is classified in the genus *Hepacivirus*. The HCV genome encodes 10 proteins, including an RNA-dependent RNA polymerase, proteases, and the E1 and E2 membrane glycoproteins. The viral RNA is translated into a polyprotein of more than 3,000 amino acids, which is then cleaved into the individual components by the viral proteases. Because the RNA-dependent RNA polymerase is error-prone and lacks the ability to proofread, mutations arise, especially in the E2 protein hypervariable regions. This region contains the neutralization epitope, and thus mutants can escape recognition by the existing immunity.

HCV cell entry involves cellular factors that facilitate virus uptake into hepatocytes. The virion is coated with low-density lipoprotein and very-low-density lipoprotein, enabling it to utilize cell surface receptors for these proteins on hepatocytes to infect the cells. The receptors include the scavenger receptor class B type I (which is also a receptor for high-density lipoprotein), tetraspanin CD81, and the tight junction proteins claudin-1 and Occludin. The virus also uses tyrosine kinases associated with receptors, such as the epidermal growth factor receptor and the ephrin receptor A2, as entry regulators. After endocytosis, the viral membrane undergoes fusion with the endosome membrane in a low pH–dependent manner. Uncoating of the nucleocapsid releases the RNA into the cytoplasm, and the RNA-dependent RNA polymerase mediates the generation of the negative-strand and then the positive-strand RNA for packaging into new virions. The virus assembly starts when viral components bud into the endoplasmic reticulum lumen and are taken through the secretory pathway. However, the exact mechanisms of viral assembly are very complex and are still under investigation.

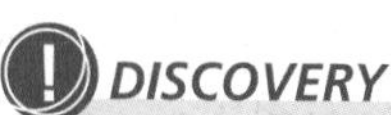

HCV was discovered by Michael Houghton and colleagues in their laboratory at Chiron Corporation in Emeryville, California, after 6 years of intense work between 1982 and 1988. To investigate the viral cause of parenterally transmitted "non-A, non-B viral hepatitis," many molecular biologic methods were used to screen hundreds of millions of cDNA clones derived from liver and plasma samples from experimentally infected chimpanzees. They isolated a single cDNA clone that they showed to be derived from a flavi-like virus. The clone was isolated using a novel, blind immunoscreening method in which antibodies derived from a clinically diagnosed non-A, non-B viral hepatitis patient were used to identify a cDNA clone encoding an immunodominant epitope within the HCV nonstructural protein 4. To ensure that the clone had a viral origin, it was tested for hybridization to a large single-stranded RNA molecule (~10,000 nucleotides) found only in non-A, non-B viral hepatitis–infected samples that shared distant sequence identity with flaviviruses. The clone was shown to be extrachromosomal and to encode a protein that elicited antibody seroconversion only in infected chimpanzees and humans. Virus-encoded enzymes essential to its life cycle are currently the targets of drug development. The chimpanzee model has been used to show the feasibility of successful vaccination strategies. Michael Houghton's essential collaborators in this endeavor were George Kuo at Chiron; Dan Bradley, a non-A, non-B viral hepatitis expert at the CDC, who provided chimpanzee samples; and Qui-Lim Choo, who worked in Houghton's laboratory, providing essential molecular biology expertise.

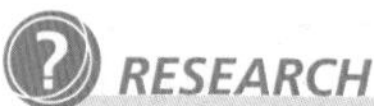

Because it appears to be impossible to isolate free HCV virions, alternative methods to study the fusion of HCV with host cells must be developed. How would you investigate the fusion of a cell expressing the HCV envelope proteins E1 and E2 with a hepatocyte expressing the CD81 receptor?

Clinical syndromes and diagnosis

Hepatitis C is the most common blood-borne infection in the United States. Acute HCV infection can result in recovery and clearance in 15% of patients, rapid progression to cirrhosis in 15% of patients, and chronic infection in 70% of patients. Acute HCV infection is usually asymptomatic. In cases where symptoms occur (20% to 30% of those newly infected persons), they include fatigue, loss of appetite, nausea and abdominal pain, and jaundice. Chronic, persistent disease presents as chronic fatigue and progresses to chronic active hepatitis within 10 to 15 years. After 20 years, this leads to cirrhosis in 20% of patients, and of these patients 20% develop liver failure. Up to 5% of chronically infected individuals develop hepatocellular carcinoma after 30 years.

Clinical diagnosis involves the exclusion of other hepatitis agents. Laboratory diagnosis includes testing for elevated ALT levels in blood, detection of anti-HCV antibodies by enzyme-linked immunosorbent assay (ELISA) or enhanced chemiluminescence immunoassay, and quantitative tests to detect the amount of viral RNA by polymerase chain reaction. HCV infection can be detected by anti-HCV screening tests 4 to 10 weeks after infection. Anti-HCV antibodies can be detected in more than 97% of infected individuals by 6 months after exposure, and HCV RNA can be detected 2 to 3 weeks following infection.

Pathogenesis and epidemiology

HCV infects T and B lymphocytes and monocytes and then infects liver cells. The HCV replication rate in hepatocytes is about 10^{12} virions per day; this high replication rate produces viral mutants that can escape detection by the immune system. Liver pathogenesis is most likely mediated by cytotoxic T cells attaching to hepatocytes that express viral antigens. Nevertheless, a direct cytopathic effect of viral replication in hepatocytes is also possible. Cytokines and interferon are produced by the innate immune response, but the viral core protein can bind the tumor necrosis factor-alpha (TNF-α) receptor and curb the stimulation of cytotoxic T cells. Nonstructural proteins of the virus can also interfere with interferon-mediated pathways. The envelope glycoproteins E1 and E2 elicit humoral and cell-mediated immune responses. Mutations in E1 and E2, however, can enable the virus to evade detection. Anti-HCV antibodies can form immune complexes that can lead to tissue damage, including vasculitis, arthritis, and glomerulonephritis. $CD8^+$ cytotoxic T cells are essential for the elimination of virally infected cells. In chronically infected patients, the release of the helper T (T_h1) cytokine TNF-α can cause a "cytokine storm" that can cause liver damage.

Hepatocellular carcinoma may be caused by the chronic damage to the liver, followed by tissue regeneration involving rapid hepatocyte proliferation, interaction of HCV proteins with cellular processes such as oncogene upregulation, disruption of cell-cycle control, and inhibition of tumor suppressor genes.

HCV is spread via blood, blood-derived products, sexual contact, and from mother to child. Blood transfusion and organ transplantation, and the administration of factors VIII and IX to patients with hemophilia, create a high risk for transmission of HCV. Before blood testing became standard practice, between 80% and 90% of post-transfusion hepatitis was caused by HCV. HIV-infected individuals who have also used intravenous drugs are highly likely to have been infected with HCV. There is an association between nonsexual household contact and HCV infection, including the use of infected toothbrushes, razors, and other items contaminated with blood. Health workers with a history of accidental needlesticks are at risk for having acquired HCV.

Treatment and prevention

Treatment of HCV infections involves the administration of pegylated interferon-α with or without ribavirin. Conjugation of poly(ethylene glycol) to interferon increases its circulation time in blood. Ribavirin is a prodrug that is transformed by cellular kinases into the 5′ triphosphate nucleotide, which interferes with RNA synthesis. Patients with HCV genotypes 2 and 3 are about three times more likely than patients with genotype 1 to respond to interferon-α therapy or interferon-α/ribavirin combination therapy. The duration of treatment also depends on the HCV genotype: A 24-week combination treatment is recommended for infection with genotypes 2 and 3, whereas a 48-week course is recommended for genotype 1. Recently developed HCV protease inhibitors telaprevir and boceprevir may be useful adjuncts to the presently used regimen.

Newer drugs that can be used without interferon have been developed. Sofosbuvir (Sovaldi, Gilead) inhibits the NS5B RNA-dependent RNA polymerase. Simeprevir (Olysio, Janssen) is an inhibitor of the NS3/4A protease. Daclatasvir (Daklinza, Bristol-Myers Squibb) is an inhibitor of the NS5A replication complex. ABT-450 inhibits the NS3 protease.

Hepatitis D Virus

HDV can be considered a "viral parasite" because it requires the presence of HBV to replicate. HDV has a single-stranded, circular RNA comprising 1,700 bases that encodes a small (24-kDa) or large (27-kDA) delta antigen that constitutes the nucleocapsid. An envelope that incorporates the HBV surface antigen HBsAg surrounds the capsid (Fig 32-7). After entry into the host cell, the RNA polymerase II in the nucleus replicates the viral RNA in a highly unusual reaction. RNA polymerase can recognize regions of viral RNA that form base pairs. The RNA forms a loop structure with enzymatic activity called a ribozyme, which cleaves the viral genome to produce mRNA that encodes the small delta antigen. A cellular enzyme, double-stranded RNA-activated adenosine deaminase, induces a mutation in the delta antigen gene to produce the large delta antigen. The large delta antigen facilitates the association of viral RNA with HBsAg and the formation of viral particles.

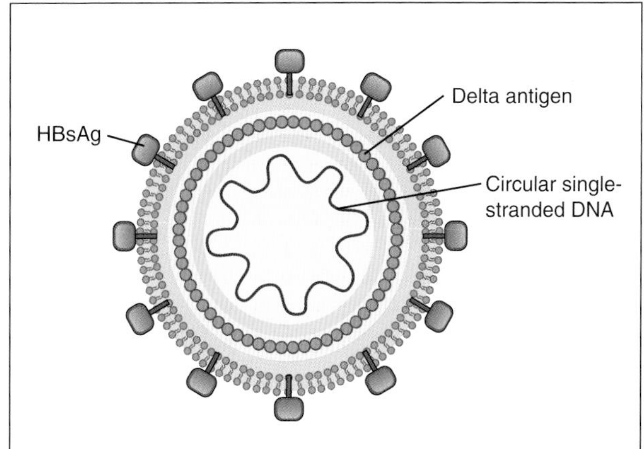

Fig 32-7 The schematic structure of HDV.

Clinical syndromes and diagnosis

The range of clinical presentation varies from mild disease to fulminant liver failure. Co-infection with HBV and HDV results in disease very similar to hepatitis B. Superinfection with HDV in persons with chronic hepatitis B results in relapses of jaundice and is more likely to cause chronic cirrhosis. Fulminant hepatitis can cause hepatic encephalopathy with altered brain function and massive hepatic necrosis; this disease is fatal in 80% of cases.

HDV is diagnosed by the presence of IgM and IgG antibodies to the HBsAg and the identification of the RNA genome.

Pathogenesis and epidemiology

HDV can replicate immediately following superinfection of a person with HBV; thus, the disease progresses more rapidly than in the case of co-infection, where the HBV has to first establish infection and replicate. HDV replication leads to cytotoxicity, which contributes to liver damage as well as the immunopathology due to infection.

Persons who are infected with both HDV and HBV are a source of infection. It is estimated that there are 25 million persons infected with HDV. The disease is endemic in parts of Africa, the Middle East, Southern Italy, and the Amazon basin. The prevalence of HDV is increasing in Northern and Central Europe because of immigration. Epidemics of delta hepatitis have been seen in populations with a high prevalence of hepatitis B.

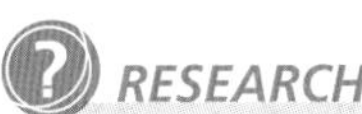

What might be the reasons for the low prevalence of HDV in Southeast Asia and China, while the prevalence of chronic HBV in this region is among the highest?

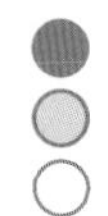

Treatment and prevention

The only treatment for HDV infection is pegylated interferon; however, the response rates are less than 30%. The HBV vaccine will prevent infection with HDV. Blood, organs, tissues, or semen should not be donated by individuals infected with HDV or HBV. Transmission can be reduced by the practice of safe sex, the use of clean needles by injection drug users, and the employment of needle safety devices by health care providers.

Hepatitis E Virus

HEV resembles HAV in that it is spread by the fecal-oral route and is a naked capsid, positive-strand RNA virus. It is an icosahedral virus with a diameter in the range of 27 to 34 nm. The incubation period is about 40 days. Most infections are subclinical, but when symptomatic, HEV causes fulminant hepatitis that may be fatal. The mortality rate in pregnant women is about 20%. HEV should be considered in any patient with raised ALT levels, regardless of age or travel history. Most HEV infections have been observed in Asia and Africa in regions with poor sanitation. Cases have been seen in the United States, most of them originating from immigrants or visitors from endemic locations. Nevertheless, locally acquired HEV (genotypes 3 and 4) does occur in developed countries, pigs being the primary host. Mother-to-child transmission has also been observed. Acute symptomatic hepatitis E seems to occur mostly in middle-aged and elderly men and causes higher mortality in patients with underlying chronic liver disease. Chronic HEV infection occurs in immunosuppressed individuals and may cause rapidly progressive cirrhosis if untreated. Hepatitis E may also cause extrahepatic manifestations, including neurologic syndromes.

Ribavirin monotherapy for 3 months appears to be effective in the treatment of chronic HEV infection. Surprisingly, immune serum globulin is not protective. For seriously ill patients, liver transplantation may be the only "therapy." The safety of blood products needs to ascertained, because blood donors are not currently screened for HEV.

Hepatitis G Virus

HGV was discovered in two patients in 1995. It is an RNA virus that is in the Flavivirus family and hence is similar to HCV. However, it replicates in lymphocytes and not hepatocytes. HGV has been detected in 2% of blood donors and 35% of HIV-seropositive individuals. Between 10% and 20% of patients infected with HCV are also infected with HGV. The clinical outcome of these patients does not appear to be different than that of individuals infected only with HCV. HGV and HIV co-infection appears to prolong the survival of HIV/AIDS patients, and some studies indicate that HGV inhibits HIV replication.

Bibliography

Bauman RW. Microbiology with Diseases by Taxonomy, ed 4. Boston: Pearson, 2014.

Centers for Disease Control and Prevention. Hepatitis B FAQs for the Public. http://www.cdc.gov/hepatitis/hbv/bfaq.htm. Accessed 28 July 2015.

Centers for Disease Control and Prevention. Hepatitis C FAQs for Health Professionals. www.cdc.gov/hepatitis/HCV/HCVfaq.htm#-section2. Accessed 28 July 2015.

Dalton HR, Hunter JG, Bendall RP. Hepatitis E. Curr Opin Infect Dis 2013;26:471–478.

Gerlich WH. Medical virology of hepatitis B: How it began and where we are now. Virol J 2013;10:209.

Greenwood D, Barer M, Slack R, Irving W. Medical Microbiology, ed 18. Edinburgh: Churchill Livingstone/Elsevier, 2012.

Houghton M. Discovery of the hepatitis C virus. Liver Int 2009;29 (suppl 1):82–88.

Hughes SA, Wedemeyer H, Harrison PM. Hepatitis delta virus. Lancet 2011;378:73–85.

Kim CW, Chang KM. Hepatitis C virus: Virology and life cycle. Clin Mol Hepatol 2013;19:17–25.

Mosby's Dictionary of Medicine, Nursing and Health Professions, ed 9. Philadelphia: Mosby/Elsevier, 2012.

Murray PR, Rosenthal KS, Pfaller MA. Medical Microbiology, ed 7. Philadelphia: Mosby/Elsevier, 2013.

National Library of Medicine. Entecavir. livertox.nlm.nih.gov/Entecavir.htm. Accessed 28 July 2015.

Ryan KJ, Ray CG. Sherris Medical Microbiology, ed 5. New York: McGraw-Hill, 2010.

Schäfer G, Blumenthal MJ, Katz AA. Interaction of human tumor viruses with host cell surface receptors and cell entry. Viruses 2015;7:2592–2617.

Zhu YZ, Qian XJ, Zhao P, Qi ZT. How hepatitis C virus invades hepatocytes: The mystery of viral entry. World J Gastroenterol 2014;20:3457–3467.

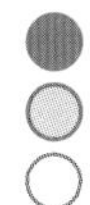

Take-Home Messages

- HAV is a naked capsid picornavirus with a positive-sense, single-strand RNA; it causes abdominal pain, poor appetite, and jaundice.
- HBV is an enveloped DNA virus that is a major cause of chronic liver disease. Hepadnaviruses are the only viruses that produce a DNA genome by reverse transcription of an intermediate RNA.
- The symptoms of hepatitis due to HBV are jaundice, pain in the upper right quadrant of the abdomen, pale stools, and dark urine.
- Between 5% and 10% of adults and 20% to 50% of children younger than 6 years of age who experienced acute HBV infection develop a chronic HBV infection. Persistent carriage of HBV is associated with primary hepatocellular carcinoma.
- HBsAg can be detected during acute or chronic HBV infection, and its presence indicates that a person can pass the virus to others. Donated blood is screened for HBsAg. The presence of the core antigen (HbcAg) is the best indicator for the presence of infectious virus.
- Liver necrosis, inflammation, and fibrosis are observed in chronic hepatitis, leading to the development of cirrhosis. Liver damage results from immune system attack on hepatocytes expressing viral antigens.
- HBV is transmitted through transfusion of blood and blood products, accidental injection of contaminated blood, exchange of fluids, and transplantation.
- Chronic hepatitis B can be treated with pegylated interferon, 3TC, adefovir, entecavir, and tenofovir.
- The HBV vaccine is based on recombinant HBsAg produced in yeast.
- HCV is an enveloped, positive-strand RNA virus with an icosahedral capsid.
- Acute HCV infection is usually asymptomatic. However, it can lead to rapid progression to cirrhosis in 15% of patients and chronic infection in 70% of patients.
- Liver pathogenesis is most likely mediated by cytotoxic T cells attaching to hepatocytes that express viral antigens.
- HCV is spread via blood, blood-derived products, sexual contact, and from mother to child.
- Treatment of HCV infections involves the use of pegylated interferon-α with or without ribavirin. The protease inhibitors telaprevir and boceprevir can be added to this regimen. Newer drugs include sofosbuvir, simeprevir, and daclatasvir.
- HDV is an RNA virus that requires the presence of HBV to replicate. The range of clinical presentation varies from mild disease to fulminant liver failure.
- HEV resembles HAV. Most infections are subclinical, but when symptomatic, the virus causes fulminant hepatitis that may be fatal.
- HGV is a flavivirus, similar to HCV. It replicates in lymphocytes and not hepatocytes and may inhibit HIV replication.

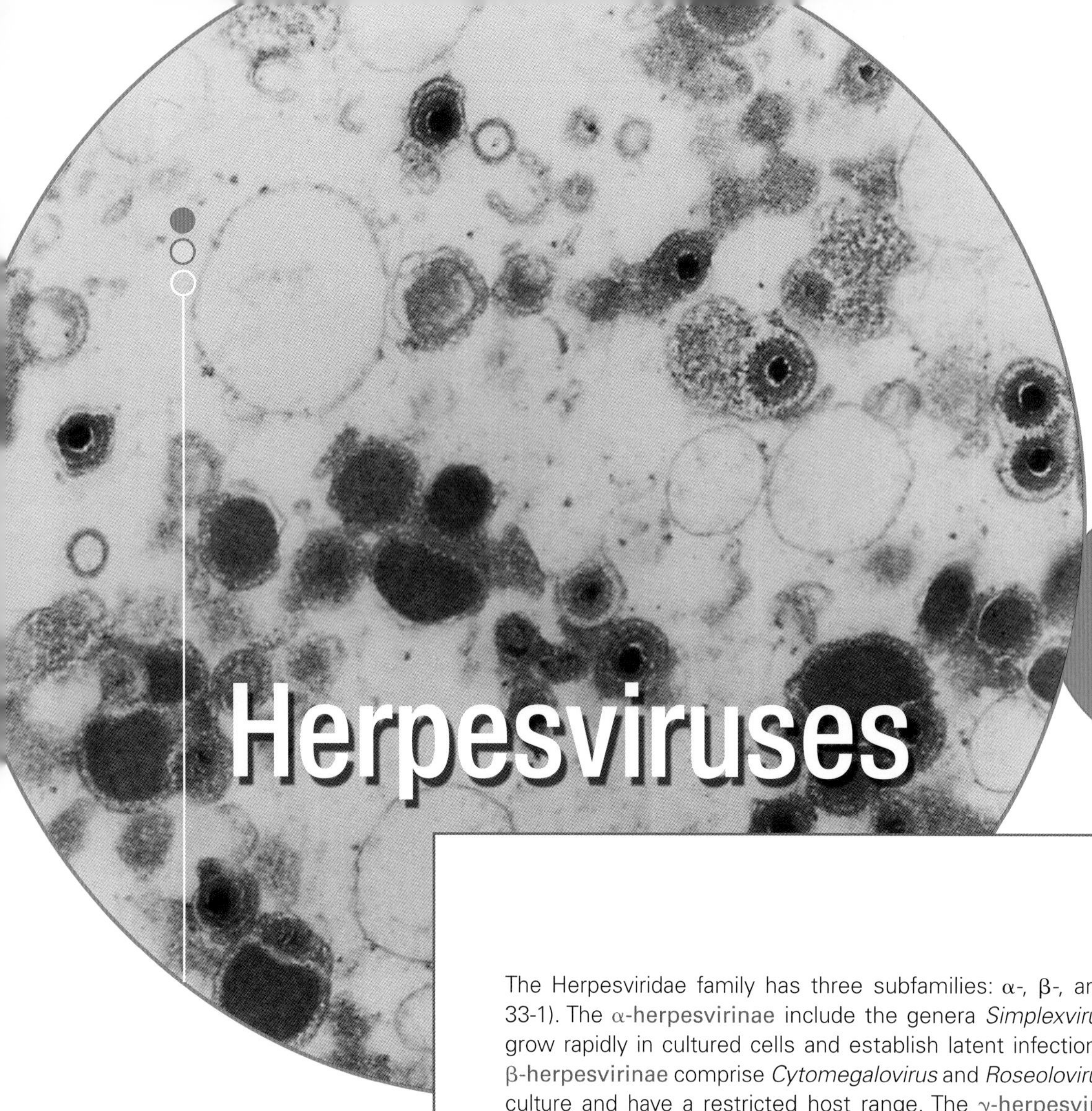

33 Herpesviruses

The Herpesviridae family has three subfamilies: α-, β-, and γ-herpesvirinae (Table 33-1). The **α-herpesvirinae** include the genera *Simplexvirus* and *Varicellovirus* that grow rapidly in cultured cells and establish latent infection in sensory ganglia. The **β-herpesvirinae** comprise *Cytomegalovirus* and *Roseolovirus* that grow slowly in cell culture and have a restricted host range. The **γ-herpesvirinae** comprise the genera *Lymphocryptovirus* and *Rhadinovirus* (Kaposi sarcoma–associated herpesvirus or HHV8). The simian virus herpes B can accidentally infect humans.

Structure and Replication

Herpesviruses are enveloped viruses, approximately 200 nm in diameter, with double-stranded DNA packed inside an icosahedral capsid. The capsid, which is about 100 nm in diameter, consists of 162 hollow hexagonal and pentagonal subunits. The space between the capsid surface and the inner aspect of the membranous envelope is called the **tegument** and contains viral proteins and enzymes. The genome is linear, double-stranded DNA, ranging in length from 125 kbp for varicella zoster virus (VZV) to 248 kbp for cytomegalovirus (CMV).

RESEARCH

What are the enzymes found in the herpesvirus tegument?

Herpesviruses bind to specific receptors on the surface of host cells and inject their nucleocapsid by membrane fusion at the plasma membrane. The nucleocapsid docks onto the nuclear membrane. The DNA is delivered into the nucleus, where it is circularized. Transcription of mRNA takes place sequentially (Fig 33-1): *(1)* Immediate early genes encode proteins involved in the initiation and regulation of viral transcription. *(2)* Early genes code for DNA polymerase, DNA-binding proteins and thymidine kinase, and minor structural proteins. *(3)* Late genes encode major structural proteins such as capsid proteins and envelope glycoproteins.

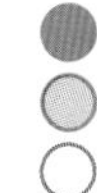

Table 33-1 Human herpesviruses

Approved name	Common name	Abbreviation	Subfamily	Tropism
HHV1	Herpes simplex virus type 1	HSV-1	α-herpesvirinae	Neurotropic
HHV2	Herpes simplex virus type 2	HSV-2	α-herpesvirinae	Neurotropic
HHV3	Varicella zoster virus	VZV	α-herpesvirinae	Neurotropic
HHV4	Epstein-Barr virus	EBV	γ-herpesvirinae	Lymphotropic
HHV5	Cytomegalovirus	CMV	β-herpesvirinae	Lymphotropic
HHV6	Human herpesvirus 6	HHV6	β-herpesvirinae	Lymphotropic
HHV7	Human herpesvirus 7	HHV7	β-herpesvirinae	Lymphotropic
HHV8	Kaposi sarcoma–associated herpesvirus	KSHV	γ-herpesvirinae	Tropic for skin

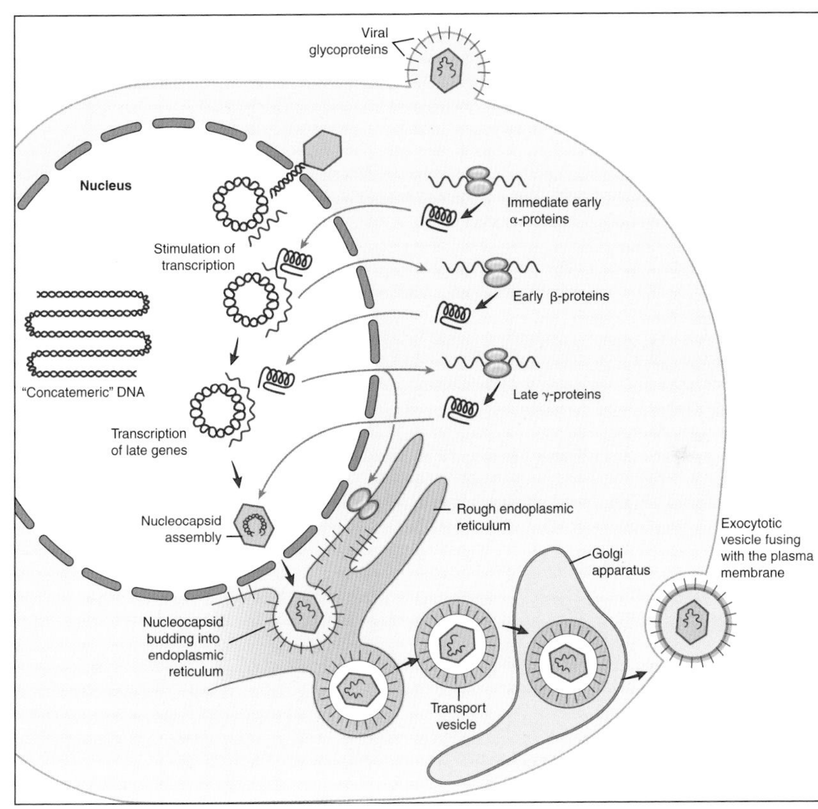

Fig 33-1 The replication cycle of herpes simplex virus type 1. (Adapted from Ryan and Ray.)

Viral DNA replication takes place in a "rolling circle" process and results in the formation of multiple tandem copies of the genome, called concatemers. These structures are cleaved into genome-sized DNA pieces that then complex with the late gene products that are transported back into the nucleus, forming the new nucleocapsid. The envelope of the virus is obtained from the inner lamella of the (double) nuclear membrane, which buds into the endoplasmic reticulum while acquiring membrane proteins. The virion is then moved via transport vesicles to the Golgi apparatus, where the membrane proteins become glycosylated. It is then packaged into an exocytotic vesicle and exocytosed at the plasma membrane.

Herpesviruses have two different infection strategies: productive infection and latency. During latency, the viral genome remains in the nucleus of the host cell for long periods without producing any infectious virions and is protected from the immune system. During reactivation, the genome can initiate productive replication that results in dissemination to different hosts.

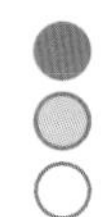

Herpes Simplex Virus

Structure and replication

Herpes simplex virus (HSV) encodes enzymes including DNA-dependent DNA polymerase, DNase, ribonucleotide reductase, and thymidine kinase. The viral glycoproteins gB, gC, gD, gH, and gE/gI are involved in attachment, and gB mediates membrane fusion. HSV-1 and HSV-2 have different versions of gB, identified as gB1 and gB2. gC, gE, and gI act as immune escape proteins, where gC binds to the C3 component of complement, which is then depleted from serum. The gE/gI complex binds the Fc region of immunoglobulin (Ig) G antibodies, thus hiding the virus from the immune system.

HSV infects most types of cells. Thus, the virus receptor must be present on most types of cells. Heparan sulfate (a proteoglycan) and an intercellular adhesion molecule, nectin-1, act as receptors for HSV-1. The major route of entry is by fusion at the plasma membrane, but endocytosis also occurs. The nucleocapsid docks with the nuclear membrane. During latent infection, replication stops after the immediate early phase. Assembly occurs in the nucleus, where capsid proteins enclose the viral DNA. The capsid buds into the endoplasmic reticulum, the membrane proteins are glycosylated in the Golgi apparatus, and the virus is released by exocytosis or cell lysis.

The main sites for HSV-1 latency are the sensory neurons of the trigeminal ganglia that innervate the lips, gingiva, and eyes. HSV-1 enters the neurons at the axon terminals, the nucleocapsid is transported to the cell body located in the ganglion, and the DNA is injected into the nucleus, where it remains as an episome. The mechanism by which latency is initiated is not understood completely. The latency-associated transcript (LAT) is the only transcript produced during the latent phase of infection; thus, it is possible that LATs promote viral latency and host cell survival. In vitro experiments with dissociated chicken ganglia indicate that the site of viral entry influences the outcome of infection. When the virus enters via the axon, latency is favored. When it enters the cell body and dendrites, productive replication is observed more often. If retrograde transport of virion-associated regulatory factors (eg, viral lytic initiator protein VP16) is not efficient, latency may ensue. When VP16 is not present, the expression of the immediate early genes is reduced.

Clinical syndromes and diagnosis

Primary HSV-1 infections are often asymptomatic. Symptomatic infections present as gingivostomatitis (or herpetic stomatitis). The lesions begin as vesicles that can become ulcerated and spread throughout the mouth on the gingiva, tongue, buccal mucosa, and pharynx, and these symptoms are accompanied by fever (Fig 33-2). Recurrent mucocutaneous HSV infections result in cold sores or fever blisters. HSV-1 may be reactivated asymptomatically and may be found in saliva. It may be isolated in saliva in 5% to 8% of asymptomatic children and in 1% to 2% of asymptomatic adults.

Herpetic keratitis may cause corneal damage and blindness. Infection of a finger or nail area results in painful vesicular lesions that pustulate, a condition known as herpetic whitlow. Eczema herpeticum is observed as vesicular lesions in areas with eczema.

In genital herpes, the initial infection with HSV-2 or HSV-1 becomes apparent after an incubation period of 2 to 20 days. Multiple small papules or vesicles coalesce into larger pustular or ulcerative lesions after 5 days. The condition usually resolves in 2 to 4 weeks. Lesions are seen on the penis, vulva, vagina, cervix, and inner thighs. Infection is accompanied by fever, malaise, myalgia, and inguinal adenitis. Recurring lesions last 7 to 8 days and are seen in 80% of patients within 12 months. Most recurrences are due to the reactivation of the virus from the dorsal root ganglion, and they usually appear in the same skin or mucosal area. The virus may be shed asymptomatically, and this may contribute to the person-to-person spread of the virus.

Infection in the newborn is often caused by HSV-2, which can disseminate to the liver, lungs, and the central nervous system, causing herpes encephalitis. Proctitis manifests with fever, anorectal pain, and inguinal adenopathy. Meningitis is a complication of HSV-2. The clinical syndromes include nuchal rigidity (neck stiffness), headache, photophobia, and nausea. Herpes encephalitis is caused primarily by HSV-1 and is the most common fatal encephalitis. It is lethal in 70% of patients if untreated and can occur at all ages. Neurons, particularly in the temporoparietal area of the brain, are damaged during viral replication, and the immune response can cause further pathology, leading to seizures and neurologic symptoms.

Cytology can be used for diagnosis. In the Tzanck test, cells are stained with Wright or Giemsa stains. Cells display giant syncytia, a ballooning cytoplasm, and eosinophilic inclusions in the nuclei. Viral antigens can be demonstrated by immunofluorescence or immunoperoxidase staining. Diagnosis of encephalitis involves polymerase chain reaction (PCR) amplification of cerebrospinal fluid samples. The cytopathic effect of the viruses can be detected in cell culture using HeLa cells and human embryonic fibroblasts.

Pathogenesis and epidemiology

HSV enters the body via mucosal surfaces or breaks in the skin. The virus replicates in cells at the base of the lesion and spreads to adjacent cells and neurons. The virus causes cytopathology at the site of infection and leads to persistent infection of lymphocytes and macrophages. A latent infection ensues in neurons. The virus can be reactivated by various stresses, including emotional stress, trauma, sunlight, upset stomach, fever, cold, menstrual cycle, and immune suppression.

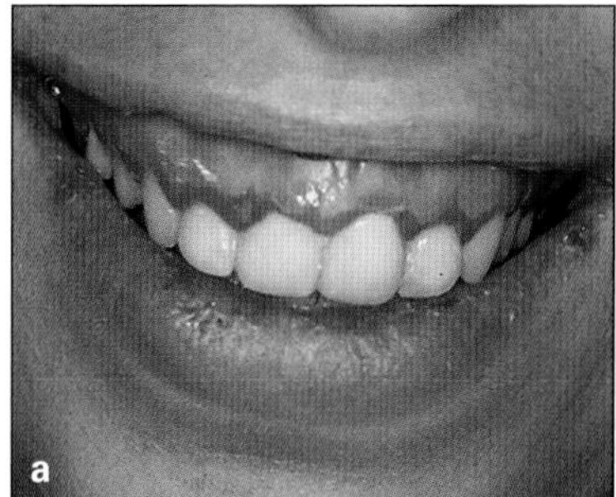

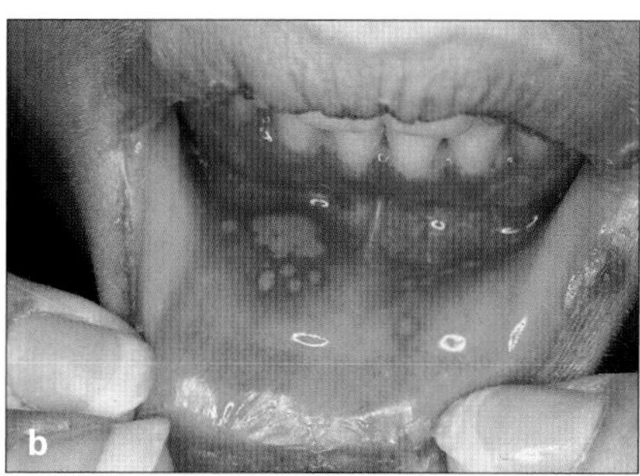

Fig 33-2 *(a)* Gingival inflammation in primary herpetic gingivostomatitis. *(b)* Clusters of ruptured vesicles, some of which have coalesced. (Reprinted with permission from Marx and Stern.)

Infection is accompanied by changes in nuclear structure, the formation of acidophilic intranuclear inclusion bodies, and syncytium formation. There is no detectable damage in neurons, which probably contain only one copy of the genome. Activation leads to production of a limited number of virions and does not kill the cell.

Infection is controlled by both humoral immunity and cell-mediated immunity. Without cell-mediated immunity, the virus can spread to the brain and other vital organs. However, the immune response can also contribute to the disease symptoms. Stress may activate the virus in nerve cells and depress immunity.

HSV-1 is present in orolaryngeal secretions and is spread via person-to-person contact, most commonly mouth to mouth. Mouth-to-skin spread can also occur, as in the case of herpetic whitlow and type 1 genital herpes.

HSV-2 is transmitted via sexual contact. Asymptomatic recurrences are likely in females, and the virus is shed in genital secretions. HSV-2 can be vertically transmitted to the fetus during delivery, by maternal viremia, or in utero.

Treatment and prevention

Oral or topical acyclovir is useful in treating first episodes but not very useful in recurrent infections. Acyclovir is indicated for severe HSV syndromes such as neonatal disease, encephalitis, and extensive disease in the immunocompromised patient. Penciclovir is a derivative of acyclovir that is used topically to treat cold sores. Famcyclovir and valacyclovir can be used in the treatment of genital herpes and in the suppression of recurrences. Valacyclovir is the valyl ester of acyclovir, and famciclovir is a derivative of penciclovir. They have improved pharmacologic properties over that of acyclovir. For example, the bioavailability of valacyclovir is 54% compared with 15% to 20% for acyclovir. These drugs do not have an effect on the latent state. Acyclovir-resistant strains of HSV have been isolated from persistent lesions in immunocompromised individuals. These strains can be treated with foscarnet.

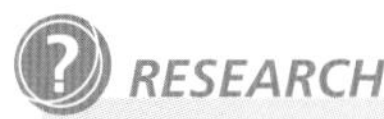

What is the mechanism of action of acyclovir?

Prevention of HSV-1 requires avoiding contact with active lesions. However, the virus may be transmitted unknowingly through oral secretions. The use of gloves may prevent herpetic whitlow. Avoidance of sexual contact during periods of active lesions is important in the prevention of HSV-2 infection. For pregnant women, having a cesarean section birth may avoid contact of the neonate with viral lesions.

Currently, there is no vaccine available. Subunit vaccines utilizing gB and gD were not efficacious.

Varicella Zoster Virus

VZV causes chickenpox, also known as varicella. Recurrence, which is the reactivation of the previously latent viral genome, causes herpes zoster (or shingles).

Clinical syndromes and diagnosis

Varicella symptoms include fever and a maculopapular rash following an incubation period of 11 to 21 days. The lesions usually start at the back of the head and ears; they then spread to the face, trunk, and extremities. The initially thin-walled vesicles become pustular within 12 hours, form a crust, and then scab over. Successive "crops" of lesions occur for 3 to 5 days, as they are at different stages of development (Fig 33-3). Mucous membrane lesions occur in the mouth, conjunctivae, and vagina. VZV causes very severe disseminated infection in immunocompromised individuals, leading to pneumonia, hepatitis, encephalitis, and nephritis. Hemorrhagic lesions are seen in thrombocytopenic patients. In 20% to 30% of adults, primary infection with VZV can lead to interstitial pneumonia, arising from the immune reaction to the virus.

Herpes zoster (shingles) occurs in people already infected with VZV (Figs 33-4 and 33-5). It is preceded by pain in a sensory nerve. The vesicular eruption involves a dermatome (an area on the surface of the body that is innervated by afferent fibers from one spinal root) and is usually unilateral. Chickenpox-like lesions appear, spaced along an erythematous base. Chronic pain syndrome occurs after herpes zoster, also called postherpetic neuralgia, and can persist for months or years. It is caused by chronic nerve irritation.

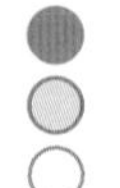

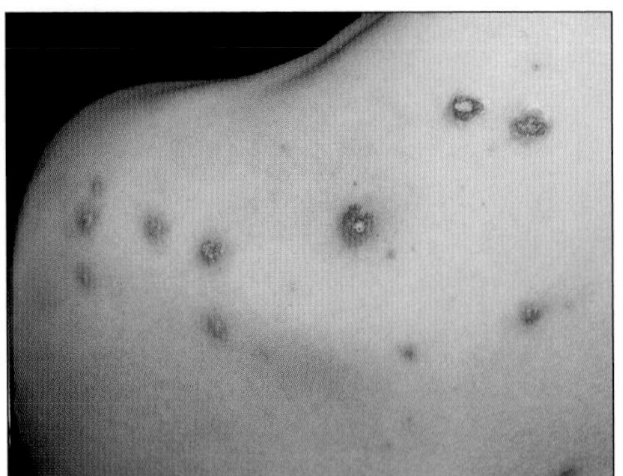
Fig 33-3 Pustules with red periphery observed in varicella zoster virus (chickenpox) infections. (Reprinted with permission from Marx and Stern.)

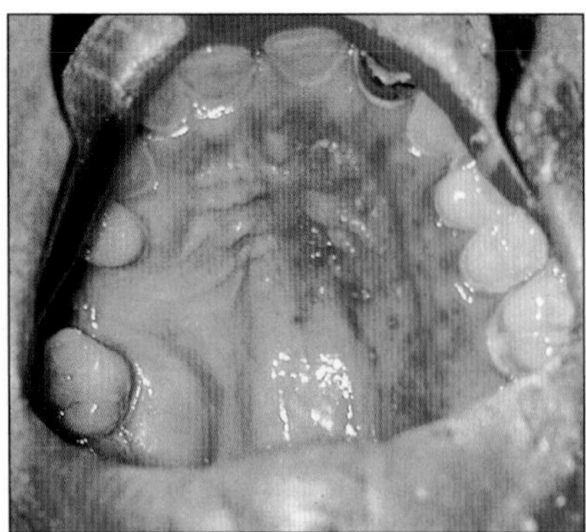
Fig 33-4 Palatal herpes zoster lesions along the greater palatine nerve, stopping at the midline. (Reprinted with permission from Marx and Stern.)

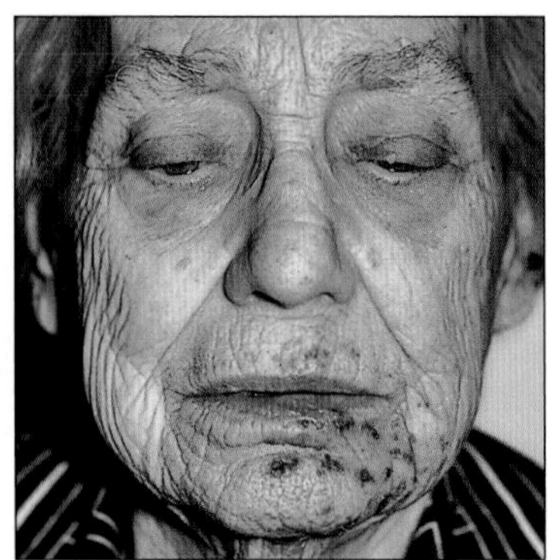
Fig 33-5 Herpes zoster lesions on the face. (Reprinted with permission from Marx and Stern.)

In congenital, drug-related, or disease-related immunosuppressed patients, the virus may disseminate to the lungs, brain, and liver and may be fatal.

VZV infection can be confirmed by cytology, which reveals intranuclear inclusions and syncytia in scrapings of the lesions. Direct fluorescent antibody is the most sensitive of the assays, particularly because the virus is labile during transportation for culturing and replicates poorly in cells in vitro. Serology is used to detect immunity (low levels of antibody) or to document active infection. PCR of cerebrospinal fluid samples is used to detect VZV encephalitis.

Pathogenesis and epidemiology

Infection begins in the mucosa of the respiratory tract. It spreads via the regional lymph nodes and primary viremia to the liver, spleen, and the rest of the reticuloendothelial system. Secondary viremia involves T lymphocytes and leads to infection of the skin, which proceeds with the formation of a dermal vesiculopustular rash. Multinucleated giant cells with intranuclear inclusions are seen in the base of the lesions. The virus becomes latent in dorsal root ganglia. It is reactivated in aged persons or in patients with impaired immunity and migrates down the sensory nerve to the skin.

VZV is readily communicable via respiratory droplets. Primary VZV infection occurs in childhood, and 90% of cases occur before age 10 years. Herpes zoster develops in 10% to 20% of the infected population.

Treatment and prevention

Acyclovir, famcyclovir, and valacyclovir can be used for varicella in adults. High-risk individuals should be protected from exposure to VZV. A live, attenuated virus vaccine (Varivax, prepared from the Oka/Merck strain) is effective in preventing varicella, but zoster can still occur in those previously infected. A vaccine for shingles (Zostavax, Merck) is recommended by the Centers for Disease Control and Prevention for use in persons 60 years and older to prevent shingles, particularly because the disease gets more severe as people age. It is very similar to the varicella vaccine but contains a higher dose of the attenuated vaccine virus.

Epstein-Barr Virus

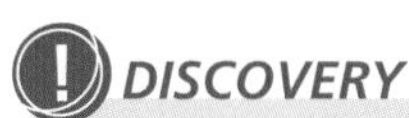

In the 1950s, Denis Burkitt described a malignant neoplasm of the jaw in African boys that appeared to be infectious. Michael Epstein and Yvonne Barr cultured specimens of the tumor. Electron microscopy of biopsies from this B-cell lymphoma revealed herpesvirus particles. Epstein-Barr virus (EBV) was the first virus shown to cause a human cancer. The association of the virus with infectious mononucleosis was discovered by chance when serum from a laboratory technician who was recovering from mononucleosis was found to interact with cells from Burkitt lymphoma. Later studies with a large population of college students verified that EBV causes mononucleosis.

EBV is the first human cancer virus to be discovered. The EBV genome has about 100 open reading frames (ie, a nucleotide sequence that begins with an initiation codon [usually ATG] and ends with a termination codon [TAA, TAG, or TGA]), some of which are expressed consistently in malignancies. These include the EBV nuclear antigen 1 and latent membrane protein 1. The virus encodes an analog of the B-cell receptor, CD40-like co-receptors, and transcription regulators. EBV also encodes microRNAs that are overexpressed in cancer and that can be transported to neighboring uninfected cells via exosomes.

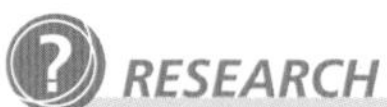

What are exosomes, and what is their significance in biology?

Clinical syndromes and diagnosis

Infectious mononucleosis is characterized by exudative pharyngitis, lymphadenopathy, hepatosplenomegaly, fever, and malaise. Complicatons of infectious mononucleosis are rare but can be serious. They include laryngeal obstruction and neurologic disorders, including meningoenceph-

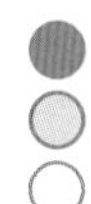

Table 33-2 Diseases associated with EBV infection and their relationship to the strength of cellular immunity

State of cellular immunity	Diseases of EBV
Lacking (HIV/AIDS)	Oral hairy leukoplakia
Poor (malaria)	Burkitt lymphoma
	Nasopharyngeal carcinoma
Normal	Asymptomatic (children)
Vigorous	Infectious mononucleosis

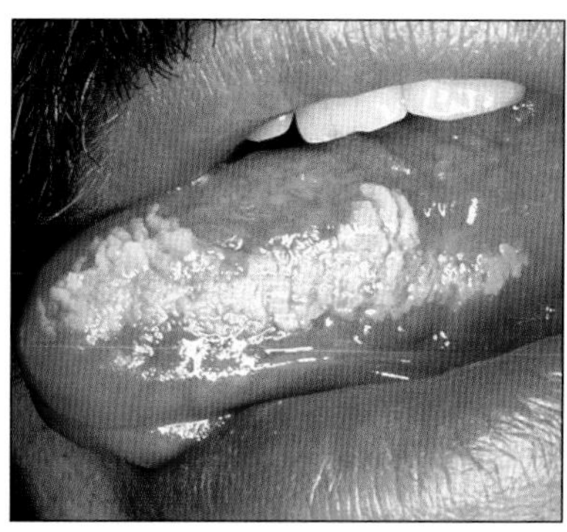

Fig 33-6 Advanced oral hairy leukoplakia on the lateral border of the tongue in an HIV-seropositive patient resulting from EBV infection and immunosuppression. (Public Health Image Library image 6061, courtesy of J. S. Greenspan, BDS, and Sol Silverman, Jr, DDS.)

alitis, facial nerve palsies, optic neuritis (swelling of the eye nerve), transverse myelitis (swelling of the spinal cord), and Guillain-Barré syndrome (an immune system disease in which nerve damage occurs). EBV infections in children are much milder and often subclinical (Table 33-2).

EBV-induced lymphoproliferative disease occurs in immunocompromised individuals. Patients with human immunodeficiency virus (HIV) may develop EBV-induced lesions in the mouth called hairy leukoplakia, characterized by raised white patches usually seen on the tongue (Fig 33-6). Patients with congenital deficiency of T-lymphocyte function may develop invasive lymphomas.

EBV can cause Burkitt lymphoma, a tumor of the jaw and face resulting from the immortalization of B cells, which is caused by the translocation of the *C-myc* oncogene next to a very active promoter. Co-infection with the malaria parasite *Plasmodium falciparum* promotes the involvement of EBV with Burkitt lymphoma. EBV infection can also result in nasopharyngeal carcinoma, in which the tumor cells are of epithelial origin. This cancer is endemic in Asia and is seen in adults. Other cancers associated with EBV infection are Hodgkin disease and non-Hodgkin lymphoma.

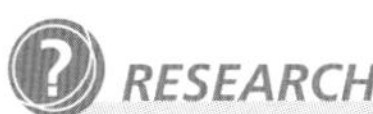

RESEARCH

Why does EBV cause nasopharyngeal carcinoma in an Asian population but not in other infected people?

Hematologic examination shows elevated lymphocyte and monocyte levels with atypical lymphocytes called Downey cells, which have a basophilic and vacuolated cytoplasm and an unusual nuclear shape. A nonspecific test used often to diagnose infectious mononucleosis is the heterophile antibody test. These antibodies are produced by the activation of B cells and include an IgM "heterophile" antibody that recognizes the Paul-Bunnell antigen on sheep and bovine erythrocytes. There are also specific antibody tests for *(1)* IgG antibodies to the viral capsid antigen, which appear early in the illness; *(2)* antibodies to the early antigen, which are found during the active phase of infection (weeks to months after onset); and *(3)* antibodies to EBV nuclear antigen, which are found 3 to 6 weeks after onset and persist for life.

Pathogenesis and epidemiology

EBV establishes productive infection of the epithelial cells of the oropharynx and the nasopharynx. The virus is shed into the saliva and accesses B cells in the lymphatic tissue and blood. It acts as a B-cell mitogen and prevents apoptosis. T cells can limit the proliferation of these B cells. Infectious mononucleosis results from the activation and proliferation of immune effector cells, particularly suppressor CD8 cells, which appear as atypical lymphocytes called *Downey cells*. The T-cell response to infection causes the swollen lymph glands, spleen, and liver that are characteristic for the disease and help with diagnosis.

EBV is shed into saliva and is acquired by close contact between persons through saliva. More than 90% of EBV-infected persons shed the virus even when they are asymptomatic. Children can acquire the virus from contaminated cups, toothbrushes, and utensils. Infectious mononucleosis is known as "kissing disease," as saliva is often shared between adolescents and young adults by kissing. Disease in children is usually subclinical.

EBV-associated Burkitt lymphoma is associated with immunosuppression caused by malaria, which may be a co-factor in this neoplasm. Nasopharyngeal carcinoma occurs primarily in southeast China, suggesting a genetic component of disease onset or environmental factors.

Treatment and prevention

There is no effective treatment or vaccine for EBV infection. Infection elicits life-long immunity. Treatment with acyclovir or ganciclovir has not shown any significant effects on the progression of infectious mononucleosis.

Cytomegalovirus

The name of the virus is derived from its cytopathic effect on infected cells, resulting in swelling, hence "cytomegaly." CMV carries not only its DNA but also four species of mRNA transcribed from one immediate early gene, two early genes, and one late gene. These mRNAs are most likely localized in the tegument (the amorphous layer of protein located between the capsid and the envelope).

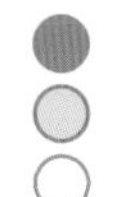

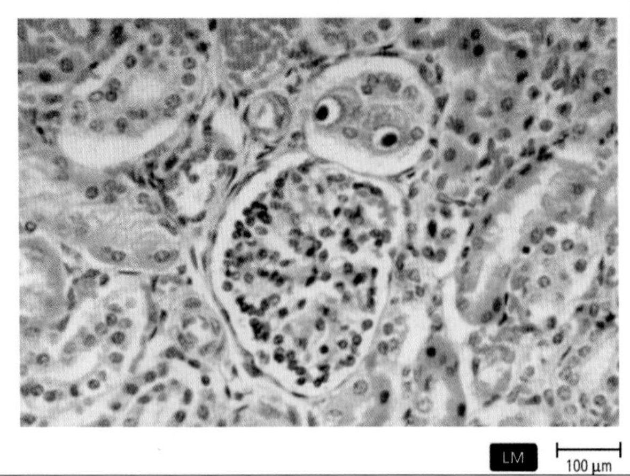

Fig 33-7 CMV-infected cells with "owl's eye" nuclear inclusion bodies. CMV infects mononuclear leukocytes, bone marrow myeloid precursors, and vascular endothelial cells. (Copyright Dr P. Marazzi.)

Clinical syndromes and diagnosis

In immunocompetent individuals, CMV infection rarely results in symptomatic disease. In some persons, CMV can cause mononucleosis that is less severe than that caused by EBV, with pharyngitis and lymphadenopathy. In immunocompromised patients, it can cause retinitis, blurred vision, central nervous system lesions, and pulmonary disease. CMV infection is the most common viral cause of congenital defects. It can cause hepatosplenomegaly, jaundice (due to hepatitis), thrombocytopenia, intrauterine growth retardation, microcephaly, encephalitis, and myocarditis.

Infection can be diagnosed by cytology, showing cytomegalic cells and basophilic intranuclear inclusions called owl's eye inclusion bodies (Fig 33-7), after staining with basic dyes such as methylene blue. Infected cells can be identified with fluorescent antibody staining.

Pathogenesis and epidemiology

CMV establishes latent infection in mononuclear leukocytes (T cells and macrophages) and bone marrow myeloid progenitor cells. It is reactivated by immune suppression caused by steroids or HIV infection. It establishes productive infection in mucosal epithelial cells in the lungs. CMV pneumonia is most likely the result of a potent immune reaction to infected cells in the lungs.

Congenital abnormalities are more common when the fetus is infected during the first trimester. Death of infected precursor cells at this stage can result in organ defects. Congenital infections occur through the cervix or mother's blood, and perinatal infections can result from breastfeeding. In children, transmission is via saliva. In older individuals, transmission is via kissing, unprotected sexual activity, or organ transplantation.

Treatment and prevention

Intravenous ganciclovir (Cytovene, Genentech) is the most commonly used antiviral, but it can cause bone marrow toxicity and loss of spermatogenesis. It has been successful in treating CMV hepatitis, colitis, and encephalitis. Its prolonged use controls CMV retinitis in HIV/AIDS. Foscarnet is an alternative drug that does not require phosphorylation in infected cells; however, it is nephrotoxic. Prophylaxis with antiviral drugs reduces CMV disease and CMV-associated mortality in organ transplant patients. Orally administered valganciclovir provides systemic ganciclovir levels similar to that obtained intravenously. Fomivirsen (Vitravene, Isis) is the only antisense oligodeoxynucleotide drug used in the treatment of the disease.

Prevention of transmission involves screening of blood and organ donors and the use of safe sexual practices.

Human Herpesvirus 6

Human herpesvirus 6 (HHV6) replicates in lymphoid tissue, especially $CD4^+$ T lymphocytes, where it establishes a latent infection. The cellular receptor for HHV6 is CD46, which is expressed on all nucleated cells. The virus can infect the brain, liver, tonsils, and salivary glands. HHV6 type B causes exanthem subitum (or roseola infantum), which is a benign febrile (about 39°C) illness of early childhood. The rapid-onset fever is followed by a faint maculopapular rash that starts on the trunk and face and spreads to the extremities. The virus is shed in the throats of 70% of infants by 12 months. HHV6 may cause mononucleosis and lymphadenopathy in adults.

Active viral infection can be diagnosed by culture or PCR detection of DNA in blood.

HHV6 can be treated with ganciclovir. In severe cases, foscarnet or cidofovir can be used.

Human Herpesvirus 7

HHV7 was first isolated in 1990 from activated helper T cells of a healthy individual. The virus is found frequently in saliva, and it is most likely transmitted by close contact. HHV7 infection is often asymptomatic, but it can cause fever without rash, febrile convulsions, exanthem subitum, and hemiplegia (paralysis of one side of the body).

Human Herpesvirus 8

HHV8 was discovered by genetic analysis of Kaposi sarcoma (KS) tissue, which indicated genetic homology to EBV and *Herpesvirus saimiri*. KS in AIDS patients is a malignancy of vascular endothelial cells, which transform into elongated, spindle-like cells. The lesions are dark purple and often occur on the skin, in the oral cavity, and on the soles of the feet.

The virus is also called Kaposi sarcoma–associated herpesvirus (KSHV). In early studies, KSHV DNA was detected in saliva from 75% of 24 HIV-positive patients with KS, 15% of HIV-positive patients without KS, and 0% of uninfected individuals. Resistance of KSHV DNA from saliva to DNase treatment was consistent with the presence of virions. These data suggest that KSHV can replicate in the oropharynx and that salivary contact could contribute to KSHV transmission. It may also be transmitted sexually.

HHV8 infects preferentially B cells. It also infects endothelial and epithelial cells, sensory nerve cells, and monocytes. It appears to be a necessary but not a sufficient cause of KS. Ganciclovir and foscarnet have activity against HHV8.

B virus *(Herpesvirus simiae)*

B virus is related to HSV and is found in macaques. It is transmitted to humans via bites or saliva. Vesicles and redness occur at the infection site. In the absence of treatment, 70% of the ensuing encephalopathy is fatal. Treatment involves thorough cleansing of the wound with soap, povidone-iodine, concentrated detergent, chlorhexidine, and water, followed by ganciclovir or acyclovir administration.

Bibliography

Bauman RW. Microbiology with Diseases by Taxonomy, ed 4. Boston: Pearson, 2014.

Caselli E, Di Luca D. Molecular biology and clinical associations of Roseoloviruses human herpesvirus 6 and human herpesvirus 7. New Microbiol 2007;30:173–187.

Centers for Disease Control and Prevention. About Epstein-Barr Virus (EBV). www.cdc.gov/epstein-barr/about-ebv.html. Accessed 29 July 2015.

Centers for Disease Control and Prevention. B Virus (herpes B, monkey B virus, herpesvirus simiae, and herpesvirus B). www.cdc.gov/herpesbvirus/index.html. Accessed 29 July 2015.

Centers for Disease Control and Prevention. Public Health Image Library. phil.cdc.gov. Accessed 4 August 2015.

Centers for Disease Control and Prevention. Shingles Vaccination: What You Need to Know. www.cdc.gov/vaccines/vpd-vac/shingles/vacc-need-know.htm. Accessed 29 July 2015.

De Bolle L, Naesens L, De Clercq E. Update on human herpesvirus 6 biology, clinical features, and therapy. Clin Microbiol Rev 2005;18:217–245.

Dittmer DP, Damania B. Kaposi sarcoma associated herpesvirus pathogenesis (KSHV)—An update. Curr Opin Virol 2013;3:238–244.

Greenwood D, Barer M, Slack R, Irving W. Medical Microbiology, ed 18. Edinburgh: Churchill Livingstone/Elsevier, 2012.

Lieberman PM. Epstein-Barr virus turns 50. Science 2014;343:1323–1325.

Marx RE, Stern D. Oral and Maxillofacial Pathology: A Rationale for Diagnosis and Treatment, ed 2. Chicago: Quintessence, 2012.

Mosby's Dictionary of Medicine, Nursing and Health Professions, ed 9. Philadelphia: Mosby/Elsevier, 2012.

Murray PR, Rosenthal KS, Pfaller MA. Medical Microbiology, ed 6. Philadelphia: Mosby/Elsevier, 2009.

Ryan KJ, Ray CG. Sherris Medical Microbiology, ed 5. New York: McGraw-Hill, 2010.

Shin H, Iwasaki A. Generating protective immunity against genital herpes. Trends Immunol 2013;34:487–494.

Wilson AC, Mohr I. A cultured affair: HSV latency and reactivation in neurons. Trends Microbiol 2012;12:604–611.

Take-Home Messages

- Herpesviruses have two different infection strategies: productive infection and latency.
- Symptomatic primary HSV-1 infections present as gingivostomatitis. Recurrent mucocutaneous HSV-1 infections result in cold sores.
- HSV-1 is present in orolaryngeal secretions and is spread via person-to-person contact.
- In genital herpes, initial infection with HSV-2 or HSV-1 becomes apparent after 2 to 20 days. Five days later, multiple small papules or vesicles coalesce into larger pustular or ulcerative lesions.
- HSV-2 is transmitted via sexual contact.
- Varicella (chickenpox) symptoms include fever and a maculopapular rash following an incubation period of 11 to 21 days. Successive "crops" of lesions occur for 3 to 5 days, as they are at different stages of development.
- Herpes zoster (shingles) occurs when VZV is reactivated, with vesicular eruptions along a dermatome.
- EBV causes infectious mononucleosis, characterized by exudative pharyngitis, lymphadenopathy, hepatosplenomegaly, fever, and malaise.
- EBV is the first human cancer virus to be discovered. It can cause Burkitt lymphoma and nasopharyngeal carcinoma.
- CMV can cause retinitis, blurred vision, central nervous system lesions, and pulmonary disease in immunocompromised patients. CMV infection is the most common viral cause of congenital defects.
- HHV6 can infect the brain, liver, tonsils, and salivary glands, and type B causes exanthem subitum (roseola infantum).
- HHV8 is associated with Kaposi sarcoma, a malignancy in which endothelial cells are elongated and spindle-shaped.

Orthomyxoviruses: Influenza Virus 34

Orthomyxoviridae are lipid-enveloped RNA viruses, and influenza A, B, and C viruses are the only members of the family. Only influenza A and B viruses cause significant acute respiratory disease in humans, characterized by fever, malaise, headache, and myalgia, as well as a nonproductive cough. Influenza pandemics (worldwide epidemics) can occur unpredictably as a result of the emergence of new subtypes of influenza A viruses.

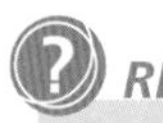

RESEARCH

What subtype of influenza is the "swine flu" that emerged in 2009?

Structure and Replication

Influenza virus is a negative-strand RNA virus that has a segmented genome consisting of eight different molecules associated with the nucleoprotein (NP) and RNA polymerase (PB1, PB2 and PA). In this respect, it differs from paramyxoviruses (eg, mumps, measles), which have a single RNA genome. The envelope contains the glycoproteins hemagglutinin (HA) and neuraminidase (NA) and is lined on the inside by the matrix (M_1) protein (Figs 34-1 and 34-2). The M_1 protein is thought to facilitate the assembly of the virus. The M_2 protein is an integral membrane protein that acts as a proton (H^+) channel (see Fig 34-2); this function is important for the survival of the virus.

RESEARCH

How does the M_2 protein aid the survival of the virus? What would happen if this channel were blocked by a drug?

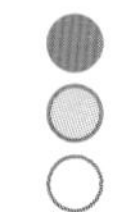

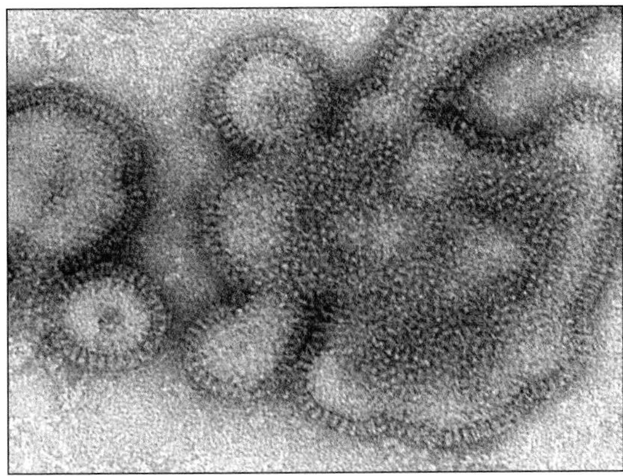

Fig 34-1 Transmission electron micrograph of H3N2 influenza virus. Note the spikes on the membrane; these are the envelope glycoproteins NA and HA. Note the irregular ("pleiomorphic") shape of some virions. (Public Health Image Library image 13470, courtesy of Dr Michael Shaw and Doug Jordan, MA.)

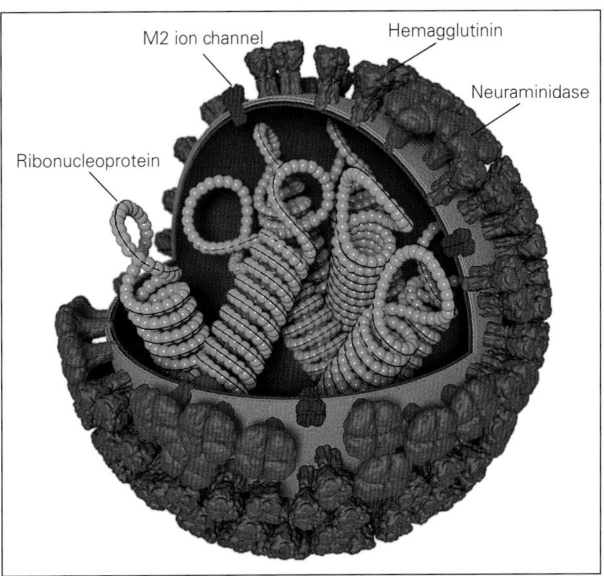

Fig 34-2 Schematic structure of influenza virus. (Public Health Image Library image 17346, courtesy of Dan Higgins).

The HA acts as the viral attachment protein that binds to sialic acid–containing glycoproteins or glycolipids on epithelial cells. HA also mediates the fusion of the viral membrane with the membrane of the endosome, following endocytosis and mild acidification (pH ~5) of the endosome lumen.

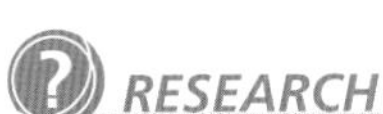

RESEARCH

How is the endosome acidified?

Mutations in the HA and NA cause antigenic drifts if the changes are minor and antigenic shifts if the changes are substantial. Antigenic shifts also occur as a result of reassortment of the segmented viral genome when avian and human influenza viruses co-infect swine cells. When virions bud from the surface of these cells, they may package some RNAs from human influenza and some from the avian virus. The shifts in HA occur only in the case of influenza A and are designated H1, H2, etc. There are 16 variants of HA that have been designated.

NA cleaves sialic acids on proteins, including the cell receptor for influenza virus. It appears to facilitate the release of virions from infected cells. The antigenically changed NA molecules are designated N1, N2, etc. There are currently nine variants of NA that have been identified.

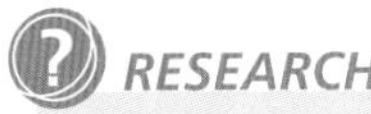

RESEARCH

What would happen to influenza virus if an inhibitor of NA were administered to virus-infected cells?

Strains of influenza are classified by the type (A, B, or C), place of original isolation, date of original isolation, and antigen type (HA and NA), separated by virgules (slashes). For example, the strain of virus that caused the Hong Kong influenza pandemic is designated as A/Hong Kong/1968/H3N2. The most recent pandemic strain of "swine flu" was caused by the virus designated as A/California/09/H1N1.

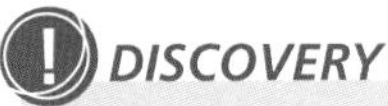

DISCOVERY

The HA, NP, and NS genes (about one-third of the total genome) of the A/California/09/H1N1 influenza virus are homologous to classical North American swine flu strains. The PB2 and PA genes (about one-third of the genome) are from North American avian flu strains. The remaining third of the genome (NA, MP, and PB1 genes) are similar to Eurasian swine flu and human flu strains. Ruben Donis, chief of the molecular virology and vaccines branch of the Centers for Disease Control and Prevention, has proposed the following hypothesis for the origin of the A/California/09/H1N1 strain: "The virus may have originated in a US pig that traveled to Asia as part of the hog trade. The virus may have infected a human there, who then traveled back to North America, where the virus perfected human-to-human spread, maybe even moving from the United States to Mexico."

Influenza virus enters host cells by first binding to sialic acid–containing glycoproteins and glycolipids on the cell surface (Fig 34-3). The virus is internalized in coated vesicles, which then mature into endosomes. Acidification of the endosome lumen causes a large conformational change of the HA and of the HA trimer. Exposure of the hydrophobic fusion-promoting peptide at the N-terminus of HA and its insertion into the lipid bilayer of the endosome membrane mediate the fusion of the viral and host cell membrane (Fig 34-4). Because the viral NP is bound to

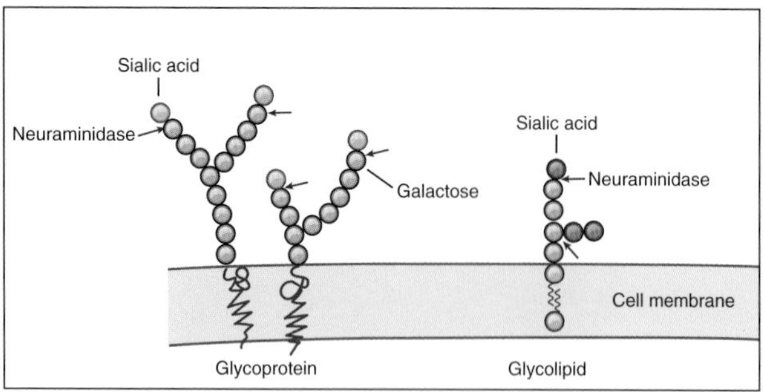

Fig 34-3 Influenza virus binds to sialic acid–containing glycoproteins or glycolipids on the host cell plasma membrane.

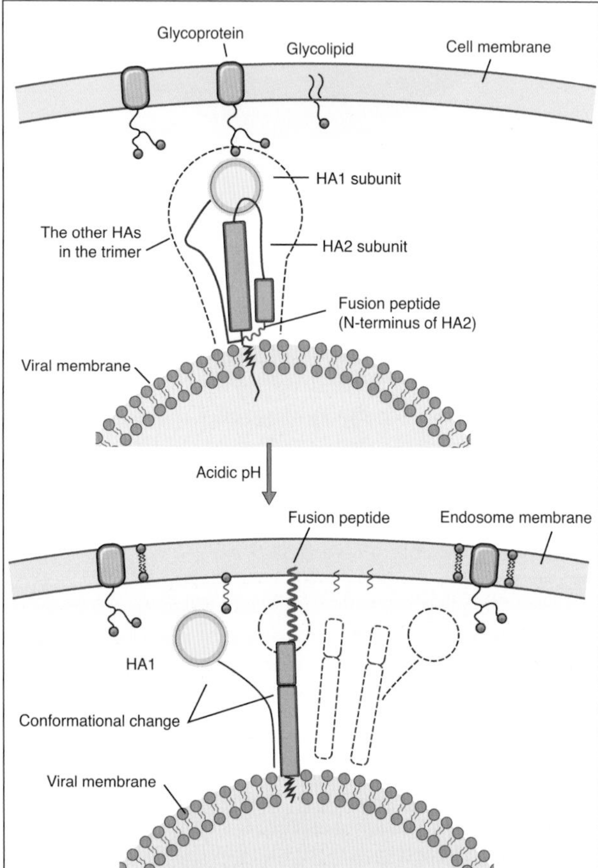

Fig 34-4 The viral HA undergoes a conformational change following endocytosis and endosome acidification and mediates the fusion of viral and cellular membranes. At neutral pH, the HA1 subunit initially binds to sialic acid on glycoproteins and glycolipids. The fusion peptide *(green)* of HA2 is hidden near the viral membrane. The low pH–induced conformational change results in the insertion of the fusion peptide into the endosome membrane, bringing the two membranes closer. The molecular details of how this step leads to membrane fusion are not well understood.

the M_1 matrix protein, its entry into the cytoplasm is initially hindered. The influx of protons through the M_2 channel into the virion appears to disrupt the M_1-NP interaction, thereby enabling the cytoplasmic entry of the NP.

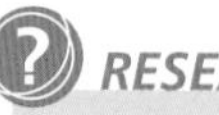

RESEARCH

How could one show that the M_2 protein functions as described? Are there any specific inhibitors of M_2?

The M_1-free nucleocapsid is transported to the nucleus, where the negative-strand RNA is transcribed into the positive strand. The positive-strand mRNA migrates to the cytoplasm, where it is translated into protein. The viral proteins are produced in the endoplasmic reticulum, and HA and NA are glycosylated in the Golgi apparatus. The transmembrane M_2 protein prevents the acidification of the Golgi apparatus by enabling protons to leak into the cytoplasm. This has the important function of enabling HA to maintain its neutral-pH conformation. If HA were to encounter a low-pH environment during viral biosynthesis, it would undergo an irreversible conformational change and become nonfunctional.

Vesicles with HA and NA incorporated in their membrane bud from the Golgi apparatus and transport the proteins to the cell surface. M_1 proteins bind to the cytoplasmic tails of HA and NA, help assemble these proteins, and line the cytoplasmic side of the plasma membrane. Meanwhile, the negative-strand RNA is generated from the positive-strand mRNA in the nucleus and is transported into the cytoplasm (Fig 34-5). This genomic RNA associates with the nucleocapsid and polymerase proteins; these complexes also bind to the M_1 protein. The assembled virus produces an outward protrusion on the surface of the cell and buds from the plasma membrane. Extracellular trypsin-like proteases cleave the HA into HA1 and HA2 subunits that now become fusion ready. One of the reasons for the confinement of influenza virus replication to the respiratory tract is that such enzymes are localized in this tissue.

Clinical Syndromes and Diagnosis

The incubation period for influenza virus is 1 to 4 days. The initial indications of infection are malaise and headache. This is usually followed by an abrupt onset of fever, severe myalgia, and a nonproductive cough. The illness persists for about 3 days. If there are no complications, recovery is complete.

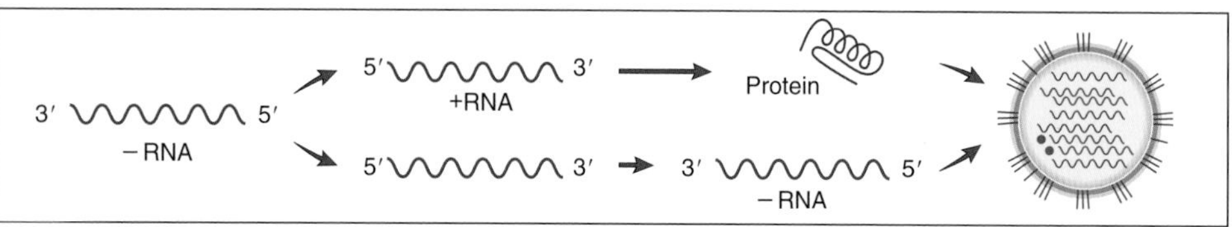

Fig 34-5 A simplified scheme for the replication of influenza virus. (Adapted from Flint et al.)

The complications following influenza infection include bacterial pneumonia (caused by *Streptococcus pneumoniae*, *Haemophilus influenzae*, or *Staphylococcus aureus*), myositis (inflammation of muscle), central nervous system involvement (encephalopathy), or Reye syndrome. Reye syndrome is an acute encephalitis in children and occurs after a variety of febrile viral infections (varicella, influenza A and B). Salicylates (aspirin) increase the likelihood of the development of this syndrome and thus should be avoided.

Influenza virus causes a cytopathic effect in cultured cells that they can infect. The Madin-Darby canine kidney cells are used often for this purpose. Because infected cells express HA on their surface before virus budding, and because erythrocytes can bind to HA, hemadsorption can be used as a method to detect influenza virus. Furthermore, immunofluorescence or enzyme-linked immunosorbent assay (ELISA) can be used to detect viral antigens. Because influenza virus causes the agglutination of erythrocytes, the presence of antibodies against influenza virus can be detected by the inhibition of hemagglutination.

Pathogenesis and Epidemiology

Following inhalation of influenza virus, NA cleaves sialic acid components of the mucus layer, facilitating access to the ciliated respiratory epithelial cells. Infection interferes with protein and nucleic acid synthesis and can result in desquamation (shedding) of mucus-secreting and ciliated cells, which interferes with the ciliary clearance mechanism of the respiratory tract. Apoptosis (programmed cell death) of the infected cells results in the generation of local inflammatory mediators that attract mononuclear leukocytes to the infection site. Infection, and the resulting production of double-stranded RNA as a replication intermediate, causes the induction of interferon-α by leukocytes and interferon-β by fibroblasts. These cytokines activate natural cytotoxic (or *natural killer*) cells that recognize and kill virally infected cells. As the respiratory epithelium is compromised, bacterial superinfection can occur. Presentation of influenza antigens by dendritic cells to CD4$^+$ and CD8$^+$ T cells results in the generation of cytotoxic T cells. These cells recognize viral antigens attached to major histocompatibility class I molecules and presented by infected cells and cause the lysis of virus-infected cells. T-cell responses are important both for resolution and for immunopathogenesis. The production of antibodies against defined epitopes of HA and NA is important for future protection of the host from influenza virus.

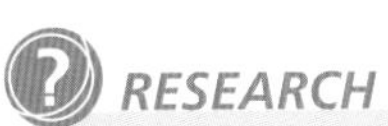
RESEARCH

Why was the 1918 Spanish flu so deadly?

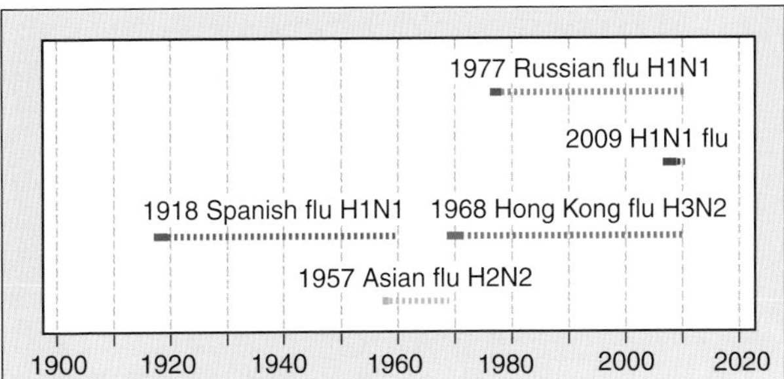

Fig 34-6 The emergence of new influenza subtypes.

Influenza infection is spread via small airborne droplets released during talking, breathing, and coughing. The virus can also sit on countertops as long as a day. Children, immunosuppressed individuals (including pregnant women), the elderly, and individuals with heart and lung ailments (including smokers) are at highest risk for more serious disease, pneumonia, and other complications.

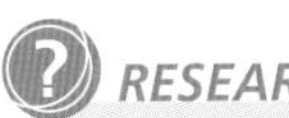
RESEARCH

Why is it important to wash hands often to prevent influenza infection?

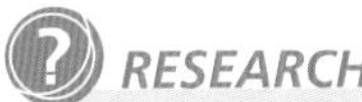
RESEARCH

About 36,000 people die every year of influenza in the United States, although this is not publicized in the press. What could health authorities, including the US government, do to reduce the number of these deaths? What could the general public do to prevent them?

Reassortment of genomic fragments of influenza A virus can cause pandemics by generating completely new virus strains to which the population does not have immunity because it has not been exposed previously to a similar strain. Reassortment usually involves pigs that get co-infected with a duck influenza virus and a human influenza virus. During virus assembly, viral genome segments from the different viruses in the same cell can be incorporated into a particular virion, which now has properties different from those of the original co-infecting viruses, and can infect humans. This type of reassortment is thought to be the source of pathogenic human strains (Fig 34-6). In 1997, an influenza virus designated as A/Hong Kong/156/97 (H5N1) was isolated from 18 people in Hong Kong and caused 6 deaths. The virus resembled A/Chicken/Hong Kong/258/97, leading to the destruction of all 1.6 million chickens in Hong Kong. An H5N1 "bird flu" emerged in 2006, with 383 cases and 241 deaths until the end of May 2008. This was an alarming 63% mortality rate.

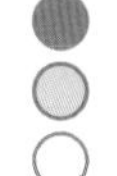

Treatment and Prevention

To relieve symptoms, acetaminophen (and not aspirin) can be given. The first anti-influenza drugs developed were amantadine and rimantadine, which block the M_2 channel. They may be useful if administered within 24 to 48 hours of the onset of influenza symptoms. However, many strains of influenza virus have developed resistance against these drugs.

The NA inhibitors oseltamivir (Tamiflu, Gilead; oral) and zanamivir (Relenza; GlaxoSmithKline; inhalation) bind to the conserved active site of NA. Because HA on newly formed virions binds to sialic acid residues on the cell surface, the NA is necessary to cleave off the sialic acid and to facilitate the release of the virus. Thus, NA inhibitors are thought to work by inhibiting the release of viruses from infected cells and their subsequent spread to adjacent cells.

The best method for controlling infection is immunization. The vaccine usually incorporates the antigens of the A and B strains that are likely to be prevalent during the approaching winter. The vaccine is recommended for elderly people and those with chronic medical conditions that predispose them to severe illness after infection with influenza virus. Vaccination is also recommended for medical care providers and others who might transmit the virus to those at risk.

To produce vaccines, the strains of influenza are propagated in embryonated eggs, inactivated in formaldehyde, and purified in a sucrose gradient; then the virus is disrupted with the detergent Triton X-100. The necessity to use eggs for this production may limit the speed with which new vaccines can be produced for a new flu season. Thimerosal is added to the vaccine preparation as a preservative (25 µg Hg/dose). Pediatric vaccines are prepared without thimerosal because of concerns regarding the total dose of Hg that infants and children may be exposed to as a result of numerous pediatric vaccinations.

A live attenuated virus vaccine, FluMist (MedImmune), is also available. The virus is temperature sensitive, with limited replication at 38°C to 39°C. It is cold adapted to replicate efficiently at 25°C and is administered via intranasal spray. This vaccine is approved for healthy persons in the age range 5 to 49 years.

Bibliography

Centers for Disease Control and Prevention. Public Health Image Library. phil.cdc.gov. Accessed 4 August 2015.

Düzgüneş N, Pedroso de Lima MC, Stamatatos L, et al. Fusion activity and inactivation of influenza virus: Kinetics of low pH-induced fusion with cultured cells. J Gen Virol 1992;73:27–37.

Flint SJ, Enquist LW, Racaniello VR, Skalka AM. Principles of Virology, ed 3. Washington, DC: ASM, 2009.

Influenza Specialist Group. Influenza Viruses. www.isg.org.au/index.php/about-influenza/influenza-viruses/. Accessed 30 July 2015.

Lanzrein M, Schlegel A, Kempf C. Entry and uncoating of enveloped viruses. Biochem J 1994;302(pt 2):313–320.

Murray PR, Rosenthal KS, Pfaller MA. Medical Microbiology, ed 6. Philadelphia: Mosby/Elsevier, 2009.

Pedroso de Lima MC, Ramalho-Santos J, Düzgüneş N, Flasher D, Nir S. Entry of enveloped viruses into host cells: Fusion activity of the influenza hemagglutinin. In: Pedroso de Lima MC, Düzgüneş N, Hoekstra D (eds). Trafficking of Intracellular Membranes: From Molecular Sorting to Membrane Fusion. Berlin: Springer, 1995:131–154.

Pedroso de Lima MC, Ramalho-Santos J, Flasher D, Slepushkin VA, Nir S, Düzgüneş N. Target cell membrane sialic acid modulates both binding and fusion activity of influenza virus. Biochim Biophys Acta 1995;1236:323–330.

Short KR, Veldhuis Kroeze EJ, Reperant LA, Richard M, Kuiken T. Influenza virus and endothelial cells: A species specific relationship. Front Microbiol 2014;5:653.

Sonnberg S, Webby RJ, Webster RG. Natural history of highly pathogenic avian influenza H5N1. Virus Res 2013;178:63–77.

Sun J, Braciale TJ. Role of T cell immunity in recovery from influenza virus infection. Curr Opin Virol 2013;3:425–429.

Take-Home Messages

- Influenza viruses are negative-strand RNA viruses. They bind to sialic acid–containing receptors on epithelial cells.
- Following endocytosis, the viral membrane fuses with the endosome membrane at low pH and releases the nucleocapsid into the cytoplasm.
- The symptoms include malaise, headache, an abrupt onset of fever, severe myalgia, and a nonproductive cough.
- Influenza infection may lead to complications such as bacterial pneumonia, myositis, encephalopathy, and Reye syndrome.
- Mutations in the HA cause antigenic drifts. Antigenic shifts are primarily the result of reassortment of the segmented genome in cells co-infected with different strains.
- Treatment has to be started soon after the onset of symptoms. The most effective drugs against influenza are zanamivir and oseltamivir.
- The strains used for the current vaccination are H1N1, H3N2, and Influenza B.

Paramyxoviruses: Measles, Mumps, and Respiratory Syncytial Viruses

35

Diseases

Paramyxoviruses include measles, parainfluenza, mumps, respiratory syncytial, Nipah, and Hendra viruses. Measles virus causes a generalized infection with a maculopapular rash that spreads throughout the body. Disease caused by parainfluenza virus is characterized by pharyngitis, bronchitis, pneumonia, and croup. Mumps virus causes systemic infection as well as parotiditis (or *parotitis*). Infection by respiratory syncytial virus is localized in the respiratory tract and results in rhinitis, pharyngitis, bronchiolitis, and pneumonia. Newly discovered members of the paramyxoviruses are Nipah virus, which causes encephalitis and respiratory disease, and Hendra virus, which also causes respiratory disease.

Structure and Replication

Paramyxoviruses are lipid-enveloped viruses containing a single negative-strand RNA that forms a helical nucleocapsid in association with nucleoproteins (Figs 35-1 and 35-2). The virion contains an RNA-dependent RNA polymerase to transcribe the negative-strand genome into mRNA. The pleomorphic lipid envelope includes the membrane proteins hemagglutinin/neuraminidase (HN), which facilitates binding to cell surface receptors, and the F (fusion) protein, which mediates the fusion of the viral and cellular membranes at neutral pH. The other proteins of the virus include nucleoprotein (NP) and the matrix (M) protein (see Fig 35-1). Recent studies indicate that the matrix protein in measles virus may be attached to the nucleocapsid.

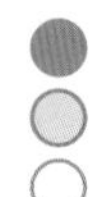

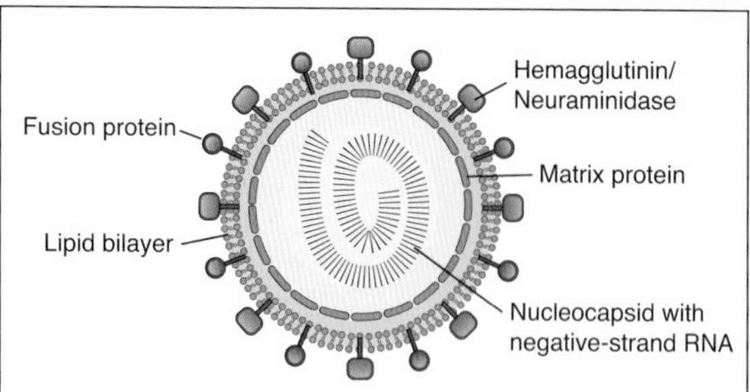

Fig 35-1 Schematic structure of a paramyxovirus. The nucleocapsid contains negative-strand RNA with the associated P protein, nucleoprotein, and large protein and has RNA-dependent RNA polymerase activity. Viral attachment is mediated by the glycoproteins hemagglutinin/neuraminidase, hemagglutinin, and/or G protein, and membrane fusion with the host cell plasma membrane is achieved by the fusion protein.

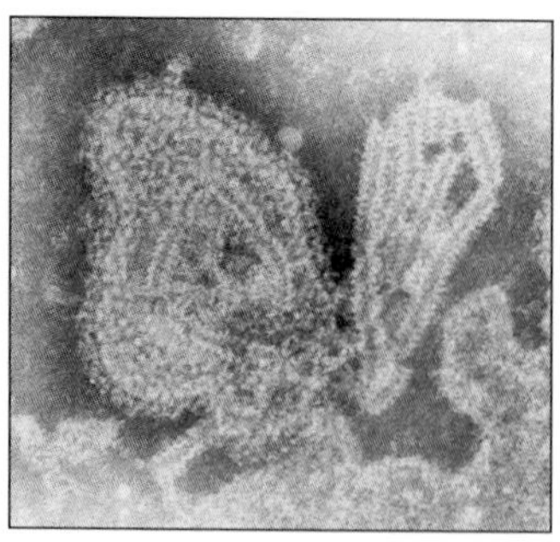

Fig 35-2 Negative-staining transmission electron micrograph of mumps virus. (Public Health Image Library image 1874, courtesy of Dr F. A. Murphy.)

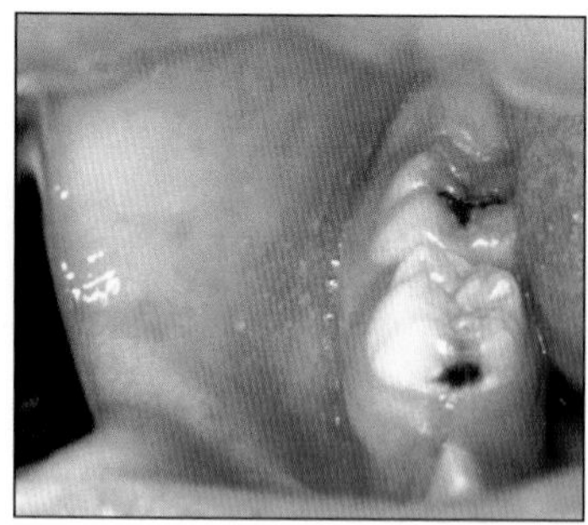

Fig 35-3 A measles patient with Koplik spots on the buccal mucosa, on the third pre-eruptive day, indicative of the onset of the disease. (Public Health Image Library image 6111, courtesy of the Centers for Disease Control and Prevention.)

After binding to a cell surface receptor (sialic acid, CD46, CD150), the virus fuses with the plasma membrane and releases its nucleocapsid into the cytoplasm. Transcription, translation, and replication take place in the cytoplasm. All of the components assemble at the plasma membrane of the host cell, and the completed virion buds from the cell surface, taking with it part of the host cell membrane.

Measles Virus

Infection by measles virus (rubeola virus) may be fatal. It is the most significant cause of death in children between 1 and 5 years old. Before the introduction of a vaccine, there were annually about 3 to 4 million cases of measles in the United States, with about 48,000 hospitalizations and 400 to 500 deaths. An inactivated virus vaccine was used between 1963 and 1967, reducing the cases per thousand from about 400 to 50. However, some recipients exposed to the measles virus developed "atypical measles" with more severe symptoms. A live attenuated virus vaccine was introduced in 1971 as part of the MMR (measles, mumps, rubella) vaccine, and it nearly eliminated measles cases. Between 1989 and 1991, however, an epidemic of measles resulted in 55,000 cases, 11,000 hospitalizations, and more than 120 deaths, primarily among children. In 2009, there were only 71 cases of measles in the United States. Worldwide, 344,000 deaths were reported to the WHO in 2010, with 139,000 estimated deaths.

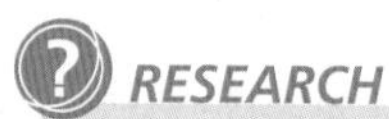

RESEARCH

What were the causes of the measles outbreak in 1989 in the United States?

More recent outbreaks of measles in the United States have affected 173 individuals in 2015 and more than 600 people in 2014. Most of the patients had not been vaccinated against measles. The increase in the number of recent cases is attributable to a troubling decrease in the rate of vaccination of school-age children, resulting from parents' fears of potential side effects.

Clinical syndromes and diagnosis

The prodrome (symptom indicative of an approaching disease) starts with high fever, cough, coryza (acute inflammation of the nasal mucous membrane accompanied by profuse nasal discharge), and conjunctivitis. The incubation period is 7 to 13 days. Following 2 days of illness, bright red lesions with a white, central dot appear on mucous membranes, most commonly on the buccal mucosa; these are known as Koplik spots (Fig 35-3). They may also appear on mucous membranes of the conjunctivae and vagina. Within a day of the appearance of Koplik spots, the typical maculopapular rash (exanthema) of measles appears first on the head and then spreads over the body. The rash persists for 3 to 5 days and then begins to disappear.

Encephalitis is one of the most feared complications of measles that occurs in 0.1% to 0.5% of those infected and may be fatal in 15% of such cases. Bacterial pneumonia can develop in some patients and is responsible for most of the deaths associated with measles. Atypical measles, a more intense presentation of measles, occurs in people who received the older inactivated virus vaccine and were subsequently exposed to the wild measles virus. Subacute sclerosing panencephalitis is a very serious neurologic complication of measles virus that may lead to blindness, spasticity, and changes in personality, behavior, and memory.

Measles may be confused with Rocky Mountain spotted fever, meningococcemia, scarlet fever, and varicella. The virus may be isolated from the oropharynx or urine within the first 5 days of the onset of symptoms; when added to susceptible cell cultures, it produces multinucleated syncytia. Rapid diagnosis is possible by the direct fluorescent antibody test on pharyngeal cells or urinary sediment. The

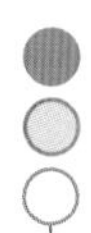

RNA genome of the virus can be identified by the reverse transcription polymerase chain reaction (RT-PCR). Antibodies to measles virus may be detected by hemagglutination inhibition or indirect fluorescent antibody tests.

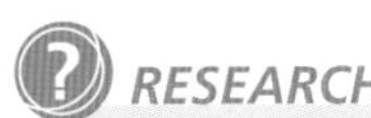

What is a direct fluorescent antibody test, and how does it differ from the indirect fluorescent antibody test?

Pathogenesis and epidemiology

Measles is transmitted via respiratory droplets and is highly contagious. Measles virus infection causes cell-cell fusion and cell lysis. Persistent infection is observed in brain cells. After infection of respiratory epithelial cells, it spreads to the lymphatic system, conjunctiva, urinary tract, and central nervous system. Infection of endothelial cells lining small blood vessels and the immune reaction of T cells cause the characteristic maculopapular rash. Infection can result in encephalitis of several forms, including subacute sclerosing panencephalitis caused by a defective form of the virus.

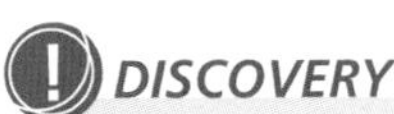

The measles virus hemagglutinin protein facilitates initial binding to host cell surface receptors, and the F protein mediates membrane fusion between the viral and cell membranes. The cellular receptor was identified by using a monoclonal antibody against the surface glycoprotein CD46; the antibody blocked viral infection. This was further confirmed by expressing this protein in nonpermissive murine cells by transfecting the gene encoding the protein into these cells and showing that the virus could bind these cells and produce infectious virus. CD46 is a member of the "regulators of complement activation" superfamily of proteins, which normally help in preventing the binding of complement components on host tissues.

Treatment and prevention

Although there are no treatments for measles once the illness sets in, the vaccine can be administered to nonimmunized individuals within 3 days of exposure (postexposure prophylaxis), resulting in milder symptoms. Immune serum globulin may be given to pregnant women and immunocompromised individuals within 6 days of exposure. This measure can prevent measles or result in less severe symptoms. Giving high doses of vitamin A may reduce the severity of the disease.

For prevention of measles, the MMR vaccine is administered to infants between 12 and 18 months of age and then again at 4 to 6 years old. The vaccine includes live attenuated virus strains. Outbreaks of measles may occur because of some parents' refusal to vaccinate their children, as in the 2014–2015 outbreak.

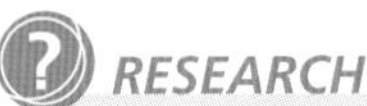

How did Finland reduce the incidence of measles from 105 per 100,000 in 1982 to 0.1 per 100,000 in 1995?

Parainfluenza Viruses

Clinical syndromes and diagnosis

Laryngotracheal bronchitis (croup) results in swelling and endangers the airways. Croup involves a barking cough, difficulty breathing, and laryngeal spasms. Other symptoms include hoarseness, "seal bark" cough, tachycardia, and tachypnea. Cell culture, hemadsorption, and RT-PCR tests can be used to detect the virus.

Pathogenesis and epidemiology

Parainfluenza virus types 1 to 3 cause severe lower respiratory tract infections. The host immune response may contribute to the pathogenesis. These viruses are transmitted via respiratory droplets and person-to-person contact. Outbreaks can occur in hospitals, nurseries, and pediatric wards.

Treatment and prevention

Nebulized hot or cold steam is used to relieve symptoms, but the airways should be monitored. There are no antivirals or vaccines effective against parainfluenza viruses.

Mumps Virus

Clinical syndromes and diagnosis

Mumps virus causes parotitis, painful swelling of the salivary glands. Other symptoms include fever, headache, muscle aches, fatigue, and loss of appetite. Complications resulting from mumps virus infection include orchitis (inflammation of the testis), oophoritis (inflammation of the ovary), pancreatitis, meningoencephalitis, and central nervous system involvement (in 50% of patients).

The virus can be detected by hemadsorption that is inhibited by mumps-specific antibody. It can also be detected by RT-PCR or real-time PCR.

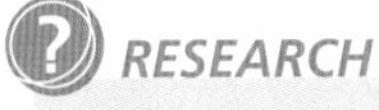

What is real-time PCR?

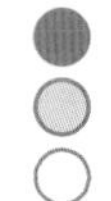

Pathogenesis and epidemiology

Mumps virus causes lytic infection of cells in the respiratory tract. It multiplies in the ductal epithelial cells of the parotid gland and causes swelling due to inflammation. It is transmitted via respiratory droplets. The virus is present in respiratory secretions in infected persons 7 days before the onset of symptoms.

Treatment and prevention

Treatment is symptomatic. The live attenuated virus vaccine, MMR, is effective in preventing mumps infection.

Respiratory Syncytial Virus

Respiratory syncytial virus (RSV) is the most frequent cause of fatal acute respiratory infection in infants and young children. Almost everyone carrying the virus is infected by age 4 years, and re-infections occur, even among older people. RSV is classified as a pneumovirus within the paramyxovirus family, and it has been named as such because it mediates cell-cell fusion in cell culture, forming multinucleated giant cells called *syncytia*. The G glycoprotein in the envelope mediates attachment to host cells, and the F glycoprotein causes the fusion of the viral and cellular plasma membranes.

Clinical syndromes and diagnosis

The symptoms range from the common cold to pneumonia. Bronchiolitis (a lower respiratory tract illness) may occur in infants, and rhinorrhea (runny nose) is seen in older children. The infection is accompanied by low-grade fever, tachypnea (abnormally rapid breathing), and tachycardia (rapid heartbeat, greater than 100 bpm). Other clinical syndromes include hypoxemia (low oxygen levels in the blood), hypercapnia (retention of carbon dioxide), and hyperexpansion of the lungs.

RSV infection can be diagnosed by antigen detection using immunofluorescence or enzyme immunoassay or by PCR. The virus can also be identified by inoculation of respiratory secretions on cultured cells and detection of syncytia within a few days. A four-fold increase in titer of antibodies against the virus indicates a recent infection.

Pathogenesis and epidemiology

RSV infection results in the necrosis of epithelial cells, bronchi, and bronchioles; interstitial infiltration of mononuclear cells; and blockage of the smaller airways with necrotic cells, mucus, and fibrin. Syncytia with cytoplasmic inclusion bodies are observed occasionally among the epithelial cells of the upper respiratory tract. Vaccination with a killed virus vaccine appears to increase the severity of subsequent disease. This may be explained by a heightened immunologic response at the time of exposure to the wild-type virus. Natural infection does not prevent re-infection. Patients with more severe disease have helper T (T_h2) $CD4^+$ cells (rather than T_h1 $CD4^+$ cells found in patients with mild disease) that produce interleukin-4 (IL-4), IL-5, IL-6, and IL-10.

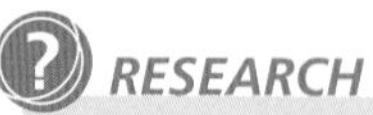

RESEARCH

Why does natural infection not prevent re-infection with RSV?

Between 25% and 40% of infants and children exposed to RSV for the first time will have signs or symptoms of bronchiolitis or pneumonia. A small percentage of the children (0.5% to 2%) will require hospitalization, most of them being younger than 6 months of age. Infections occur every year in the winter. RSV is a serious nosocomial pathogen; the introduction of the virus into a nursery can be devastating. The virus is transmitted on hands, by fomites, and to some degree by respiratory droplets.

Treatment and prevention

Supportive treatment includes oxygen, intravenous fluids, and nebulized cold steam. Aerosolized ribavirin is approved for the treatment of patients predisposed to a more severe course (eg, premature or immunocompromised infants). Passive immunization with an anti-RSV immunoglobulin is available for premature infants. Vaccination with an experimental killed virus vaccine appears to increase the severity of subsequent disease.

Control measures to prevent spread of the virus include hand washing and wearing gowns, goggles, and masks.

Nipah Virus

A paramyxovirus has been identified as the etiologic agent of an outbreak of severe encephalitis and respiratory illness in people with close-contact exposure to pigs in Southeast Asia. Together with Hendra virus, Nipah virus has been classified in the genus *Henipavirus* in the Paramyxoviridae family. The virus persists in low numbers in fruit bats and when passed to pigs replicates very rapidly and causes severe disease. The infected pigs develop a peculiar loud cough, which facilitates transmission to humans. Of the 269 human cases in 1999, 108 were fatal.

Although generally considered to be a zoonotic virus, transmitted from animals to humans, half of the cases reported in Bangladesh between 2001 and 2008 were the result of human-to-human transmission. In India, 75% of cases occurred among hospital staff and visitors, indicating human-to human transmission.

Initial symptoms are influenza-like, such as myalgia, fever, headache, vomiting, and sore throat. Subsequent symptoms include drowsiness, altered consciousness, and encephalitis and seizures in severe cases. Currently there are no vaccines or treatment available.

Hendra Virus

This *Henipavirus* caused outbreaks of severe respiratory infections in horses in Australia. Between 1994 and 2013, seven human cases were reported, some cases presenting with encephalitis. The mortality rate is 57%. Hendra virus has also been isolated from a fruit bat, suggesting a reservoir for the virus.

Bibliography

Bryan C. Upper respiratory tract infections and other infections of the head and neck. Microbiology and Immunology On-line, University of South Carolina School of Medicine. http://www.microbiologybook.org/Infectious%20Disease/Upper%20respiratory%20tract.htm. Accessed 31 July 2015.

Centers for Disease Control and Prevention. Measles Cases and Outbreaks. www.cdc.gov/measles/cases-outbreaks.html. Accessed 31 July 2015.

Centers for Disease Control and Prevention. Public Health Image Library. phil.cdc.gov. Accessed 4 August 2015.

Centers for Disease Control and Prevention. Respiratory Syncytial Virus Infection (RSV). www.cdc.gov/rsv/about/infection.html. Accessed 31 July 2015.

Enders G. Paramyxoviruses. In: Baron S (ed). Medical Microbiology, ed 4. Galveston, TX: University of Texas Medical Branch at Galveston, 1996.

Loney C, Mottet-Osman G, Roux L, Bhella D. Paramyxovirus ultrastructure and genome packaging: Cryo-electron tomography of Sendai virus. J Virol 2009;83:8191–8197.

Mosby's Dictionary of Medicine, Nursing and Health Professions, ed 9. Philadelphia: Mosby/Elsevier, 2012.

Murray PR, Rosenthal KS, Pfaller MA. Medical Microbiology, ed 6. Philadelphia: Mosby/Elsevier, 2009.

Ryan KJ, Ray CG. Sherris Medical Microbiology, ed 5. New York: McGraw-Hill, 2010.

Tortora GJ, Funke BR, Case CL. Microbiology: An Introduction, ed 10. San Francisco: Benjamin Cummings, 2010.

World Health Organization. Hendra Virus (HeV) Infection. http://www.who.int/csr/disease/hendra/en/. Accessed 31 July 2015.

World Health Organization. Immunizaton surveillance, assessment and monitoring. http://www.who.int/immunization/monitoring_surveillance/en/. Accessed 31 July 2015.

World Health Organization. Nipah Virus (NiV) Infection. http://www.who.int/csr/disease/nipah/en/. Accessed 31 July 2015.

Take-Home Messages

- Paramyxoviruses are negative-strand RNA viruses.
- The symptoms of measles virus infection include a rash that starts on the head and spreads throughout the body. Other symptoms include cough, coryza, conjunctivitis, and the appearance of Koplik spots on the buccal mucosa.
- The symptoms of mumps virus infection include parotiditis, orchitis, and oophoritis.
- RSV is the most frequent cause of fatal acute respiratory infection in infants and young children. Aerosolized ribavirin is approved for the treatment of patients predisposed to a more severe course.

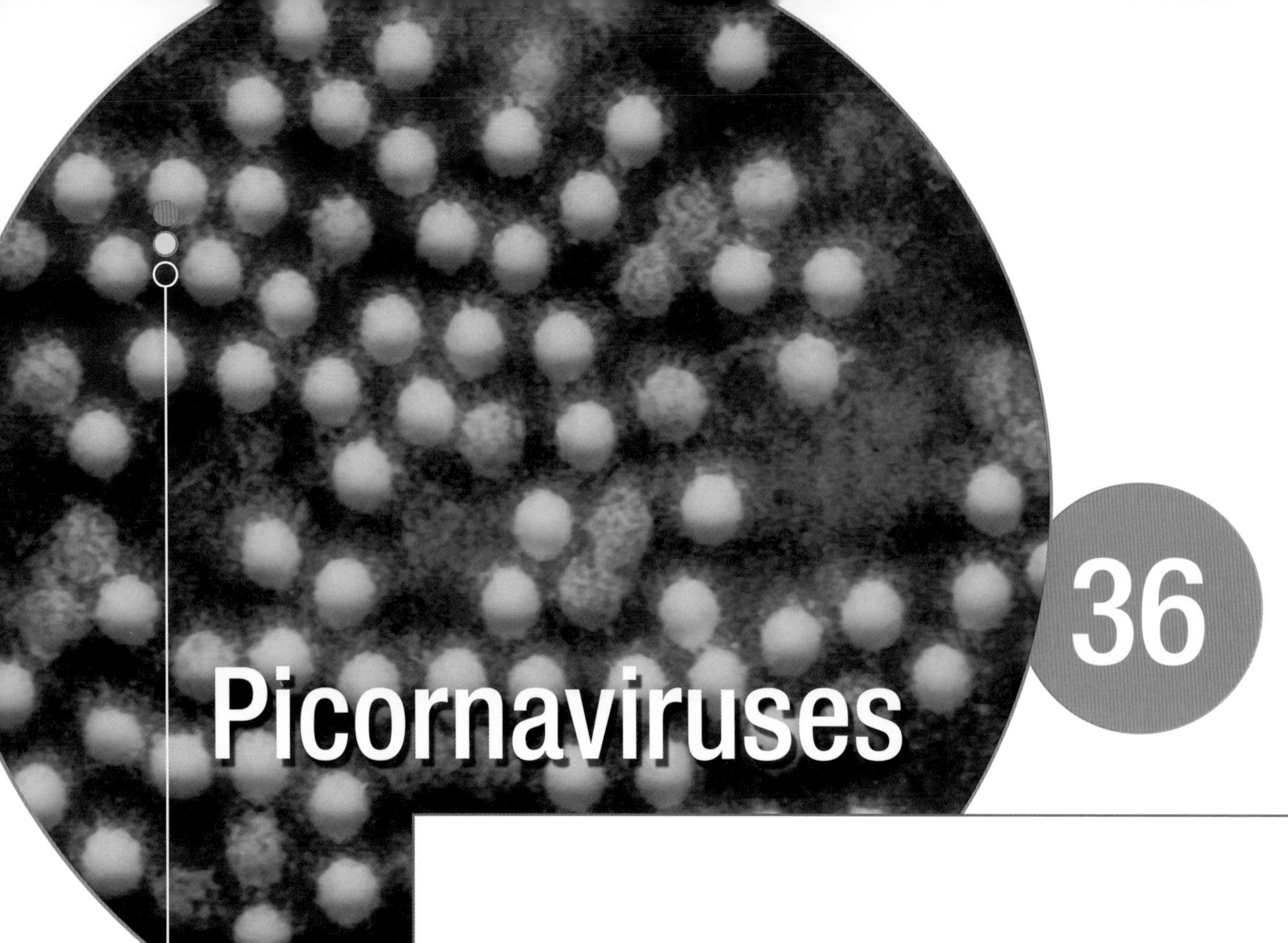

36 Picornaviruses

Structure and Replication

Picornaviruses are small, non-enveloped, single-stranded, positive-strand RNA viruses 30 nm in diameter (Fig 36-1). **Enteroviruses** are resistant to pH in the range 3 to 9, detergents, mild sewage treatment, and heat. They include **poliovirus**, **Coxsackievirus A**, **Coxsackievirus B**, **echovirus** (enteric, cytopathic, human, orphan), and **enterovirus**. Enterovirus 72 is also known as **hepatitis A virus** and is now classified as a hepatovirus. **Rhinoviruses** are labile at acidic pH, and their optimum growth temperature is 33°C.

Picornaviruses have an icosahedral capsid. The 12 vertices are each composed of five **protomers**, and each protomer is composed of four nonglycosylated polypeptides: VP1, VP2, VP3, and VP4. The VP1 protein contains a "canyon" structure that binds to the cellular receptor. For most rhinoviruses and some Coxsackieviruses, the receptor is intercellular adhesion molecule-1 (ICAM-1), which is found on epithelial cells, endothelial cells, and fibroblasts. Many enteroviruses bind to the **CD55** molecule ("decay accelerating factor" involved in the degradation of complement proteins). Poliovirus binds to CD155, a member of the immunoglobulin superfamily, also called the *poliovirus receptor*. Coxsackievirus B binds to the **CAR** (Coxsackievirus and adenovirus receptor) molecule.

Early electron micrographs of poliovirus-infected cells showed virions directly penetrating the plasma membrane, giving rise to the belief that viral entry occurs directly at the cell surface. Inhibition of infectivity in the presence of the ionophore monensin to dissipate the proton gradient in endosomes implicated a pH-dependent route. Poliovirus appears to expose hydrophobic "fusion domains" of its proteins at low pH,

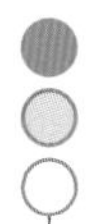

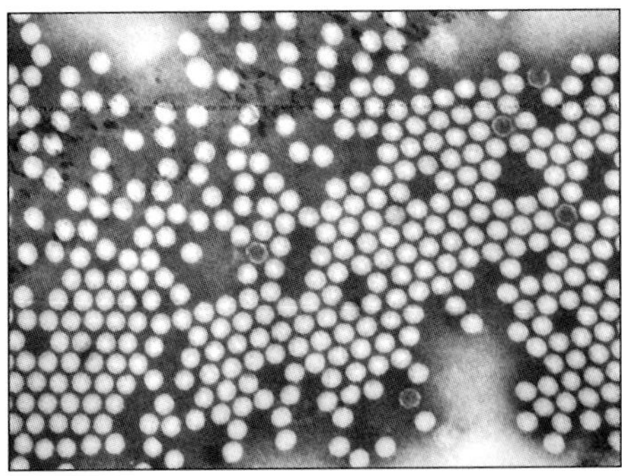

Fig 36-1 Electron micrograph of poliovirus. (Public Health Image Library image 1875, courtesy of Dr Fred Murphy and Sylvia Whitfield.)

Fig 36-2 Poliovirus entry into cells. (Reprinted with permission from Flint et al.)

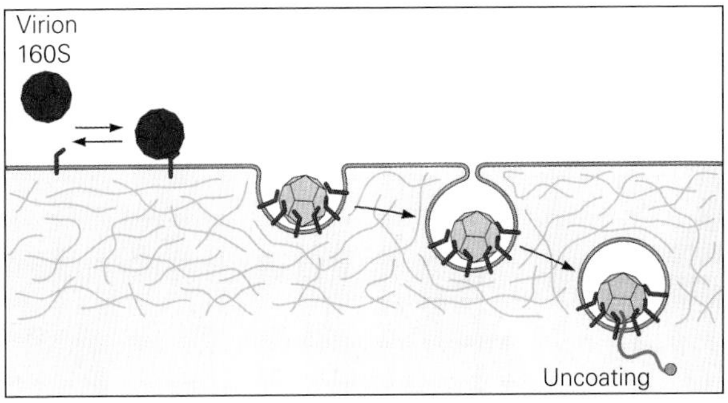

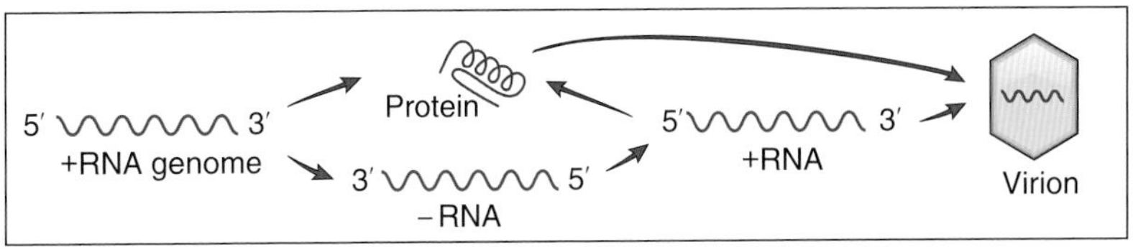

Fig 36-3 Replication of picornaviridae.

suggesting that it enters cells via an acidic intracellular vesicle. Inhibition of actin polymerization also inhibits infection. However, classical coated-pit endocytosis and caveolin-mediated pathways do not seem to be involved in internalization of poliovirus.

Upon virus binding to the receptor, the VP4 molecule is released, thereby weakening the virion structure. The VP1 protein then forms a channel in the plasma membrane through which the RNA genome enters the cytoplasm (Fig 36-2). Although RNA does not have a 5′-methylated cap, it recognizes the ribosomes by means of its internal ribosome entry site RNA loop. The RNA is translated into a polyprotein, which is then cleaved into individual proteins by virus-encoded proteases. The RNA-dependent RNA polymerase also encoded by the virus makes a negative-strand RNA copy, which serves as a template for the genomic RNA (Fig 36-3). The number of viral RNA molecules may reach 400,000 copies per cell. The viral proteins and RNA associate to form as many as 100,000 viral particles per cell within 3 to 4 hours of infection.

Viral tactics to inhibit cellular protein synthesis

Picornaviruses use a number of tactics to render the intracellular environment advantageous for themselves:

- A viral protease cleaves the ribosomal cap-binding protein (EIF4-G), thereby inhibiting the binding of most cellular mRNAs to the ribosome.
- A viral protease also cleaves the cellular transcription factor CREB.
- The membrane permeability changes induced by viral infection impair the ability of cellular mRNA to bind ribosomes.
- The abundant viral RNA can compete with cellular mRNA for molecular factors involved in translation.

Poliovirus

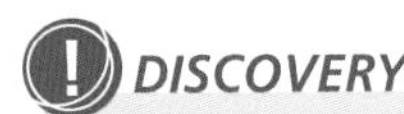

DISCOVERY

At a meeting of the Royal and Imperial Association of Physicians in Vienna on December 18, 1908, Dr Karl Landsteiner reported that poliomyelitis could be transferred experimentally from humans to apes in a study he performed with Erwin Popper. Soon after the meeting, Landsteiner published a paper in which he stated that "the poliomyelitis virus belongs to the group of filterable micro-organisms" that are known to be viruses. His results were soon confirmed by others. Landsteiner declared during a congress in Washington in 1912 that a vaccine against poliomyelitis should be possible, although it might prove to be difficult. The first polio vaccine became available 43 years later, in 1955.

Clinical syndromes and diagnosis

Paralytic poliomyelitis is the major illness and occurs in 0.1% of infected children and in about 1.3% of infected adults. The severity of the paralysis depends on the extent of the neuronal infection and the neurons affected. The extent of paralysis is variable, and some functions may be restored within 6 months. During the incubation period of about 14 days, increased muscular activity can lead to the paralysis of the limbs that were exercised, possibly resulting from increased vascularity, facilitating the spread of the virus to nerve endings.

Bulbar (cranial) poliomyelitis may involve the muscles of the pharynx, vocal cords, and those involved in respiration. If untreated, this disease results in death in 75% of patients. "Iron lungs" were used in the 1950s to enable patients to breathe. Persons whose tonsils have been removed are more likely to develop bulbar poliomyelitis, possibly because of the reduced levels of secretory immunoglobulin (Ig) A in the pharynx and the subsequent reduction in antiviral protection.

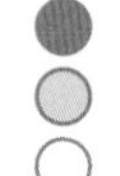

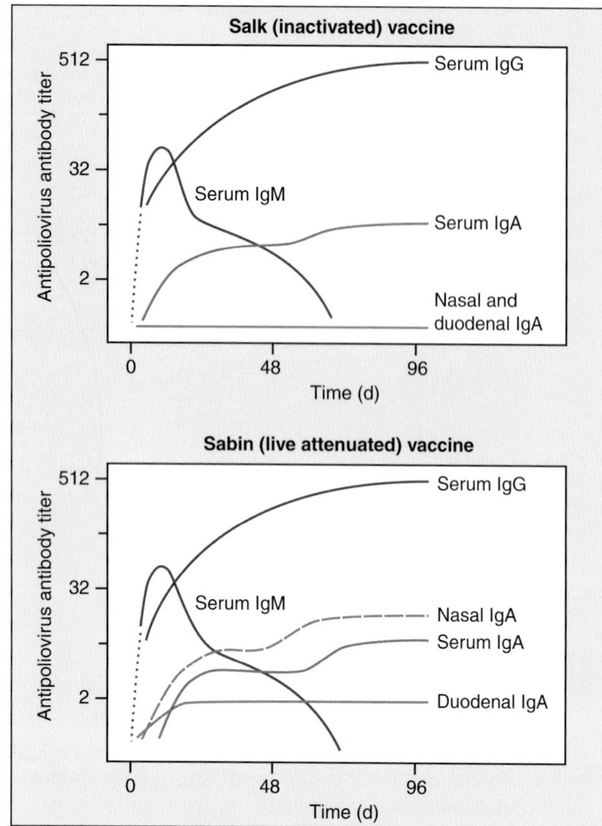

Fig 36-4 Serum and secretory antibody responses to the Salk and Sabin polio vaccines. (Adapted from Murray et al.)

Abortive poliomyelitis (the minor illness) is a mild, febrile illness, with sore throat, malaise, and vomiting observed in 5% of infected individuals.

Nonparalytic poliomyelitis is seen in 1% to 2% of infected individuals who develop aseptic meningitis, with symptoms including fever, headache, stiff neck, and photophobia. The patients recover completely within 10 days.

Post-polio syndrome can manifest itself decades after the initial infection, although no poliovirus is detected, and involves the deterioration of the muscles where the nerves were damaged initially.

Poliovirus can be recovered from a patient's pharynx early in the infection and in the feces up to 30 days after infection and can be grown in monkey kidney cells. Reverse transcription polymerase chain reaction (RT-PCR) can be used to detect the 5′ untranslated region of the viral RNA in the cerebrospinal fluid. This method can also be used for the detection of other enteroviruses.

Pathogenesis and epidemiology

Poliovirus is transmitted by the fecal-oral route. It multiplies in the lymphoid tissue of the tonsils and Peyer's patches and spreads to the central nervous system through the bloodstream. Poliovirus replicates preferentially in motor neurons in the anterior horn of the spinal cord. The paralytic effect of the virus results from the death of these cells and the paralysis of the muscles innervated by these neurons. Cell damage also elicits an immune response, resulting in edema that can also affect cells in addition to the infected ones. Resolution of the edema can result in the apparent improvement in level of paralysis several weeks after the acute infection phase.

Poliovirus is transmitted from person to person and via the fecal-oral route. The virus can survive in the feces for many weeks and contaminate food and water, especially under unsanitary conditions.

Treatment and prevention

The development and use of the killed virus vaccine by Jonas Salk in the 1950s drastically reduced the incidence of polio. This vaccine is indicated for the initial vaccination of nonimmunized adults, because the risk of disease from the live vaccine is higher in adults than in children, and for the vaccination of immunodeficient individuals. The Salk vaccine is now being used for childhood immunization to avoid the risk of reversion of the live Sabin vaccine, which happens at a rate of one in 4 million doses. The vaccine is administered at 2, 4, and 6 to 18 months as well as at 4 to 6 years.

The live attenuated polio vaccine developed by Albert Sabin interrupts fecal-oral transmission by inducing high levels of secretory IgA in the gastrointestinal tract, since it replicates there (Fig 36-4). The much less virulent vaccine was generated by passage of the virus in cell culture, resulting in a virus that could replicate in the oropharynx and the intestinal tract but not in neuronal cells. It is given orally, and thus it is accepted more readily. The attenuated vaccine virus can be transmitted from person to person, and thus it can indirectly immunize more people. It also prevents the spread of the virus by stopping the excretion of the virus in stools.

The number of polio cases in the world has fallen from an estimated 350,000 in 1988 to 407 in 2013. The Americas, Europe, Southeast Asia, and the Western Pacific are currently polio free. Afghanistan, Nigeria, and Pakistan are the only countries that have not eradicated polio.

Coxsackieviruses

Coxsackievirus is named after the town in New York where the viruses were first isolated. There are at least 24 serotypes of Coxsackievirus A and 6 serotypes of Coxsackievirus B. They are transmitted by the fecal-oral route and by aerosols. One of the diseases caused by Coxsackievirus A is herpangina. The disease is not related to herpesvirus infection. The clinical syndromes include fever, sore throat, pain on swallowing, anorexia, and vomiting. Vesicular, ulcerated lesions are seen around the soft palate and uvula. The disease requires only symptomatic management.

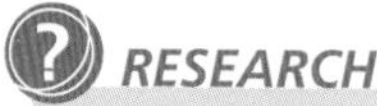

What other microorganisms are named after the town or region where they were first observed?

Hand-foot-and-mouth disease is caused by Coxsackievirus A16, although other Coxsackieviruses have also been associated with the disease. It usually affects infants and children younger than age 5 years, but it is sometimes seen in adults. The symptoms include mild fever, blisterlike sores in the mouth, and a skin rash. Lesions appear initially in the oral cavity and then develop within 1 day on the palms and soles. Hand-foot-and-mouth disease is sometimes confused with foot-and-mouth disease, which is a disease of cattle, sheep, and swine caused by a different virus. Coxsackievirus B (Fig 36-5) is responsible for myocardial and pericardial infections that may be especially severe in newborns and may lead to heart failure. Acute benign pericarditis is seen mostly in young adults but also in older persons. Infection of pancreatic beta cells with Coxsackievirus B can cause destruction of the islets of Langerhans and subsequent insulin-dependent diabetes.

Pleurodynia (Bornholm disease) is caused by Coxsackievirus B. Its symptoms include sudden onset of fever and unilateral low thoracic, pleuritic chest pain, also known as "the devil's grip." It lasts for about 4 days but may relapse.

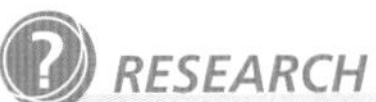

What are pleuritic chest pain and pleurisy?

Viral, or aseptic, meningitis is caused by either Coxsackieviruses or echoviruses. It is an acute, febrile illness accompanied by headache, rigid neck, and skin rash. It is an inflammation of the tissues covering the brain and spinal cord.

Echoviruses

Certain echoviruses cause respiratory disease, aseptic meningitis, maculopapular rash, and paralysis. Echovirus 9 epidemics have been observed in Europe and North America, with clinical syndromes including sore throat and rash on the face, neck, and chest. Some patients have clinical signs of meningitis. Patients with echovirus 16 infections present with fever, abdominal pain, and mild sore throat, followed by a pink macular or maculopapular rash on the face, back, and chest. This disease is also referred to as Boston fever. Echoviruses 4, 6, and 30 can cause aseptic meningitis in children and adults. Echoviruses 13, 18, and 30 have caused outbreaks of viral meningitis in the United States. Echoviruses 6, 9, and 11 are most likely transmitted to neonates during birth or postnatally from the mother or nursery attendants and can cause hepatitis, meningoencephalitis, and circulatory collapse.

Enteroviruses

Most people who get infected with a non-polio enterovirus do not get sick or only have mild coldlike symptoms. Enterovirus 70 has caused outbreaks of acute hemorrhagic conjunctivitis, which resolves within about a week. Neurologic complications of this infection include polio-like paralysis. Outbreaks of enterovirus 71 have caused fatal myocarditis in Malaysia. Enterovirus 71 has also caused large outbreaks of hand-foot-and-mouth disease worldwide, especially in children in Asia. Some enterovirus 71 infections have been linked to brainstem encephalitis.

In 2014, an outbreak of enterovirus D68 caused severe respiratory infections in infants and children in the United States, with 1,153 confirmed cases.

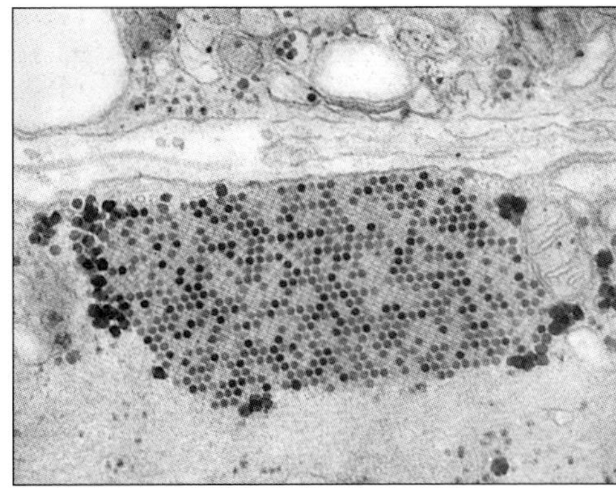

Fig 36-5 Electron micrograph of Coxsackievirus B in muscle tissue. (Public Health Image Library image 10204, courtesy of Dr Fred Murphy and Sylvia Whitfield.)

Rhinoviruses

Human rhinoviruses, which were discovered in the 1950s, are responsible for more than 50% of coldlike illnesses. There are three genetically distinct groups (A, B, and C) within the genus *Enterovirus* and the family Picornaviridae and about 115 serologic types. They cause upper respiratory tract infection, sinusitis, and otitis media. The use of PCR assays in clinical laboratories has led to the realization that rhinoviruses are also lower respiratory tract pathogens, particularly in patients with asthma, immunocompromised individuals, infants, and elderly patients. They can be distinguished from other enteroviruses by the fact that they do not infect the gastrointestinal tract and are sensitive to acid. Some rhinoviruses can survive heating to 50°C and are stable at room temperature on environmental surfaces for several days. Their optimal growth temperature is 33°C, explaining their preference for the nasal mucosa. Infected cells release bradykinin and histamine, which cause increased secretions (runny nose), vasodilation, and sore throat. The release of cytokines during inflammation can promote the spread of the virus by enhancing the expression of ICAM-1 receptors for the virus. Whether the clinical symptoms of rhinovirus infections are a direct consequence of viral pathogenicity or the result of the host immune response is still being investigated. Coronaviruses, adenoviruses, influenza C virus, and Coxsackieviruses also cause the "common cold."

Rhinoviruses are transmitted by respiratory droplets or by contaminated fingers touching the eye or nasal mucosa. The incidence is high in preschool-aged children, who can then infect their families.

Currently, there are no approved antiviral therapies for rhinoviruses, and treatment is supportive (eg, inhaling hot, humid air to help with nasal drainage). Experimental drugs include pleconaril, arildone, and disoxaril that contain a chemical group (3-methylisoxazole) that inserts into the base of the receptor-binding canyon of the viral capsid and blocks uncoating of the virus. Enviroxime is an inhibitor of the viral RNA-dependent RNA polymerase. There are no vaccines against rhinoviruses, primarily because of the multiple serotypes and antigenic drift of the virus.

Bibliography

Centers for Disease Control and Prevention. Global Health – Polio: Our Progress Against Polio. www.cdc.gov/polio/progress/index.htm. Accessed 31 July 2015.

Centers for Disease Control and Prevention. Hand, Foot and Mouth Disease (HFMD). www.cdc.gov/hand-foot-mouth/about/index.html. Accessed 31 July 2015.

Centers for Disease Control and Prevention. Non-Polio Enterovirus: Enterovirus D68. www.cdc.gov/non-polio-enterovirus/about/EV-D68.html. Accessed 31 July 2015.

Centers for Disease Control and Prevention. Non-Polio Enterovirus: Outbreaks & Surveillance. www.cdc.gov/non-polio-enterovirus/outbreaks-surveillance.html. Accessed 31 July 2015.

Centers for Disease Control and Prevention. Public Health Image Library. phil.cdc.gov. Accessed 4 August 2015.

Flint SJ, Enquist LW, Racaniello VR, Skalka AM. Principles of Virology, ed 3. Washington, DC: ASM, 2009.

Greenwood D, Barer M, Slack R, Irving W. Medical Microbiology, ed 18. Edinburgh: Churchill Livingstone/Elsevier, 2012.

Jacobs SE, Lamson DM, St George K, Walsh TJ. Human rhinoviruses. Clin Microbiol Rev 2013;26:135–162.

Levinson W. Review of Medical Microbiology and Immunology, ed 11. New York: McGraw-Hill, 2010.

Murray PR, Rosenthal KS, Pfaller MA. Medical Microbiology, ed 7. Philadelphia: Mosby/Elsevier, 2013.

Ryan KJ, Ray CG. Sherris Medical Microbiology, ed 5. New York: McGraw-Hill, 2010.

Schwick HG. Poliomyelitis in Landsteiner's time and today. Wien Klin Wochenschr 1991;103:136–140.

Thorley JA, McKeating JA, Rappoport JZ. Mechanisms of viral entry: Sneaking in the front door. Protoplasma 2010;244:15–24.

Take-Home Messages

- Picornaviruses are non-enveloped, single-stranded, positive-strand RNA viruses 30 nm in diameter.
- Among the picornaviruses, the detergent- and low pH–resistant enteroviruses include poliovirus, Coxsackievirus A, Coxsackievirus B, echovirus, and enterovirus.
- Poliovirus is transmitted by the fecal-oral route.
- The severity of the paralysis in paralytic poliomyelitis depends on the extent of the neuronal infection and the neurons affected. This illness occurs in only 0.1% of infected children.
- Bulbar (cranial) poliomyelitis may involve the muscles of the pharynx, vocal cords, and respiration; if untreated, it results in death in 75% of patients.
- The killed virus Salk vaccine and the attenuated virus Sabin vaccine are highly effective in preventing polio. The Salk vaccine is used currently for childhood immunizations in the United States to avoid the risk of reversion of the live Sabin vaccine.
- Coxsackievirus A can cause herpangina, with vesicular, ulcerated lesions around the soft palate and uvula.
- Hand-foot-and-mouth disease is caused by Coxsackievirus A16, with symptoms including mild fever, blisterlike sores in the mouth, and a skin rash.
- Coxsackievirus B causes myocardial and pericardial infections that may be especially severe in newborns and may lead to heart failure. This virus also causes pleurodynia.
- Coxsackieviruses can cause aseptic meningitis.
- Certain echoviruses cause respiratory disease, aseptic meningitis, maculopapular rash, and paralysis.
- Rhinoviruses cause upper respiratory tract infection (the common cold), sinusitis, and otitis media.

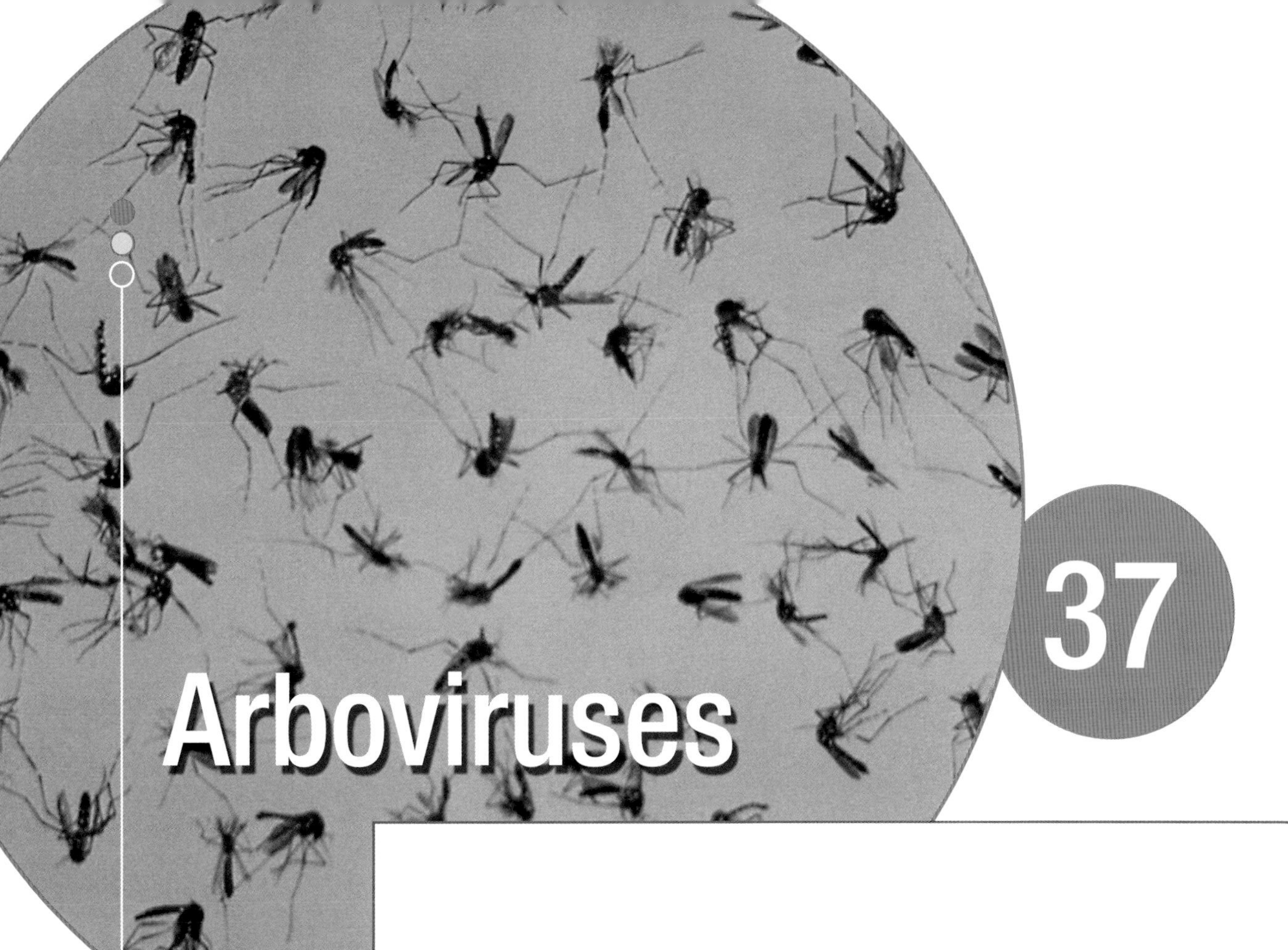

37 Arboviruses

Alphaviruses (except for the rubivirus, ie, rubella virus), flaviviruses (except for hepatitis C and G viruses), and bunyaviruses (except for hantaviruses) are grouped together as arboviruses, an acronym for arthropod-borne viruses. Transmission occurs when mosquitos or other arthropods inject infected saliva into blood vessels or extravascular tissues while blood-feeding.

Alphaviruses

There are eight alphaviruses that infect humans. These are Eastern equine encephalitis virus (EEEV) (Fig 37-1), Western equine encephalitis virus (WEEV), Venezuelan equine encephalitis virus (VEEV), Sindbis virus, Semliki Forest virus, Ross River virus, Chikungunya virus, and O'nyong-nyong virus.

Structure and replication

Alphaviruses (family Togaviridae) are enveloped, single-stranded, positive-strand RNA viruses with an icosahedral capsid and a lipid envelope and a diameter of about 60 to 70 nm. The envelope is held tightly and conforms to the shape and symmetry of the capsid. The membrane contains two or three glycoproteins that form a single spike on the viral surface. The viral envelope fuses with the membrane of an endosome following acidification, delivering the capsid into the cytoplasm.

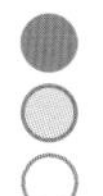

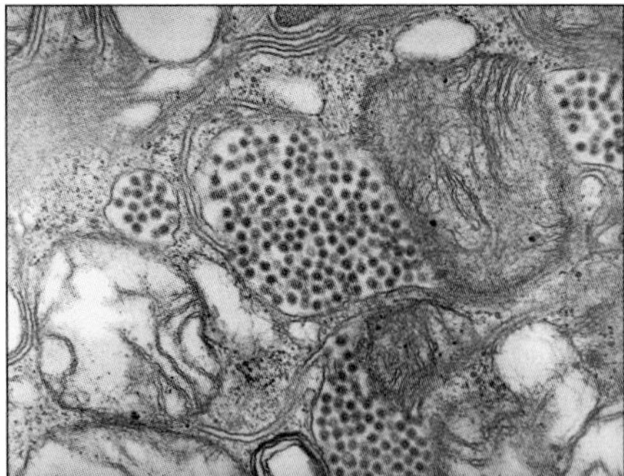

Fig 37-1 Electron micrograph of Eastern equine encephalitis virus in a mosquito salivary gland. (Public Health Image Library image 1868, courtesy of Dr Fred Murphy and Sylvia Whitfield.)

The alphavirus genome acts as mRNA, two-thirds of which is translated into a polyprotein that is then cleaved by a viral protease (part of the polyprotein) into the nonstructural proteins (NSP1–NSP4). These proteins assemble as the RNA-dependent RNA polymerase to replicate the viral genome. The remaining one-third of the mRNA is copied from the negative-strand template and encodes the capsid and envelope proteins E1, E2, and E3. The genomic RNA combines with 240 capsid proteins to form the nucleocapsid, which then associates with the E2 protein at the plasma membrane. The membrane buds off to form the mature virion.

Clinical syndromes and diagnosis

Alphaviruses cause a flulike syndrome and encephalitis. Group I of the four EEEV strains is endemic in North America and the Caribbean and is the cause of most cases of infection. Most EEEV infections in humans are either not apparent or cause a low-grade fever, followed by arthralgia, myalgia, and malaise. If EEEV crosses the blood-brain barrier, it causes severe, acute encephalitis that kills 50% to 75% of infected humans and causes serious neurologic sequelae in survivors. Initial symptoms of EEE may often progress to confusion, feeling sleepy, or coma.

WEEV usually causes subclinical infection but can cause serious complications in infants and children. The mortality rate of WEE is about 4% and occurs mostly in the elderly. VEEV infects humans and horses and is prevalent in the northern countries of South America and the Southern United States. In humans, VEEV causes headache, fever, chills, nausea, vomiting, and myalgia and may progress to encephalitis.

Of the alphaviruses, EEEV most closely resembles WEEV and may have been a genetic predecessor of WEEV. The complete nucleotide sequence for WEEV revealed 11,508 nucleotides with an 84% concordance of protein similarity with EEEV. The virus probably originated as a recombinant of EEEV and Sindbis virus. The capsid and nonstructural genes are derived from EEEV, while the envelope protein genes are derived from a Sindbis-like virus.

Diagnosis is via reverse transcription polymerase chain reaction (RT-PCR) of the viral genome of the mRNA in blood or other samples. Cytopathologic effects and immunofluorescence may also aid in diagnosis. Individual species or strains can be distinguished by means of monoclonal antibodies.

RESEARCH

What are the clinical syndromes of infections due to Sindbis virus, Semliki Forest virus, Ross River virus, Chikungunya virus, and O'nyong-nyong virus?

Pathogenesis and epidemiology

Alphaviruses are transmitted by mosquitos and can infect humans, horses, monkeys, reptiles, birds, and amphibians. EEEV and WEEV are transmitted from birds by the *Culiseta* mosquito. VEEV is transmitted from rodents by *Culiseta* and *Aedes* mosquitos.

Different viruses can infect different tissues, resulting in unique symptoms. Most EEEV infections in humans are without symptoms or produce a low-grade fever followed by malaise, arthralgia, and myalgia. However, in some cases, EEEV crosses the blood-brain barrier and causes a severe, and often fatal, acute encephalitis that kills 50% to 75% of infected humans and leaves many survivors with serious neurologic sequelae. EEEV infection in children generally has a more rapid onset and is more severe. The disease is also more severe in elderly patients. Histologic examination shows diffuse meningoencephalitis, neuronal necrosis, perivascular accumulation of neutrophils and mononuclear cells, and blood vessel occlusion. The virulence of EEEV may be the result of its ability to avoid nonspecific immunity via interferon-α and interferon-β production.

EEEV infections occur in the Eastern United States, South America, and the Caribbean. There are about 12 to 17 cases per year in the United States; the most recent epidemic was in North Carolina in 2003 and involved 26 cases. EEEV occurs more often in the summer, in wooded areas next to stagnant freshwater. The mosquito vector usually dies off in the winter.

WEEV is seen primarily west of the Mississippi River and in South America. The worst epidemic occurred in the Western United States and Canada in 1941, with 3,336 cases in humans. Since 1964, there have been fewer than 700 confirmed cases in the United States, with only a few cases annually. It is spread by the *Culex* mosquito, which is found on the West Coast of the United States, and finds a reservoir in birds.

Studies in experimental animals have indicated that VEEV replicates primarily in dendritic cells in lymphoid tissues and spreads by viremia. It infects the central nervous system, causing encephalitis. The virus appears to infect particular parts of the peripheral nervous system, replicate in olfactory and dental tissues, and disseminate into the brain, causing meningoencephalitis. VEEV is transmitted primarily via mosquitos, but infection via aerosols can also occur.

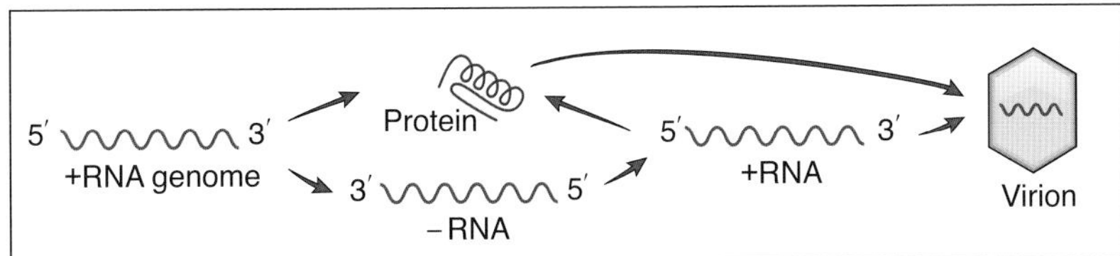

Fig 37-2 The replication cycle of flaviviruses.

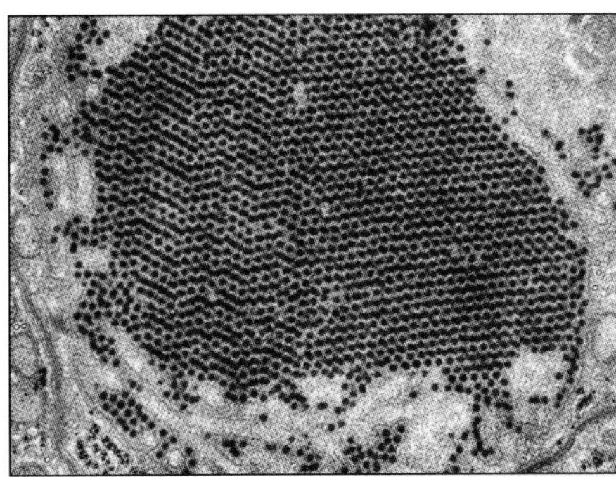

Fig 37-3 Electron micrograph of St Louis encephalitis virions in the salivary gland of a mosquito. (Public Health Image Library image 10228, courtesy of Dr Fred Murphy and Sylvia Whitfield.)

Treatment and prevention

There is no vaccine, preventive drug, or specific treatment for infections caused by alphaviruses. Encephalitis patients are managed supportively, such as with anticonvulsive treatment, temperature reduction with ice packs, and ventilation.

Flaviviruses

The family Flaviviridae includes St Louis encephalitis virus (SLEV), West Nile virus (WNV), Japanese encephalitis virus, Murray Valley encephalitis virus, and Russian spring-summer encephalitis virus. It also includes the hemorrhagic viruses dengue and yellow fever viruses.

Structure and replication

Flavivirus structure is similar to that of alphaviruses, but the diameter of the virions is only 40 to 50 nm. The capsid (C) proteins cover the genomic RNA complexed with small basic proteins. The membrane contains the glycosylated E protein and the matrix (M) protein. Following endocytosis of the virus and fusion via the E protein, the positive-sense RNA that enters the cytoplasm is translated into a polyprotein, which is then cleaved by a protease encoded by the virus (Fig 37-2). The prM protein, a precursor to the M protein, forms a heterodimer with the E protein. The pr segment of the prM protein is cleaved at the cell membrane by the cellular protease furin, forming the mature virion.

Clinical syndromes and diagnosis

SLEV (Fig 37-3) can cause headache, neck stiffness, fever, disorientation, tremors, convulsions, spastic paralysis, and coma. However, many people infected with SLEV may show no symptoms, and those with mild illness may only develop a headache and fever. The disease is more severe in the elderly.

WNV causes West Nile fever in about 20% of infected people. The clinical syndromes include fever, vomiting, diarrhea, headache, and body aches, sometimes with a skin rash and swollen lymph glands that last a few days. Fatigue and weakness can continue up to several months. In about 1% of infected individuals, encephalitis or meningitis is seen, and the risk increases with age.

Dengue and yellow fever viruses cause disease outside the United States; however, imported cases occur as a result of travel to and from tropical areas. Classic dengue, also called *breakbone fever*, has flulike symptoms, with severe pains in muscles and joints, lymphadenopathy, leukopenia, and maculopapular rash. The incubation period is 5 to 11 days, and the illness lasts about 7 days but relapses. It is estimated that there are 100 million cases of dengue fever annually.

Dengue hemorrhagic syndrome is the result of infection with a serotype of dengue virus after an initial infection by a different serotype. It starts abruptly, with a fever of 40°C, anorexia, vomiting, petechiae, and enlarged liver lasting 5 to 10 days. Recovery ensues in most cases. Occasionally, this second infection leads to dengue shock syndrome, resulting from the increase in vascular permeability.

Yellow fever starts with a sudden headache and fever, accompanied by nausea, vomiting, and myalgia. Jaundice is caused by the involvement of the liver. Gastrointestinal hemorrhage (hematemesis or "black vomit") may occur. The mortality rate during epidemics is as high as 50%.

Pathogenesis and epidemiology

Flaviviruses are cytolytic and establish systemic infection. Monocytes and macrophages are the primary targets of flaviviruses. Flavivirus infection is enhanced up to 1,000-fold by non-neutralizing antibody that binds to the Fc receptors on these cells and facilitates cellular uptake. The double-stranded RNA replicative intermediate produced during the replication of flaviviruses induces interferon-α and interferon-β, which limit the replication of the viruses. However, interferons also stimulate the immune system, with the induction of flulike symptoms.

SLEV and WNV are transmitted to humans via infected mosquitos, primarily the *Culex* species. Infection with SLEV is thought to provide lifelong immunity against re-infection. In the United States, an average of 102 cases have been reported to the Centers for Disease Control and Prevention annually, and the range has been between 2 and 1,967. The geographic range of the virus extends from Canada to Argentina. However, most cases are seen in the United States.

The first WNV cases in the United States were seen in 1999 in the New York City area. In 2002, the virus had spread to Colorado, and there were 4,000 cases and 274 deaths. By 2003, the virus had spread to California, with a total of 7,700 cases and 166 deaths.

Dengue hemorrhagic syndrome occurs as a result of the production of large amounts of cross-reacting antibodies when a second infection with another serotype occurs. There are two possible mechanisms for the ensuing events: *(1)* Non-neutralizing antibodies mediate uptake into monocytes and macrophages, which then activate memory T cells. Large amounts of cytokines are released. *(2)* The virus-antibody immune complexes activate the complement system, causing increased vascular permeability and thrombocytopenia. The vasculature may rupture, causing internal bleeding, loss of plasma, and shock. There are about 500,000 cases of dengue hemorrhagic syndrome a year, mostly in South Asia, and the fatality rate is about 10%. Dengue virus and its vector are found in parts of South America, and cases have been seen in Texas, Florida, and Puerto Rico.

Yellow fever is caused by yellow fever virus infections, which cause liver, kidney, and heart degeneration and upper gastrointestinal tract hemorrhage. It occurs primarily in the tropical areas of South America and Africa.

Japanese encephalitis virus has caused epidemics of encephalitis in India, Korea, China, Southeast Asia, and Indonesia, mostly affecting children and with a fatality rate of 20%.

Preliminary diagnosis of arboviral infections is often based on the patient's clinical presentation, the places and dates of travel, and the epidemiologic history of the place where infection occurred. Specific viruses are usually diagnosed by testing the serum or cerebrospinal fluid for virus-specific immunoglobulin M and neutralizing antibodies.

Treatment and prevention

There is a live vaccine against yellow fever that was developed in the 1930s. Live and inactivated viral vaccines against Japanese encephalitis virus are available. Mosquito bites should be prevented by insect repellent containing DEET, picaridin, IR3535, or oil of lemon eucalyptus on skin and clothing. Permethrin can be used on clothing to protect against mosquitos even through several washes. In severe cases, patients need to be hospitalized to receive supportive treatment, including intravenous fluids, pain medication, and nursing care.

Bunyaviruses

The family Bunyaviridae includes the genera *Orthobunyavirus* (La Crosse encephalitis virus), *Phlebovirus* (Rift Valley fever virus), *Hantavirus* (Sin Nombre virus), *Tospovirus*, and *Nairovirus* (Crimean-Congo hemorrhagic fever virus). The family comprises over 300 species, making it the largest family of viruses.

Bunyaviruses are enveloped, negative-strand RNA viruses. Some bunyaviruses have icosahedral symmetry, some have locally ordered capsids, and others have no detectable symmetry. They enter cells via coated-pit endocytosis or phagocytosis and undergo fusion with the endosome membrane at acidic pH. The genome is segmented, with the large (L) RNA encoding the RNA-dependent-RNA polymerase, which is thought to be cleaved from a polyprotein also encoded by the L RNA. The medium (M) RNA encodes two envelope glycoproteins, and the small (S) RNA encodes a nucleocapsid protein. The virus assembles by budding through Golgi vesicles, disrupting the Golgi structure in the process, and is transported to the plasma membrane.

La Crosse encephalitis virus (LCEV) is transmitted via the *Aedes triseriatus* mosquito. Initial viremia may cause flulike symptoms. It causes encephalitis by neuronal and glial damage, as well as cerebral edema. Approximately 80 to 100 neuroinvasive cases of LCEV are reported each year. LCE presents with fever lasting 2 to 3 days, headache, fatigue, lethargy, nausea, and vomiting. Seizures during the acute illness are common, but the infection is fatal in less than 1% of cases. In some cases, there are neurologic sequelae of varying duration, including recurrent seizures, hemiparesis, and cognitive and neurobehavioral abnormalities.

Hepatic necrosis can occur in Rift Valley fever infections. In Crimean hemorrhagic fever and *Hantavirus* infections, the primary lesion is leakage of plasma and erythrocytes through the vascular endothelium.

Hantaviruses are not arboviruses but are discussed here as members of Bunyaviridae. They are transmitted via contact with aerosols of infected rodent urine. Hantaan virus was first detected in 1951 in soldiers during the Korean war. This virus causes hemorrhagic fever with renal syndrome in Japan, Korea, and China. Puumala virus causes a similar condition in Scandinavia. Sin Nombre virus causes hantavirus pulmonary syndrome and is transmitted from deer mice. It was first encountered in May 1993 in the Southwestern United States and has also caused disease elsewhere in the United States, Canada, and South America. It was identified by RT-PCR amplification of samples from the lungs and livers of the victims using primers corresponding to sequences in other hantaviruses.

Bibliography

Atkins GJ. The pathogenesis of alphaviruses. ISRN Virology 2013: 861912.

Centers for Disease Control and Prevention. Eastern Equine Encephalitis. www.cdc.gov/EasternEquineEncephalitis/tech/virus.html. Accessed 31 July 2015.

Centers for Disease Control and Prevention. La Crosse Encephalitis. www.cdc.gov/lac/. Accessed 31 July 2015.

Centers for Disease Control and Prevention. Public Health Image Library. phil.cdc.gov. Accessed 4 August 2015.

Centers for Disease Control and Prevention. Saint Louis Encephalitis. www.cdc.gov/sle/. Accessed 31 July 2015.

Centers for Disease Control and Prevention. West Nile virus. www.cdc.gov/westnile. Accessed 31 July 2015.

Greenwood D, Barer M, Slack R, Irving W. Medical Microbiology, ed 18. Edinburgh: Churchill Livingstone/Elsevier, 2012.

Guu TS, Zheng W, Tao YJ. Bunyavirus: Structure and replication. Adv Exp Med Biol 2012;726:245–266.

Levinson W. Review of Medical Microbiology and Immunology, ed 11. New York: McGraw-Hill, 2010.

Murray PR, Rosenthal KS, Pfaller MA. Medical Microbiology, ed 7. Philadelphia: Mosby/Elsevier, 2013.

Ryan KJ, Ray CG. Sherris Medical Microbiology, ed 5. New York: McGraw-Hill, 2010.

Vogel P, Kell WM, Fritz DL, Parker MD, Schoepp RJ. Early events in the pathogenesis of eastern equine encephalitis virus in mice. Am J Pathol 2005;166:159–171.

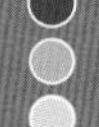

Take-Home Messages

- Certain alphaviruses, flaviviruses, and bunyaviruses are grouped together as arthropod-borne viruses (or arboviruses).
- Alphaviruses cause a flulike syndrome and encephalitis.
- If EEEV crosses the blood-brain barrier, it causes severe encephalitis that kills 50% to 75% of infected humans and causes serious neurologic sequelae in survivors.
- SLEV, WNV, and Japanese encephalitis virus are in the family Flaviviridae.
- West Nile fever is seen in about 20% of infected people and is characterized by fever, vomiting, diarrhea, headache, and body aches, sometimes with a skin rash and swollen lymph glands.
- Classic dengue presents with flulike symptoms, including severe muscle and joint pain, lymphadenopathy, leukopenia, and maculopapular rash.
- Dengue hemorrhagic syndrome is seen following infection with a serotype of dengue virus after an initial infection by a different serotype.
- The syndromes of yellow fever include sudden headache and fever, nausea, vomiting, myalgia, jaundice, and gastrointestinal hemorrhage.
- Bunyaviruses are enveloped, negative-strand RNA viruses and include LCEV and Rift Valley fever virus. Sin Nombre virus is a *Hantavirus* and is not transmitted by arthopods; it causes hantavirus pulmonary syndrome.

Rhabdoviruses, Poxviruses, and Coronaviruses

38

Rabies virus was first described in Mesopotamia in 2300 BC, and it causes fatal disease in humans and animals unless the host is vaccinated. Evidence for smallpox infections was found in Egyptian mummies dating back 3,000 years. In the 20th century, smallpox caused hundreds of millions of deaths. Coronaviruses are one of the causes of the common cold, but an emerging strain caused severe disease in 2003.

Rhabdoviruses

The name Rhabdovirus is derived from the word *rhabdos*, meaning "rod" in Greek. The Rhabdoviridae family includes the genera *Vesiculovirus*, which infects cattle, horses, and pigs, and *Lyssavirus* (derived from the Greek word for "frenzy"), which includes rabies virus. Other Lyssaviruses include Lagos bat virus, Mokola virus, Duvenhage virus, European bat lyssavirus types 1 and 2, Australian bat lyssavirus, and West Caucasian bat virus.

Structure and replication

The Rhabdoviruses are bullet-shaped, enveloped, negative-strand RNA viruses with a diameter of 50 to 95 nm and a length of 130 to 380 nm (Fig 38-1). They encode only five proteins: nucleoprotein (N), phosphoprotein (P), matrix protein (M), membrane glycoprotein (G), and polymerase (L). The exact mechanism of cellular tropism of rabies virus and other lyssaviruses is not known. The nicotinic acetylcholine receptor, the p75 nerve growth factor receptor, and the neural cell adhesion molecule may facilitate entry into neurons. However, these viruses infect many other types of cells, which must have other receptors. The G protein of vesicular stomatitis virus has been used to produce pseudotype viruses that encapsulate the human immunodeficiency virus (HIV) genome to introduce the HIV genome into different types of cells. The N protein protects the RNA from ribonuclease digestion.

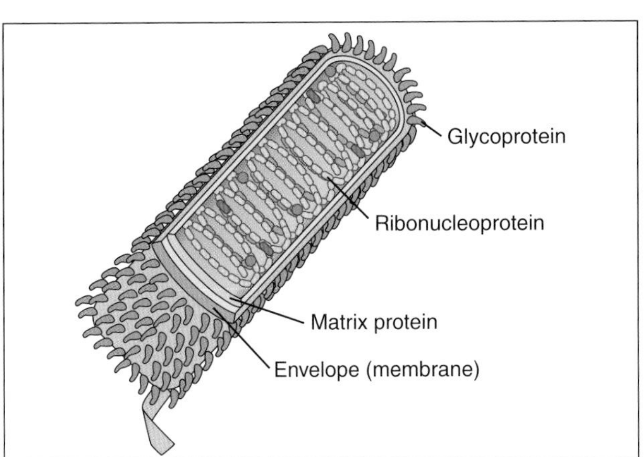

Fig 38-1 Schematic diagram of rabies virus. (Adapted from Public Health Image Library image 970, courtesy of the Centers for Disease Control and Prevention.)

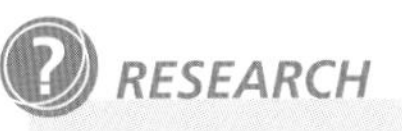

RESEARCH

How can one determine the cellular receptors for a virus?

Rabies virus is endocytosed, and the G protein mediates the fusion of the viral membrane with the endosome membrane upon acidification of the endosome lumen by an H^+-adenosine triphosphatase. The nucleocapsid is released into the cytoplasm.

Viral RNA-dependent RNA polymerase transcribes the viral RNA into five mRNAs, which are then translated into the viral proteins. New viral genomes are generated via a positive-strand RNA template. Newly synthesized G protein is transported to the cell membrane. The M protein surrounds the newly synthesized ribonucleoprotein and associates with the G protein in the plasma membrane, and the virus buds off.

Clinical syndromes and diagnosis

Infection by rabies virus, for example through a bite by a rabid animal, is followed by a highly variable incubation period of 10 days to 1 year, with an average of 20 to 90 days. During the ensuing prodrome phase of 2 to 10 days, malaise, headache, nausea, vomiting, fever, upper respiratory distress, insomnia, and pain and itching at the site of the bite are observed. Virus is detected in the central nervous system. The next phase is the acute neurologic phase, which lasts 2 to 7 days and presents as hyperactivity, disorientation, hallucination, hydrophobia (resulting from the pain experienced when trying to swallow water), convulsions, and lethargy. The patient then goes into a coma, with respiratory arrest, hypotension, and cardiac arrest.

The preferred methods of diagnosis are *(1)* detection of viral antigens by direct immunofluorescence and *(2)* detection of the viral genome by the reverse transcription polymerase chain reaction. Samples can be obtained from saliva, serum, and spinal fluid. Viral infection of neuronal tissue in 70% to 90% of cases results in the formation of cytoplasmic inclusions containing aggregates of viral nucleocapsids called *Negri bodies*.

Pathogenesis and epidemiology

Rabies-infected animals secrete the virus in their saliva, and the virus is usually transmitted from the bite of the animal. However, the virus can also be transmitted via the inhalation of aerosolized virus generated, for example, by bats in caves and via intact mucosal membranes. The virus replicates in muscle tissue at the site of infection for days to months, then moves on to the central nervous system and travels to the dorsal root ganglia and the spinal cord by retrograde axoplasmic transport. The virus progresses to the brain (the hippocampus, cerebral cortex, and cerebellum), from which it descends to the salivary glands, eyes, adrenal medulla, and other tissues. Infection of the central nervous system results in encephalitis, with infiltration of lymphocytes and plasma cells, and neuronal degeneration. The incubation period for rabies virus depends on the amount of viral inoculum, the amount of affected tissue, the innervation of the site, and the distance between the site of infection and the central nervous system.

Neutralizing antibodies appear after the onset of clinical disease. The virus is most likely hidden from the immune response. Post-exposure immunization most likely prevents the spread of the virus from the infected muscle tissue to the nervous system.

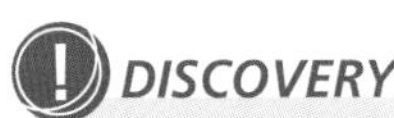

DISCOVERY

Louis Pasteur noted in the late 1800s that rabies had a long incubation period before the onset of disease, and he hypothesized that vaccination soon after infection might prevent the disease. In 1885, a 9-year-old boy named Joseph Meister was bitten severely by a rabid dog and was brought to Pasteur with the hope of preventing disease. Pasteur had not used the vaccine successfully on a human. At the time, the idea of using attenuated viruses and bacteria as vaccines was very new. Thus, injecting a person with even an attenuated disease agent was controversial. Moreover, Pasteur was not a medical doctor and might have faced serious consequences. Pasteur was certain that the boy would die from rabies if nothing was done. Therefore, he began a course of 13 injections of a "vaccine" made from the dried spinal cord of an infected rabbit. Meister did not develop rabies, and the treatment was considered a success. Many years later, Meister worked as caretaker of Pasteur's tomb at the Pasteur Institute in Paris.

It is estimated that there are 70,000 deaths per year from rabies in the world. Most of the cases are the result of dog bites, especially in India and Latin America. In the United States, more cats than dogs were reported to have rabies in the years 2000 to 2004. Most of these cases were "spillover infections" from raccoons in the eastern United States. Different strains of the virus have been identified in raccoons, skunks, foxes, and coyotes. Several species of insectivorous bats are reservoirs for certain strains of rabies virus. In Western Europe, badgers and foxes are also major carriers of rabies. According to the World Health Organization (WHO), about 10 million people receive treatment every year after exposure to animals suspected of carrying the rabies virus.

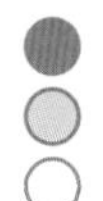

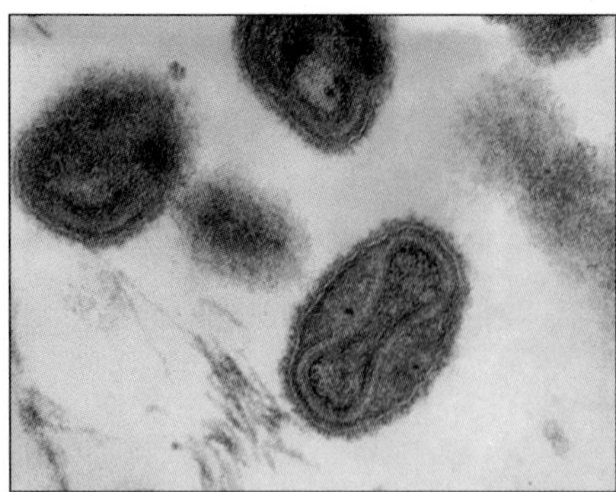

Fig 38-2 Electron micrograph of smallpox virus. (Public Health Image Library image 1849, courtesy of Dr Fred Murphy and Sylvia Whitfield.)

Treatment and prevention

The wound of the infectious bite should be cleaned right away with soap and water or a substance that is known to inactivate the virus (such as povidine-iodine). Antirabies serum may also be placed around the wound, as recommended by the WHO. Post-exposure prophylaxis is essential to prevent the onset of rabies. Around 20,000 people a year receive the rabies vaccine in the United States. Individuals exposed to the saliva of an infected animal by a bite or via an open wound or mucous membrane should receive the vaccine. The bites of bats may be inconspicuous, and anyone exposed to a bat even without an obvious bite wound, for example while sleeping, should undergo post-exposure prophylaxis. This includes the administration of both human rabies immune globulin (passive immunity) and the vaccine (active immunity).

The currently used vaccines are the human diploid cell vaccine and the purified chick embryo cell vaccine. Independent of the interval between exposure and beginning of treatment, the following regimen is recommended for any kind of exposure. Individuals who have been vaccinated previously or are receiving pre-exposure vaccination for rabies should receive only the vaccine. The schedule of intramuscular administration of the human diploid cell vaccine is on the day of exposure and then on days 3, 7, 14, and 28. No changes should be made to the recommended schedule of administration of the vaccine.

Poxviruses

The family Poxviridae includes the subfamily Chordopoxvirinae, which includes the genera *Orthopoxvirus*, *Parapoxvirus*, *Molluscipoxvirus*, and *Yatapoxvirus*, all of which can infect humans. Variola (smallpox), vaccinia, cowpox, and monkeypox viruses are classified under the *Orthopoxvirus* genus. Variola virus has two variants: variola major and variola minor. Bovine papular stomatitis, Orf, and pseudocowpox viruses are included in the genus *Parapoxvirus*.

Structure and replication

Smallpox is in the shape of an ellipsoid, with the small "diameter" about 200 nm and the oblong "diameter" in the range of 240 to 300 nm (Fig 38-2). The DNA genome is packaged within an hourglass- or dumbbell-shaped core membrane. Next to the core are the lateral bodies that contain viral DNA-dependent RNA polymerase and transcription factors that enable the virus to replicate entirely in the cytoplasm. These structures are wrapped inside a protein shell, termed the *outer membrane*. The newly synthesized virus is assembled in inclusion bodies and released primarily by cell disruption. Some virions are wrapped in Golgi-derived membranes and are released "naturally," without causing cell disruption. During biosynthesis, the virus causes the irreversible inactivation of host cell RNA molecules, leading to cytotoxicity.

Clinical syndromes and diagnosis

Of the two clinical forms of smallpox, variola major is more common and more severe, with higher fever and extensive rash. It has an overall fatality rate of about 30%. Variola minor is less common and much less severe, with a death rate of 1% or less.

At the end of an incubation period of 7 to 17 days, high fever, malaise, head and body aches, and sometimes vomiting are observed. This prodrome phase may last for 2 to 4 days. In the early rash period (about 4 days), a rash appears as small red spots on the tongue and in the mouth. The spots become sores that spread large quantities of virus into the mouth and throat, rendering the patient most contagious. A rash appears on the face and spreads to the arms, legs, hands, and feet. At this point, the fever subsides. The rash becomes raised bumps by the third day of appearance.

The bumps fill with a thick fluid on the fourth day and display a depression in the center. At this point, fever rises again and stays elevated until the lesions are covered with scabs. The bumps become pustules, which then begin to form a crust and scab. By the end of the second week after the rash appears, most of the sores have scabbed over. By about the 20th day after the onset of the rash, the scabs fall off; when all the scabs are cleared, the patient is no longer contagious. The lesions leave scars, which are most evident on the face, and arise from the destruction of sebaceous glands followed by shrinking of granulation tissue and fibrosis.

Diagnosis can be confirmed by growing the virus in cell culture and by detecting viral antigens in samples from vesicles by immunofluorescence.

Pathogenesis and epidemiology

Smallpox virus is transmitted via inhalation and initially replicates in the upper respiratory tract. It spreads via the lymphatics and by viremia to internal and dermal tissues. It also replicates in the spleen, bone marrow, and lymph nodes. The virus has mechanisms to inhibit the interferon, complement, and other immune responses. Death, which usually occurs in the second week of disease, is most likely caused by circulating immune complexes and soluble variola antigens.

The spread of smallpox from one person to another requires direct and prolonged face-to-face contact. Smallpox can also be transmitted by direct contact with infected bodily fluids or contaminated objects. Humans are the only natural hosts of smallpox virus.

Smallpox was probably first used as a biologic weapon during the French and Indian Wars by British soldiers in North America. Soldiers distributed blankets that had been used by smallpox patients with the intent of initiating outbreaks among American Indians. Concerns have arisen in recent years about the possibility of the use of smallpox as a biologic weapon.

The last case of smallpox in the United States occurred in 1949. The WHO campaign to eradicate smallpox worldwide began in 1967. The last case in the world was in Somalia in 1977. Routine vaccination against smallpox was stopped after this.

Treatment and prevention

There is no specific treatment for smallpox. However, potential treatments being investigated as bioterrorism countermeasures are cidofovir, HPMPA, Cyclo HPMPC, ribavirin, tiazofurin, carboxylic 3-deazaadenosine, and tecovirimat. Before 1972, smallpox vaccination was recommended for all US children at age 1 year. Individuals vaccinated once may not have lifelong immunity. Those vaccinated at birth and at ages 8 and 18 years have maintained stable antibody levels for 30 years.

The ACAM2000 smallpox vaccine (Sanofi Pasteur) is a live vaccinia virus vaccine licensed in the United States by the Food and Drug Administration for active immunization for persons determined to be at high risk for smallpox infection, for example, first responders in case of a bioterrorism attack. An exposed individual can be immunized up to 4 days following exposure and be protected. ACAM2000 is the majority of the US government's smallpox vaccine stockpile; there are more than 196 million doses of the vaccine in the Strategic National Stockpile.

Molluscum contagiosum

Molluscum contagiosum virus produces nodular, wartlike skin lesions. It is transmitted by sexual contact, wrestling, or fomites. The lesions disappear within 2 to 12 months. They may be removed surgically. Histologic examination of the lesions indicates hyperplasia, ballooning degeneration, thickening of the skin, and eosinophilic inclusions called *molluscum bodies*.

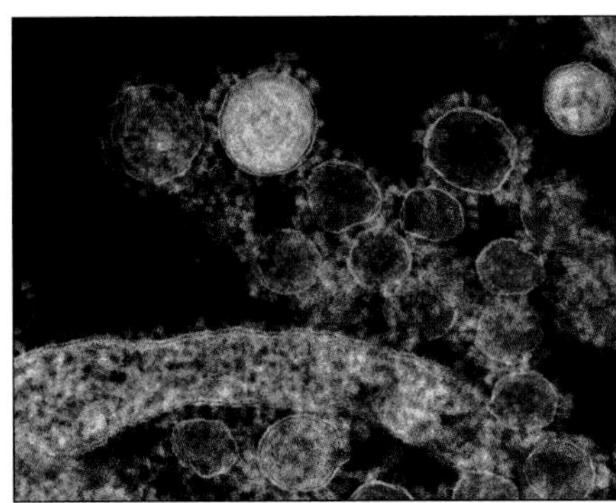

Fig 38-3 Digitally colorized transmission electron micrograph of Middle East respiratory syndrome coronavirus. (Public Health Image Library image 18111, courtesy of the National Institute of Allergy and Infectious Diseases.)

Vaccinia

Vaccinia virus is derived from the cowpox virus originally used by Edward Jenner in the 1790s. It is used as a vaccine and has been instrumental in the eradication of smallpox. However, in some cases it may cause complications, including encephalitis, eczema vaccinatum, myocarditis and pericarditis, and progressive infection, especially in immunocompromised individuals. Vaccinia virus can be used as an expression vector for the production of live recombinant vaccines, including vaccines against HIV and a vaccinia–rabies G protein vaccine left on bait food to vaccinate raccoons, foxes, and other mammals.

Coronaviruses

In early 2003, a highly infectious disease called severe acute respiratory syndrome (SARS) appeared in Southeast Asia and infected 8,421 people worldwide and caused 784 deaths. The etiologic agent was identified as a coronavirus that was different from the previously known human coronaviruses OC43 and 299E. Blood samples from SARS patients had antibody that reacted with cells infected with the suspected SARS coronavirus virus. The sequence of the SARS-associated coronavirus was determined within 3 months of the outbreak of the epidemic. Identical sequences of the virus were found in 12 patients from different locations. This observation is consistent with a point-source outbreak.

The virus-specific serologic response can be detected by indirect immunofluorescence and enzyme-linked immunosorbent assay (ELISA).

A new coronavirus called Middle East respiratory syndrome coronavirus emerged in Saudi Arabia in 2012 (Fig 38-3). It has caused severe illness and death in people from several countries.

Coronaviruses are named for the solar corona-like surface projections of the virions (see Fig 38-3). The nucleocapsid consists of a positive-strand RNA and the nucleocapsid protein. The viral membrane is derived from intracellular membranes and contains the glycoprotein S, with S1 and S2 subunits. The tropism of coronavirus is determined by the interaction of S1 with the cell surface receptor; this leads to a conformational change in the S2 that exposes the fusion peptide, which then inserts into the cell membrane. Coronaviruses are different from orthomyxoviruses and paramyxoviruses in that they do not have a negative-strand genomic RNA and have a different mechanism of replication. The genome is translated to produce an RNA-dependent RNA polymerase (L), which transcribes the genomic RNA into a negative-sense template RNA. The L protein then produces the positive-sense genomic RNA and five to seven mRNAs that encode the different viral proteins. These individual mRNAs may recombine during viral assembly to produce new strains. The genome associates with the rough endoplasmic reticulum modified by viral proteins and buds into the lumen. Viral particles inside vesicles are released by exocytosis. Coronavirus infection induces a reticulovesicular network of modified membranes thought to be the site of virus replication.

Coronaviruses infect the epithelial cells of the upper respiratory tract and replicate best at 33°C to 35°C. It is spread via aerosols and large droplets. The incubation period is 3 days. The infection may exacerbate a preexisting chronic pulmonary disease, such as asthma or bronchitis, and may lead to pneumonia.

Coronaviruses cause 10% to 15% of upper respiratory tract infections and pneumonias. They are the second most common cause of the "common cold." They are also linked to gastroenteritis.

The control of transmission of coronaviruses is difficult. No specific antiviral therapy is available, nor a vaccine. Reinfection can occur despite the presence of serum antibodies.

Bibliography

Albertini AAV, Baquero E, Ferlin A, Gaudin Y. Molecular and cellular aspects of rhabdovirus entry. Viruses 2012;4:117–139.

Centers for Disease Control and Prevention. Public Health Image Library. phil.cdc.gov. Accessed 4 August 2015.

Centers for Disease Control and Prevention. Rabies. www.cdc.gov/-rabies/symptoms/index.html. Accessed 3 August 2015.

Centers for Disease Control and Prevention. Smallpox Disease Overview. www.bt.cdc.gov/agent/smallpox/overview/disease-facts.asp. Accessed 3 August 2015.

The College of Physicians of Philadelphia. The History of Vaccines. www.historyofvaccines.org/content/timelines/pasteur. Accessed 3 August 2015.

Fung TS, Liu DX. Coronavirus infection, ER stress, apoptosis and innate immunity. Front Microbiol 2014;5:296.

Greenwood D, Barer M, Slack R, Irving W. Medical Microbiology, ed 18. Edinburgh: Churchill Livingstone/Elsevier, 2012.

Levinson W. Review of Medical Microbiology and Immunology, ed 11. New York: McGraw-Hill, 2010.

Murray PR, Rosenthal KS, Pfaller MA. Medical Microbiology, ed 7. Philadelphia: Mosby/Elsevier, 2013.

Perlman S, Netland J. Coronaviruses post-SARS: Update on replication and pathogenesis. Nat Rev Microbiol 2009;7:439–450.

Ryan KJ, Ray CG. Sherris Medical Microbiology, ed 5. New York: McGraw-Hill, 2010.

Take-Home Messages

- Rhabdoviruses are bullet-shaped, enveloped, negative-strand RNA viruses.
- The rabies virus is usually transmitted from the bite of an infected animal. It can also be transmitted through the inhalation of aerosolized virus generated by bats in caves and via intact mucosal membranes.
- Post-exposure prophylaxis is essential to prevent the onset of rabies. Around 20,000 people a year receive the rabies vaccine in the United States.
- Smallpox, an enveloped DNA virus, is one of the largest and most complex viruses.
- Of the two clinical forms of smallpox, variola major is more common and more severe, with higher fever and extensive rash.
- Coronaviruses are enveloped, positive-strand RNA viruses named for the solar corona-like surface projections of the virions.
- Coronaviruses are the second most common cause of the "common cold."
- A coronavirus strain that emerged in 2003 caused severe acute respiratory syndrome (SARS).

Rubella Virus, Filoviruses, Reoviruses, and Noroviruses

39

Rubella virus is an alphavirus, but unlike other alphaviruses, it is not an arthropod-borne virus. Filoviruses include the deadly Ebola and Marburg viruses. The name reovirus is based on the first letters of respiratory, enteric, and orphan viruses and was coined by Albert Sabin, who is best known for having developed the live attenuated polio vaccine. Reoviruses include orthoreoviruses, orbivirus, coltivirus, and rotaviruses. Noroviruses were previously termed Norwalk-like viruses and belong to the Caliciviridae family.

Rubella Virus

Rubella ("little red") virus is a respiratory togavirus that causes German measles. It is the only member of the genus *Rubivirus*. It has a positive-strand RNA genome and a nucleocapsid that are surrounded by an envelope (Fig 39-1). The virus is 60 to 70 nm in diameter and is pleomorphic. The virus encodes an RNA-dependent RNA polymerase that mediates the replication of the RNA genome. Replication and assembly take place in the cytoplasm, and the virus buds from the plasma membrane.

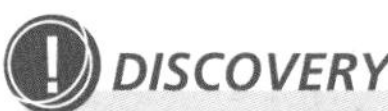

Two German physicians in the middle of the 18th century described a disease now known as *rubella* or *German measles*. Because it is a mild disease with few complications, little attention was paid to it until 1941. The Australian ophthalmologist Sir Norman Gregg discovered the connection between congenital abnormalities in the infant, such as congenital cataracts, and maternal rubella infection during pregnancy.

The virus is transmitted via respiratory droplets and transplacentally in pregnant women. The incubation period for rubella is 12 to 21 days. The virus may be shed in the pharynx for about a week before and after the characteristic rash. Symptoms of infection include a macular rash that starts on the face and progresses to the extremities, malaise, fever, and lymphadenopathy. Arthralgia is not common in children

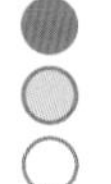

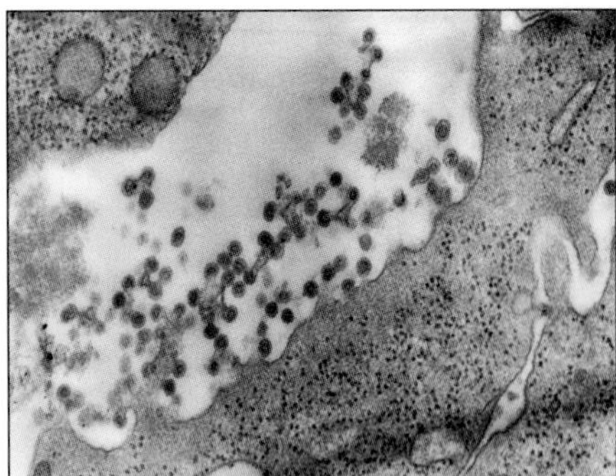

Fig 39-1 Rubella virus budding from an infected cell. (Public Health Image Library image 10221, courtesy of Dr Fred Murphy and Sylvia Whitfield.)

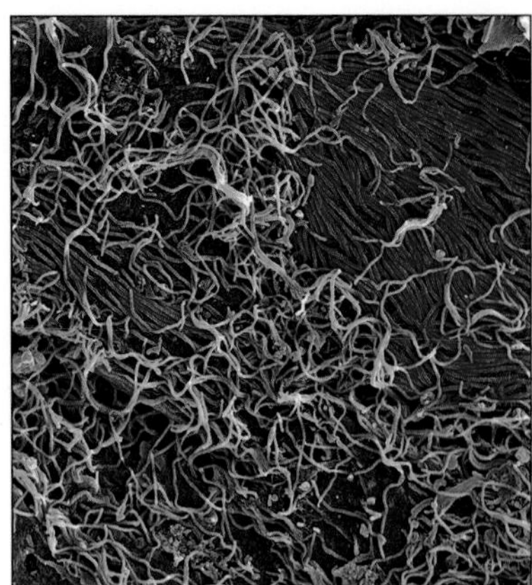

Fig 39-2 Digitally colored scanning electron micrograph of filamentous Ebola virions budding from a chronically infected Vero cell. (Public Health Image Library image 17779, courtesy of the National Institute of Allergy and Infectious Diseases.)

but may be seen in a majority of adults. More severe adult forms of rubella are caused by immunopathology. In rare cases, postinfectious encephalitis can occur, but recovery is usually complete. Natural infection confers lifelong immunity.

Maternal rubella infections can cause congenital cataracts, heart defects, deafness, improper development, and intellectual disability and is termed congenital rubella syndrome.

Infection with rubella virus can be diagnosed by its ability to interfere with echovirus cytopathology in cell culture. A rise in antibody titer from the acute phase to the convalescent phase (detected by hemagglutination inhibition or enzyme-linked immunosorbent assay [ELISA]), or the presence of immunoglobulin M (IgM) in an acute-phase serum sample, indicates a positive diagnosis. In pregnant women, the presence of IgM antibody indicates a recent infection. An IgG titer at or greater than 1:8 indicates immunity and that the fetus will be protected.

Rubella can be prevented by a live attenuated vaccine that is part of the MMR vaccine. It is first administered at 15 months of age and then again at 4 to 6 years.

Filoviruses

Filoviruses include Marburg and Ebola viruses. They are filamentous, enveloped, negative-strand RNA viruses about 80 nm in diameter and 800 to 14,000 nm in length (Fig 39-2). The Ebola virus glycoprotein causes cytotoxicity to vascular endothelial cells. Its receptor appears to be the Niemann-Pick C1 protein. It replicates in the cytoplasm.

Filoviruses cause severe or fatal hemorrhagic fevers, edema, and hypovolemic shock. The viruses cause tissue necrosis in parenchymal cells of the liver, spleen, lymph nodes, and lungs.

The *ebolavirus* species was discovered in 1976, near the Ebola River, in a region currently part of the Democratic Republic of the Congo. There are five subspecies of *Ebolavirus*: *(1)* Ebola virus or *Zaire ebolavirus*, *(2)* Sudan virus or *Sudan ebolavirus*, *(3)* Taï Forest virus or *Taï Forest ebolavirus*, *(4)* Bundibugyo virus or *Bundibugyo ebolavirus*, and *(5)* Reston virus or *Reston ebolavirus*. The first four of these subspecies have caused disease in humans. The fifth has caused disease only in nonhuman primates.

The illness begins with flulike symptoms, and within a few days, nausea, vomiting, and diarrhea ensue. Then hemorrhage begins, which can result in death in as many as 90% of patients with clinically evident disease.

Ebola virus has caused epidemics in the Democratic Republic of the Congo (formerly Zaire), Gabon, and the Sudan. The most recent and severe outbreak occurred in Guinea, Sierra Leone, and Liberia in 2014. In Guinea by July 2014, there were 460 suspected and confirmed cases of Ebola virus disease, including 339 fatalities. By January 2015, there were 2,920 cases and 1,913 deaths. In Sierra Leone by July 2014, of the 533 suspected and confirmed cases, 233 resulted in death. These numbers increased to 10,561 cases and 3,216 deaths by January 2015. In Liberia, there were 329 suspected and confirmed Ebola cases and 156 deaths by July 2014, and by January 2015 there were 8,643 cases and 3,700 deaths. The virus has 97% homology to *Z ebolavirus*. The mechanisms of natural transmission are unknown. It may be endemic in bats and wild monkeys and can be spread to humans and between humans via infected blood or secretions.

Eighteen percent of the population in rural areas of central Africa have antibody to this virus, suggesting that subclinical infections result in antibody production without causing disease. In preclinical studies, successful *ebolavirus* vaccine candidates have been identified. Gene-based vaccines were shown to be immunogenic in human clinical trials.

When an outbreak occurs, it is important to quarantine the patients. Health care providers need to use extensive protective gear. Standard treatment for Ebola hemorrhagic fever consists of supportive therapy, involving *(1)* proper maintenance of the patient's fluids and electrolytes, *(2)* controlling the patient's oxygen availability and blood pressure, and *(3)* treating any secondary infections. Experimental therapeutics include monoclonal antibodies, hyperimmune serum, a nucleoside analog (BCX4430), recombinant human activated protein C, and interferon.

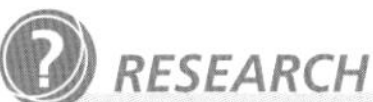

RESEARCH

What is the function of protein C?

Marburg hemorrhagic fever is a rare but severe disease that affects humans as well as nonhuman primates. It is caused by Marburg virus, which was first recognized in 1967, when outbreaks occurred in laboratories in Marburg, Frankfurt, and Belgrade. The source of the infection was traced to African green monkeys and their tissues used for research. The reservoir for Marburg virus is the African fruit bat, which does not show any symptoms. Marburg hemorrhagic fever has been reported in Uganda, Zimbabwe, the Democratic Republic of the Congo, Kenya, Angola, and South Africa, with many of the outbreaks starting with mine workers working in bat-infested mines.

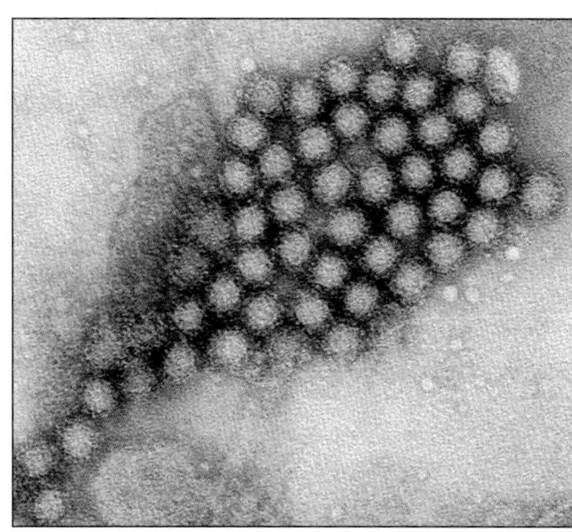

Fig 39-3 Digitally colored transmission electron micrograph of rotavirus. (Public Health Image Library image 178, courtesy of Dr Erskine Palmer.)

Reoviruses

Reoviruses have a double-layered protein capsid containing 10 to 12 double-stranded RNA segments. Reoviridae were first recovered from both respiratory secretions and feces but were not associated with a particular disease and were thus considered to be "orphan" viruses. Orthoreoviruses cause meningitis and encephalitis in mice, but they do not appear to cause disease in humans. Orbivirus is transmitted by ticks and mosquitos and can cause fever, rashes, leukopenia (in two-thirds of cases), and meningitis and encephalitis (in 3% to 7% of cases). Coltivirus is also transmitted by ticks and mosquitos and causes a febrile disease with gastroenteritis (in 20% of cases), rash (in 10%), and meningitis or encephalitis (in 3% to 7%).

Rotaviruses are the most common cause of serious diarrhea in young children. In developing countries, rotavirus diarrhea is a severe life-threatening disease. About 2 million children under 5 years old die from diarrheal diseases, and 40% of these deaths are caused by rotavirus. In industrial countries, 40% to 50% of hospitalizations due to diarrheal disease are the result of rotavirus infection. Rotaviruses are spread via the fecal-oral route. They can survive on hands, furniture, and toys. Rotavirus has seven different groups, from A to G. Rotavirus A causes the majority of infections in infants and young children. It may also cause disease in adults. Rotaviruses may be transmitted to humans from infected animals.

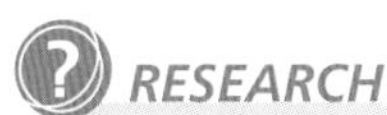

RESEARCH

What are the diseases caused by rotavirus B and rotavirus C?

The outer surface of rotavirus has 132 channels and 60 spikes, each composed of VP4 trimers (Fig 39-3). The viral diameter is 75 nm. It has 11 RNA segments. The virus attaches to host cell sialic acid and $\alpha2\beta1$ integrin via its VP4 protein. $\alpha2\beta1$ integrin, other integrins, and heat shock protein 70 act as post-binding receptors. The outer capsid is removed by proteolytic digestion when crossing the cell membrane, producing an intermediate infectious subviral particle, which still contains the RNA. The RNA is transcribed into mRNA by the RNA-dependent RNA polymerase of the virus, and the mRNA exits through channels in the viral capsid. The replication of the virus takes place in electron-dense structures called viroplasms near the nucleus and endoplasmic reticulum. The newly synthesized virions enter the endoplasmic reticulum, acquiring a transient membrane, which then carries the virus to the apical membrane of the infected enterocytes, where it is released into the gastrointestinal tract.

Rotavirus infects differentiated epithelial cells at the ends of intestinal villi. The virus causes cytotoxicity of the villi and mononuclear cell infiltrates in the lamina propia. Infection prevents the absorption of water and causes secretion of water and loss of ions in a watery diarrhea, resulting in severe dehydration. Supportive therapy to replace fluids is essential to restore the blood volume and electrolyte balance. A typical oral rehydration solution recommended by the World Health Organization contains 2.6 g/L NaCl, 1.5 g/L KCl, 2.9 g/L trisodium citrate, and 13.5 g/L anhydrous glucose. Rotavirus can be detected by electron microscopy and antigen detection assays, such as ELISA.

Two rotavirus vaccines are available: *(1)* RotaTeq (Merck) is a reassortant bovine rotavirus expressing the VP4 and VP7 of five different human rotaviruses. *(2)* RotaRix (GlaxoSmithKline) is a single-strain attenuated human rotavirus.

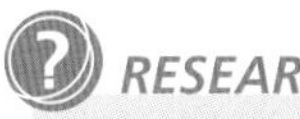

RESEARCH

How are attenuated rotavirus vaccines obtained in the laboratory?

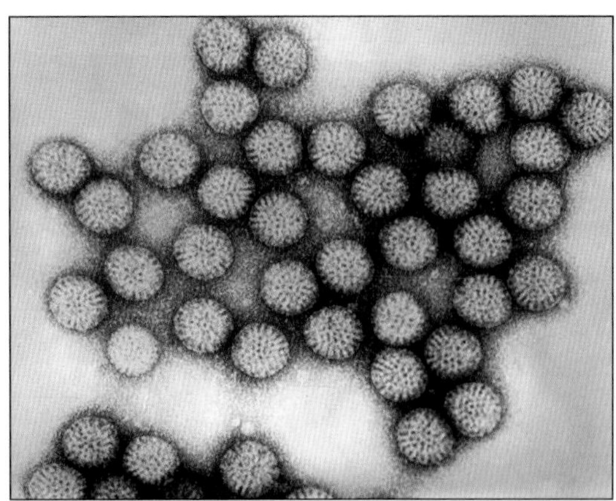

Fig 39-4 Transmission electron micrograph of norovirus. (Public Health Image Library image 10706, courtesy of Charles D. Humphrey, PhD.)

Noroviruses

Noroviruses are named after the original Norwalk strain, which was first identified in Norwalk, Ohio, in 1968. Noroviruses belong to the family Caliciviridae, which also includes sapoviruses. Both viruses cause acute gastroenteritis. Noroviruses have a positive-strand RNA genome and a naked capsid 27 nm in diameter (Fig 39-4). Only 18 virions are estimated to be able to initiate disease. They are resistant to heat (60°C), pH 3, and detergent. They damage the intestinal brush border.

Norovirus causes about 20 million cases of acute gastroenteritis in the United States, resulting in 400,000 emergency room visits, 1.7 to 1.9 million outpatient visits, 56,000 to 71,000 hospitalizations, and 570 to 800 deaths, mostly among young children and the elderly. There are six recognized norovirus genogroups, three of which (GI, GII, and GIV) affect humans. The symptoms of disease caused by norovirus are acute onset of vomiting, watery diarrhea with abdominal cramps, and nausea. In some cases, a low-grade fever, headaches, and myalgias may develop. The symptoms may last 24 to 72 hours. Complications include severe dehydration, especially in young children and older adults.

Norovirus is transmitted through close personal contact with an infected person, by touching contaminated surfaces, and through the consumption of contaminated water, shellfish, or salad. A careless infected food handler can spread the disease. Reverse transcription quantitative polymerase chain reaction (RT-QPCR) is used to detect viral RNA as well as to provide estimates of the viral load. Enzyme immunoassays may also be used to detect viral antigens, but their sensitivity is poor.

Bibliography

Centers for Disease Control and Prevention. 2014 Ebola Outbreak in West Africa: Case Counts. www.cdc.gov/vhf/ebola/outbreaks/2014-west-africa/case-counts.html. Accessed 3 August 2015.

Centers for Disease Control and Prevention. Ebola (Ebola Virus disease). www.cdc.gov/vhf/ebola/. Accessed 3 August 2015.

Centers for Disease Control and Prevention. Marburg hemorrhagic fever (Marburg HF). www.cdc.gov/vhf/marburg/. Accessed 3 August 2015.

Centers for Disease Control and Prevention. Norovirus. www.cdc.gov/norovirus. Accessed 3 August 2015.

Centers for Disease Control and Prevention. Public Health Image Library. phil.cdc.gov. Accessed 4 August 2015.

Fausther-Bovendo H, Mulangu S, Sullivan NJ. Ebolavirus vaccines for humans and apes. Curr Opin Virol 2012;2:324–329.

Gatherer D. The 2014 Ebola virus disease outbreak in West Africa. J Gen Virol 2014;95:1619–1624.

Greenwood D, Barer M, Slack R, Irving W. Medical Microbiology, ed 18. Edinburgh: Churchill Livingstone/Elsevier, 2012.

Levinson W. Review of Medical Microbiology and Immunology, ed 11. New York: McGraw-Hill, 2010.

Metcalf P, Cyrklaff M, Adrian M. The three-dimensional structure of reovirus obtained by cryo-electron microscopy. EMBO J 1991;10:3129–3136.

Murray PR, Rosenthal KS, Pfaller MA. Medical Microbiology, ed 7. Philadelphia: Mosby/Elsevier, 2013.

Ryan KJ, Ray CG. Sherris Medical Microbiology, ed 5. New York: McGraw-Hill, 2010.

Take-Home Messages

- Rubella ("little red") virus is a respiratory togavirus that causes German measles, characterized by a macular rash, malaise, fever, lymphadenopathy, and arthralgia in adults.
- Maternal rubella infections can cause congenital cataracts, heart defects, deafness, improper development, and intellectual disability.
- Filoviruses include Marburg and Ebola viruses, which are filamentous, enveloped, negative-strand RNA viruses.
- Filoviruses cause severe or fatal hemorrhagic fevers, edema, and hypovolemic shock.
- Rotaviruses are the most common cause of serious diarrhea in young children, especially in underdeveloped countries.
- Noroviruses are naked capsid, positive-strand RNA viruses.
- Norovirus causes about 20 million cases of acute gastroenteritis in the United States every year.

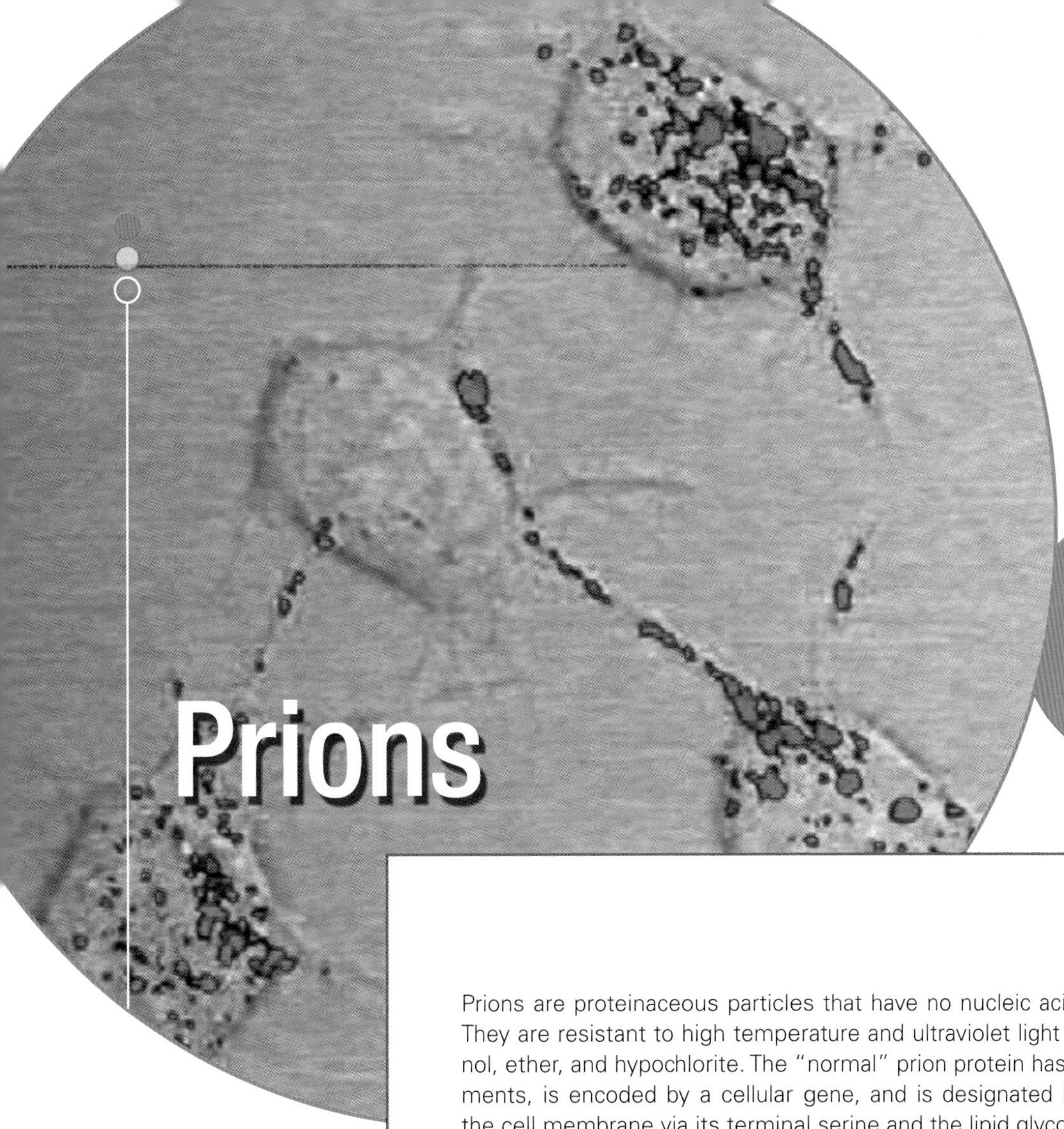

40

Prions

Prions are proteinaceous particles that have no nucleic acid associated with them. They are resistant to high temperature and ultraviolet light but are sensitive to phenol, ether, and hypochlorite. The "normal" prion protein has significant α-helical segments, is encoded by a cellular gene, and is designated PrP^{C}. PrP^{C} is attached to the cell membrane via its terminal serine and the lipid glycophosphatidylinositol. The protein can undergo a conformational change to a β-pleated sheet structure, for unknown reasons, and the modified protein can interact with the normal protein and alter its conformation to the modified one (Fig 40-1). The altered protein, called PrP^{Sc} for *scrapie-like prion protein*, forms filaments called *scrapie-associated fibrils* that are birefringent and cell free. The fibrils are morphologically and histochemically identical to amyloid, which is found in the brains of persons with diseases of the central nervous system (Fig 40-2).

RESEARCH

How does PrP^{Sc} become cell free, when PrP^{C} is membrane associated?

Because PrP^{Sc} has the same amino acid sequence as its normal counterpart, there is no immune response against the prion, although it is surprising that different conformational epitopes are not recognized by the immune system. No inflammatory response is seen in infected brain tissue.

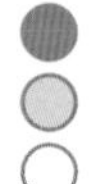

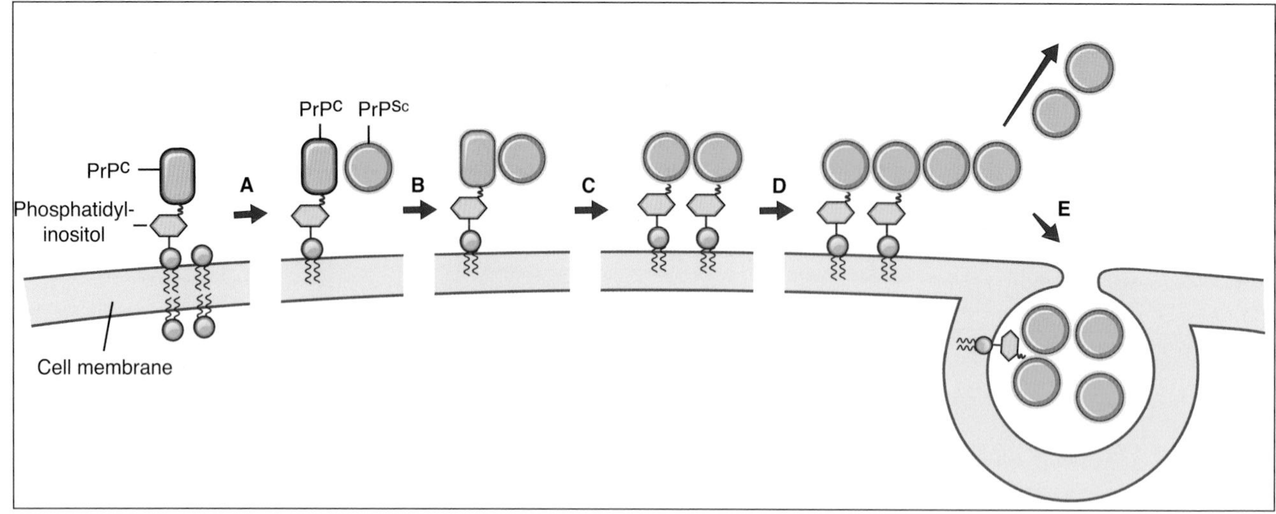

Fig 40-1 A model for the proliferation of prions. The normal PrP^C is anchored to the cell membrane by phosphatidylinositol. The scrapie prion, PrP^{Sc}, interacts with PrP^C on the cell surface (A), forcing the PrP^C to change its conformation to that of PrP^{Sc} (B). Newly synthesized PrP^C forms chains of PrP^{Sc} along the cell surface (C). Some of the PrP^{Sc} chains break off and initiate the PrP^C to PrP^{Sc} conversion on other cells (D). Some PrP^{Sc} proteins are internalized by neuronal cells (E).

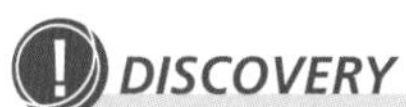

DISCOVERY

Stanley Prusiner was probably the first scientist to suspect that a protein, with no genetic material that allows it to replicate, could cause disease. The hypothesis was controversial, and many in the scientific community dismissed Prusiner's work as heretical. As one of his mentors explained, "Nobody believed in the existence of prions for many years, but with his dogged persistence and wonderful integrity he went on until he unlocked the cause of mad cow disease and the rest of the prion diseases." Prusiner started this work in 1972 when one of his patients died of Creutzfeldt-Jakob disease, a type of dementia. Previous researchers had shown that similar brain diseases, including kuru and scrapie, a disease affecting sheep, could be transmitted by injecting extracts of an infected brain into a host. Prusiner undertook research to identify the infective agent and in 1982 claimed that the agent was a single protein. He called the protein a *prion* (pronounced *pree-on*). These proteins are a natural component of human and animal brains. In their physiologic form, they do not cause problems. Prusiner found that prions sometimes change shape, become defective, and then interact with normal prions to change them into the defective form. This change results eventually in the death of entire regions of brain tissue as they accumulate the abnormal proteins. Prusiner also showed that prion diseases are transmitted from one species to another. Feeding cows the edible internal organs of sheep infected with the scrapie agent will transmit the disease.

Stanley Prusiner was awarded the Nobel Prize in Physiology or Medicine in 1997, citing the discovery of the prion, a rogue protein that is totally unlike anything else previously known to cause infectious disease.

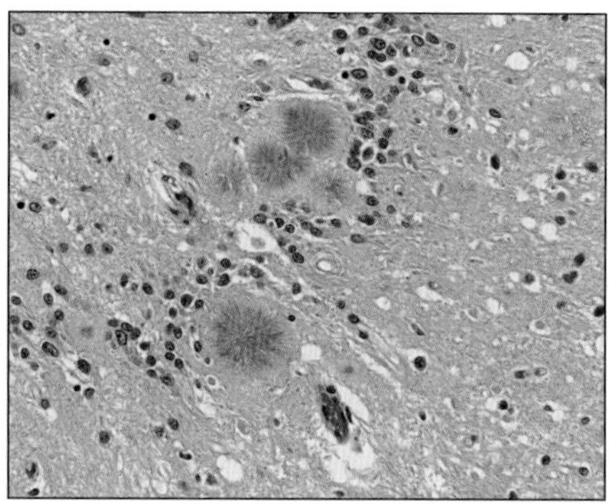

Fig 40-2 Amyloid plaques in the brain tissue of a patient with variant Creutzfeldt-Jakob disease. The plaques have a hyaline (transparent) eosinophilic core, with a peripheral margin of radiating fibrils, circumscribed by a pale halo. (Public Health Image Library image 10130, courtesy of Sherif Zaki, MD, and Wun-Ju Shieh, MD, PhD, MPH.)

Prions cause **transmissible spongiform encephalopathies**, which are characterized by the spongy holes seen in the brain parenchyma caused by neuronal death, without indicators of inflammation. The main human encephalopathies are kuru, Creutzfeldt-Jakob disease, variant Creutzfeldt-Jakob disease, Gerstmann-Sträussler-Scheinker syndrome, sporadic fatal insomnia, and fatal familial insomnia. The primary animal diseases are scrapie, bovine spongiform encephalopathy (also known as *mad cow disease*), transmissible mink encephalopathy, and chronic wasting disease seen in mule, deer, and elk.

In spongiform encephalopathies, PrP^{Sc} is taken up by neurons and phagocytotic cells; however, it is difficult to degrade. Prion uptake may induce autophagy, which may be involved in vacuolization, but this hypothesis needs to be evaluated. The high concentration of prions in the brain may also contribute to tissue damage.

Kuru

Kuru is a disease involving tremors and ataxia (lack of muscle control during voluntary movements, such as walking) and occurred only among the Fore tribes of New Guinea. *Kuru* means to shiver from fever cold, and the disease was related to the cannibalistic practices of the tribes. The tribespersons would eat the brains of their dead, and the women and children who prepared the food could also be infected via the conjunctivae or cuts in the skin. This tribal practice has stopped, and kuru has almost disappeared.

Creutzfeldt-Jakob Disease

Creutzfeldt-Jakob disease (CJD) is a progressive, fatal illness of the central nervous system. It can present as a psychiatric disorder, forgetfulness, disorientation, involuntary movement, and seizures, occurring mostly in the sixth or seventh decade of life. After running its course of 4 to 7 months, it leads to paralysis, pneumonia, and death. The brains of patients suffering from CJD have a spongiform appearance (see Fig 40-2), similar to that observed in sheep with scrapie. Prions have been found in the brains of CJD patients. The incidence of CJD throughout the world is one in 1 million per year, and there is no evidence of person-to-person transmission. However, infection can occur via corneal transplants, electrodes used for neurosurgery, and human growth hormone derived from the pituitary gland.

There is no therapy for CJD. Treatment is supportive to make the patient comfortable.

Bovine Spongiform Encephalopathy and Variant Creutzfeldt-Jakob Disease

Two cases of bovine spongiform encephalopathy (BSE), or mad cow disease, in cattle were identified in the United Kingdom in 1986. Two probable cases had occurred in the 1970s. The disease was most likely caused by feeding cattle contaminated animal byproducts (meat and bone meal) obtained from a spontaneously originating BSE or scrapie-infected sheep products. The symptoms included incoordination, apprehension, increased sensitivity to stimuli (hyperesthesia), tremors, and weight loss. The epidemic peaked with 40,000 cases in 1992, but new infections have been averted through tight controls on cattle feed.

The prion that causes BSE apparently can survive the cooking of processed meat from infected animals; it has infected and killed more than 200 people. This infection is called variant Creutzfeldt-Jakob disease (vCJD), and it afflicted 175 people in the United Kingdom and 49 people in other countries from October 1996 to March 2011. vCJD mostly affected young adults who presented with psychiatric issues that progressed to dementia.

In addition to infection, prion diseases can also be familial (genetic) or sporadic, with no known history of exposure. Gerstmann-Sträussler-Scheinker disease syndrome and fatal familial insomnia are familial prion diseases.

Gerstmann-Sträussler-Scheinker Disease

Gerstmann-Sträussler-Scheinker disease is a mostly inherited neurodegenerative brain disorder that causes ataxia and dementia, occurring primarily in the age range 35 to 55 years. It rarely occurs sporadically (ie, without familial involvement). The infectious agent can be transmitted to experimental animals.

Fatal Familial Insomnia

This is a familial prion disease that causes sleeping difficulties, followed by dementia and death within 1 to 2 years. The age range within which this disease occurs is 35 to 61 years. The infectious agent causes disease in experimental animals.

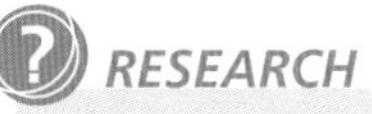

What types of experimental therapies might be developed for prion diseases?

Bibliography

Centers for Disease Control and Prevention. Public Health Image Library. phil.cdc.gov. Accessed 4 August 2015.

Levinson W. Review of Medical Microbiology and Immunology, ed 11. New York: McGraw-Hill, 2010.

Murray PR, Rosenthal KS, Pfaller MA. Medical Microbiology, ed 7. Philadelphia: W. B. Saunders, 2013.

National Center for Advanced Translational Sciences. Gerstmann-Straussler-Scheinker disease. rarediseases.info.nih.gov/gard/7690/gerstmannstrausslerscheinker-disease/resources/1. Accessed 4 August 2015.

Penn Arts and Sciences. Nobel Prize in medicine awarded to Stanley Prusiner, C'64, M'68. www.sas.upenn.edu/sasalum/newsltr/fall97/Prusiner.html. Accessed 4 August 2015.

Ryan KJ, Ray CG. Sherris Medical Microbiology, ed 5. New York: McGraw-Hill, 2010.

World Health Organization. Variant Creutzfeldt-Jakob disease. www.who.int/mediacentre/factsheets/fs180/en/. Accessed 4 August 2015.

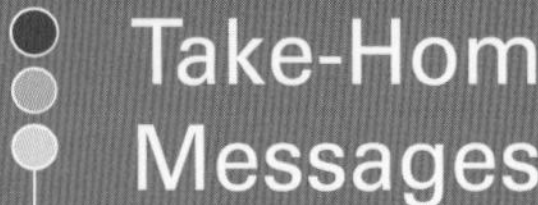

Take-Home Messages

- Prions are proteinaceous particles that have no nucleic acid associated with them.
- The "normal" prion protein, designated PrP^C, has significant α-helical segments.
- The prion protein is altered to a β-pleated sheet structure, PrP^{Sc} for scrapie-like prion protein, that forms filaments called *scrapie-associated fibrils*.
- Prions cause transmissible spongiform encephalopathies, which are characterized by the spongy holes seen in the brain parenchyma caused by neuronal death.
- Creutzfeldt-Jakob disease is a progressive, fatal illness of the central nervous system.
- The prion that causes bovine spongiform encephalopathy can be transmitted to people, causing variant Creutzfeldt-Jakob disease.

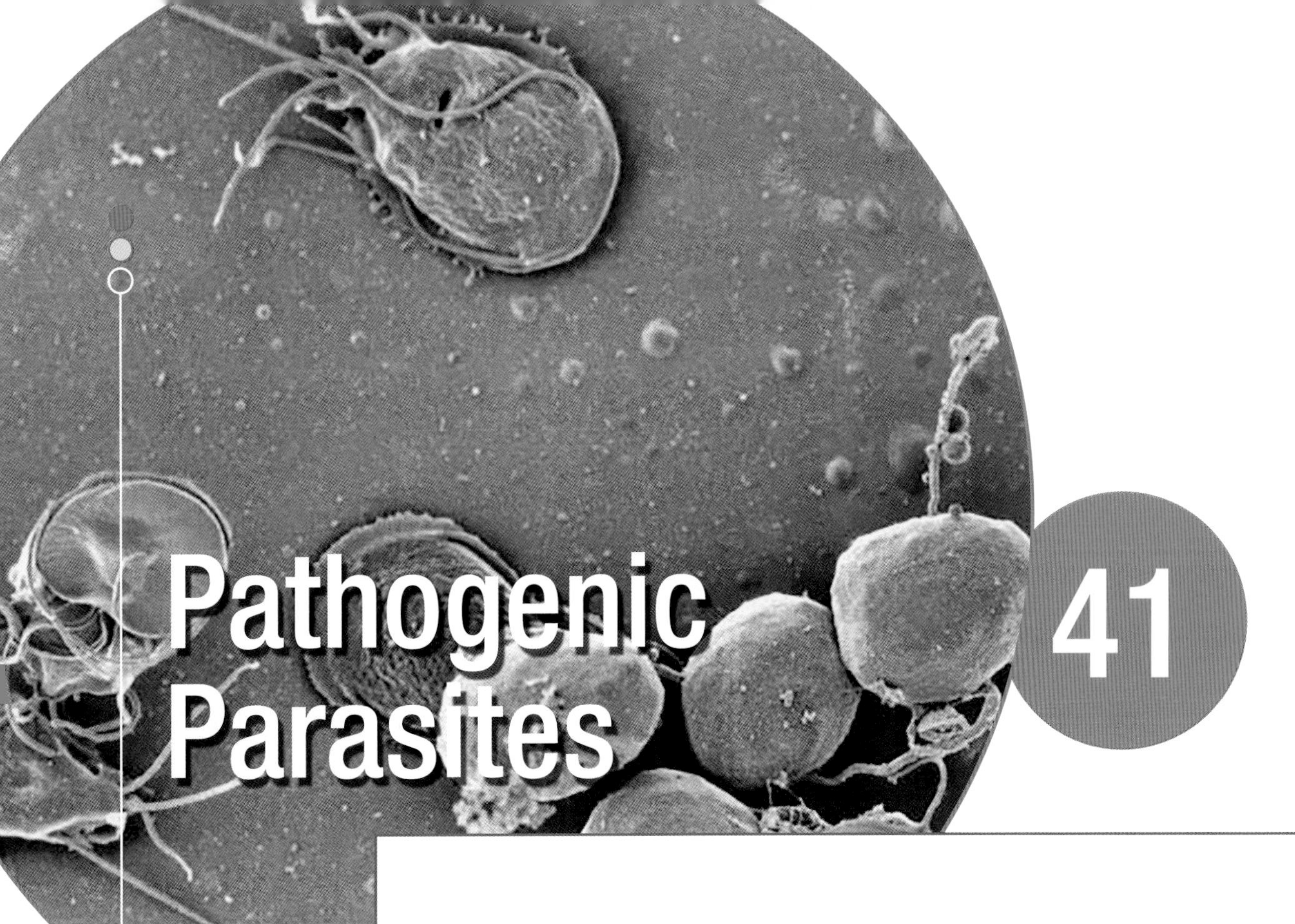

Pathogenic Parasites

The number of parasite-infected individuals and the number of associated deaths worldwide are enormous and must be a concern to all health care workers (Table 41-1). Although tropical diseases are not endemic to the United States, it is likely that travelers to tropical areas and refugees from developing countries may present with parasitic diseases. As evident with the advent of West Nile virus in the United States, it is possible that vectors of parasitic diseases can also appear in Northern climates, particularly as climate change results in warmer and more humid conditions.

Parasites may be classified into protozoa, which include amoeba, flagellates, ciliates, and microsporidia, and metazoa, which include roundworms, flatworms, flukes, and tapeworms. Protozoa are simple microorganisms. Their protoplasm is enclosed by a cell membrane and contains the membrane-bound nucleus, endoplasmic reticulum, and food storage granules. Motility is achieved by pseudopods or by complex structures like flagella or cilia. Amoebae, amoeboflagellates, and some other protozoa pinocytose soluble nutrients and phagocytose particulate organic matter. Intracellular microsporidia assimilate nutrients by diffusion. Many parasitic protozoa develop a cyst form that is less metabolically active and has a thick external cell wall that protects the organism against harsh environmental conditions. The cyst facilitates the transmission of the organism from host to host.

Metazoa include helminths and arthropods. Helminths are complex multicellular organisms. The surface of some worms is covered with a protective cuticle. They have elaborate attachment structures such as hooks, suckers, teeth, or plates. Nematodes are roundworms and include *Trichinella spiralis*. The Platyhelminthes are flatworms with ribbon segments and include *Schistosoma* species.

This chapter covers intestinal and urogenital protozoa as well as blood and tissue protozoa.

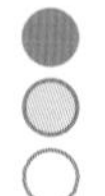

Table 41-1 Estimated number of individuals infected by parasites and the annual mortality from these infections

Infection	Number infected	Annual deaths
Malaria	198 million	584,000
Chagas disease	7–8 million	20,000
Leishmaniasis	1.3 million/year	20,000–30,000
Schistosomiasis	240 million	200,000
African trypanosomiasis	100,000/year	50,000

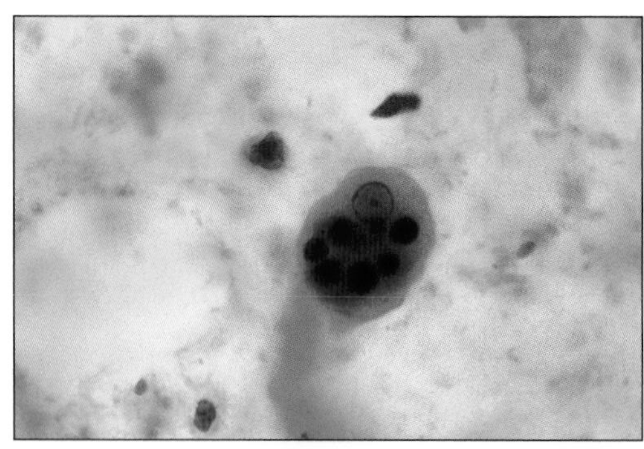

Fig 41-1 An *Entamoeba histolytica* trophozoite containing a single nucleus with its centrally placed karyosome and six ingested erythrocytes. (Public Health Image Library image 546, courtesy of the Centers for Disease Control and Prevention.)

Intestinal and Urogenital Protozoa

Intestinal and urogenital protozoa include amoebae associated with abdominal pain and cramping; flagellates including *Giardia* (diarrhea, abdominal cramps) and *Trichomonas* (vaginitis); coccidia including *Cryptosporidium* (enterocolitis, watery diarrhea) and *Cyclospora* (nausea, anorexia, cramping); and microsporidia, which some taxonomists consider as fungi (diarrhea, ocular pain, hepatitis).

Amoebae: *Entamoeba histolytica*

Entamoeba histolytica has two forms: *(1)* the actively feeding stage, the trophozoite, and *(2)* the quiescent, resistant, and infective stage, the cyst (Fig 41-1). When cysts are ingested, they release the pathogenic trophozoites in the duodenum. Trophozoites can move via the generation of pseudopods. The trophozoites cause local necrosis in the large intestine. An ionophore-like cytotoxin, proteases, and phospholipase A2 may be involved in necrosis. The trophozoites can spread to the peritoneal cavity, liver, lungs, brain, and heart.

E histolytica is transmitted via water and food contaminated with cysts passed by asymptomatic carriers, sewage, infected insects, and anal sexual intercourse.

The clinical syndromes include abdominal pain, cramping, and colitis with diarrhea. Extraintestinal amoebiasis causes fever, chills, and leukocytosis (transient increase in the number of leukocytes). Amoebic abscess of the liver causes pain over the liver, hepatomegaly, fever, and weight loss.

E histolytica infections can be treated with metronidazole, followed by iodoquinol. To prevent infection, water in endemic areas should be boiled, and fruits and vegetables should be cleaned thoroughly before consumption. Raw vegetables, unboiled water (including ice cubes), and unpeeled fruits should be avoided.

Flagellates

Giardia lamblia

The cyst form of *Giardia* is acquired by drinking inadequately treated contaminated water, by ingesting contaminated, uncooked vegetables or fruits, or person to person by the fecal-oral route (Fig 41-2). It is found in streams and lakes, and beavers and muskrats act as reservoirs. Outbreaks can occur in day-care centers. Gastric acid stimulates excystation. The released trophozoites can attach to the intestinal villi, causing inflammation, but they do not invade the mucosa nor enter the blood. Tissue necrosis does not occur.

Infection is asymptomatic in about 50% of infected people. In others, mild diarrhea to severe malabsorption syndrome is observed. Inflammation of the duodenal mucosa causes malabsorption of protein and fat. Other symptoms include abdominal cramps, gas (flatulence), and excess fat in feces. Recovery is spontaneous in 10 to 14 days, but chronic disease may develop.

Treatment involves metronidazole or nitazoxanide, but other alternatives exist. The mechanism of action of metronidazole and other nitroimidazoles involves the reduction of their nitro groups by bacterial nitroreductase, generating a cytotoxic compound that interacts with parasitic guanine and cytosine, causing the loss of helical structure and breakage of DNA strands.

Prevention of *Giardia* infections involves the avoidance of contaminated water and the use of proper filtration systems in municipal water supplies.

Trichomonas vaginalis

Trichomonas causes urogenital infections (Fig 41-3). It exists only as a trophozoite and is found in the urethras and vaginas of infected women and urethras and prostate glands of infected men. It is transmitted via sexual intercourse. Infants may be infected during birth if the mother is infected. It is estimated that 3.7 million individuals are infected in the United States.

Clinical symptoms range from mild irritation to severe inflammation. However, most infected women are asymp-

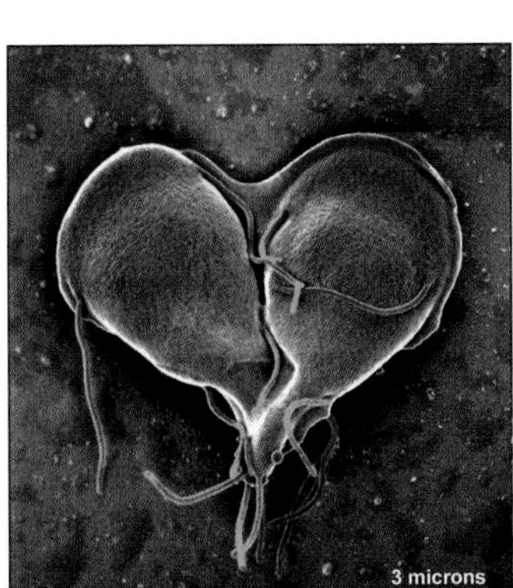

Fig 41-2 Scanning electron micrograph of *Giardia lamblia* in the process of cell division. (Public Health Image Library image 11652, courtesy of Dr Stan Erlandsen.)

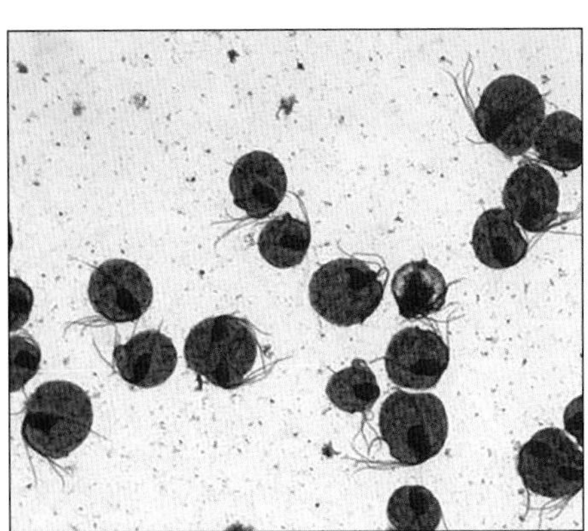

Fig 41-3 *Trichomonas vaginalis* parasites.

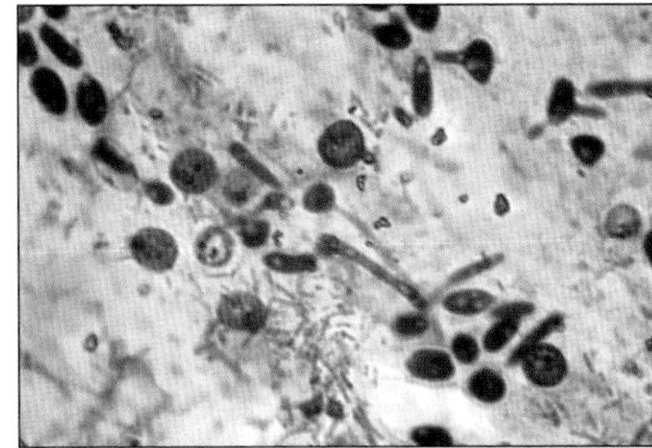

Fig 41-4 Micrograph of *Cryptosporidium* oocysts stained with a modified cold Kinyoun acid-fast staining technique and under an oil immersion lens. The oocysts stain red, and yeast cells, which are not acid-fast, stain green. (Public Health Image Library image 5242, courtesy of the Centers for Disease Control and Prevention.)

tomatic. Infection can result in extensive inflammation and erosion of the epithelial lining, causing itching, burning, and painful urination. Genital inflammation may facilitate human immunodeficiency virus (HIV) infection via unprotected sexual intercourse.

The drugs of choice are metronidazole and tinidazole. Metronidazole was originally introduced for the treatment of *Trichomonas* vaginitis. Drug-resistant organisms may require treatment with higher doses.

Coccidia: *Cryptosporidium parvum*

Cryptosporidia attach to the brush border of intestinal epithelium and replicate. They are covered with a double membrane derived from microvilli and are considered intracellular microorganisms. Oocysts mature to include four sporozoites, and their cell wall stains red with acid-fast staining (Fig 41-4).Cryptosporidia can spread from animal reservoirs as well as person to person by the fecal-oral route. After ingestion, the sporozoites are released from the oocysts and transform into trophozoites, which undergo both asexual (schizogony) and sexual (gametogony) reproduction.

Cryptosporidia are resistant to chlorination and ozone treatment. Cryptosporidiosis can be transmitted via contaminated water, as exemplified by the outbreak of cryptosporidiosis in Milwaukee in 1993 that infected around 300,000 people. This outbreak was the result of the contamination of the municipal water supply by runoff of local waste and surface water.

Clinical syndromes include watery diarrhea without blood, nausea, anorexia, vomiting, and low-grade fever. The infection resolves spontaneously in about 10 days. In immunocompromised or AIDS patients, extensive fluid loss occurs, with 50 or more stools per day; this condition can last for months to years.

There is no broadly effective treatment that has been established in controlled studies. Preventive measures include avoidance of contaminated water supplies.

Blood and Tissue Protozoa

Medically important blood and tissue protozoa (and the major diseases they cause) include *Plasmodium* (malaria), *Babesia* (hemolytic anemia, renal failure), *Toxoplasma* (lung, heart, and central nervous system infection), *Sarcocystis* (muscle infection), *Acanthamoeba* (encephalitis, eye and skin infection), *Balamuthia* (encephalitis), *Naegleria* (meningoencephalitis), *Leishmania* (leishmaniasis), and *Trypanosoma* (sleeping sickness, Chagas disease).

Plasmodium

Plasmodia are coccidian parasites (a subclass of parasitic protozoa) requiring two hosts: the mosquito for sexual reproduction and humans and other animals for the asexual reproductive stage. Humans are infected by the bite of an Anopheles mosquito. The sporozoites introduced into the bloodstream enter the parenchymal cells of the liver (exoerythrocytic cycle). Some species (*Plasmodium vivax* and *Plasmodium ovale*) establish a dormant infection in the liver with no division of the hypnozoites. The latter can be eventually released, causing disease months to years after initial infection. Hepatocytes rupture to release the plasmodia, called merozoites at this stage, which then attach to erythrocytes and enter them, starting the erythrocytic cycle (Fig 41-5). After reproduction, the erythrocytes lyse and release up to 24 merozoites. Some merozoites develop into male and female gametocytes, which can then start the sexual reproductive cycle if ingested by a mosquito. The parasite can also be transmitted via transfusion, needle sharing, and congenitally.

There are four major species of *Plasmodium*:

1. *P vivax* causes benign tertian malaria, characterized by attacks of fever, chills, and malarial rigors every 48 hours.
2. *P ovale* causes benign tertian or ovale malaria, where erythrocytes become oval in shape.

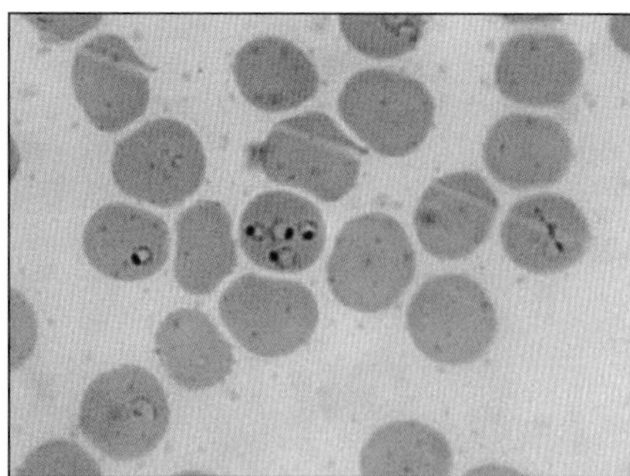

Fig 41-5 Intraerythrocytic *Plasmodium falciparum* ring-form trophozoites (rings). The erythrocyte in the center has four trophozoites. Rings may possess one or two chromatin dots. There is usually no enlargement of infected erythrocytes. (Public Health Image Library image 612, courtesy of Dr Mae Melvin.)

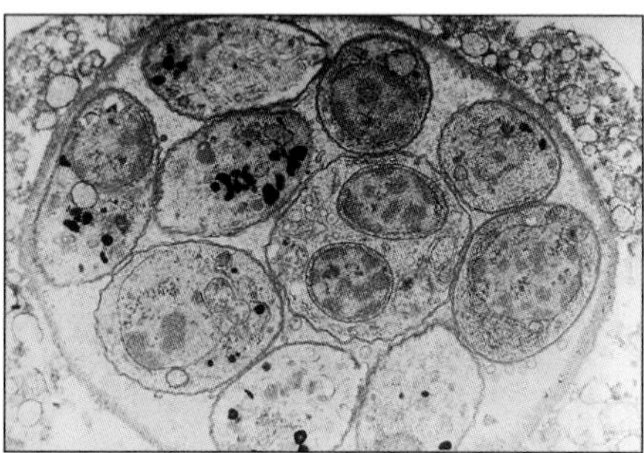

Fig 41-6 Transmission electron micrograph of a *Toxoplasma gondii* tissue cyst, within which bradyzoites are developing. In the human host, the *T gondii* parasites form cysts in skeletal muscle, the myocardium, the brain, and the eyes, and these cysts may remain throughout the life of the host. (Public Health Image Library image 14380, courtesy of the Centers for Disease Control and Prevention.)

3. *Plasmodium malariae* causes quartan or malarial malaria, with fever patterns every 72 hours.
4. *Plasmodium falciparum* causes malignant tertian malaria. The symptoms include chills, fever, headache, myalgias, arthralgias, splenomegaly, and anemia. *P falciparum* infection results in high levels of parasitemia, because it can infect red cells of all ages, unlike *P vivax*, which infects reticulocytes, or *P malariae*, which infects only mature red cells. Heterozygotic sickle cell trait red cells have too little adenosine triphosphatase activity to support the growth of *P falciparum*, and people with this trait are protected against malaria.

P falciparum is the most likely *Plasmodium* species to cause death if left untreated. Infected and destroyed red cells adhere to the vascular endothelium, and capillaries can be plugged by red cells, platelets, leukocytes, and malarial pigment. These can result in cerebral malaria, leading to delirium, convulsions, coma, and death. Kidney damage can result in blackwater fever, characterized by hemoglobinuria, acute renal failure, and tubular necrosis, which can lead to death.

The parasite makes a protein called PfEMP1 that mediates its adherence to walls of blood vessels. The parasite can make different versions of this protein, thereby avoiding neutralization by host antibodies.

There are a number of alternatives for the treatment of malaria. Chloroquine or parenteral quinine is used if the origin of the disease is not from an area where chloroquine resistance has developed. If resistant, other agents such as mefloquine with or without artesunate, quinidine, Fansidar (pyrimethamine-sulfadoxine, a folic acid antagonist; Roche), and doxycycline can be used.

Artemisinins can reduce the parasite biomass by 10^8-fold within 3 days. The remaining organisms can be reduced by a second drug (eg, mefloquine or lumefantrine). Artemether from the *Artemisia annua* plant is the first artemisinin class drug approved in the United States.

Chloroquine accumulates preferentially in parasitized red blood cells and may interfere with DNA replication, bind ferriprotoporphyrin IX released from hemoglobin to form a toxic complex, or raise the pH of the parasite's intracellular vesicles, interfering with its ability to degrade hemoglobin.

Primaquine can be used against extraerythrocytic parasites. Other antimalarial drugs include phenanthrenemethanols (halofantrine) that affect mitochondrial function and sesquiterpenes (artemisinin) that react with heme and cause free-radical damage to parasite membranes.

Prevention measures include chemoprophylaxis and prompt eradication of infections, control of mosquito breeding, and protection of individuals by netting, protective clothing, and insect repellents.

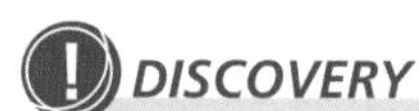

The symptoms of malaria were described in ancient Chinese medical writings such as *Nei Ching*, the Canon of Medicine (2700 BCE). Hippocrates in ancient Greece noted the principal symptoms. The Qinghao plant (*A annua*) was described in the medical treatise *52 Remedies* in the 2nd century BCE. The antifever properties of Qinghao were described by Ge Hong in 340 CE, and the active ingredient, known as *artemisinin*, was isolated by Chinese scientists in 1971. Derivatives of artemisinin, known as *artemisinins*, are effective antimalarial drugs, particularly in combination with other drugs. Spanish Jesuit missionaries in the New World learned from Native American tribes of a medicinal bark that was effective against fevers. The medicine from this bark is now known as *quinine*, which is used to treat malaria, along with artemisinins.

The parasites in the blood of a patient suffering from malaria were first noticed by Charles Laveran, a French army surgeon in Constantine, Algeria, in November 1880. Laveran was awarded the Nobel Prize in 1907 for this discovery. The Italian neurophysiologist Camillo Golgi found that there were at least two forms of the disease, one with tertian periodicity and one with quartan periodicity. He also found that fever coincided with the release of merozoites into blood.

Ronald Ross, a British officer in the Indian Medical Service, demonstrated in 1897 that malaria parasites could be transmitted from infected patients to mosquitoes and that mosquitoes could transmit the parasites from bird to bird. Ross was awarded the Nobel Prize in 1902 for this discovery.

Toxoplasma gondii

Toxoplasma gondii is a coccidian intracellular parasite whose essential reservoir host is the cat. Human infection with *T gondii* is common; however, immunocompromised individuals such as AIDS patients are more likely to have severe manifestations. It is estimated that 23% of the population over the age of 12 years in the United States have been infected with *Toxoplasma*. Toxoplasma cysts (Fig 41-6) are acquired by eating undercooked contaminated meat or other foods contaminated with objects that were in touch with contaminated meat, by animal-to-human transmission, or by congenital transmission. The cysts rupture in the small intestines, and the released tachyzoites infect a large variety of cells. As the immune system limits the infectious forms, the microorganism differentiates into bradyzoites (see Fig 41-6).

The clinical syndromes include chills, fever, headaches, myalgia, lymphadenitis, and fatigue, occasionally resembling infectious mononucleosis. Infection is characterized by cell destruction, reproduction of more organisms, and eventual cyst formation. *T gondii* can infect cells in the lungs, heart, lymphoid organs, and the central nervous system, including the eye.

In normal hosts, the infection resolves spontaneously. In immunocompromised patients, pyrimethamine plus sulfadiazine are given. Pyrimethamine is teratogenic and should not be used in the first trimester of pregnancy. The macrolide spiramycin can be substituted in such cases.

Prevention involves avoiding uncooked meat and exposure to cat feces. Pregnant women should be especially careful to avoid *Toxoplasma* infection.

Leishmania

Leishmania species are flagellated protozoa transmitted via sandflies. The promastigote, which is a long, slender form with a flagellum, is present in the saliva of infected sandflies and is transmitted via a bite (Fig 41-7). The microorganism then transforms into the amastigote stage, which invades cells of the reticuloendothelial system. The cells rupture, resulting in tissue destruction.

Leishmania donovani causes "kala-azar," "dumdum fever," or visceral leishmaniasis, characterized by chills and sweating resembling malaria, enlargement of the liver and spleen, weight loss, and emaciation. Kidney damage can also occur. If untreated, it can lead to death. There are about half a million new cases per year, a great majority of which are seen in Bangladesh, India, Nepal, Brazil, and the Sudan.

Leishmania tropica and *Leishmania major* are associated with cutaneous leishmaniasis, which presents as a red papule that becomes pruritic and ulcerates.

Treatment involves the use of pentavalent antimonial compounds, such as stibogluconate (Pentostam, GlaxoSmithKline), which inhibit glycolytic and Krebs cycle enzymes. These are toxic to the host, but the therapeutic value is due to enhanced uptake by the parasite and the intense metabolic activity of the parasite. Potential new therapies include amphotericin B liposome formulation, miltefosine, paromomycin, and sitamaquine.

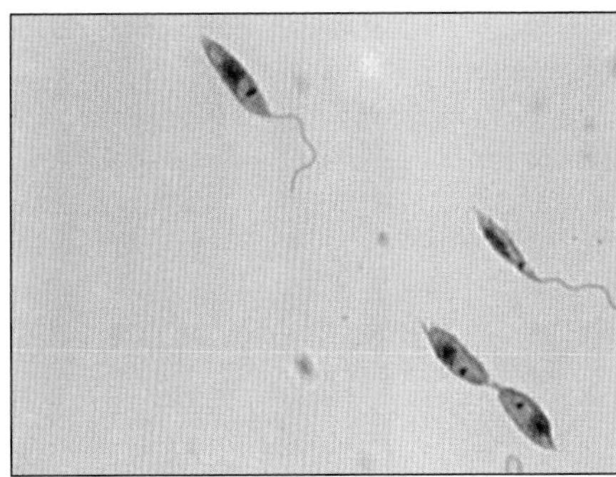

Fig 41-7 Promastigote-stage *Leishmania* microorganisms. (Public Health Image Library image 11072, courtesy of Dr Mae Melvin.)

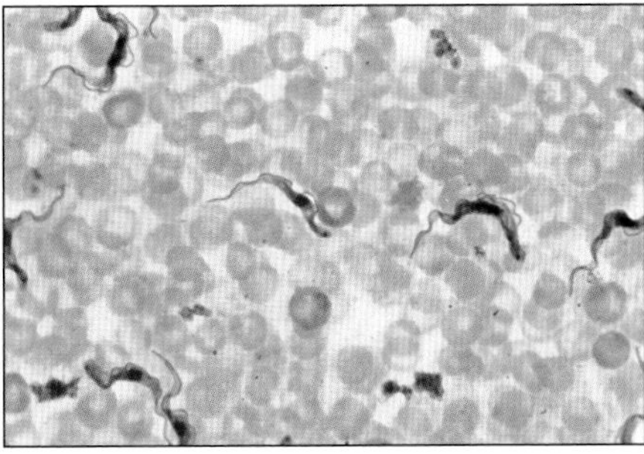

Fig 41-8 Light micrograph of Giemsa-stained thin film blood smear with *Trypanosoma brucei gambiense* parasites. (Public Health Image Library image 10167, courtesy of Dr Mae Melvin.)

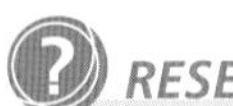

RESEARCH

What type of antimicrobial drugs are amphotericin B liposome formulation, miltefosine, paromomycin, and sitamaquine?

Trypanosoma

Trypanosoma brucei gambiense causes African trypanosomiasis, or sleeping sickness. It is transmitted by tsetse flies. The infective stage is the trypomastigote (Fig 41-8). It causes an ulcer at the site of the fly bite. As lymph nodes are invaded, fever, myalgia, and arthralgia develop. Chronic disease progresses to the central nervous system, causing lethargy, tremors, meningoencephalitis, and general deterioration. This parasite can change the molecules on its surface to avoid host immune attack. At the early stages of disease, suramin and pentamidine are drugs of choice. At later stages, melarsoprol, which can penetrate the blood-brain barrier, can be used. Difluoromethylornithine has activity against both acute and late forms of the disease.

Trypanosoma cruzi causes American trypanosomiasis, or Chagas disease, and is transmitted by the reduviid bug ("kissing bug"). It is seen most often in South and

Central America. The infectious typomastigotes migrate to the heart, brain, and liver and become intracellular amastigotes, which multiply and destroy the host cell. The disease is characterized by an erythematous area called a chagoma around the bite, rash and edema around the eyes and face, and central nervous system involvement. It is most severe in children younger than 5 years. Drugs used for treatment include nifurtimox, allopurinol, and benznidazole.

Bibliography

Centers for Disease Control and Prevention. The History of Malaria, an Ancient Disease. www.cdc.gov/malaria/about/history/index.html. Accessed 4 August 2015.

Centers for Disease Control and Prevention. Parasites - *Giardia*. www.cdc.gov/parasites/giardia/. Accessed 4 August 2015.

Centers for Disease Control and Prevention. Parasites - Toxoplasmosis (*Toxoplasma* infection). www.cdc.gov/parasites/toxoplasmosis/. Accessed 4 August 2015.

Centers for Disease Control and Prevention. Public Health Image Library. phil.cdc.gov. Accessed 4 August 2015.

Centers for Disease Control and Prevention. Trichomoniasis. www.cdc.gov/std/trichomonas/STDFact-Trichomoniasis.htm. Accessed 4 August 2015.

Engleberg NC, DiRita V, Dermody TS. Schaechter's Mechanisms of Microbial Disease. Baltimore and Philadelphia: Lippincott Williams & Wilkins, 2007.

Levinson W. Review of Medical Microbiology and Immunology, ed 11. New York: McGraw-Hill, 2010.

Maya JD, Orellana M, Ferreira J, Kemmerling U, López-Muñoz R, Morello A. Chagas disease: Present status of pathogenic mechanisms and chemotherapy. Biol Res 2010;43:323–331.

Murray PR, Rosenthal KS, Pfaller MA. Medical Microbiology, ed 7. Philadelphia: Mosby/Elsevier, 2013.

Ryan KJ, Ray CG. Sherris Medical Microbiology, ed 5. New York: McGraw-Hill, 2010.

World Health Organization. Chagas disease (American trypanosomiasis). www.who.int/mediacentre/factsheets/fs340/en/. Accessed 4 August 2015.

World Health Organization. Factsheet on the World Malaria Report. http://www.who.int/malaria/media/world_malaria_report_2014/en/. Accessed 4 August 2015.

World Health Organization. Leishmaniasis. www.who.int/mediacentre/factsheets/fs375/en/. Accessed 4 August 2015.

World Health Organization. Schistosomiasis. www.who.int/schistosomiasis/en/. Accessed 4 August 2015.

Take-Home Messages

- *E histolytica* infections cause abdominal pain, cramping, and colitis with diarrhea. Extraintestinal amoebiasis causes fever, chills, and leukocytosis.
- *G lamblia* can cause mild diarrhea to severe malabsorption syndrome in about half of infected people.
- *T vaginalis* causes urogenital infections, with symptoms ranging from mild irritation to severe inflammation.
- Infection with *C parvum* causes watery diarrhea without blood, nausea, anorexia, vomiting, and low-grade fever. AIDS patients are especially vulnerable.
- *P falciparum* causes malignant tertian malaria. The symptoms include chills, fever, headache, myalgias, arthralgias, splenomegaly, and anemia.
- If left untreated, *P falciparum* can destroy red blood cells, which can then obstruct capillaries, resulting in cerebral malaria and kidney damage.
- Drug resistance is a very significant problem in the control of malaria.
- *T gondii* can infect cells in the lungs, heart, lymphoid organs, and the central nervous system, including the eye. It can cause myalgia, lymphadenitis, and fatigue.
- *Leishmania* species are flagellated protozoa transmitted via sandflies. *L donovani* causes visceral leishmaniasis that resembles malaria. *L tropica* and *L major* are associated with cutaneous leishmaniasis.
- *T brucei gambiense* causes African trypanosomiasis, or sleeping sickness, and is transmitted by tsetse flies.
- *T cruzi* causes American trypanosomiasis, or Chagas disease, and is transmitted by the reduviid bug.

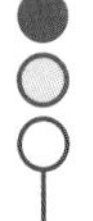

Cases in Medical Microbiology

This chapter is intended as an exercise to test the reader's newfound knowledge in medical microbiology. Each case description should lead the reader to a particular diagnosis. All diagnoses are presented at the end of the chapter.

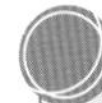

CASE 1

A 4-year-old child experienced a rapid onset of fever that lasted for 3 days and then suddenly returned to normal. Two days later, a maculopapular rash appeared on the trunk and spread to other parts of the body.

CASE 2

A neonate exhibited microcephaly, hepatosplenomegaly, and rash. A radiograph indicated intracerebral calcification. The mother had symptoms similar to mononucleosis during the third trimester of her pregnancy.

CASE 3

A 23-year-old college student developed malaise, fatigue, fever, swollen glands, and pharyngitis. Heterophile antibodies and atypical lymphocytes were detected in blood.

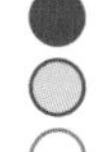

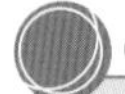

CASE 4

A 5-year-old boy had an ulcerative rash with vesicles around the mouth. Vesicles and ulcers were also present within the mouth. Results of a Tzanck smear showed multinucleated giant cells. The lesions resolved after 18 days.

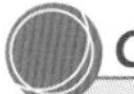

CASE 5

A 40-year-old man with multisystem failure following bilateral pneumonia was taken to the hospital. He had presented to his local physician 3 days previously complaining of fever, malaise, and some respiratory symptoms. He was given amantadine for suspected influenza. His condition worsened, with shortness of breath and a fever reaching 41°C. A laboratory examination revealed abnormal liver and kidney function. He was treated with Timentin (ticarcillin-clavulanic acid) and trimethoprim-sulfamethoxazole. Bronchoscopic examination revealed mildly inflamed airways containing thin, watery secretions. Gram staining of the bacteria grown on buffered charcoal-yeast extract agar indicated weakly staining Gram-negative microorganisms.

CASE 6

A 4-month-old girl was admitted to the hospital with severe respiratory distress. She had developed a cough and rhinitis a few days before admission. Then she began to wheeze and developed a fever. She became lethargic and was brought to the hospital. One sibling was reported to be coughing, and her father had a "cold." She had a fever of 39°C, tachycardia (pulse of 220/min), and tachypnea (respirations of 80/min). A chest radiograph revealed interstitial infiltrates. She was placed in respiratory isolation. Blood and nasopharyngeal cultures were sent to the bacteriology and virology laboratories. Some of the suspected causes were parainfluenza virus, respiratory syncytial virus, *Mycoplasma pneumoniae*, and influenza virus. A rapid diagnostic test was positive, and aerosolized ribavirin was administered. She was given a bronchodilator to treat the bronchospasm that caused her wheezing. She was discharged on day 8.

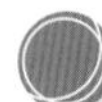

CASE 7

A 40-year-old woman brought her daughter to the pediatrician with the complaint of a rash. The daughter's face had rosy cheeks, but she had no fever or other notable symptoms. The mother reported that her daughter had had a mild cold within the previous 2 weeks, and that she herself was currently having more joint pain than usual and was very tired.

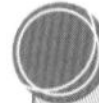

CASE 8

A boy attending summer camp complained of a sore throat, headache, cough, red eyes, and fatigue and was sent to the infirmary. His temperature was 40°C. Soon afterward, other campers and counselors came to the infirmary with similar symptoms. The symptoms lasted for about a week. All the patients had gone swimming in the camp pond, and many other people in the camp complained of similar symptoms.

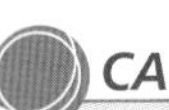

CASE 9

A 32-year-old woman presented with a cough lasting several weeks and a 15-lb weight loss. She also had night sweats and fevers and felt fatigued. Despite erythromycin treatment for suspected pneumonia given by her family physician, her fever and cough got progressively worse. She complained about coughing blood-tinged sputum. She had emigrated from India to the United States several years ago, but she often returned to India to visit her relatives. The physical examination indicated a temperature of 39°C and bilateral rales and lymphadenopathy. A chest radiograph revealed infiltrates in the right upper lobe. Some of the likely causes of illness are *Legionella pneumophila*, *Histoplasma capsulatum*, *Mycoplasma pneumoniae*, *Mycobacterium tuberculosis*, and *Actinomyces* species.

CASE 10

A 31-year-old woman presented with low-grade fever, malaise, and a rash. She recalled having painful ulcers, which appeared on the vulva 1 month before this new episode. She did not seek medical attention at that time, and the ulcers resolved spontaneously in 10 days. She had had four sexual partners in the month preceding the development of ulcerative lesions. Physical examination revealed inguinal lymphadenopathy, a generalized rash on palms and soles, and pustular cutaneous lesions and condylomata lata (wartlike outgrowths) on her face. Some of the potential sources of these symptoms are Herpes simplex virus, *Treponema pallidum*, *Chlamydia trachomatis*, and *Haemophilus ducreyi*.

CASE 11

A 60-year-old man came to the emergency room with a 6-day history of fever, moderate headache, generalized myalgia, arthralgias, and fatigue. He had noticed a rash under the armpit that had spread rapidly, prompting him to seek medical attention. He had moved recently to a cottage in a wooded area. He noted multiple tick bites following a walk in the woods. He had an expanding erythematous skin lesion on his leg with a central area of clearing. These symptoms may be related to ehrlichiosis, Lyme disease, and *Rickettsia ricketsii* infection.

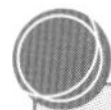

CASE 12

A 24-year-old woman developed fever, headache, and a gradually progressive dry cough. Her cough worsened over the next 2 days, becoming productive of small amounts of clear sputum. She had been in good health before this episode. Her 19-year-old brother had had similar symptoms 2 weeks earlier. The patient appeared slightly pale. Mild pharyngeal erythema was noted with minimal cervical adenopathy but no exudates. A chest radiograph revealed bilateral patchy infiltrates. The likely causes of illness include *Chlamydophila pneumoniae*, adenoviruses, influenza A and B, *Mycoplasma pneumoniae*, and *Streptococcus pneumoniae*.

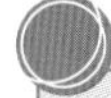

CASE 13

A 50-year-old man was hospitalized with severe watery ("rice water") diarrhea. He had just returned from a visit to Ecuador, and the symptoms appeared the day after his return. He was dehydrated and suffering from an electrolyte imbalance. Fluid and electrolyte replacement was instituted to compensate for the losses resulting from the watery diarrhea, and the patient recovered in a few days. The stool cultures were positive for a Gram-negative, flagellated bacterium.

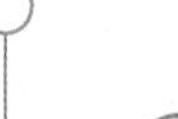

CASE 14

An 8-year-old girl presented with a 2-day history of fever, headache, earache, and swelling and tenderness at the parotid and submaxillary areas. She also found it difficult to open her jaws, to talk, or to eat. The child had been in good health; nevertheless, the parents reported that she had received only one dose of the usual childhood vaccinations because the family had moved when she was very young, and she was lost to follow-up. Some of the likely causes of illness are Coxsackievirus, mumps virus, suppurative parotitis due to *Staphylococcus aureus*, and parainfluenza virus. The patient was given analgesics for pain and recommended to drink fluids.

CASE 15

A 6-year-old girl came home from school feeling sick on a cold day. She had a high fever and complained of an itchy throat. She had difficulty swallowing food, refused to eat, and cried almost all evening. The next day she was taken to her family physician. Several children from her school had also reported sore throats. The child had received all childhood vaccinations. Physical examination revealed a red throat (pharyngeal erythema) on the soft palate and grayish-whitish tonsillar exudates. The anterior cervical lymph nodes were enlarged and tender. The patient was not coughing. The rapid antigen detection test (RADT) was positive. A throat culture on a sheep blood agar plate produced β-hemolysis. The patient was given penicillin V. The potential causes of illness include adenovirus; rhinovirus; Epstein-Barr virus; influenza A, B, and C viruses; *Streptococcus pyogenes* (Group A streptococcus); and coronavirus.

CASE 16

A 65-year-old man presented with fever, abdominal cramping, and frequent diarrhea over the last few days. Three weeks before the current episode, he was rehabilitating in an orthopedic unit after a hip replacement; there he developed nosocomial pneumonia. Cefuroxime and clindamycin were prescribed. He was discharged after improving, a week before the current episode, with maintenance oral antibiotics. His wife had no similar symptoms. His oral mucosa was dry. Sigmoidoscopy revealed an erythematous colon mucosa. A stool specimen was positive for a toxin. Some of the likely causes of this condition are antibiotic-associated diarrhea or colitis due to *Clostridium difficile*, *Campylobacter jejuni*, *Salmonella* Enteritidis, and viral gastroenteritis.

CASE 17

A 24-year-old man presented with a nonproductive cough, shortness of breath, fever, and malaise. He also had thrush. He had been infected with HIV and was taking antiretroviral medication. However, side effects of the medications forced him to stop his therapy. A chest radiograph showed consolidation of the airspace on both sides of the lungs. Sputum and bronchoalveolar lavage samples were taken for acid-fast and Gram staining. A direct fluorescent antibody test was positive for a microorganism that is seen in immunocompromised patients, especially those with AIDS. Likely microorganisms in this case are *Histoplasma capsulatum*, *Cryptococcus neoformans*, *Pneumocystis jirovecii*, and *Mycoplasma pneumoniae*.

CASE 18

An 18-year-old woman presented with fever, chills, skin rash, malaise, and arthralgia. She had been sexually active and reported a yellowish discharge in the vagina. She had erythematous maculopapular rashes on her forearm and thigh. Her knee and ankle were inflamed. She had an elevated leukocyte count. Cultures of her cervix showed Gram-negative diplococci, but her skin lesions and synovial fluid had no microorganisms. She was treated with penicillin G for 2 weeks and recovered.

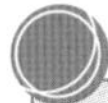

CASE 19

A 24 year-old man was admitted to the hospital with a history of a fever that was not reduced with the administration of amoxicillin or ibuprofen, an enlarged liver, and abdominal pain. He remembered eating undercooked chicken a few days ago. The blood culture indicated Gram-negative rods. The patient responded to ciprofloxacin.

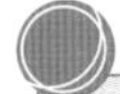

CASE 20

A 28-year-old woman presented with dysuria, fevers, and chills during the previous 5 days, lower abdominal pain, and a vaginal discharge. She indicated having sexual intercourse with three partners during the past year and did not have her partners use condoms consistently. Pelvic examination with a vaginal speculum revealed a reddened cervical os with a mucopurulent exudate. She also had cervical motion tenderness. Pelvic inflammatory disease, potentially caused by *Neisseria gonorrhoeae*, *Chlamydia trachomatis*, *Streptococcus agalactiae*, or *Mycoplasma hominis*, was considered as the cause of the symptoms. Gram stains of the secretions did not show any Gram-negative diplococci. However, the secretions contained numerous neutrophils. When the secretions were cultured under anaerobic conditions, three different species were identified. An endometrial biopsy showed reticulate bodies in cells. The patient was treated with a combination of cefoxitin and doxycycline, because this was a polymicrobial infection.

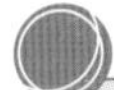

CASE 21

A 70-year-old man presented in February with an abrupt onset of fever (40°C), nonproductive cough, headache, severe sore throat, nausea, and myalgia. The patient had not been vaccinated in the past 5 years against any infectious diseases and had received several visits from younger family members. The chest radiograph was normal, and there were no abnormal sounds during breathing in a pulmonary examination. The likely causes of illness include *Streptococcus pneumoniae*, *Legionella pneumophila*, *Mycoplasma pneumoniae*, influenza virus, parainfluenza virus, adenovirus, and severe acute respiratory syndrome (SARS) coronavirus.

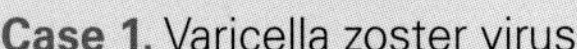

Diagnoses

Case 1. Varicella zoster virus
Case 2. Cytomegalovirus
Case 3. Epstein-Barr virus
Case 4. Herpes simplex virus
Case 5. *Legionella pneumophila*
Case 6. Respiratory syncytial virus
Case 7. Parvovirus B19
Case 8. Adenovirus
Case 9. *Mycobacterium tuberculosis*
Case 10. *Treponema pallidum*
Case 11. Lyme disease (*Borrelia burgdorferi*)
Case 12. *Mycoplasma pneumoniae*
Case 13. *Vibrio cholerae*
Case 14. Mumps virus
Case 15. *Streptococcus pyogenes*
Case 16. *Clostridium difficile*
Case 17. *Pneumocystis jirovecii* (formerly *P carinii*)
Case 18. *Neisseria gonorrhoeae*
Case 19. *Salmonella enterica* serovar Typhi
Case 20. *Chlamydia trachomatis* plus anaerobic bacteria
Case 21. Influenza virus

Bibliography

Carey RB, Schuster MG, McGowan KL. Medical Microbiology for the New Curriculum: A Case-Based Approach. Hoboken, NJ: Wiley, 2008.

Gilligan PH, Smiley ML, Shapiro DS. Cases in Medical Microbiology and Infectious Disease. Washington, DC: American Society for Microbiology, 1997.

Murray PR, Rosenthal KS, Pfaller MA. Medical Microbiology, ed 6. Philadelphia: Mosby/Elsevier, 2009.

Nath SK, Revankar SG. Problem-Based Microbiology. Philadelphia: Saunders-Elsevier, 2006.

Index

Page numbers followed by "f" indicate figures; those followed by "t" indicate tables; those followed by "b" indicate boxes

D

E

F

G

H

M

N

O

P

T

Notes

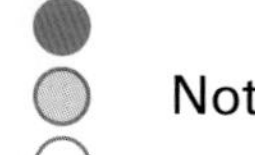

Notes

Notes

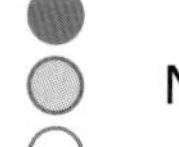

Notes

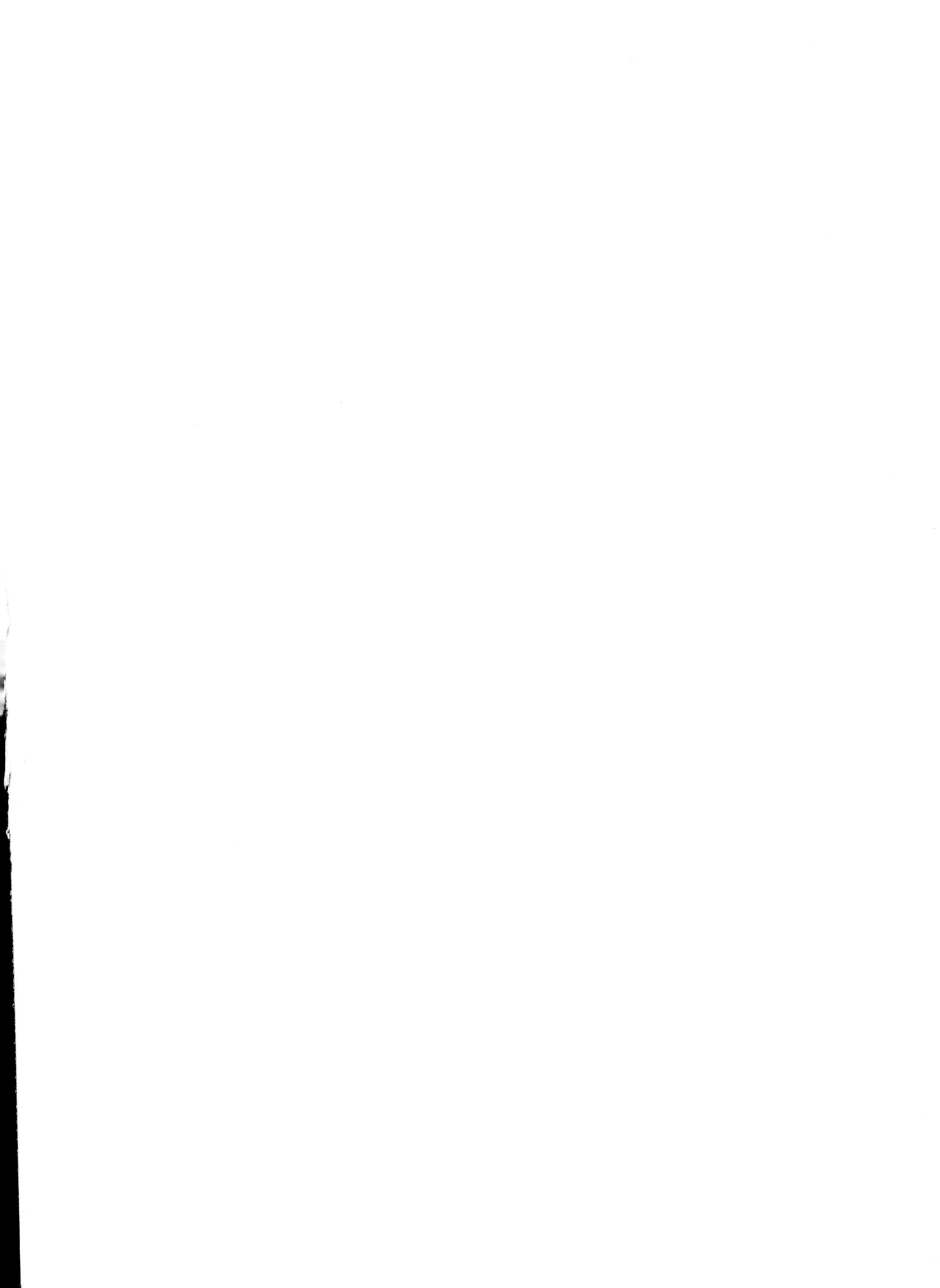